Environmental Health in Nursing

3rd Edition

Edited by:

Ruth McDermott-Levy, PhD, MPH, RN, FAAN
Professor
Co-Director, Mid-Atlantic Center for Children's Health and the Environment
Villanova University
M. Louise Fitzpatrick College of Nursing

Kathryn P. Jackman-Murphy, EdD, MSN, RN, CHSE
Director, RN/BSN Program
Charter Oak State College

Jeanne Leffers, PhD, RN, FAAN
Professor Emeritus
University of Massachusetts Dartmouth
College of Nursing and Health Sciences

Adelita G. Cantu, PhD, RN, FAAN
University of Texas Health San Antonio
School of Nursing

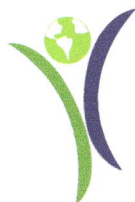

Alliance of Nurses for
Healthy Environments

Title: Environmental Health in Nursing, 3rd Edition

Publisher: Alliance of Nurses for Healthy Environments www.enviRN.org

Editors: Ruth McDermott-Levy, PhD, MPH, RN, FAAN, Kathryn P. Jackman-Murphy, EdD, MSN, RN, CHSE, Jeanne Leffers, PhD, RN, FAAN, Adelita G. Cantu, PhD, RN, FAAN

Acknowledgements: We would like to acknowledge all of our environmental health nursing leaders and experts who willingly contributed to Environmental Health in Nursing, 3rd edition. We also would like to acknowledge our reviewers and copy editor:

Reviewers:

Cara Cook, MS, RN, AHN-BC
Director of Program, Alliance of Nurses for Healthy Environments

Katie Huffling, DNP, RN, CNM, FAAN
Executive Director, Alliance of Nurses for a Healthy Environments

Claudia Smith, EdD, MPH, RN-BC
Community/Public Health Nursing Educator and Consultant, retired

Copy Editors:

Eric Bullock
Pixelpusherz

Emily Hennessee, MPH

Cover photos (clockwise starting at left, top row): ANHE nurse Lillian Jensen at a press conference at the EPA in Washington, DC; a new electric bus in Atlanta, GA; ANHE Environmental Health Nurse Fellows Felix J. Roman Hernandez and Erika Alfaro; ANHE nurses (from right) Shanda Demorest, Rachel Kerr, and Teddie Potter at a climate protest in Minneapolis, MN; ANHE Environmental Health Nurse Fellow Mia McPherson; Indigenous nursing students at Universidad Cooperativa de Colombia

ISBN: 978-0-9998123-3-4

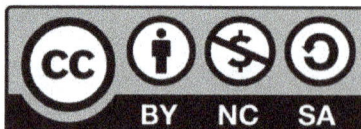

Dedication

The third edition of Environmental Health in Nursing is dedicated to the 50 nurses leaders, representing many of the major US nursing organizations, nursing unions, and environmental health, who gathered together in December of 2008 in Oracle, AZ to plan the future of environmental health nursing. Through their courage and visionary work in Oracle, the Alliance of Nurses for Healthy Environments was born and from that point on the environmental health movement within nursing grew exponentially. Thank you for your amazing vision and leadership as we work together in support of healthier environments for all.

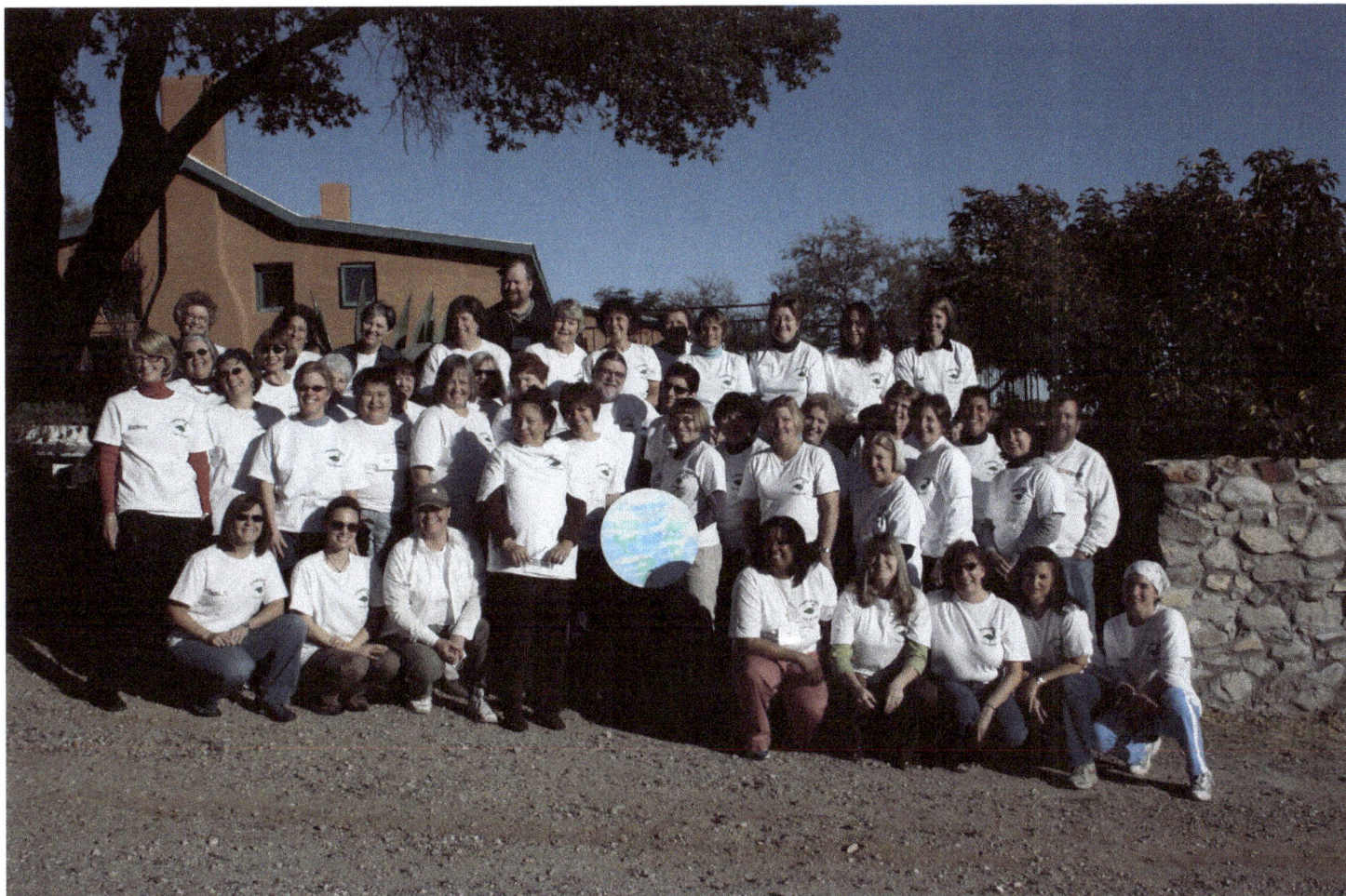

Front Row (kneeling): Denise Choiniere, Rebecca Clouse, Laura Anderko, Deirdre Walton, Corrine Mohnasky, _____, Kathi Randall, Robyn Gilden

Second Row: Brenda Afzal, Liz Blackburn, Betty Bekemier, Norma Martinez Rogers, Chris Bartholomew, Maria Amaya, Anita Nager, Katie Huffling, Sharon Rainier, Evie Bain, Kathy Hall, Patti Gates Smith

Third Row: Mary Jane Williams, Karen Duderstadt, Lill Mood, Sandy Worthington, Joanne McAuliffe?, Gingy Harshey-Meade?, Tom Engle, Catherine Ruhl, Lenore Resick, _____, _____, _____, Ann Converso, Ed Fishel

Fourth Row: Beth Lamanna, Kathy Curtis, Pat Butterfield, Catherine Dodd, Wade Hill, Jeanne Leffers, Barbara Sattler, Karen Ballard, Ginni Hall, Carolyn Graff?, Lisa Hartmyer, Jenny Edwards

*Using the magnifying glass on this old picture only got us so far. If you can identify those not listed or correct any who are misidentified, please let us know.

CONTENTS

Note: The e-text does not have an Index, we recommend using the word find feature on the pdf version of this text to find topics of interest, available at https://envirn.org/e-textbook/.

The editors of Environmental Health in Nursing, 3rd edition would like to sincerely thank the authors who generously contributed their time, knowledge, and expertise to this edition. Without our dedicated authors we would not be able to share the quality of important environmental health information that is contained in the e-text. This work was a labor of love. Love of Earth's people, families, communities, and the planet that sustains us. We hope that you find this information useful to expand your nursing practice to include environmental health.

With gratitude,

Ruth McDermott-Levy, PhD, MPH, RN, FAAN

Kathryn P. Jackman-Murphy, EdD, MSN, RN, CHSE

Jeanne Leffers, PhD, RN, FAAN

Adelita Cantu, PhD, RN, FAAN

INTRODUCTION:

The Alliance of Nurses for Healthy Environments (ANHE) is thrilled to release our 3rd edition of the Environmental Health in Nursing e-textbook in time to celebrate our 15th birthday. The idea for ANHE began at a meeting in Oracle, AZ in December 2008, where leading environmental health nurses and representatives from many of the major nursing organizations and unions came together to brainstorm how nursing could collectively work together in support of healthier environments for all. From this meeting of nurse leaders ANHE was born.

It has been such a gift to watch ANHE grow — from a couple hundred nurses to now over 7000 around the globe. Every day more and more nurses recognize that in order to truly provide the holistic, preventive care that is the foundation of nursing, we must include environmental health in our practice. More schools of nursing are incorporating environmental health throughout their curricula and more students are clamoring for this content in their programs.

ANHE nurses are spreading our wings and pushing boundaries, as we work together to address some of the most urgent public health issues of our time, like climate change. We are standing up to corporate greed and pushing for safer products over profits. We are participating in acts of civil disobedience to elevate the issue of our climate emergency. Nurses are coming together at the United Nations climate negotiations, the Conference of Parties (COP), to push for health to be a core facet of the climate negotiations and treaties.

Building upon the leadership shown during the COVID-19 pandemic, we are growing into our power as nurses and enthusiastically invite all to join us as ANHE heads into our next 15 years. Let us work together to build a world where every person has the opportunity to reach their full potential and live and thrive in a healthy environment.

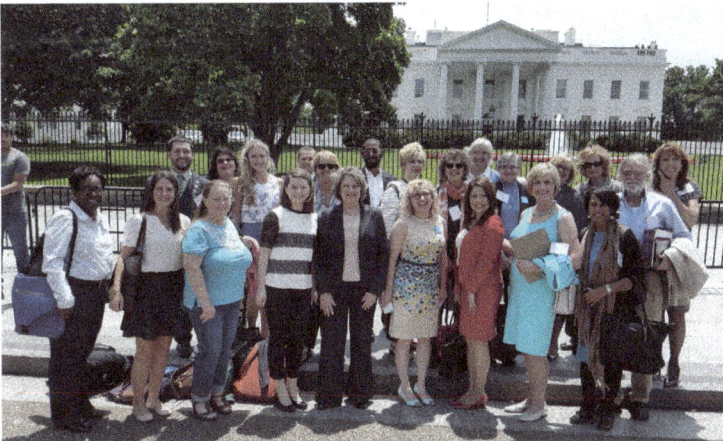

2016 Climate, Health, and Nursing White House Roundtable

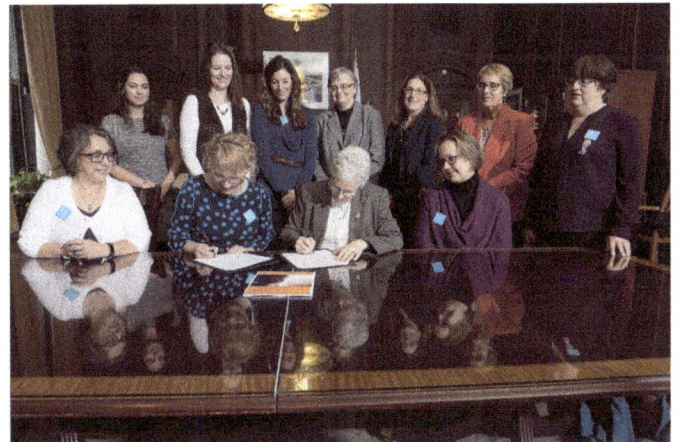

ANHE and EPA MOU signing with Gina McCarthy (2016)

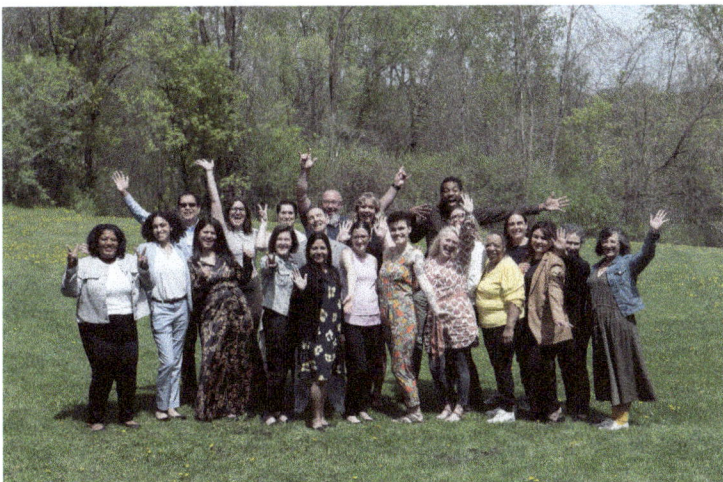

ANHE Environmental Health Nurse Fellows (2023)

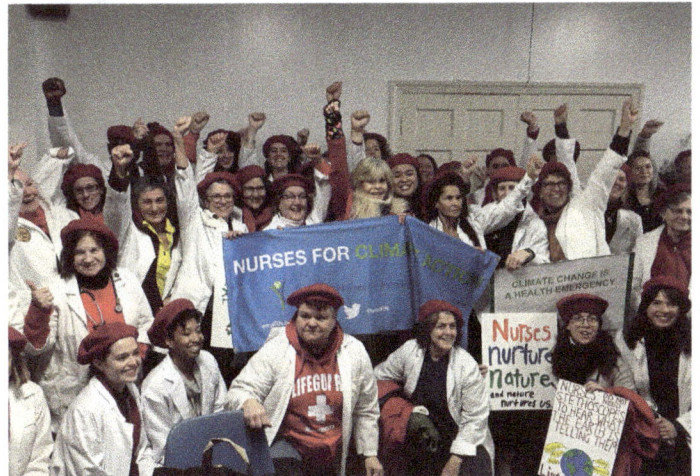

ANHE Nurses at Fire Drill Friday protest (2019)

Unit I Why Nursing? serves to inform the reader of the relevance of environmental health content for nursing practice as well as mandates from not only the 1995 IOM report but also inclusion of the ANA Scope and Standards of Practice (2020), Standard 17: Environmental Health.

Unit II Harmful Environmental Exposures and Vulnerable Populations provides an overview of populations across the lifespan and their specific vulnerabilities as well as specific populations such as workers, immigrants and persons with alterations in cognitive and physical abilities.

Unit III Environmental Health Sciences includes information about sciences that inform environmental health such as ecology, toxicology, epidemiology and risk assessment.

Unit IV Practice Settings addresses hazardous exposures in healthcare, Green Teams, green cleaning in hospitals, and pharmaceutical waste.

Unit V Sustainable Communities provides environmental health content that looks at communities. This includes information on green building initiatives, green cleaning in homes, transportation, Brownfields, food, antibiotic use in agriculture and environmental justice.

Unit VI Climate Change informs the reader about the impact of climate change on health and its implications for nursing practice.

Unit VII Advocacy includes information about advocacy for nursing practice, coalitions, legislative meetings and chemical policy reform.

Unit VIII Theory and Research In this revised, 3rd edition, this section covers models for environmental health research and interviews with cutting-edge nurse environmental health scientists.

The 3rd edition of Environmental Health in Nursing reflects how the nursing profession has moved forward since the 1995 IOM report and the important role that nurses play in protecting and caring for the environment, advocating, and advancing the science of environmental health nursing and the patients and communities we serve.

Unit 1:
Why Nursing?

ENVIRONMENTAL HEALTH IN ALL NURSING PRACTICE

Environment is one of four traditional concepts in nursing: nurse, patient/client, health, and environment. All nurses practice in one or more places that we can call an environment. Patients/clients live, work, learn, play, and worship in various environments. Nurses are to assist in creating healthy environments in which individuals, families, groups, and communities can thrive (American Nurses Association, 2020).

This first unit of the e-text describes environmental health, why nurses are involved in environmental health, and principles of environmental health in nursing. Environmental health nursing in homes/families, schools, communities, and faith communities is introduced. In this Unit, you will be introduced to some contemporary nurse luminaries and pioneers in environmental health. Also, the environmental health competencies expected of all nurses are presented. See Unit IV for details of environmental health for nurses in hospital and institutional practice settings.

REFERENCE

American Nurses Association. (2020). *Nursing: Scope and standards of practice* (4th ed). American Nurses Association.

WHY NURSES ARE INVOLVED WITH ENVIRONMENTAL HEALTH

Claudia M. Smith, PhD, MPH, RN-BC
Retired Assistant Professor
University of Maryland Baltimore
School of Nursing

Jeanne Leffers, PhD, RN, FAAN
Professor Emeritus
University of Massachusetts Dartmouth
College of Nursing and Health Sciences

WHAT IS ENVIRONMENTAL HEALTH?

"The environment is one of the fundamental determinants of individual and community health" (Institute of Medicine, 1995, p. 1). The environment along with human behavior, genetics/biology, and the health care system contribute to the health and illness among human populations (Dever, 1991).

Environmental health may be defined as that aspect of human health determined by physical, chemical, biological, and psychosocial factors in the environment (WHO, 1993, cited in Sattler & Lipscomb, 2003, p. xiii). Others define environmental health as the freedom from illness or injury...[due] to exposure to toxic agents and other [hazardous] environmental conditions" (Institute of Medicine, 1995, p. 15).

Environmental health may be defined also as "the theory and practice of assessing, correcting, controlling, and preventing factors in the environment" that negatively affect health (WHO, 1993, cited in Sattler & Lipscomb, 2003, p. xiii). Environmental factors that negatively affect health are often called environmental hazards.

"The environment is everything around us - the air we breathe, the water we drink and use, and the food we consume. It's also the chemicals, radiation, microbes, and physical forces with which we come into contact. Our interactions with the environment are complex and are not always healthy" (Centers for Disease Control & Prevention, National Center for Environmental Health, 2009).

Not only do we come in contact with our environment. our environment becomes us through the air, water, food, and other exposures. Obviously, we are dependent upon our environment for our development, growth, and survival. For example, food provides nutrients for development, growth, and energy; water composes many of our body fluids. When the physical environment is polluted, pollution is not only around us, but in us! Watch this video (22 minutes long) from the Environmental Working Group to learn eye-opening information about body burden [of chemicals] in children.

So, what are we to do to reduce environmental hazards? How can we reduce human exposure to environmental hazards? What are we to do to promote healthier environments? We can respond as nurses, workers, students, parents, family members, group members, and citizens. Why are nurses especially equipped to address environmental health?

TOP TEN REASONS THAT NURSES & ENVIRONMENTAL HEALTH GO TOGETHER

1. Nurses provide healing and safe environments for people.

2. Nurses are trusted sources of information.

3. Nurses are the largest healthcare occupation.

4. Nurses work with persons from a variety of cultures.

5. Nurses effect decisions in their own homes, work settings, and communities.

6. Nurses are trusted sources of information for policy makers.

7. Nurses translate scientific health literature to make it understandable.

8. Nurses with advanced degrees are engaged in research about the environment and health.

9. Health organizations recognize nurses' roles in environmental health.

10. Nursing education and standards of nursing practice require that nurses know how to reduce exposures to environmental health hazards (ANA, 2020).

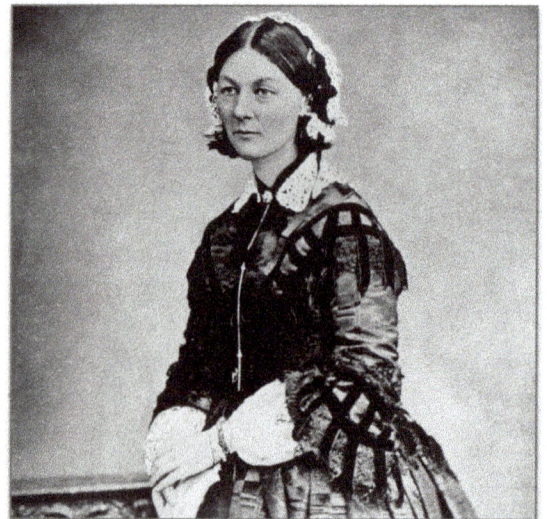

Nurses have always been leaders in providing healing and safe environments for people. Nurses protect their patients and their communities. (See Florence Nightingale's Notes on Nursing published in 1860.) Nurses are everywhere that other people are. We work in hospitals and other health care settings, homes, schools and occupational sites. Each of these places has hazards that can cause illness, injury, or premature death. Nurses work to protect people from hazards by eliminating or reducing the harms from hazards and by reducing or eliminating the hazards.

Nurses advocate for environments in which people cannot only survive, but thrive (ANA, 2007). Nurses are trusted sources of information. The most recent Gallup Poll of US residents shows that for the eighteenth year, nurses are ranked the most honest and ethical profession. When nurses speak, people listen. Nurses provide information to patients and the public about healthy and safe environments. These environments promote human health. They help prevent illness, disability, and premature death.

Registered Nurses (RNs) are the largest healthcare occupation. (See Department of Health and Human Services, 2020) One in every one hundred Americans is a Registered Nurse. (ANA, 2020). Therefore, most residents of the United States come in contact with nurses.

Nurses have experience working with persons from various racial, ethnic, cultural, and socio-economic backgrounds. We also work with persons across the lifespan, from pregnant people and newborns to those at the end of their life. Nurses build on these deep and broad communication networks to protect and improve human health.

Nurses have the capacity to effect decisions in their own homes, their work settings, and their communities. Nurses influence decisions in work settings---schools, clinics, homes, nursing homes, and hospitals. Health Care Without Harm is an international coalition of 473 organizations in more than 50 countries, working to transform the health care sector so it is safer for patients and workers. Nurses also help make decisions about health as members of community groups such as PTAs, churches, and other faith-based institutions. The numbers of nurses and their personal influence creates a unique opportunity to make change.

Nurses are uniformly viewed as trusted, un-biased sources of information by policymakers and the public (Sattler & Lipscomb, 2003). Nurses partner with professional and citizen groups that are addressing a wide range of environmental hazards which affect human health. Some nurses are actively involved in policy and advocacy work at the state and federal government level. Safer Chemicals Healthy Families is a campaign that includes nurse advocates who are working to improve U.S. federal policies that protect us from toxic chemicals.

Nurses are translators of scientific health literature. Nurses help patients, families, and members of their community to understand studies about environmental health. The Research Forum of the Alliance of Nurses for Environmental Health (ANHE) is creating a library of nursing research articles on environmental health. This will better identify evidence-based practices that nurses can implement with individuals, families, and communities.

Nurses with advanced degrees are engaged in research about the environment and health. ANHE also is promoting nurse researchers and sharing information about funding sources for research. The Research Forum of ANHE has surveyed nurses to explore the priorities for research related to environmental health and nursing. Nurses with a research-focused doctorate usually have a Doctor in Philosophy (PhD) degree and are leading this research.

KEEPING PATIENTS SAFE

Health organizations recognize nurses' roles in environmental health. The World Health Organization states that it is essential for nurses to promote healthy environments, especially homes (Adams, Bartram, & Chartier, 2008). The International Council of Nurses (2007) asserts that nurses should help reduce environmental hazards and promote clean water. In 2004, the Institute of Medicine (IOM) published the report, *Keeping patients safe: Transforming the work environment of nurses*. This report advocates for making hospitals and health care facilities safer for both patients and nurses. Nurses are to "create a safe care environment that results in high quality patient outcomes" (AACN, 2008, p. 31).

In 2010, the American Nurses' Association (ANA) added an environmental standard to Nursing: Scope and Standards for all RNs. This standard advocates that "the registered nurse integrates the principles of environmental health for nursing in all areas of practice" (ANA, 2010, p. 57). Most recent editions of the Scope and Standards have continued to develop the nurses' role in environmental health.

This standard requires every nurse to have the knowledge and skills to integrate environmental health information into their daily practice. No matter what the level of nursing education, no matter what our nursing experience, each nurse needs to be current with the expanding evidence about environmental health (AACN, 2006, 2008; NLNAC, 2008). (See Principles of Environmental Health for Nursing Practice later in this document.)

Nursing education organizations require nurses' roles in environmental health. All nurses are to serve as positive role models within healthcare settings and their community (National League for Nursing, NLN, 2000). All nurses need to know how to reduce exposure to environmental health hazards and provide safe physical environments. "Nurses use evidence-based decisions to deliver client care and [help] move clients toward positive health outcomes" (NLN, 2000, p. 14). Nurses with a diploma or an associate degree are focused primarily on the health of individuals and families (NLN). Every individual and every family have some environmental hazards.

Nurses with baccalaureate education expand their focus to include communities and population health (American Association of Colleges of Nursing, AACN, 2008; Association of Community Health Nursing Educators, ACHNE, 2010). Population health includes health promotion and disease/injury prevention with groups, communities, and populations (AACN, 2008; ACHNE, 2010).

Graduates with a master's degree in a nursing specialty or a Doctor of Nursing Practice (DNP) degree are educated to be leaders in nursing practice. As leaders in the practice arena, "DNPs provide a critical interface between practice, research, and policy" (AACN, 2006, p. 14). "The DNP graduate has a foundation in clinical prevention and population health" (AACN, 2006, p. 15). This foundation includes the nurses' ability to analyze occupational and environmental data to plan, implement, and evaluate their practice for clinical prevention and population health.

PRINCIPLES OF ENVIRONMENTAL HEALTH FOR NURSING

All nurses are to be aware of the principles of environmental health for nursing and integrate these principles into our practice, education, and research.

ANA'S PRINCIPLES OF ENVIRONMENTAL HEALTH FOR NURSING PRACTICE

1. Knowledge of environmental health concepts is essential to nursing practice.

2. The precautionary principle guides nurses in their practice to use products and practices that do not harm human health or the environment and to take preventive action in the fact of uncertainty.

3. Nurses have a right to work in an environment that is safe and healthy.

4. Healthy environments are sustained through multidisciplinary collaboration.

5. Choice of materials, products, technology, and practices in the environment that impact nursing practice are based on the best available evidence.

6. Approaches to promoting a healthy environment reflect a respect for the diverse values, beliefs, cultures, and circumstances of patients and their families.

7. Nurses participate in assessing the quality of the environment in which they practice and live.

8. Nurses, other health care workers, patients, and communities have the right to know relevant and timely information about the potentially harmful products, chemicals, pollutants, and hazards to which they are exposed.

9. Nurses participate in research of best practices that promote a safe and healthy environment.

10. Nurses must be supported in advocating for and implementing environmental health principles in nursing practice.

Source: ANA's principles of environmental health for nursing practice with implementation strategies. (2007). American Nurses' Association: Silver Spring, MD. (May be purchased in booklet form at nursebooks.org)

Finally, the Alliance of Nurses for Healthy Environments has a large collection of Podcasts with environmental health nurses created by Dr. Elizabeth Schenk, PhD, RN now into Season 4. They can be viewed on the ANHE website at New Podcasts and through the years at Podcast series. The podcasts provide evidence of the impact nurses are making to advance healthier environments.

REFERENCES

Association of American Colleges of Nursing (AACN). (2006). *The essentials of doctoral education for advanced practice nurses.* AACN.

Association of American Colleges of Nursing (AACN). (2008). *The essentials of baccalaureate education for professional nursing practice.* AACN.

Association of Community Health Nursing Educators (ACHNE), Education Committee. (2010). *Essentials of baccalaureate nursing for entry level community/public health nursing.* ACHNE.

Adams, J., Bartram, J., & Chartier, Y. (Eds.). (2008). *Essential environmental health standards in health care.* World Health Organization (WHO). http://www.who.int/water_sanitation_health/hygiene/settings/ehs_health_care.pdf.pdf

American Nurses Association (ANA). (2007). *Public health nursing: Scope & standards of practice.* American Nurses Association.

American Nurses Association (ANA). (2021). *Nursing: Scope and standards of practice* (4th ed.). American Nurses Association.

American Nurses Association. (2020). *What is Nursing?* https://www.nursingworld.org/practice-policy/workforce/what-is-nursing

Centers for Disease Control & Prevention, National Center for Environmental Health. (2009). *About National Center for Environmental Health, 2009.* http://www.cdc.gov/nceh/Information/about.htm

Dever, G.E.A. (1991). *Community health analysis: Development of global awareness at the local Level (2nd ed.).* Aspen.

Institute of Medicine (IOM). (1995). *Nursing, health, & environment.* National Academy Press.

Institute of Medicine (IOM). (2004). *Keeping patients safe: Transforming the work environment of nurses.* National Academy Press. http://www.nap.edu/openbook.php?isbn=0309090679

International Council of Nurses. (ICN) (2007). *Position statement: Reducing environmental and related lifestyle hazards.* ICN.

National League for Nursing (NLN). (2000). *Educational competencies for graduates of associate degree nursing programs.* NLN.

National League for Nursing Accrediting Commission (NLNAC). (2020). *NLNAC 2017 standards and criteria. [Includes diploma, associate, baccalaureate, masters, and post-masters certificates.]* https://www.acenursing.org/acen-accreditation-manual/

Nightingale, F. (1860). *Notes on nursing.* D. Appleton & Company. http://digital.library.upenn.edu/women/nightingale/nursing/nursing.html

Sattler, B. & Lipscomb, J. (Eds.). (2003). *Environmental health and nursing practice.* Springer Publishing Company.

US Bureau of Labor Statistics. (2020). *Occupational Labor Statistics.* https://bit.ly/3lccYfd

U.S. Department of Health and Human Services, Health Resources and Services Administration, National Center for Health Workforce Analysis. 2019. *Brief Summary Results from the 2018 National Sample Survey of Registered Nurses, Rockville, Maryland.* https://bhw.hrsa.gov/health-workforce-analysis/data/national-sample-survey-registered-nurses

ENVIRONMENTAL HEALTH AND FAMILIES/HOMES

Judith Focareta, RN, MEd
Medical Policy Clinician
Highmark Health
Pittsburgh, PA

Environmental Health is important throughout the life cycle. From preconception to aging populations, the environment is a contributor to health and illness. Childbearing families are particularly at risk. This is because babies developing in the womb and growing children are quite vulnerable to assaults from air pollution and chemicals present in water, food, and products.

For example,

- Epidemiological studies show that children whose parents work in the farming communities of California have a higher incidence of childhood leukemia (Wigle, Turner, & Krewski, 2009). It is suspected that exposure to pesticides is responsible.

- Air pollution has been linked to a number of adverse health effects such as preterm labor and most recently autism in children.

- The phthalate DEHP has been eliminated from many newborn nurseries and neonatal intensive care units because of evidence implicating this chemical in male reproductive changes.

- Bbisphenol A (BPA), a component of many plastic products including children's toys, has been shown to be an endocrine disruptor and is linked to cancer and developmental delays.

CRITICAL WINDOWS

Critical windows of vulnerability have been defined in the literature as the following: "Periods during life when an exposure causes a stronger deficit in health later in life compared with other periods when exposure (could have) occurred" (Sanchez, Hu, & Tellez-Rojo, 2011, p. 1).

"Key developmental or reproductive life stages where the body can be more biologically vulnerable or influenced by exposures to chemicals in the environment" (Scott, 2015, p. 395).

Many of these critical windows occur as the fetus develops in utero. In this prenatal environment even small doses of chemicals can cause harm. Exposure to low-doses of chemicals rarely causes gross abnormalities that are obvious at birth. A more likely scenario is that they interfere with the programming that occurs during development, thus creating disease susceptibilities later in life.

According to the American Academy of Pediatrics, children also have unique vulnerabilities to environmental exposures because of their different metabolism, body structure, daily behavior, and lifestyle (Davis, 2007).

During puberty and adolescence the brain is still developing. Chemical exposures during this time can bioaccumulate and be passed to the baby during pregnancy and/or breastfeeding.

HOME EXPOSURES

Exposures to chemicals of concern often occur in the home. It has been estimated that Americans spend 90% of their time indoors. It then becomes important to recognize and decrease environmental stressors in the home environment. Harmful chemicals can be introduced through the foods that we eat, the water we drink, the products that we utilize, and the air that we breathe.

The foods we consume may contain pesticide residues. Plastic food wrap may expose families to phthalates such as bisphenol A (BPA). High fat foods such as meat and dairy may contain chemicals that are lipophilic such persistent organic pollutants (POPs). Fish may be contaminated with mercury, a known neurotoxin.

Petroleum products, pesticides and fertilizers may contaminate water, especially wells. Water filtration devices may not be adequate to eliminate chemicals of concern from the water supply for safe consumption.

Phthalates are chemicals that appear in everyday household products including personal care items and cleaning products as added fragrance. They are also components of many plastic products and may show up in children's toys. These chemicals are endocrine disruptors (EDCs). EDCs have the capacity to interfere with hormone regulation and this may cause permanent disruption of metabolic processes.

Lead is a heavy metal that was present in interior paints before it was gradually phased out in the 1970's. It may still be detectable in older homes built before 1978. It is a potent neurotoxin and can accumulate in dust. Because chemicals such as lead accumulate in dust, be sure to damp clean regularly. Other possible sources for lead especially for children may include toys, jewelry, and lead in plumbing pipes (CDC, 2020).

Indoor air pollution is linked to volatile organic compounds or VOCs. Common sources of indoor VOC exposure include building materials, paints, household cleaning products, furniture made from particle board, and carpets. All of these products have the capacity to "off gas" chemicals such as formaldehyde and benzene.

NURSE RESPONSIBILITIES

Nurses must have the knowledge and skills to protect themselves, their families, and their communities, and influence others by leading by example. Nurses who work with childbearing families have a special opportunity to educate and influence choices that can have an impact for a lifetime. Evidence shows that reducing exposures to products that contain toxic chemicals can reduce body burden.

No one can completely eliminate chemicals from their lives. But making small changes especially in the home can reduce exposures. No one can do everything. But everyone can adopt at least one change (large or small) to create a healthier environment..

Studies have shown that making simple changes results in a lower body burden of chemicals of concern. Research results document that when children's diets change from conventional to organic, pesticide metabolites are reduced. Other studies show that avoiding canned foods and other dietary sources of BPA reduce levels of that chemical in the body. And simple dietary changes can also decrease exposure to phthalates.

Changes do not have to be complicated. For example, taking your shoes off at the door can help to avoid bringing offending chemicals such as lead and pesticides into the home. Keep the house well ventilated and open windows to let in fresh air even in the winter. Purchase fresh foods and buy local and organic when possible to reduce exposure to pesticide residues.

Meal planning provides another opportunity to decrease exposure to chemicals of concern. Utilize the Environmental Working Group pesticide ratings of fruits and vegetables to decide where to spend money on organics. For example apples consistently have detectable levels of pesticide residue when tested. This is a fruit to consider buying organic or locally grown. Consider planting a "kitchen garden" or favorite vegetables and herbs. This will have the added benefit of teaching children where their food comes from. Children who are assisting with the garden will enjoy partaking of the produce as well. Eat foods with less animal fat since harmful chemicals are stored in fat. This means eating more fruits and vegetables and less meat and dairy.

Because household cleaning products can be sources of indoor air pollution it is best to avoid those that contain bleach and ammonia. Many green cleaning products are plant based or you can make your own using such common items as baking soda and vinegar. The Environmental Working Group's (EWG) Guide to Healthy Cleaning is a great resource for "greener cleaners" including vinegar. EWG gives vinegar a grade of A+ for no health concerns with use (EWG, 2020). The National Institute for Occupational Safety and Health (NIOSH) suggests using vinegar to clean windows, floors, and as a drain cleaner (NIOSH, 2014), Vinegar is naturally bacteriostatic and bactericidal (Entani et al. 1998).

Consider purchasing furniture and flooring composed of real wood. Wood composite materials off-gas VOC's as they are held together with toxic glues. Wood floors such as bamboo are also more environmentally friendly than composite or vinyl flooring and are economical as well. Look for flooring labeled no or low-VOC. Purchase paints that are labeled "low VOC" and use water-based glues.

To reduce mercury exposures, refer to the EPA/FDA guidelines which suggest eating smaller fish which contain less mercury like salmon, light tuna, and shellfish.

Don't use pesticides in your home or garden. Keep out pests by sealing cracks and holes around doors and windowsills, screens and baseboards. Vinegar can be used in a spray bottle to repel ants, mosquitos, fruit flies and other pests (Kumar, 2021). Choose plants that grow well where you live so you won't need harmful chemicals and learn about organic gardening.

Re-think your personal care products and learn to read labels. Some toothpaste contains triclosan, a chemical that is in the pesticide family. This chemical is added as a preservative to reduce bacterial contamination (FDA, n.d.). Formaldehyde and toluene are often added to nail polishes and both are linked to cancer. Buy nail formulations that are free of these additives. Avoid cosmetics that contain added fragrance. Fragrance generally contains phthalates, which are known to be endocrine disruptors. There are many "green" personal care products on the market that are cost effective. This is especially true in baby care products.

Nurses are powerful. We have the potential to change exposures for ourselves and for those we care.

REFERENCES

Barr Jr, M., DeSesso, J. M., Lau, C. S., Osmond, C., Ozanne, S. E., Sadler, T. W., ... & Sonawane, B. R. (2000). Workshop to identify critical windows of exposure for children's health: cardiovascular and endocrine work group summary. *Environmental Health Perspectives, 108*(suppl 3), 569-571.

Center for Disease Control and Prevention (CDC). (2020).*Childhood lead prevention in children.* https://www.cdc.gov/nceh/lead/prevention/sources/consumer-products.htm

Davis, A., (2007). Home environmental health risks. *OJIN: The Online Journal of Issues in Nursing, 12*(2), Manuscript 4.

Entani, E., Asai, M., Tsujihata, S., Tsukamoto, Y., & Ohta, M. (1998). Antibacterial action of vinegar against food-borne pathogenic bacteria including Escherichia coli O157:H7. *Journal of Food Protection, 61*(8), 953–959. https://doi.org/10.4315/0362-028x-61.8.953

Food and Drug Administration (n.d.). *5 things to know about triclosan.* https://www.fda.gov/consumers/consumer-updates/5-things-know-about-triclosan

Kumar, K. (2021). *Is vinegar a good bug repellent?* MedicineNet. https://www.medicinenet.com/is_vinegar_a_good_bug_repellent/article.htm

National Institute of OccupationalSafety and Health (NIOSH) (2014). *Caring for yourself while caring for others.* U.S. Department of Health and Human Services, Centers for Disease Control and Prevention, National Institute for Occupational Safety and Health, DHHS (NIOSH) Publication No. 2015–103.

Sanchez, B., Hu, H., Litman, H., & Tellez-Rojo, M. (2011). Statistical methods to study timing of vulnerability with sparsely sampled data on environmental toxicants. *Environmental Health Perspectives, 119,* 409-415. http://dx.doi.org/10.1289/ehp.1002453

Scott, D (Ed.). 2015. *Our Chemical Selves: Gender, Toxics, and Environmental Health.* UBC Press.

Selevan, S. G., Kimmel, C. A., & Mendola, P. (2000). Identifying critical windows of exposure for children's health. *Environmental Health Perspectives, 108*(Suppl 3), 451–455.

West, J. (2002). Defining critical windows in the development of the human immune system. *Human Exposure Toxicology, 21*(9-10), 499-505.

Wigle, D. T., Turner, M. C., & Krewski, D. (2009). A systematic review and meta-analysis of childhood leukemia and parental occupational pesticide exposure. *Environmental Health Perspectives, 117*(10), 1505-13.

ENVIRONMENTAL HEALTH NURSING AT THE COMMUNITY LEVEL

Jessica Castner, PhD, RN, CEN, FAAN
President and Principal Investigator
Castner Incorporated

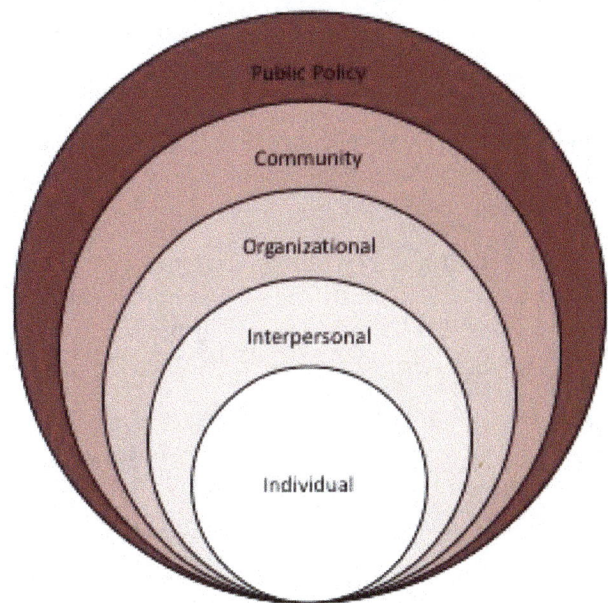

Figure 1: The Socio-Ecological Model

INTRODUCTION

Human health is influenced by an interconnected dynamic of factors from the individual's biology and genetics to the public policy that establishes access to health services. The Socio-Ecological Model (Figure 1) depicts the context of individual health within interpersonal, organizational or institutional, community, and public-policy factors (McLeroy, Bibeau, Steckler, & Glanz, 1988; Stokols, 1996).

Nurses are engaged in applying the nursing process to improve environmental health at all levels of the Socio-Ecological Model. For example, at the individual and interpersonal level, the nurse may assess a patient and family's environmental exposure history. Based on the assessment, the nurse may provide individualized education and strategies to enhance a family member's asthma control by reducing personal environmental exposures. At the organizational level, nurses may work to reduce medical waste burning practices (https://noharm-uscanada.org/issues/us-canada/waste-management) in their employing agency. This section introduces environmental health nursing at the community level

COMMUNITY

A population is a group of people who share at least one common characteristic. Communities include one or more populations and their shared goals over time (Maurer & Smith, 2013). Most commonly, communities refer to people living in the same geographical location, like a town or county. However, communities can be formed around a purpose or profession (e.g. medical community), education (e.g. online learning community), economic interest (e.g. small business community), a faith community (e.g. Catholic community), or other common characteristics or special interests (e.g. lesbian community). More information on describing and understanding the community can be found at the Community Toolbox Website. The community health nurse applies the nursing process to the overall aggregate health of their community of focus (ANA, 2013). Most nurses who provide nursing care at the community level are educated at the baccalaureate level of nursing or higher.

Community health nurses have a focus on the systems context that is broader than direct delivery of care to patients and families alone. One of the key determinants of health (http://healthypeople.gov/2020/about/DOHAbout.aspx) at the community level is the physical environment, including environmental pollution. Often, exposures to pollutants in the water, air, soil, and food supply are beyond the control of any one individual. In these circumstances, applying the nursing process at the community-level is necessary to improve health. The Nursing Practice Chapter of this eTextbook has more information on applying the nursing process at the community level.

The following video is a case example of environmental health nursing at the community level, entitled *Holding Polluters Accountable: A Community-Nurse Collaboration* (2014).

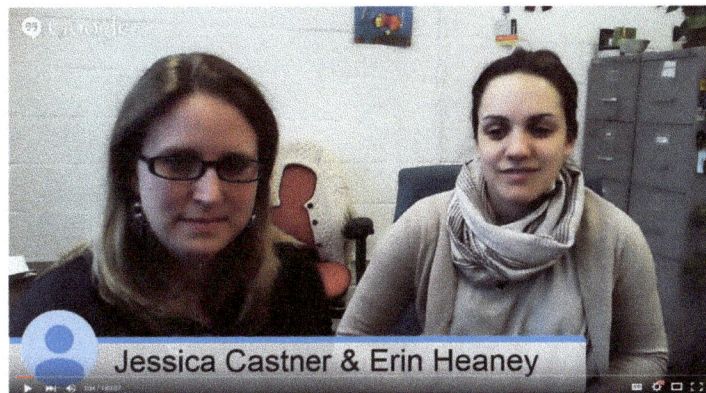

Holding Polluters Accountable: A Community-Nurse Collaboration Success Story

https://www.youtube.com/watch?v=HGzBLpZmGyM
(63:07 minutes)

REFERENCES

American Nurses Association (ANA). (2013). *Public health nursing: Scope and standards of practice* (2nd ed.). American Nurses Association.

Maurer, F., & Smith, C.M. (2013). Community assessment. In F. Maurer & C.M. Smith (Eds.), *Community/public health nursing practice: Health for families and populations* (5th ed, pp. 393-426). Elsevier.

McLeroy, K.R., Bibeau, D., Steckler, A., & Glanz K. (1988). An ecological perspective on health promotion programs. *Health Education Quarterly, 15*(4), 351–377. doi: 10.1177/109019818801500401.

Stokols, D. (1996). Translating social ecological theory into guidelines for community health promotion. *American Journal of Health Promotion, 10*, 282–298. doi: 10.4278/0890-1171-10.4.282.

FAITH COMMUNITY: AN ENVIRONMENTAL PARTNER

Ruth McDermott Levy, PhD, MPH, RN
Professor
Co-Director, Mid-Atlantic Center for Children's Health
and the Environment
Villanova University
M. Louise Fitzpatrick College of Nursing

*"Creation is not a property, which we can rule over at will;
or, even less, is the property of only a few: Creation is a gift,
it is a wonderful gift that God has given us, so that we
care for it and we use it for the benefit of all, always with
great respect and gratitude."* Pope Francis, May 21, 2014.

Partnering with the faith community is a natural fit for nurses when educating community members about environmental health risks and advocating for improved environmental regulations with policy makers. The faith community and the nursing profession share several environmental interests that could be developed into mutual programs to improve the health of individuals, families and communities. Some of the shared interests are:

• Stewardship of the earth

• Common good

• Climate change

• Justice/ Environmental Justice

• Sustainable practices

• Solidarity with marginalized groups

• Workers' rights

While the scope of this text does not permit covering each faith practice in detail, a general description of faith practices relative to the environment offers the nurse a basic understanding. The Abrahamic faiths of Judaism, Christianity, and Islam include an imperative to care for the earth and also acknowledge that the earth's resources are a gift from the Creator that must be appreciated (Green Prophet, 2008). Eastern religions, such as Hinduism and Buddhism, do not make a distinction between the person and the natural environment; people and the natural environment are all part of an interconnected web of life that must be cared for (Green Faith, n.d.). Like Eastern religions, Native American and indigenous peoples view themselves as part of the earth and their connectedness to the earth has influenced their survival throughout history (Sherrer & Murphy, 2006). The list of faith-based environmental organizations later in this section provides web links so you can learn more detail

and perspectives of specific faith traditions related to the environment.

Some churches and other faith groups enlist the services of a parish nurse to meet the spiritual and health needs of their congregation (Whisnant, 1999). The parish nurse could be a valuable partner in collaborating to develop congregation wide environmental initiatives. If a faith community does not have a parish nurse, nurses could volunteer within their own faith communities to influence the environmental health of the congregation as well as the faith community's environmental impact. Partnering with the clergy and the leadership of the faith community can promote trust of the nurse within the congregation. Most faith communities also have resources that can assist them in serving as a center for environmental health outreach. For example churches, synagogues, mosques, and temples have meeting rooms, office space, and frequently volunteers to support environmental health initiatives. Furthermore, the faith community has a moral structure from which nurses can frame an environmental discussion (Green Prophet, 2008) to the congregation, the larger community, or policy makers.

There are many environmental faith based organizations. Some are single faith and others are multi-faith organizations. Here is a list of some faith based environmental organizations and their web sites.

Organization Name	Web Site	Organization Purpose
Catholic Climate Covenant	catholicclimatecovenant.org/about/story	Catholic teaching related to care for creation and climate change
Coalition on the Environment and Jewish Life (COEJL)	www.coejl.org/	Strengthening stewardship of the Earth through outreach, activism and Jewish learning
Green Faith	greenfaith.org	Teach & mobilize people of diverse religious backgrounds for environmental leadership
Interfaith Power and Light	www.interfaithpowerandlight.org/	Interfaith group with a focus on climate change
Islamic Foundation for Ecology & Environmental Sciences	www.ifees.org.uk/green-guide-for-muslims	U.K. based organization. Provides a "Green Guide for Muslims"

Organization Name	Web Site	Organization Purpose
National Religious Partnership for the Environment	www.nrpe.org/	Partnership of faith based environmental organizations. Good resources for various religions' environmental perspective
Pachamama Alliance	www.pachamama.org/	Influencing society to have environmentally sustainable partnerships with indigenous people
Quaker Earth Care Witness	www.quakerearthcare.org/	Network of Quakers addressing ecological and social world crises
Tribal P2: Pollution Prevention Network	tribalp2.org/	Collaborates with U.S. tribes to reduce environmental & health risks on tribal lands
Evangelical Environmental Network	www.creationcare.org/	A ministry for Evangelical Christians in the U.S. that educates, inspires, and mobilizes them in their effort to care for God's creation

REFERENCES

Green Faith. (n.d.). *Religious teachings on the environment.*

Green Prophet. (2008). *Faith & the environment: Multi-faith perspectives.* http://www.greenprophet.com/2008/07/faith-the-environment/

Sherrer, N., & Murphy, T. (2006). Probing the relationship between Native Americans and ecology. *Joshua: Journal of Science and Health at the University of Alabama, 4,* 16-18.

Whisnant, S. (1999). The parish nurse: Tending to the spiritual side of health. *Holistic Nursing Practice, 14*(1), 84-6.

SPOTLIGHT ON NURSES

MY ROAD TO ENVIRONMENTAL HEALTH
Lill Mood, RN, MPH, FAAN
Retired, South Carolina Department of Health and
Environmental Control
Columbia, SC

When I am asked how I got involved in environmental health, my first impulse is to talk about the day in 1993 when Lewis Shaw, the engineer in charge of Environmental Quality Control (EQC) at the South Carolina Department of Health & Environmental Control (DHEC) approached me. We had been colleagues on the State Health Commissioner's Executive staff for several years where he was a Deputy Commissioner and I was Assistant Commissioner and State Director of Public Health Nursing.

I will never forget his words: "I think we need a nurse." He was asking me to transfer into his deputy area which carried responsibility for the state and federally-delegated programs of Air Quality, Water, Solid & Hazardous Waste, and the Environmental Laboratory. He saw the need for someone who could be a bridge between his staff of environmental scientists and engineers and communities that were impacted by environmental events and hazards.

At that time, I had been a public health nurse for more than 20 years and from my position on the Commissioner's staff had a broad understanding of the interconnectedness of the agency's responsibility for public health and environmental protection. I also had working relationships of long-duration in most of the working units of the agency. The thought of creating a new job that would strengthen the link between health and environment as well as letting me spend time in local communities was very appealing.

For the next eight years, calls were directed to my office from citizens who were concerned about something in their environment:

- something looked unusual, smelled strange, tasted odd

- too many people around them were ill, especially with cancer

- they were uneasy about the industry nearby

- there were rumors that a landfill was coming to their neighborhood.

The list was long, and my job was to listen, to go and let them show me and talk with me about their worries. I spent a lot of my working hours at kitchen tables, country churches, and neighborhood meetings all across the state. Then I was to follow-through to assure that our staff made an appropriate response.

Sometimes the follow-up was supplying them with the information we had and they did not, and providing for interpretation of data unfamiliar to them. Sometimes the problem called for an environmental investigation, often combined with analysis of health data for the area, particularly data from the cancer registry. Sometimes we provided public forums, with participation of experts in their issues of concern, to discuss and clarify and decide on a course of action. In these situations, I worked with the community to plan for where and when to meet and how to keep them informed over the course of resolving the issue.

Often my calls were from front-line staff in our environmental programs and district offices. There may be need to let a community know of an industry's application for an environmental permit. We may be involved in cleaning up a spill or other source of environmental contamination. In that case, my job was to alert the community, with the necessary information for them to protect themselves and/or become actively involved in the permitting or enforcement process. Sometimes the staff just wanted me to go with them to meet with some upset citizens.

My job also carried responsibility for risk communication —helping staff to understand that risk was a combination of "hazard and outrage" and our job included addressing both! (Peter Sandman's work in this area was invaluable to me. www.psandman.com) Over time, our staff came to understand how people react to risk and how we can prevent and allay fears by how we respond and communicate. Community meetings, which I often moderated, went from being situations filled with angry crowds where our staff felt they deserved "hazardous duty pay", to collaborative events. We all learned what valuable assets watchful citizens, who care about their environment, are to our work of surveillance and protection.

I was involved in planning and delivering continuing education for staff—in orientation sessions, in workshops, in immersion environmental learning experiences for local health department professionals, and in developing materials to aid the staff in responding to frequently occurring questions.

My work began to extend from a focus on our agency staff to lecturing to university classes in schools of nursing and public health. I was asked to chair the Institute of

Medicine Study of Nursing, Health & Environment (1995) and then was often invited to speak about the resulting report to numerous groups in many states. With some pioneering colleagues at the University of Maryland, we developed a chapter on Environmental Health for Stanhope & Lancaster's Public Health Nursing text. Diana Mason asked that I contribute an environmental vignette for her book on Policy and Politics in Nursing and Health Care. I served on the Enforcement Subcommittee for EPA's National Environmental Justice Advisory Council, and that lead to involvement with other EPA and environmental justice initiatives, including organizing and implementing a Future Search conference in South Carolina. Being a part of the Alliance of Nurses for Healthy Environments (ANHE) has been an exciting and joy-filled experience, with new opportunities and relationships.

My career and world expanded in ways I had never imagined. I realize that my environmental health journey did not really begin with that conversation with Lewis Shaw. I began heading in this direction from my days as a nursing undergraduate when my public health nursing professor and life-long mentor, Virginia Phillips, taught me the multi-disciplinary nature of public health, modeled it in her practice and made it an integral part of my concept of the breadth of public health and my approach to solving public health problems. My graduate program in the School of Public Health at the University of SC included required course work in environment as well as multi-discipline practice seminars addressing real issues in our state. The connections between health and environment and the necessity of a variety of expertise to prevent and address problems in each domain were cemented into my DNA!

My commitment to protecting and improving our environment did not end with retirement. I am still actively involved, especially in issues of the built environment—public transportation, more livable communities with safe spaces for walking and biking, community design and development that considers access to goods and services for all of the population, and public policy decision-making that supports community involvement and sustainable living. I am active in my church's efforts to be a more "green congregation", rooted in our calling to "tend and care for all of creation."

My community knows me as an avowed "tree-hugger", and I have confirmed that again with the wonderful opportunity to work with high school students planting sequoia trees!

The first principle I learned in environmental health is that "everything is connected to everything else." That is a basic principle for the environment and health and for life itself.

ADVOCATING FOR ENVIRONMENTAL JUSTICE

Dorothy Lewis Powell, RN, EdD, FAAN
Professor Emeritus
Duke University
School of Nursing

I grew up in a small southern town in Vance County, North Carolina in the 1950s and 60s. My family lived within the city limits about 100 yards from the city dump where the town's trash was burned in open space each afternoon. I vividly recall the dark smoke that would rise and the darkness and ash that would float overhead and descend over neighboring communities of African-American families. On wash day, we had to be sure to get the clothes off the line before the tall pile of trash was ignited. In the summertime, it was difficult to sit outdoors because of the dust and dirt on our street. Occasionally, a city truck would drive by and spray a solution on the street, giving us temporary relief from the dusty particles.

As a young child, I did not understand the nature of these problems. This was the way of life, and like my family, I adapted and co-existed with these environmental assaults. As I grew older and learned about the environment in secondary school, college, and beyond, I would revisit these childhood memories and be appalled by how our health and wellbeing had been threatened by such exposure.

During the 1970s, the State of North Carolina routinely dumped polychlorinated byphenyls (PCB)-laced oil, a highly toxic carcinogenic compound, on the roadbeds in certain areas of the state. After many years of protests and court action, the state removed the worn PCB-laced residue with the intention of burying it in a landfill in Warren County, NC, adjacent to Vance County. Opponents of that plan argued that Warren County was selected because the area was rural and the majority of the residents were poor, black and politically unable to determine their fate. My uncle, a well-regarded civic-minded local leader, joined other local and national civil rights leaders, community activists, and environmental groups from around the nation in protesting the intended burial of the toxic waste in the Warren County landfill. These accounts of environmental injustice stimulated my personal and professional ambitions. My interest in community health nursing and the impact of environmental, economic, political, and racially-linked exposure of toxic substances on vulnerable populations was the stimulus that increasingly matured my interest and commitment to environmental and population health.

I served as Dean of the Howard University College School of Nursing for 18 years. During that time, a small group of public/community health-minded faculty and I became involved in the Mississippi Delta Project, funded by Agency for Toxic Substances and Disease Registry. The aim of the project was to increase awareness of environmental health concepts and practices in nursing curricula in schools of nursing in the Mississippi Delta. The Delta is a geographical area comprised of 219 counties over seven states where a plethora of corporate farms, industrial factories, petroleum refineries, and other "dirty industries," posed hazardous exposure to the area's residents, who were largely poor, under-educated, African-American and politically unengaged. Our work led to the development of a modular curriculum, Environmental Health and Nursing: The Mississippi Delta Project (1999), comprised of six modules: demographics of the Delta, culture, toxicology, environmental justice, community assessment, and community engagement and advocacy. I authored the environmental justice module which, along with other modules, continued to evolve and opened doors for collaboration with other schools of nursing, invited presentations around the county with nursing and non-nursing groups, and led to other publications and to my appointment to the EPA National Environmental Justice Advisory Committee.

MY JOURNEY AS AN ADVOCATE FOR ENVIRONMENTAL HEALTH IN NURSING
Barbara Sattler, RN, DrPH, FAAN
Professor Emeritus
University of San Francisco

It takes a village to get good things done. I have been one of many nurses who have discovered environmental health and decided to do something about it. My particular strengths are that I am enthusiastic, creative, and persuasive. That alone would never be enough to sustain forward motion - that required a great many patient, detail oriented, highly organized, and dedicated colleagues who followed through with the sometimes tedious efforts required to integrate environmental health into nursing education, practice, research and policy/advocacy. I salute us all.

There are a couple of things that have been motivators to me for as long as I can remember – social justice, the environment, learning, and having fun. My interest in human health was something that developed later in my 20s when I entered nursing school. I went to a hospital-based diploma nursing program that no longer exists and early in my nursing career I was a critical care nurse first in San Francisco and then in Baltimore – ICU, CCU, ER,

and Burn Unit which I really loved. At the same time, I also was very involved in my nursing union and became part of the contract negotiation team. I learned a lot about the importance of collective action, the power of organizing, and how to work strategically to accomplish goals.

I don't actually have any degrees in nursing, just my Diploma that allowed me to sit for the Boards and become a Registered Nurse. My degrees are BS in Political Science, and both a master's and Doctorate in Public Health from the Johns Hopkins School of Public Health. In between my two graduate degrees, I was the Executive Director of a small non-profit, MaryCOSH (Maryland Committee on Occupational Safety and Health) that worked on a variety of occupational health issues. My main focus was helping to pass a statewide worker right to know law so that workers could find information about the toxic chemicals that they were working with. Our success was largely a function of the diversity of the coalition that we created which included unionized workers, firefighters, health professionals, and non-profit organizations like Clean Water Action and the American Lung Association. Learning to play with folks who have different agendas and yet finding a common one that we could all agree upon was a critical skill for future work.

Then I worked for the United Steelworkers Union. During that time, I went to many different kinds of worksites where I began to understand how poorly we were protecting workers from toxic exposures and, by extension, their families and communities.

My first job after graduate school was directing the National Center for Hazard Communication where I did research and worked with labor, industry, and the government on developing the best tools to train and educate people (workers, community members, health professionals) about hazardous chemicals. As early as 1991, we developed a completely on-line degree on environmental management.

I left that Center, which was at the College Park Campus of the University of Maryland and joined the faculty at the School of Medicine in the Baltimore Campus where I started the Environmental Health Education Center. My first center grants were from the U.S. Environmental Protection Agency to work on lead poisoning prevention. This work expanded into a more comprehensive healthy homes initiative and continued to grow into healthy schools and then healthy hospitals.

I was struck by a 1985 report by the Institute of Medicine (IOM) that showed how physicians did not learn about occupational and environmental health – which was equally true for nurses. Two colleagues and I made an appointment and met with Andrew Pope at the Institute of Medicine to ask for a similar study to be created to look at what nurses learned about occupational and environmental health. We were able to compel him and the IOM. A committee was created that was chaired by Lillian Mood, a brilliant public health nurse from South Carolina who continues to do great environmental health work in her retirement.

The report, Nursing, Health, and the Environment, created a framework for thinking about how to integrate environmental health into the nursing profession. This framework has consistently guided my environmental health and nursing work ever since. It calls for nursing to integrate environmental health into nursing education (our own education and our patient/community education), practice (by both integrating environmental assessments into our clinical care and attending to the environmental healthiness of our health care settings), research, and policy/advocacy. Later, when we created the Alliance of Nurses for Healthy Environments (ANHE), these four domains became our standing committees. An overarching value that is applied to all four domains is environmental justice.

After six or so years on the faculty at the Medical School, the Dean of the University of Maryland, School of Nursing asked me to bring the Environmental Health Education Center to nursing and help to develop the first environmental health and nursing program in the country. I did this with the help of Brenda Afzal, who was my associate and "partner in crime" for many years. There were also a great many other key players at Maryland like Claudia Smith who is an active member of ANHE's Education Work Group, Robyn Gilden who now heads up the Center, and Katie Huffling who is now the Executive Director of ANHE.

At about the same time, I was able to secure a very generous grant ($1.4 million) from the Kellogg Foundation to work with nursing faculty from Howard University to develop and deliver faculty development training on the integration of environmental health into nursing education. We trained over 200 faculty in 17 states and then provided them with two additional years of support. This helped to seed a new crop of environmental health champions within schools of nursing. Pat Butterfield did similar workshops in Montana with funding from the Agency for Toxic Substances and Disease Registry (ATSDR).

While the IOM report was clear that all nurses should learn about environmental health, it became clear to me that some nurses needed to dig deeply into this area. With a grant from the Health Services Resources

Administration (HRSA), I started the first master's degree program in Environmental Health and Nursing. This was a fabulous program that helped to train some of today's nursing leaders. The nursing students who studied with me over the years went on to become executive sustainability officers in hospitals, directors in non-profit organizations, and faculty in environmental health nursing. Many of them expressed their leadership within their nursing specialty professional organizations, helping to bring educational programs and presentations to their national meetings. Though the program was a generalist program, the students often gained significant expertise in environmental topics, for example, Brenda Afzal on drinking water and Robyn Gilden on pesticide use and children's health.

In the late 1990s I was involved in the creation of a national campaign called Health Care Without Harm (HCWH). In one of the early meetings in California, we gathered environmentalists from a variety of organizations – Greenpeace, Environmental Working Group, the Center for Environmental Health, and others – along with a couple of physicians and a small group of nurses, including Charlotte Brody who is a brilliant strategist. It was brought to our attention that one of the biggest contributors to mercury in our air was medical waste incinerator emissions. There were over 3,000 incinerators in the country at the time. Together, we ran a successful campaign that eliminated mercury thermometers in health care (and essentially everywhere else in the U.S.). and we suggested health care facilities close all but fewer than 100 medical waste incinerators.

For a few years I chaired the HCWH Nurses Work Group with my good friend and nursing colleague Susan Wilburn who was then a senior staff at the American Nurses Association in the Center for Occupational and Environmental Health. (The ANA closed that center down and changed their focus to nurses' wellness. I think they should have added wellness instead of eliminating health and safety.) We organized workshops all over the country called RN-NoHarm, helping to launch another cadre of nurses into the realm of environmental health. In this case they were often focused on greening their hospitals. The HCWH campaign morphed into a non-profit organization that spawned a range of exceptional programs like Practice Green Health and the Global Green and Healthy Hospitals.

For several years, the Beldon Fund supported a collaborative nursing approach to green hospitals and address chemical policies in the U.S. The key players were the ANA's Center for Occupational and Environmental Health, HCWH's Nurses Workgroup, and the

Environmental Health Education Center at the University of Maryland. This work included educational efforts and training of nurses in advocacy skills. Nurses worked closely with environmental and public health organizations in their state houses and capitals to advocate for sorely needed comprehensive chemical policy reform. Nurses also worked on many policies that addressed individual chemicals such as BPA and categories of products such as safe cosmetics. We worked with staff at the National Library of Medicine to include training on searching their databases for the best evidence regarding toxic chemicals. We remained scrupulous about being evidence-based in our assertions and in our writings.

We sponsored a half dozen writers' retreats/workshops for nurses who wanted to write articles about environmental health. These were both great fun and very productive and continued to build a "community" of nurses from around the country who were interested in and working on environmental health. These retreats often took place in extraordinary locations like the Northern California Coast and Martha's Vineyard at times in retreat centers, but often at ANHE member's homes.

With Beldon Funds, we organized a group of unions that represent nurses around the country to talk about how to use collective bargaining to better protect nurses from potentially toxic chemicals in hospital settings. The result was a compendium of model language that could be negotiated and inserted into contracts, thus adding another legal framework for protecting nurses (and by extension other employees and patients) from unnecessary harmful exposures in health care.

In 2008, there were a number of nurses around the country that were doing environmental health activities, but they were poorly coordinated. We were not yet building a movement. With funding from the Kendeda Fund, we organized a 4-day retreat in Oracle, AZ, with 50 nursing leaders from around the country. At the end of the retreat we decided to create a national organization, which became an official non-profit organization, called the Alliance of Nurses for Healthy Environments (ANHE). I was a founding Board member and have since then been on and off the Board. This organization has created a wealth of resources, workshops, webinars, a website, a virtual eTextbook, and has effectively engaged in political advocacy. ANHE has helped support the community of nurses who are interested in environmental health.

There are many ways that ANHE is now seen as the voice of environmental health nursing in the country. The ANA defers environmental health questions and efforts to ANHE. We helped to get the first "Environmental Standard" into the 2010 Scope and Standards of Professional Nursing Practice. After ANHE members visited with the head of the National Institute of Nursing Research and the National Institute of Environmental Health Science, these two NIH institutes put out a joint request for nursing research in environmental health. The major national and state environmentalist organizations seek ANHE to help support policy efforts in our state houses and capitals.

Until 2014, ANHE was a US and Canada-based organization. After a working trip to Australia to meet with nursing unions on greening their hospitals and on "fracking", I realized that they were wrestling with the same issues we were in the U.S. and that we should communicate with each other and share resources. We expanded ANHE's scope and created an international Climate Change Committee that incorporates work on fracking and other fossil fuel issues, with monthly calls and nurses from the UK, Australia, Canada and the US.

After retiring from the University of Maryland in 2012, I moved to California, where I am currently a full-time Professor at the University of San Francisco. I continue to be a Board member of ANHE. I am working with the Jonas Nursing Center to develop a scholarship program for doctoral (PhD and DNP) students who are interested in environmental health. With colleagues in Australia and with Susan Wilburn of Global Green and Healthy Hospitals, I am developing a Global Environmental Health Nursing Certificate.

There are some things that "I" did regarding environmental health and nursing, but the vast majority of things "we" did. We have had some very generous funders over the years and a great many supporters. We have helped to birth nursing environmental health champions. I've been involved in 3 decades of work that is helping to form the next generation of nurses who we hope will consider environmental health a critical component of the nursing profession.

"The best way to predict the future is to design it."
Buckminster Fuller

Unit II:

Harmful Environmental Exposures and Vulnerable Populations

INTRODUCTION

Unit I highlighted various roles of the nursing profession where knowledge of environmental exposures is central to practice. In Unit II, the focus is upon populations who are most vulnerable to harmful environmental exposures. While risks to adverse health outcomes can vary according to geography, housing, and location of environmental exposures, some people are at greater risk due to their biophysical and sociopolitical vulnerability. Unit II explains risk and vulnerability across the lifespan with a focus upon specific vulnerabilities and harmful effects at various developmental stages. The chapters in this unit highlight the unique vulnerabilities such as pesticide exposures to children, dental amalgams, and environmental vulnerabilities for immigrants and refugees. The influence of the social determinants of health are considered throughout Unit II, which are commonly referred to as factors where people live, learn, work, play and pray. Social determinants at neighborhood and community levels impact individual level exposures.

HARMFUL ENVIRONMENTAL EXPOSURES AND VULNERABLE POPULATIONS

Jeanne Leffers, PhD, RN, FAAN
Professor Emeritus
University of Massachusetts Dartmouth
College of Nursing and Health Sciences

All humans are at risk for harmful effects of environmental hazards. For certain human populations the risks of harm are greater due to biologic, social, economic, or other factors. Such population groups are often referred to as vulnerable populations. A vulnerable person or group has "aggravating factors that place them at greater risk for ongoing poor health status than other at-risk persons" (Maurer, 2013, p. 528). Some vulnerable groups include children, the poor, those without homes, refugees, people living with disabilities and those with mental illness. These vulnerable populations have been identified through epidemiological studies as having poorer health outcomes. This paper will discuss various factors that make specific populations across the life span more vulnerable to poor health outcomes from environmental stressors.

RISK AND VULNERABILITY

Risk is the likelihood that a harmful health event will occur in a given population during a specific time period. Our knowledge of risk emerges from the science of epidemiology. Epidemiology is the study of health and illness in human populations. Epidemiological studies show that environmental hazards can cause poorer health.

Environmental hazards can increase human risk of illness, disability and premature death. The Environmental Protection Agency (EPA) defines risk as the "chance of harmful effects to human health or to ecological systems resulting from exposure to an environmental stressor" (EPA, 2021b). An environmental hazard is any physical, chemical, or biological entity that causes harm. The EPA also provides information on risk assessment for such hazards.

Some common factors that affect the risk of harmful health events cannot be changed. Such factors include age, gender, race or ethnicity. Other factors that affect the risk of harmful health events can be changed. These factors result from biophysical, environmental, psychosocial and sociopolitical circumstances (Leffers et al, 2004). When environmental threats to health are examined, all humans are at risk in relation to global climate change and the increasing use of untested and toxic chemicals.

Vulnerability can be defined as "a varying state of weakness or strength that can be mobilized when one encounters a threatening event" (Leffers et al, 2004, pg 19). This definition includes individual and experiential factors that result in variability of outcomes across populations.

Risk and vulnerability are related to each other. Some describe vulnerability as a series of threshold factors that increase or amplify risk and lead to poorer health outcomes. Others argue that vulnerability can vary according to the capacity of the individual and may not lead to poorer health outcomes. This view says that positive attributes of those identified as vulnerable can enable them to overcome risk and vulnerability, leading to better outcomes (Leffers et al, 2004). The North Carolina Preparedness and Emergency Response Research Center (NCPERRC) makes a similar distinction between risk and vulnerability. They note that risk is directly affected by a hazard while the degree of vulnerability is defined as "the characteristics of a person or group and their situation that influences their capacity to anticipate, cope with, and resist and recover from the impact of an emergency" (NCPERRC, 2012).

The notion of "windows of vulnerability" refers to specific times during human development that have been identified for higher risks to health. For example, at times a child can have better recuperative capacity than adults. In other situations, children are at far greater risk for the detrimental effects of chemicals of concern on their developing organs (Brent, Tanski, & Weitzman, 2004; Sanchez, Hu, Litman & Tellez-Rojo, 2011; Suk & Sly, 2016; EPA, 2021a).

Various populations have been identified as more vulnerable to environmental hazards. Further, this concern has been explained in documents assessing risk for the harmful effects of climate change such as the Climate and Health Assessment of the US Global Change Research Program. As stated earlier, individual and experiential factors can lead to different vulnerability across populations. These factors include those whose biophysical characteristics make them more vulnerable such as the developing fetus, infants, children and older adults. People with acquired biophysical factors such as chronic illness, those with differences in functioning due to trauma, and those with altered immunity also become more vulnerable to poor health outcomes. Additionally those born with congenital anomalies and with variations in cognitive and physical abilities may be at more risk from specific toxic exposures.

Behavioral factors such as developmental age appropriate behavior, activities, hobbies and occupational exposures all raise vulnerability. Social factors such as where a person lives, works or spends a great deal of time can also make them more vulnerable. Recently, there is mounting concern for the impact of environmental degradation as part of a social-ecological dimension of risk and vulnerability (Depietri, 2020).

The following discussion will address biophysical, behavioral and social factors that increase vulnerability. For each of the areas, the topic will be addressed across the lifespan from fetal development through the older adult population.

EMBRYONIC AND FETAL DEVELOPMENT
Biophysical Factors

Healthy fetal development requires precise timing and feedback for cells to divide and mature properly for necessary cell replication and differentiation. For this to occur there is an interaction between genetic and environmental factors (Brent, Tanski & Weitzman, 2004; Schettler, Solomon, Valenti and Huddle, 1999; Zheng et al, 2016). For the developing fetus the risks are acquired through exposures across the placenta from the pregnant person. In fact, any exposure to the fetus from the mother is considered environmental ("Environmental Factors in Birth", 2009). So, while the only exposure pathway for fetal toxic exposures is placental, the fetus is particularly sensitive to the broad range of all environmental toxins that the pregnant person is exposed to before and during their pregnancy. As will be discussed later, the pregnant person's exposure risk varies throughout pregnancy due to the variations in maternal physiology during pregnancy. Toxins may affect both the structural development and biochemical function of cells in fetal organ systems. Fetal sensitivity to toxins occurs as a result of the flexibility of the cell and the capacity for changes during embryonic development (Schettler et al., 1999). For each specific exposure, many things interact to create the risk and health outcomes. The magnitude of the exposure, the dose of the toxin, the embryonic stage, and metabolism of the mother and embryo all interact to vary the risk and the outcomes. The embryo is particularly sensitive to structural damage due to these mechanisms. Additionally, the blood brain barrier is not fully developed in the embryo allowing neurotoxins greater access to the fetus (Schettler et al, 1999; CDC, 2019). Often the person is unaware that they are pregnant during this critical period when she may be exposed to toxins. Additionally, many chemicals have not been tested for toxicity to human development (Tanner, et al, 2020). Due to the stage of fetal development the impact of these risks can be very serious and harmful, resulting in life long impairments (Dietrich, et al, 2005). The study of what are referred to as windows of vulnerability or critical developmental periods is complex and requires sophisticated data analysis (Sanchez, Hu,

Litman & Tellez-Rojo, 2011; Selevan, Kimmel & Mendola, 2000).

The healthy development of children must be a priority. Tickner & Hoppin (2000) argue that children are generally more vulnerable to environmental exposures and have less control of those environments than do adults. In addition, the risks to susceptible children are not well understood scientifically. Therefore, in the absence of clear evidence the Precautionary Principle must be followed (Tickner and Hoppin, 2000).

Many adverse health outcomes for the developing fetus are referred to as birth defects. Genetic factors as well as environmental exposures interact in ways to create problems with organ structure or function. While scientists agree that environmental exposures are not well understood, those exposures that are known require more action and those that are not known require more research ("Environmental Factors in Birth", 2009). Reported adverse health outcomes from environmental health threats such as toxic chemicals include low birth weight infants, congenital anomalies, pregnancy loss from miscarriage, and neurodevelopmental problems (See Table 1).

Also endocrine disrupting chemicals (EDCs) have been linked to altered gender development and sexual organ malformations. Common environmental estrogens that mimic estradiol and attach to estrogen receptors are certain polychlorinated biphenyls (PCBs), Bisphenol A (BPA), phthalates, and pharmaceutical estrogens. High-level exposures have been confirmed for their role in gender related effects and scientists fear that even low level exposure can also result in these birth defects ("Are EDCs blurring", 2005). For more information about EDCs see the chapter in Unit 3 Environmental Health Sciences.

Another feature of exposure is bioaccumulation. Bioaccumulation is a process by which toxins accumulate as they move up the food chain. Humans are at the top of the food chain, absorbing chemicals from meat, fish and produce consumed in the diet and as a result carry more concentrated levels of chemicals in the body. Consequently, the pregnant person may have large amounts of toxins in her body that are passed on to the very small fetus. Due to its small size, the developing fetus can be exposed to a greater proportion of the toxin, which can result in life-long neurological deficits (Schettler, Soloman, Valenti, & Huddle, 1999; Zenker, Cicero, Prestinaci, Bottoni, Carere, 2014)).

Scientists examine the relationship between in-utero development and adult health. Mounting evidence supports the argument that prenatal exposures lead to lifelong consequences in adulthood. These consequences include congenital anomalies, risk for hypertension, insulin resistance, kidney disease and other health conditions. Recent studies in the area of epigenetics indicate that prenatal exposure to environmental contaminants can adversely affect the fetal epigenome and put the fetus at risk of diseases and disorders throughout the lifespan and transgenerationally (Perera & Herbstman, 2011).

Finally, studies examine the likelihood of preterm birth resulting from exposures to environmental toxicants, though no consistent evidence has been found to date, there are indications that future studies might document such evidence (Ferguson, O'Neill, & Meeker, 2013).

INFANTS
Biophysical Factors

Once delivery occurs, the newborn must transition from the life sustaining physiology of the fetus to an independent process of functioning that includes respiration, nutrition and elimination. The resting respiratory rate in infants is twice that of adults; this means that infants are exposed to 2 times more toxins per body weight than are adults. Nutritionally, infants take in 2 ½ times more water and 3 to 4 times more food per body weight than adults. This increases infant exposures to pesticides and other toxins in food and water much greater than exposures in adults. Infants have less developed brain, respiratory, gastrointestinal, immune, reproductive and metabolic systems than older children and adults (Bearer, 1995; Wigle, 2003). Their gastrointestinal tract is more permeable making it easier for toxins to be absorbed. Common exposures to toxins include pesticides, heavy metals, persistent organic pollutants and phthalates.

Social Factors

Most infants are delivered in hospitals where they are exposed to chemicals used in the nursery and hospital settings, particularly Polyvinyl Chloride (PVC), di 2-ethylhexyl phthalate (DEHP) and Bisphenol A (BPA). PVC is used in medical products as a plasticizer for tubing and other devices. Most PVC medical devices are from 20-40% DEHP and are commonly used in hospital nurseries. Neonatal intensive care units often use PVC medical products for IV solutions, enteral feedings and other necessary treatments. These chemicals are known to leach out of the medical device into lipid containing fluids contained in the solutions. As reproductive and developmental toxins these chemicals can expose infants at the time when they are adjusting to extrauterine life and have immature organ systems. Due to their small size and variety of exposures, newborns in NICUs can be exposed to chemicals of concern at far greater levels comparative to adult exposures (Schettler, 2002). While nursing initiatives such as Green Birthdays by the American College of Nurse Midwives seek to improve health care settings, referred to as Green Nursing, infants continue to be exposed to environmental hazards from the moment of their birth. For many newborns the time spent in the NICU can be weeks or months increasing their exposure to these hazards. See Unit 4: Hazards in the NICU.

Additionally infants spend most of their time in a single environment for prolonged periods, such as a crib, where the exposures do not vary. However, if hazardous materials are present, they become more concentrated in this single environment (Bearer, 1995). Infants attending day care are confined to the same environment all day where they may be susceptible to indoor air contaminants. Indoor air quality in homes is often 10-50 times more hazardous than outdoor air where infants are exposed to carcinogens, neurotoxins and pesticides. While breastfeeding is considered the best nutrition for infants, chemicals such as polybrominated diphenyl ethers (PBDEs), PCBs, organochloride pesticides and dioxins that accumulate in human fat tissue in the breast have been shown to be transmitted to the infant during breastfeeding. These chemicals can also be found in formulas made from cow's milk. Further, the skin of a newborn is a highly absorptive surface and infants are exposed to a number of toxic chemicals in the personal care products that are applied to their skin (Bearer, 1995). See Unit 4: Personal Care and Safer Cleaning Products.

CHILDREN
Biophysical Factors

Children are more susceptible to environmental toxins because their ongoing physical development and physiology put them at greater risk. Tickner and Hoppin (2000) note that children are more susceptible to environmental toxins for four important reasons:

- they undergo periods of rapid growth and development (window of vulnerability);

- they have age-related differences in absorption, metabolism, detoxification and excretion of substances;

- they incur greater exposure to environmental toxins; and

- they incur exposure from the fetal period throughout life so that the cumulative effects of toxic exposures lead to greater risk.

Table 1 Commonly Identified Chemical Exposures and Birth Defects-1

EXPOSURE	BIRTH DEFECT OR LOW BIRTH WEIGHT
Arsenic	Cardiac Defects
Bisphenol A	Reproductive system anomalies
Dioxin	Neural Tube Defects Neurobehavioral Problems Hypospadias Oral Clefts
Lead	Cardiac Defects Neural Tube Defects Neurobehavioral Problems Hypospadias Oral Clefts
Methyl Mercury	Neural Tube Defects Neurobehavioral Problems
Particulate Matter in Air	Vascular Defects (Patent Ductus Arteriosis)
PCBs	Impaired hearing*
Sulphur Dioxide	Musculoskeletal defects Cardiac Defects
Environmental Tobacco Smoke	Low Birth Weight Attention Deficit Hyperactivity Disorder
Air Pollution	Low Birth Weight
Pesticides	Low Birth Weight Congenital Anomalies

(Swanson, Entriner, Buss, & Wadhwa, 2009; Kim & Cizmadia, 2010).

*Noted in animal studies

The actual specific period of vulnerability for adverse effects of the toxic chemical exposures depends upon the toxin itself and its mechanism for action, the dose of that toxin, the actual target tissue for the toxicant and the timetable for development in the child (Wigle, 2003). Other factors that affect exposure and risk are location of toxin and child, breathing zones, oxygen consumption, food consumption, water consumption and behavioral development (Bearer, 1995, NIEHS, 2020).

Children's developmental changes from infancy to adolescence affect the toxicokinetics of their exposures. For example, their body composition has greater water content and less lipid content that can affect chemicals that bind to lipids. While that may offer protection in the early months, the body lipids rise rapidly after birth for the first nine months. This rise in lipids increases the child's sensitivity to lipid binding chemicals such as dioxin, a known carcinogen. Children have a larger sized liver per body weight that can allow for hepatic metabolic clearance. But the larger liver can also allow for activation of toxic metabolites. Immature enzyme function in the liver reduces the body's ability to clear/remove environmental chemicals while immature renal function slows the elimination of chemicals and metabolites. There is a long postnatal period of development for the lungs and brain. Limited serum protein binding capacity in the birth to three month period of infancy creates the potential for more toxicants and chemicals in the body when pharmaceuticals and environmental chemicals are not bound to the serum and freely circulate in the infant's body (Ginsberg, Hattis, Miller, & Sonawane, 2004). Such physiological processes of normal development create critical periods where toxic exposures can be most harmful.

Children breathe more rapidly than adults and take in more air than adults. Toddlers generally breathe twice as fast as adults while school age children under the age of 12 years breathe about 1 ½ times as fast as adults. Children consume 3-4 times more food per body weight than adults, and drink more than 2 and ½ times more water per body weight than adults. As a result, they experience greater exposures to environmental health hazards of 2 to 5 times that of an adult.

Human development continues through childhood and the digestive, excretory and reproductive systems have not reached full development during childhood. As a result the protective mechanisms of a fully developed adult gastrointestinal tract may reduce exposures while mature kidneys and liver are better able to detoxify and eliminate toxins that affect children in greater concentrations. Additionally, toxins continue to pose risk for healthy reproductive system development and can result in decreased fertility and damage to reproductive structures and function (Silbergeld & Patrick, 2005).

Behavioral Factors

Children are more vulnerable to toxins due to behavioral factors as well due to oral, dermal and inhalation exposures specific to developmental stage behaviors (Moya, Bearer & Etzel, 2004). Children play at ground level both inside on the floor and outside in grass and other play spaces. Consequently they are exposed to materials that are tracked inside onto floors, and settle from the air. Common hazards on floors are pesticides and fertilizers, cleaning supplies, lead dust in older homes, and other household chemicals (Sattler, Afzal, Condon, Belka & McKee, 2010). Outdoor hazards include the chemicals used in lawn and garden care but also chemicals transported by water runoff that include petroleum products, automotive additives, paints, and other industrial products.

Children also use hand-to-mouth behavior to learn and explore which makes them more vulnerable to toxins on household items as well as toxins within products such as toys. Harmful chemicals such as lead, cadmium and phthalates have been found in products commonly used by children including sleep accessories such as positioners and wedges, teethers and other plastic toys. Research indicates that on average a child's hands contact contaminated surfaces up to 32 times during eating, with even more contact to food before the food enters the mouth. Approximately 20-80 % of dietary exposures come from such hand to mouth behavior (Akland et al, 2000).

While infants may spend more time in cribs and indoors, as children age they are more likely to be at play both indoors and outdoors. Indoors they are likely to sit and lay on floors while outside they are likely to play in grass or soil, which can contain harmful pesticides. These can also be tracked into the home on human and animal feet. Wood playground equipment often has been treated with creosote and arsenic, which are toxic.

Other location factors include the time a school age child spends in the school setting. Indoor air in schools has been identified as a source of carcinogens, neurotoxicants and endocrine disruptors (EDCs). These include chemicals such as lead, radon, pesticides, asbestos, and volatile organic compounds (VOCs) such as solvents and formaldehyde. Further, schools can be a source of environmental hazards such as cleaning products as well. See Unit 4: Safer Cleaning Products.

In addition, children live in families where they can be exposed to "take home toxins." This refers to toxins that their family members are exposed to in the work setting and carry home on their clothing and personal belongings. A commonly recognized take home toxin is asbestos, which is linked to the development of lung conditions, particularly mesothelioma. Decades later, children who have been exposed to chemicals in their home or from take home toxins are at risk of developing conditions such as mesothelioma, Parkinson's Disease, and various forms of cancer.

Nurses can aid families to anticipate childhood risks during various stages of development through the tools provided in the Physicians for Social Responsibility (PSR) Pediatric Environmental Health Tool Kit as well as the National Institute of Environmental Health Sciences (NIEHS) Children's Health: Why the Environment Matters.

ADOLESCENTS
Biophysical factors

During puberty the adolescent experiences changes in hormones and the metabolic interactions of neurochemicals for development. This poses a "window of vulnerability" for the adolescent whose endocrine, immune, musculoskeletal and reproductive systems are undergoing maturation and can be heavily exposed to chemicals known to affect many systems. According to the Environmental Working Group report, Teen Girls' Body Burden of Hormone-Altering Cosmetics Chemicals, an array of sex hormones present at minute levels in the body are responsible for the transition from childhood to adulthood and current research suggests that adolescents may be at particular risk for exposure to even trace levels of hormone disrupting chemicals.

Behavioral Factors

Adolescent girls are likely to increase their use of personal care products and cosmetics increasing their exposure to toxic chemicals in such products. Studies indicate that, on average, girls have up to 13 hormone altering chemicals from four chemical families - phthalates, triclosan, parabens, and musks - in their bodies. In addition to posing serious health effects as hormone disruptors, these chemicals also have the potential to cause cancer as well. Results suggest that young women are being exposed to a wide variety of cosmetic preservatives that puts them at serious risk during this important period of development (EWG, 2016).

Adolescents also are at risk due to their occupational exposures. During this phase of life they are most likely to begin employment in a variety of settings and more than 80% do work during some part of the year (Etzl & Balk, 2003). Frequently, adolescent boys go to work in the summer in lawn care services, painting and sealing driveways. At times they begin to work as entrepreneurs creating their own summer employment in such positions that are not monitored by Occupational Safety and Health Administration (OSHA). They may be unaware of the hazardous materials to which they are exposed. Adolescents employed in a variety of settings can be exposed to environmental tobacco smoke, solvents, and other cleaning agents (Etzel & Baklk, 2003). A report by OSHA noted that more than two million youth are exposed to farm-related hazards. Beyond the dangers of heavy equipment injuries are adolescents' exposures to the fertilizers and pesticides used in agricultural settings. These include chemicals known to be carcinogenic, neurotoxicants and hormone disruptors.

PREGNANT PEOPLE
Biophysical Factors

While most scientists are concerned about prenatal exposures for the fetus, there is evidence that pregnant people are also at more risk themselves for exposure to environmental toxins due to their changing physiology during pregnancy. For example, decreased motility of the gastrointestinal tract increases intestinal transit. This delay can lead to greater absorption of toxins. Due to decreased plasma albumin concentration during pregnancy, compounds that are normally bound to albumin are altered kinetically (Brent, 2004). Increased extracellular fluid volumes affect the transfer of compounds dependent upon fluid concentration. Therefore, many toxins can actually move more readily into the pregnant person. In addition during pregnancy, there are changes in renal elimination and liver metabolism and variations in uterine blood flow that affect their ability to detoxify and clear toxins from her body. Elevated blood lead levels in the pregnant person may lead to pregnancy induced hypertension, a most serious and potentially life threatening complication of pregnancy (Yazbeck et al, 2009).

ADULTS

The average weight Caucasian man is the norm to which all standards for chemical safety have been applied. As a result, the discussion of vulnerability compares the various populations across the lifespan to the healthy adult. In addition, factors that affect the overall health of an adult such as chronic illness, affect the adult's susceptibility to environmental toxins. As noted in the discussion of adolescents, the use of personal care products varies by gender, and physiologic differences between male and female genetics and hormones can alter the risk factors for men and women.

Social Factors

Where a person lives, works, attends school, worships and plays can increase the risk of toxic exposures. These are considered to be the social determinants of health and greatly impact health outcomes. These exposures can have a serious impact upon their health. The EPA Children's Health Protection Advisory Committee (CHPAC) Letter to the EPA Administrator examined the impact of the social determinants of health as a factor of increased risk and vulnerability.

Beyond the individual level issues or household residence, school and workplace, there are neighborhood effects that impact the health of poor and underrepresented groups at much higher levels of exposure. These increased exposures and negative health outcomes are commonly termed issues of environmental justice. This textbook offers a chapter on Environmental Justice for further information on that important topic. However those who live in more hazardous areas suffer injustice from their greater exposure to toxins.

In addition, the various hobbies and recreational activities that a person pursues can impact the amount of toxins they are exposed to in their lifetime. If the hobby includes paint and paint thinners, for example, an individual would be placed at a similar risk to those who are exposed occupationally. Home gardeners can be exposed to pesticides used. The person who "tinkers" on cars or motorcycles may be exposed to exhaust, degreasers, solvents, and cleaners. Often these spaces may not have adequate ventilation, further increasing the exposure of the hobbyist.

Further, various traditional remedies include toxins such as mercury, lead and other heavy metals. Folk remedies that contain lead, such as "greta" and "azarcon" are used to treat an upset stomach. In many Latino communities a form of mercury azogue is ingested to relieve empacho, a form of gastrointestinal malaise (for more information: HIDDEN DANGER Environmental Health Threats in the Latino Community). In a study of traditional Asian herbal remedies, levels of arsenic, lead and mercury were found to be at toxic levels in 49% of the products and 74% of them exceeded public health guidelines for prevention of disease (Garvey, Hahn, Lee & Harbison, 2001).

Social Factors: Occupation

Workplace exposures to hazards affect almost all categories of workers globally. The Occupational Health and Safety Administration (OSHA) reports that in 2019 more than 5,000 workers in the United States alone lost their lives in work related events. Early concerns for occupational health and safety began with identification of the hazards of coal miners and the development of pneumoconiosis or black lung disease. Common examples of occupations known for serious health effects from environmental toxins are agricultural workers who are exposed to pesticides, workers in dry cleaning establishments who are exposed to solvents such as tetracholoroethylene (PERC), shipyard workers, and those who work with insulation who are exposed to asbestos (Levy et al, 2005).

Workers exposed to chemicals such as vinyl chloride, benzene, copper sulfate, plastics and asbestos have higher rates of cancers such as lung cancer, kidney cancer and leukemia and other blood related conditions. Workers exposed to environmental tobacco smoke, carbon monoxide, or solvents are at increased risk for heart disease including arrhythmias. Since the early recognition of the link between occupation and health with coal miners, a variety of other lung conditions have been linked to workplace exposures including byssinosis (Brown lung) and those who work with cotton; silicosis and those who work in sandblasting and with ceramic and cement materials; and asthma from chemicals such as chromium, aluminum, nickel and exposure to dust. Those who work in smelters or foundries and those in the pharmaceutical industry are at greater risk of neurological disorders through workplace exposure to toluene, mercury, lead, arsenic, pesticides, plastics, and carbon monoxide. (See table 2).

Various federal agencies such as the Occupational Safety and Health Administration (OSHA) and National Institute of Environmental Safety and Health (NIOSH) study, monitor, enforce standards and provide important research and education to improve worker health. The American Association of Occupational Health Nurses supports nursing efforts in occupational and environmental health. Fundamentals of Occupational and Environmental Health Nursing. Nurses are exposed to many hazardous chemicals in their work in the hospital and other health care settings. It is known that various medical products that nurses are exposed to contain toxic substances. However, there has been little confirmation of the health burden this places upon a nurse's body. In a bio-monitoring study conducted by the organization, Physicians for Social Responsibility, nurses and physicians in 10 states were found to have levels of chemicals with known or suspected negative health outcomes. In those tested, bisphenol A (BPA), mercury, phthalates, polybrominated diphenyl ethers (PBDEs), triclosan, and perfluorinated compounds (PFCs) were among the chemicals found. All persons in the study had at least five of the six kinds of chemicals tested and all had BPA and some form of phthalates in their bodies (Wilding, B.C., Curtis, K., & Welker-Hood, K. (2009).

Further, evidence suggests that previous ethnic and racial disparities in workplace exposures to toxins persist today. Historically, black workers were shown to be disproportionately exposed to silicosis, chromate, and carcinogens from coke ovens. Latinos are shown to face disproportionate risks from pesticide, lead and mercury exposure (NRDC, 2004). More recent reports of disproportionate exposures show that Latino agricultural workers, Native American mine workers and newly immigrated Asians are among those whose workplace exposures exceed that of whites (Murray, 2003).

OLDER ADULTS
Biophysical factors

It is important to note that persons older than age 65 demonstrate great variability in physical changes that affect vulnerability. Frailty of the very old, the presence of serious health conditions and residential, behavioral, and lifestyle factors contribute to differences in susceptibility (Geller & Zenick, 2005). A priority of the National Academies of Sciences, Engineering and Medicine stress the importance of research to better understand the role of environmental exposures in the development of age related diseases such as dementia, cancer and cardiovascular disease.

Older adults are at greater risk for harmful health effects from toxic exposure for two reasons. First, they experience physiological changes related to aging. The effectiveness of their respiratory system to clear inhaled toxins is diminished due to decreased lung volume, elasticity and lowered ventilation rate. Weakened skin integrity reduces their capacity to resist dermal exposures. Liver metabolism and renal function is less effective due to reduced blood flow, effects of aging and the effect of specific age related diseases. Reduced capacity to metabolize and excrete toxins absorbed through respiratory, gastrointestinal, and dermal pathways increases the harmful effects of toxic exposures. Polypharmacy is frequent in older adults and the interaction of a large number of pharmaceutical chemicals and environmentally adsorbed chemicals puts added stress on metabolic processes. In addition, changes in immunity and other processes of aging combine with exposures earlier in their lifetime to contribute to the development of illnesses. For example, Parkinson's disease has been shown to be related to exposure to neurotoxins earlier in life.

Second, the older population experiences a greater number of chronic illnesses that can be adversely affected by exposures to environmental hazards. Conditions such as Chronic Obstructive Pulmonary Disease (COPD), asthma and other chronic lung conditions are made worse by exposure to environmental tobacco smoke, particulate matter, tobacco smoke and other criteria air pollutants. Studies indicate that air pollution and climate can have significant adverse effects on those who have cardiac disease (Gold & Samet, 2013; Di et al, 2017). For more information about the impact of climate change upon older adults see the chapter in the climate change unit following.

Behavioral factors

Older adults spend up to 90% of their time indoors exposing them to indoor air pollution, which is comprised of outdoor air contaminants as well as specific contamination in indoor settings (Davis, 2009). Outdoor air pollution includes pollutants such as sulfur dioxide, nitrogen dioxide, ozone, and particulate matter.

Most of the literature that addresses environmental risk among of people with developmental disabilities or cognitive delays examines the relationship of toxic exposures and neurodevelopment effects. More research is needed to explore the effects of toxic exposures to an individual who has some type of cognitive or developmental difference. Researchers question whether physiological factors such as alterations to the nervous system make an individual more vulnerable to added exposures. Resources are available for older adults and environmental risks to health at the Alliance of Nurses for Healthy Environments (ANHE) website.

PERSONS WITH ALTERATIONS IN COGNITIVE AND PHYSICAL ABILITIES

Environmental exposures are associated with a number of neurodevelopmental effects (EPA, 2013). Organizations such as the American Association on Intellectual and Developmental Disabilities note that the potential for cumulative effects of hazardous chemical exposure for the population with intellectual and developmental disabilities should be addressed through ongoing research (AAIDD, 2012). People with developmental differences who are able to work can be exposed to toxins in their work setting. Those living with physical and cognitive disabilities are more likely to live in community based residential homes where they are likely to be exposed to a variety of household environmental health toxins from poor indoor air quality. These pollutants include carbon monoxide, lead, mercury, radon, pesticides and cleaning products (Davis, 2009). The American Association on Intellectual and Developmental Disabilities addresses the risks for environmental exposures in their position statement (AAIDD, 2012).

GLOBAL HEALTH

Across the globe, all humans are at greater risk from climate change in terms of changes in temperature and humidity, drought, plant life, wildfires, and changes in air quality. However, some regions of the world are experiencing the harmful effects of climate change at a

Table 2 Chemical Exposure and Health Outcomes

CHEMICAL EXPOSURE	ADVERSE HEALTH OUTCOME
Vinyl Chloride	Liver Cancer Cardiovascular Disease
Benzene	Leukemia Aplastic Anemia Neutropenia
Benzidine (various chemical formulas)	Bladder Cancer
Copper Sulphate	Anemia and Blood Disorders
Plastics	Neurological Effects
Asbestos	Asbestosis Lung Cancer Mesothelioma
Particulate Matter Sulphur Dioxide	Asthma
Environmental Tobacco Smoke	Cardiovascular Effects Pulmonary Disease Asthma
Carbon Monoxide	Cardiovascular Disease, including Angina
Solvents	Arrhythmias Liver Damage
Cotton Fibers	Byssinosis
Dust From Cement; Sandblasting; Ceramics	Pneumoconiosis Bronchitis
Pesticides	Skin Cancer

greater rate. Water is becoming scarcer in many regions and the melting of the ice cap and glaciers is putting some poorer, heavily populated regions into crisis due to flooding, extreme weather events, and loss of habitat.

Researchers estimated that 25-53% of the burden of illness worldwide can be attributed to environmental health risk factors when they considered nutritional factors in food, pesticides and environmental tobacco smoke but excluded known genetic causes and behavioral factors such as smoking and diet (Smith, Corvalan & Kjellstrom, 1999). While the study was not able to confirm the estimates, the results indicate that environmental hazards contribute to disease and financial burdens worldwide (Smith, Corvalan & Kjellstrom, 1999). The World Health Organization (2015) provides methodology to quantify the disease burden attributable to environmental health risks including indoor and outdoor air pollution, lead, mercury, occupational exposures to carcinogens, environmental tobacco smoke and solar radiation. Toxins such as lead in gasoline, arsenic and high levels of fluoride in water, and DDT are exposures found in the developing world that do not occur in the United States.

Additionally, the policies of the richer countries contribute to global health disparities. Currently many pesticides banned for use in the United States and Europe are sold for use in poor tropical regions. Many developed countries have been disposing of pharmaceuticals by dumping these and electronic hazards in poorer countries (Ahsanuddin, 2012; Bradley, 2014). Currently, for example, Kenya has large electronic-waste dumps near large population centers causing exposure to many toxic chemicals including heavy metals (Schluep, Rochat,Munyea, Laissaoui,Wone, Kane, Hieronymi, 2008).

Finally, protection is more limited in many regions of the world. As developing countries adopt many of the less environmentally friendly products such as plastic bottling and bags, they are more likely to dispose of these non-recyclables by dumping and burning. Such practices increase the human risks, particularly carcinogens from air, water and soil pollution.

This overview of the vulnerability to environmental health risks by a variety of populations highlights the biophysical, behavioral and social factors that increase risk for many people. Advocacy to reduce risk of exposure to toxins and to protect health in ways the Precautionary Principle advises must be evident for all people globally. The particular needs of the vulnerable populations discussed here add evidence to the need for policy change.

REFERENCES

AAIDD: American Association on Intellectual and Developmental Disabilities. (2012). *Environmental health: Position statement of AAIDD.* http://aaidd.org/news-policy/policy/position-statements/environmental-health#.VVxurKblfV0

Ahsanuddin, S. (2012). *Apartheid of pharmacology: Priorities of pharmaceutical industry in developing countries.* Americans for Informed Democracy. http://www.aidemocracy.org/students/apartheid-of-pharmacology-priorities-of-the-pharmaceutical-industry-in-developing-countries/

Akland, G.G., Pellizzari, E.D., Hu, Y., Boberds, M., Rohrer, C.A., Leckie, J.O., & Berry, M.R. (2000). Factors influencing total dietary exposures in young children. *Journal of Exposure Analysis and Environmental Epidemiology, 10*(6 pt 2), 710-722.

Are EDCs blurring issues of gender? (2005). *Environmental Health Perspectives, 113*(10), A671-677.

Bearer, C.F. (1995). Environmental health hazards: How children differ from adults. *The Future of Children, 5*(2) 11-26.

Bradley, L. (2014). *E-waste in developing countries endangers environment, locals.* US News and World Report. http://www.usnews.com/news/articles/2014/08/01/e-waste-in-developing-countries-endangers-environment-locals

Brent, R.L., Tanski, S., & Weitzman, M. (2004). A pediatric perspective on the unique vulnerability and resilience of the embryo and the child to environmental toxicants: The importance of rigorous research concerning age and agent. *Pediatrics, 113*(4), 935-944.

Centers for Disease Control and Prevention (CDC). (2019). *National report on human exposure to environmental chemicals.* https://www.cdc.gov/exposurereport/

Children's Health Protection Advisory Committee (CHPAC). (2013). *Letter to the EPA Administrator.* https://www.epa.gov/sites/production/files/2016-01/documents/chpac_social_determinants_of_health_combined.pdf

Davis, A. D. (2009). Home environmental health risks of people with developmental disabilities living in community-based residential settings: Implications for community-health nurses. *Journal of Community Health Nursing, 26*, 183-191.

Depietri, Y. (2020). The social–ecological dimension of vulnerability and risk to natural hazards. *Sustainability Science, 15*, 587–604. https://doi.org/10.1007/s11625-019-00710-y

Di, Q., Dai, L., Wang, Y., Zanobetti, A., Choirat, C., Schwartz, J. D., & Dominici, F. (2017). Association of short-term exposure to air pollution with mortality in older adults. *JAMA, 318*(24), 2446-2456.

Dietrich, K. N, Eskanazi, B., Schantz, S., Yolton, K., Rauh, V. A, Johnson, C. B.,Alkon, A. Canfield, R. L., Pessah, & Berman, R. F. (2005). Principles and Practices of Neurodevelopmental Assessment in Children: Lessons Learned from the Centers for Children's Environmental Health and Disease Prevention Research. *Environmental Health Perspectives 113*, 1437–1446. doi:10.1289/ehp.7672

EPA: Environmental Protection Agency. (2013). *America's children and the environment.* EPA. http://www.epa.gov/ace/

EPA: Environmental Protection Agency (EPA). (2021a) *Children are not little adults.* https://www.epa.gov/children/children-are-not-little-adults

EPA: Environmental Protection Agency (2021b). *What is risk?* https://www.epa.gov/risk/about-risk-assessment#whatisrisk

Etzel, R.A., & Balk, S. J. (Eds.). (2011). *Pediatric environmental health (3rd Ed.).* Committee on Environmental Health, American Academy of Pediatrics.

Environmental Working Group (EWG). (2008). *Teen girls' body burden of hormone-altering cosmetics chemicals.* http://www.ewg.org/research/teen-girls-body-burden-hormone-altering-cosmetics-chemicals

Ferguson, K. K., O'Neill, M. S., & Meeker, J. D. (2013). Environmental contaminant exposures and preterm birth: A comprehensive review. *Journal of Toxicology and Environmental Health. Part B, Critical Reviews, 16*(2), 69–113. doi:10.1080/10937404.2013.775048

Garvey, G. J., Hahn, G., Lee, R.V., & Harbison, R. D. (2001). Heavy metal hazards of Asian traditional remedies. *International Journal of Environmental Health Research, 11,* 63-71.

Geller, A.M., & Zenick, H. (2005). Aging and the environment: A research framework. *Environmental Health Perspectives, 113,* 1257-1262.

Ginsberg, G., Hattis, D., Miller, R. & Sonawane, B. (2004). Pediatric pharmacokinetic data: Implications for environmental risk assessment for children. *Pediatrics, 113*(4), 973-983.

Gold, DR, & Samet, JM. (2013). Air pollution, climate and heart disease. *Circulation, 128,* e11-e14. doi: 10.1161/CIRCULATIONAHA.113.003988

Kim, H. & Cizmadia, P. (2010). *Adverse Birth Outcomes and Environmental Health Threats.* Physicians for Social Responsibility. http://www.psr.org/assets/pdfs/abo-fact-sheet.pdf

Maurer, F. (2009). Vulnerable populations. In F. Maurer & C. Smith (Eds.). *Community/public health nursing: Health for families and populations.* (pp 532-556). St. Louis: Elsevier/Saunders.

McDermott, M. J., Mazor, K. A., Shost, S. J., Narang, R. S, Aldous, K. M., & Storm, J. E. (2005). Tetracholorethylene (PCE, Perc) levels in residential dry cleaner buildings in diverse communities in New York City. *Environmental Health Perspectives,*113(10),11336-1343.

Messerlian, Carmen & Williams, Paige & Ford, Jennifer & Chavarro, Jorge & Mínguez-Alarcón, Lidia & Dadd, Ramace & Braun, Joseph & Gaskins, Audrey & Meeker, John & James-Todd, Tamarra & Chiu, Yu Han & Nassan, Feiby & Souter, Irene & Petrozza, John & Keller, Myra & Toth,

Messerlian, C., Williams, P. L., Ford, J. B., Chavarro, J. E., Mínguez-Alarcón, L., Dadd, R., ... & EARTH Study Team. (2018). The Environment and Reproductive Health (EARTH) Study: a prospective preconception cohort. *Human Reproduction Open, 2018*(2). 10.1093/hropen/hoy001.

Moya, J., Bearer, C. F. & Etzel, R. A. (2004). Children's behavior and physiology and how it affects exposure to environmental contaminants. *Pediatrics, 113*(4 Part 2), 996-1006.

Murray, L. (2003). Sick and tired of being sick and tired: Scientific evidence, methods, and research implications for racial and ethnic disparities in occupational health. *American Journal of Public Health, 93*(2), 221-226.

National Institute of Environmental Health Sciences (NIEHS). (2020) *Children's environmental health.* https://www.niehs.nih.gov/health/topics/population/children/index.cfm

NCPERRC. (2012). *Vulnerable and at-risk populations resource guide. Research Brief.* North Carolina Preparedness and Emergency Response Research Center. https://sph.unc.edu/wp-content/uploads/sites/112/2015/07/nciph-perrc-varp-guide.pdf

Natural Resources Defense Council. (2004). *Hidden danger: Environmental threats in the Latino Community.* http://www.nrdc.org/health/effects/latino/english/latino_en.pdf

Perera, F., & Herbstman, J. (2011). Prenatal environmental exposures, epigenetics, and disease. *Reproductive Toxicology, 31*(3), 363–373. doi:10.1016/j.reprotox.2010.12.055

Quintero-Somaini, A., & Quirindongo, M. (2004). *Hidden danger: Environmental health threats in the Latino Community.* Natural Resources Defense Council. http://www.nrdc.org/health/effects/latino/english/latino_en.pdf

Sánchez, B., Hu, H., Litman, H., and Téllez-Rojo, M.M. (2011). Statistical Methods to Study Timing of Vulnerability with Sparsely Sampled Data on Environmental Toxicants. *Environmental Health Perspectives, 119,* 409–415. doi:10.1289/ehp.1002453

Sattler, B., Afzal, B., Condon, M., Belka, E., & McKee, T. (2010). *CH EH homes and communities.* American Nursing Foundation. http://nursingworld.org/mods/mod961/cehmfullNEW.htm

Schettler, T. (2002). *DEHP exposures during the medical care of infants: A cause for concern.* Health Care without Harm. www.noharm.org/goinggreen

Schettler, T., Soloman, G., Valenti, M. & Huddle, A. (1999). *Generations at risk: Reproductive health and the environment.* MIT Press.

Selevan, S.G., Kimmel, C.A., & Mendola, P. (2000). Identifying critical windows for exposure for children's health. *Environmental Health Perspectives.* 108(supplement 3), 451-455.

Schluep, M,, Rochat, D., Munyea, AW., Laissaoui, SA, Wone, S., Kane, C., Hieronymi, K. (2008) Assessing the e-waste situation in Africa. *Electronics Goes Green 2008, 8-10.* http://ewasteguide.info/system/files/Schluep_2008_EGG.pdf

Silbergled, E. K., & Patrick, T.E. (2005). Environmental exposures, toxicologic mechanisms & adverse pregnancy outcomes. *American Journal of Obstetrics and Gynecology,* 192, (S-11-21).

Smith, K. R., Corvalan, C. F., & Kjellstrom, T. (1999). How much global ill health is attributable to environmental factors? *Epidemiology, 10,* 573-584.

Stein, J., Schettler, T., Rohrer, B., Valenti, M., & Myers, N. (2008). *Environmental threats to healthy aging: With a closer look at Alzheimer's disease and Parkinson's' Disease.* Greater Boston Physicians for Social Responsibility and the Science and Environmental Health Network. http://www.ageheatlhy.org/pdf/GBPSRSEHN_HealthyAging1017.pdf

Suk, W. A., Sly, P. D. (2016). Ensuring a bright future for children's environmental health. *Annals of Global Health,* 82(1). https://rb.gy/ik31ox

Swanson, J. M., Entriner, S., Buss, C., & Wadhwa, P. D. (2009). Developmental origins or health and disease: Environmental Exposures. *Seminars in Reproductive Medicine,* 27(5), 391-402.

Tanner, E. M., Hallerbäck, M. U., Wikström, S., Lindh, C., Kiviranta, H., Gennings, C., & Bornehag, C. G. (2020). Early prenatal exposure to suspected endocrine disruptor mixtures is associated with lower IQ at age seven. *Environment International,* 134, 105185. https://www.sciencedirect.com/science/article/pii/S0160412019314011?via%3Dihub

Tickner, J. A., & Hoppin, P. (2000). Children's environmental health: A case study in implementing the precautionary principle. *International Journal of Occupational and Environmental Health, 6,* 281-288.

Wienhold, B. (2009). Environmental factors in birth defects: What we need to know?. *Environmental Health Perspectives,* 117(10), A440-A447.

Wigle, DT. (2003). *Child health and the environment.* Oxford University Press.

Wilding, B. C., Curtis, K., & Welker-Hood, K. (2009). *Hazardous chemicals in health care: A snapshot of chemicals in doctors and nurses.* Physicians for Social Responsibility.

World Health Organization. (2015). *Quantifying environmental health impacts.* http://www.who.int/quantifying_ehimpacts/countryprofiles/en/

Yazbeck, C., Thiebaugeorges, O., Moreau, T., Goua, V., Debotte, G., Sahuquillo, J., Forhan, A. Foliguet, B., Magnin, G., Slama, R., Charles, M. & Huel, G. (2009). Maternal blood lead levels and the risk of pregnancy induced hypertension: The EDEN cohort study (2009). *Environmental Health Perspectives, 117,* 10.

Zenker A., Cicero, M. R., Prestinaci, F., Bottoni,P., Carere, M. (2014) Bioaccumulation and biomagnification potential of pharmaceuticals with a focus to the aquatic environment, *Journal of Environmental Management,133,* 378-387,

Zheng, T., Zhang, J., Sommer, K., Bassig, B. A., Zhang, X., Braun, J., ... & Kelsey, K. (2016). Effects of environmental exposures on fetal and childhood growth trajectories. *Annals of Global Health,* 82(1), 41-99. https://doi.org/10.1016/j.aogh.2016.01.008

PESTICIDES AND CHILD VULNERABILITIES
Robyn Gilden, PhD, RN
Assistant Professor, Family and Community Health,
University of Maryland School of Nursing

INTRODUCTION

Pesticides are chemical formulations that are widely used in society and may create human health threats. The US Environmental Protection Agency (EPA) (2018) defines a pesticide as "any substance intended for preventing, destroying, repelling, or mitigating any pest," including insect, plant, fungus, rodent, or bacteria. Pesticides include insecticides, herbicides, fungicides, rodenticides, and biocides and are ubiquitous in our environment. The usual biological targets of pesticides are the pests' nervous or reproductive system, although they may affect other organisms, including humans.

CHILDREN

Bearer (Bearer 1995), coined the phrase that is now the axiom, "children are not little adults." Several differences are especially important when discussing environmental exposures. For example, young children explore their world with hand-to-mouth activity (Black et al., 2005)

The research conducted by Black et al. (2005) sought to evaluate the potential exposure to pesticides based on children's activities. This study reports findings from the first phase of a 24-month longitudinal project that took place in Laredo, TX between May and August 2000. The sample included 52 children, ages 7-53 months in 29 homes. Data were collected by four hours of video taping mouthing and food handling behaviors and collecting samples of house dust, soil, hand loadings, and urine. A questionnaire was also completed by the adult in the household. The study found both object mouthing (Rs= -0.329, p=.017) and hand mouthing (Rs= -0.301, p=.030) decrease with increasing age. Playing outside differed by age (X2=8.1, p=.04) and hand washing increased with age except after playing outside. The authors conclude that the EPA's standard risk assessment estimate of 49 combined hand- and object- to mouth contacts/hour may not be protective enough of infants since 39% of less than one-year olds exceeded that limit.

Children are also closer to the ground, play outside in the dirt, eat and drink more per body weight than adults, have limited selection of food, and many of their various body systems are still developing (Bearer 1995; Black et al. 2005; Eskenazi et al. 1999; Islam et al. 2018; Reigart & Roberts 2001; Thomas 1995; Tulve et al. 2002). Children can be exposed to chemicals of concern, including pesticides in the diet, school, gardens/yards, in the home and from take-home contact with parents' work clothes (Hyland & Laribi 2017; Zahm & Ward 1998).

For example, a follow-up longitudinal study done by Lu et al (Lu et al., 2009) to assess children's exposure to pyrethroid insecticides by collecting series of urine samples during summer and fall 2003, and winter and spring 2004. A total of 1757 spot urine samples were collected from 19 out of 23 children, age 3-11. Linear mixed models analysis was used and results show two urinary metabolites common to pyrethroid insecticides were present at a significant level when controlling for season, age, gender, residential use, and dietary intake.

Children also have a longer time for the effects of exposure to impact their health. In Rohlman's cross-sectional study (Rohlman et al., 2007) researchers compared neurobehavioral (NB) performance of 119 Hispanic adolescents and adults working in agriculture to 56 Hispanic adolescents and adults not currently working in agriculture and found a significant inverse relationship between NB performance and both age and years of use (p=.04). They conclude that a future longitudinal study is needed to assess the cohort of adolescent agricultural workers to see if there is a more significant deterioration in NB performance when early use is added to the number of years used.

PREGNANT PERSON/FETUS

Even more critical periods of growth and development exist for a developing fetus with the opportunity for more permanent and debilitating results. Whyatt (2007) reported that indoor air concentrations of pesticides correlated with umbilical cord blood levels and the babies born with the highest cord blood levels of chlorpyrifos also had significantly lower weight and length at birth. The article series by Whyatt et al (2004; 2007; 2009) are all from the same Columbia Center for Children's Environmental Health (CCCEH) cohort that followed African American and Dominican women registered at two New York City Hospitals' prenatal clinics who live in either North Manhattan or South Bronx. The 2004 article presents findings from 314 mother-baby pairs including maternal personal air samples collected over the last months of pregnancy, umbilical cord blood samples, and measures of fetal growth. "Specifically, birth weight decreased by 42.6 g (95% CI, −81.8 to −3.8, p = 0.03), and birth length decreased by 0.24 cm (95% CI, −0.47 to −0.01, p = 0.04) for each log unit increase in cord plasma chlorpyrifos levels" (p. 1128-9).

Prenatal exposures to pesticides have been linked with otitis media, respiratory distress, asthma, and cancer

(Weselak et al. 2007). Exposure prior to or during pregnancy increased risk for Acute Lymphocytic Leukemia, Wilms' Tumor, and brain cancer (Daniels et al. 1997; Zahm & Ward 1998). The latest review of the literature published by Infante-Rivard (Infante-Rivard & Weichenthal 2007) updated Zahm and Ward (1998) and included 21 studies published from 1999-2004. Fifteen of these studies showed statistically significant increases for childhood cancer related to either childhood pesticide exposure or parental occupational exposure.

POTENTIAL HEALTH EFFECTS

There are many studies investigating the human health effects of pesticide exposure. There are so many possible combinations of chemicals, routes of exposures, and exposed individuals it is not surprising the results are variable. Below is a brief review of potential health effects and based on the assumptions of the Precautionary Principle (ANA, 2003), the preponderance of suggestive evidence warrants protective action.

Neurodevelopmental

Given that a main mode of action in controlling pests is targeting the nervous system, it is understandable that a high enough exposure over an extended period of time would result in neurological impact in humans. According to the National Academies of Science Report Environmental Neurotoxicology (Council 1992) less than 10% of over 70,000 chemicals in use in the US have any form of neurological testing let alone complete information. A challenge for determining neurodevelopmental effects of pesticides is that chemicals can act through a variety of mechanisms, making it difficult to confirm effects from study to study in different populations (Ray & Fry 2006).

Research indicates a link between prenatal pesticide exposure in mothers and related health effects in their children such as development attention deficit hyperactivity disorder behaviors (Yolton et al. 2014), social behavioral problems (Ribas-Fito et al. 2007), neurodevelopmental delays (Eskenazi et al. 2007; Handal et al. 2007; Ribas-Fito et al. 2003; Torres-Sanchez et al. 2007), and impaired gross and fine motor skills (Guillette et al. 1998). Additionally, research is starting to show that timing of the insult can impact outcomes, as prenatal exposure to pesticides very early on in gestation while the brain is forming neurons can lead to late-onset Parkinson disease (Iglesias et al. 2018). Prenatal and early life pesticide exposure has also been linked with difficulties in hearing (Gatto et al. 2014) and language development (Dzwilewski & Schantz 2015)

In a cross-sectional study by Handal et al (2007), the goal was to compare neurobehavioral (NB) development of children 3-61 months of age between those who did and did not live in areas of high pesticide exposure in the flower growing region in Ecuador. The sample was 219 mothers and 283 children, 154 who lived in two communities of high pesticide exposure and 129 who lived in a community not associated with industry-related pesticide use. A questionnaire to assess NB development was administered to the children and a separate questionnaire was administered to the mothers. Anthropomorphic measures were taken on the children and mothers and a blood sample was taken from the children to assess for anemia. Findings revealed that younger children (3-23 months) from the high-exposure area were significantly delayed in three out of five NB domains. Children scored 8.8 points lower on gross motor skills (p=.002, Cohen's d for effect size= .4), 5.0 points lower on fine motor skills (p=.06, d=.2) and 5.8 points lower on socio-individual skills (p=.02, d=.3). For older children (23-61 months) there was a suggestive trend with 3.8 point lower performance on gross motor skills assessment (p=.06, d=.2). The effect was much more pronounced when malnourishment was combined with high pesticide exposure, indicating a possible subpopulation at even higher risk for NB delay.

Reproductive and Endocrine

As little is known about neurodevelopmental effects, even less is known about reproductive and endocrine impacts. Investigation is also complicated by multiple chemicals capable of acting in similar ways on the hormonal systems. Several studies (Damgaard et al. 2006; Virtanen & Adamsson 2012) found boys with cryptorchidism had mothers with higher levels of organochlorine (OC) pesticide metabolites in their breast milk. In a review of the environmental and health impacts of the herbicide 2,4-Dichlorophenoxyacetic acid (2,4-D), Islam et al (Islam et al. 2018) report interference with the hormone necessary for spermatogenesis. Pesticides also have been implicated in altered thyroid function (Meeker et al. 2006a), decreased testosterone (Meeker et al. 2006b), gestational diabetes (Saldana et al. 2007), menstrual irregularities (Farr et al. 2004), and fetal death related to congenital birth defects (Bell et al. 2001; Wang et al. 2016). Additionally, pre and postnatal pesticide exposure can lead to later development of diabetes and obesity (Giulivo et al. 2016).

Immune system

A variety of pesticide-related immune system effects also have been investigated. Pesticides are suspected to lead to an increased risk for exposure to allergens and hay fever

(Weselak et al. 2007) and be a cause or trigger for multiple chemical sensitivity (Caress & Steinemann 2003).

Weselak et al (2007) conducted a cross-sectional study to investigate the possible immunotoxic effects of exposure to pesticides prenatally. The study used Ontario Farm Family Health Study data collected in 1991. It included 3405 children out of 5853 reported pregnancies. Results show a link between herbicides (OR=1.56, 95% CI 1.15-2.11), insecticides (OR=1.48, 95% CI 1.07-2.03), and fungicides (OR=1.69, 95% CI 1.15-2.47) and allergy and hay fever. More specifically for phenoxy herbicides (OR=1.43, 95% CI 1.03-1.99) and 2,4-D (OR=1.66, 95% CI 1.11-2.49). The association held true for male children and children of both genders that were 12 years old and older at the time of the questionnaire.

In a review of literature, Colosio (Colosio et al. 2005) described existing evidence that demonstrated a wide variety of pesticides can affect the immune system, but most of the studies are of high dose exposures and that data are lacking to indicate health risk from low, chronic doses. The review also stated that it is difficult to capture reversible effects.

Respiratory

There is little research available for respiratory effects in children from pesticide exposure, but the literature base is growing. Salam (Salam et al. 2004) identified increased risk of asthma related to pesticide exposure and Spencer (Spencer and O'Malley 2006) reported pesticides as an irritant and asthma trigger. Other studies support the link between prenatal and early life exposure to pesticides and increased odds of asthma symptoms and exercise-induced breathing issues, particularly if the exposure comes during the second half of pregnancy (Raanan et al. 2015; Vrijheid et al. 2016). In a systematic review and meta-analysis, Hosseini et al. (Hosseini et al. 2017), concluded support for a link between low fruit and vegetable intake and increased odds of asthma and allergies.

Salam et al. (2004) conducted a case-control study nested in a larger population-based study of children's respiratory health. One of the purposes of the research was to test the hypothesis that environmental exposures, including pesticides, led to increased occurrence of transient wheezing or persistent asthma. The sample was drawn from public school children in 12 southern California communities from the 4, 7, and 10th grades. There were 279 cases with asthma and 412 controls. Results indicate a 4.58 times (95% CI 1.36-15.43) increased risk for asthmatic children to have been exposed to herbicides during the first year of life and a 2.39 times (95% CI 1.17 – 4.89) increased risk of exposure to pesticides. As an

aside, it is interesting that the authors separate herbicides and pesticides when, in actuality, herbicides are a class under the broader category of pesticides.

Cancer

One of the most common endpoints investigated for health effects for any chemical exposure is cancer. Identification of causative mechanisms for cancer is often problematic due to multiple exposures and long latency periods.

The research thus far implicates pesticides in leukemia/lymphoma (Daniels et al. 1997; Infante-Rivard & Weichenthal 2007; Islam et al. 2018; McNally & Parker 2006; Menegaux et al. 2006; Zahm & Ward 1998). Menegaux et al (2006) conducted a hospital-based case-control study in four hospitals in France. There were 280 incident cases of acute leukemia and 288 hospitalized controls admitted between 1995 and 1999. The purpose was to analyze the relation between childhood acute leukemia and pesticide exposures. There was a significant relationship between leukemia and insecticide use at home during gestation (OR=1.8, 95% CI 1.2-2.8) and during childhood (OR=1.7, 95% CI 1.1 – 2.4). Garden pesticide use (OR=1.7, 95% CI 1.1 – 2.7), insecticide use (OR=2.4, 95% CI 1.3 – 4.3) and fungicide use (OR=2.5, 95% CI 1.0 – 6.2) were significantly associated with leukemia. Use of insecticide shampoos to treat head lice were also significantly related to leukemia (OR=1.9, 95% CI 1.1 – 3.2), especially if they contained pyrethroids (OR=2.0, 95% CI 1.1 – 3.4).

A similar national-registry based case-control study conducted in France in 2003 and 2004 (Rudant et al. 2007) had similar conclusions. Male and female cases were 764 for acute leukemia (AL), 130 Hodgkin lymphoma (HL), and 166 Non-Hodgkin lymphoma (NHL) and controls were 1,681 randomly selected from the French population using random digit dialing. Data were collected via phone interview using a structured questionnaire. Findings for maternal use of household pesticides any time during pregnancy indicate a 2.2 times increased risk for AL (95% CI 1.8 – 2.6) and 1.9 times increased risk of NHL (95% CI 1.3 – 2.6). Paternal use of insecticides during pregnancy or childhood increased risk for AL 1.4 times (95% CI 1.2 – 1.7).

Other probable cancers linked with pesticide exposure include breast (Clark & Snedeker 2005; Giulivo et al. 2016), prostate (Andreotti et al. 2009), pancreas (Andreotti et al. 2009), liver (Dharmani & Jaga 2005), kidney (Zahm & Ward, 1998; Daniels et al., 1997), lung (Zahm & Ward, 1998), brain (Daniels et al. 1997; Shim et al. 2009; Van Maele-Fabry et al. 2017; Zahm & Ward 1998), central nervous system (Georgakis 2017) and skin (Zahm & Ward, 1998).

A case-control study by Shim et al (2009) investigated the possible association between childhood brain cancer and parental exposure to pesticides at home and at work. Study participants were selected from statewide cancer registries in four east coast states as part of the Atlantic Coast Brain Cancer study during 2000-2001. Four hundred twenty-one cases and 421 controls participated. A suggestive outcome was found for astrocytoma and maternal herbicide use during the preceding two years before the child was born (OR=1.9, 95% CI 1.2-3.0).

Genetics

Genetic variations may determine how susceptible a child is to the effect of a pesticide exposure, whether prenatal or early-life. Paraoxonase-1 (PON1) is an enzyme that can detoxify several insecticides including organophosphates (OPs) and pyrethroids. Research is beginning to demonstrate that different polymorphisms in PON1 can increase the odds of health risks from exposure to the insecticides the enzyme breaks down (Marsillach et al. 2016; Yolton et al. 2013).

NURSING ACTIONS

More educational resources

- MD Pesticide Network's Pesticides and Public Health: Critical Literature on Human Health http://www.mdpestnet.org/wp-content/uploads/2012/11/MPN-07Journal-FINAL.pdf

- National Library of Medicine Environmental Health, Toxicology & Chemical Information https://envirotoxinfo.nlm.nih.gov/

Practice resources

- Health Care Without Harm Pesticide Resources: https://noharm-uscanada.org/issues/us-canada/cleaners-and-pesticides-resources#pesticides

- Californians for Pesticide Reform

- Bio-Integral Resource Center

- Northwest Coalition for Alternatives to Pesticides

- Extoxnet's Pesticide Information Profiles

- IPM Institute of North America http://ipminstitute.org/

- Integrated pest management - A more conservative and less toxic approach to pest management involves assessing the problem, making structural changes first and then using the least toxic chemical pesticide as a last resort. Structural changes include removing food

and water sources, sealing cracks and fixing holes in screens. Least toxic chemicals include boric acid and natural oils like citronella.

- NY State Health Department Reducing Pesticide Exposure https://www.health.ny.gov/environmental/pests/reduce.htm

- Prevent pests from entering your home or garden.

- Consider non-chemical methods for controlling pests.

- Select the product that best fits your needs.

- Follow label directions exactly when mixing and applying pesticides.

- Store and dispose of pesticides properly.

- Minimize environmental impacts from pesticide use.

- Pediatric Environmental Health Specialty Units, a network of experts in reproductive and children's environmental health https://www.pehsu.net/

Advocacy organizations

- American Academy of Pediatrics Council on Environmental Health https://www.aap.org/en-us/about-the-aap/Councils/Council-on-Environmental-Health/Pages/COEH.aspx

- Beyond Pesticides works with allies in protecting public health and the environment to lead the transition to a world free of toxic pesticides. https://beyondpesticides.org/

- Children's Environmental Health Network is a national multi-disciplinary organization whose mission is to protect the developing child from environmental health hazards has wonderful online resources. https://cehn.org/

- Pesticide Action Network of North America works to replace pesticide use with ecologically sound and socially just alternatives. http://www.panna.org/

REFERENCES

Andreotti, G., Freeman, L. E. B., Hou, L., Coble, J., Rusiecki, J., Hoppin, J. A., Silverman, D. T., & Alavanja, M. C. (2009). Agricultural pesticide use and pancreatic cancer risk in the Agricultural Health Study Cohort. *International Journal of Cancer, 124*(10), 2495–2500. https://doi.org/10.1002/ijc.24185

Bell, E. M., Hertz-Picciotto, I., & Beaumont, J. J. (2001) A Case-Control Study of Pesticides and Fetal Death Due to Congenital Anomalies. *Epidemiology, 12*(2), 148–156. https://doi.org/10.1097/00001648-200103000-00005

Black, K., Shalat, S. L., Freeman, N. C. G., Jimenez, M., Donnelly, K. C., & Calvin, J. A. (2004). Children's mouthing and food-handling behavior in an agricultural community on the US/Mexico border. *Journal of Exposure Science & Environmental Epidemiology*, 15(3), 244–251. https://doi.org/10.1038/sj.jea.7500398

Caress, S. M., & Steinemann, A. C. (2003). A review of a two-phase population study of multiple chemical sensitivities. *Environmental Health Perspectives*, 111(12), 1490–1497. https://doi.org/10.1289/ehp.5940

Clark, H. A., & Snedeker, S. M. (2005). Critical Evaluation of the Cancer Risk of Dibromochloropropane (DBCP). *Journal of Environmental Science and Health, Part C*, 23(2), 215–260. https://doi.org/10.1080/10590500500234996

Colosio, C., Birindelli, S., Corsini, E., Galli, C., & Maroni, M. (2005). Low levelexposure to chemicals and immune system. *Toxicology and Applied Pharmacology*, 207(2), 320–328. https://doi.org/10.1016/j.taap.2005.01.025

Claudio, L. (1993)Environmental Neurotoxicology. National Research Council. National Academy Press, Washington, DC, 1992, 154 pp. $24.95. *Environmental Research*, 62(2), 339–340. https://doi.org/10.1006/enrs.1993.1119

Damgaard, I., Skakkebæk, N., Toppari, J., Virtanen, H., Shen, H., Schramm, K.-W., Petersen, J., Jensen, T., & Main, K. (2006). Persistent pesticides in human breast milk and cryptorchidism. *Environmental Health Perspectives*, 114(7), 1133–1138. https://doi.org/10.1289/ehp.8741

Daniels, J. L., Olshan, A. F., & Savitz, D. A. (1997). Pesticides and childhood cancers.*Environmental Health Perspectives*, 105(10), 1068–1077. https://doi.org/10.1289/ehp.971051068

Dharmani, C., & Jaga, K. (2005). Epidemiology of Acute Organophosphate Poisoning in Hospital Emergency Patients. *Reviews on Environmental Health*, 20(3). https://doi.org/10.1515/reveh.2005.20.3.215

Dzwilewski, K. L., & Schantz, S. L. (2015). Prenatal chemical exposures and child language development. *Journal of Communication Disorders*, 57, 41–65. https://doi.org/10.1016/j.jcomdis.2015.07.002

Eskenazi, B., Bradman, A., & Castorina, R. (1999) Exposures of children to organophosphate pesticides and their potential adverse health effects. *Environmental Health Perspectives*, 107(suppl 3), 409–419. https://doi.org/10.1289/ehp.99107s3409

Eskenazi, B., Marks, A. R., Bradman, A., Harley, K., Barr, D. B., Johnson, C., Morga, N., & Jewell, N. P. (2007). Organophosphate Pesticide Exposure and Neurodevelopment in Young Mexican-American Children. *Environmental Health Perspectives*, 115(5), 792–798. https://doi.org/10.1289/ehp.9828

Farr, S. L., Cooper, G. S., Cai, J., Savitz, D. A., & Sandler, D. P. (2004). Pesticide Use and Menstrual Cycle Characteristics among Premenopausal Women in the Agricultural Health Study. *American Journal of Epidemiology*, 160(12), 1194–1204. https://doi.org/10.1093/aje/kwi006

Gatto, M., Fioretti, M., Fabrizi, G., Gherardi, M., Strafella, E., & Santarelli, L. (2014). Effects of potential neurotoxic pesticides on hearing loss: A review. *NeuroToxicology*, 42, 24–32. https://doi.org/10.1016/j.neuro.2014.03.009

Giulivo, M., Lopez de Alda, M., Capri, E., & Barceló, D. (2016). Human exposure to endocrine disrupting compounds: Their role in reproductive systems, metabolic syndrome and breast cancer. A review. *Environmental Research*, 151, 251–264. https://doi.org/10.1016/j.envres.2016.07.011

Guillette, E. A., Meza, M. M., Aquilar, M. G., Soto, A. D., & Garcia, I. E. (1998). An anthropological approach to the evaluation of preschool children exposed to pesticides in Mexico. *Environmental Health Perspectives*, 106(6), 347–353. https://doi.org/10.1289/ehp.98106347

Handal, A. J., Lozoff, B., Breilh, J., & Harlow, S. D. (2007). Effect of Community of Residence on Neurobehavioral Development in Infants and Young Children in a Flower-Growing Region of Ecuador. *Environmental Health Perspectives*, 115(1), 128–133. https://doi.org/10.1289/ehp.9261

Hosseini, B., Berthon, B. S., Wark, P., & Wood, L. G. (2017). Effects of Fruit and Vegetable Consumption on Risk of Asthma, Wheezing and Immune Responses: A Systematic Review and Meta-Analysis. *Nutrients*, 9(4), 341. https://doi.org/10.3390/nu9040341

Hyland, C., & Laribi, O. (2017). Review of take-home pesticide exposure pathway in children living in agricultural areas. *Environmental Research*, 156, 559–570. https://doi.org/10.1016/j.envres.2017.04.017

Iglesias, E., Pesini, A., Garrido-Pérez, N., Meade, P., Bayona-Bafaluy, M. P., Montoya, J., & Ruiz-Pesini, E. (2018, August). Prenatal exposure to oxidative phosphorylation xenobiotics and late-onset Parkinson disease. *Ageing Research Reviews*, 45, 24–32. https://doi.org/10.1016/j.arr.2018.04.006

Infante-Rivard, C., & Weichenthal, S. (2007, January). Pesticides and Childhood Cancer: An Update of Zahm and Ward's 1998 Review. *Journal of Toxicology and Environmental*

Health, Part B, 10(1–2), 81–99. https://doi.org/10.1080/10937400601034589

Islam, F., Wang, J., Farooq, M. A., Khan, M. S., Xu, L., Zhu, J., Zhao, M., Muños, S., Li, Q. X., & Zhou, W. (2018). Potential impact of the herbicide 2,4-dichlorophenoxyacetic acid on human and ecosystems. Environment International, 111, 332–351. https://doi.org/10.1016/j.envint.2017.10.020

Lu, C., Barr, D. B., Pearson, M. A., Walker, L. A., & Bravo, R. (2008). The attribution of urban and suburban children's exposure to synthetic pyrethroid insecticides: a longitudinal assessment. Journal of Exposure Science & Environmental Epidemiology, 19(1), 69–78. https://doi.org/10.1038/jes.2008.49

Marsillach, J., Costa, L. G., & Furlong, C. E. (2016). Paraoxonase-1 and Early-Life Environmental Exposures. Annals of Global Health, 82(1), 100. https://doi.org/10.1016/j.aogh.2016.01.009

Mcnally, R. J. Q., & Parker, L. (2006). Environmental factors and childhood acute leukemias and lymphomas. Leukemia & Lymphoma, 47(4), 583–598. https://doi.org/10.1080/10428190500420973

Meeker, J. D., Barr, D. B., & Hauser, R. (2006). Thyroid hormones in relation to urinary metabolites of non-persistent insecticides in men of reproductive age. Reproductive Toxicology, 22(3), 437–442. https://doi.org/10.1016/j.reprotox.2006.02.005

Meeker, J. D., Ryan, L., Barr, D. B., & Hauser, R. (2006). Exposure to Nonpersistent Insecticides and Male Reproductive Hormones. Epidemiology, 17(1), 61–68. https://doi.org/10.1097/01.ede.0000190602.14691.70

Menegaux, F. (2006). Household exposure to pesticides and risk of childhood acute leukaemia. Occupational and Environmental Medicine, 63(2), 131–134. https://doi.org/10.1136/oem.2005.023036

Raanan, R., Harley, K. G., Balmes, J. R., Bradman, A., Lipsett, M., & Eskenazi, B. (2015). Early-life Exposure to Organophosphate Pesticides and Pediatric Respiratory Symptoms in the CHAMACOS Cohort. Environmental Health Perspectives, 123(2), 179–185. https://doi.org/10.1289/ehp.1408235

Ray, D. E., & Fry, J. R. (2006). A reassessment of the neurotoxicity of pyrethroid insecticides. Pharmacology & Therapeutics, 111(1), 174–193. https://doi.org/10.1016/j.pharmthera.2005.10.003

Reigart, J. R., & Roberts, J. R. (2001, October). PESTICIDES IN CHILDREN. Pediatric Clinics of North America, 48(5), 1185–1198. https://doi.org/10.1016/s0031-3955(05)70368-0

Ribas-Fitó, N., Cardo, E., Sala, M., Eulàlia de Muga, M., Mazón, C., Verdú, A., Kogevinas, M., Grimalt, J. O., & Sunyer, J. (2003). Breastfeeding, Exposure to Organochlorine Compounds, and Neurodevelopment in Infants. Pediatrics, 111(5), e580–e585. https://doi.org/10.1542/peds.111.5.e580

Rohlman, D. S., Lasarev, M., Anger, W. K., Scherer, J., Stupfel, J., & McCauley, L. (2007). Neurobehavioral Performance of Adult and Adolescent Agricultural Workers. NeuroToxicology, 28(2), 374–380. https://doi.org/10.1016/j.neuro.2006.10.006

Rudant, J., Menegaux, F., Leverger, G., Baruchel, A., Nelken, B., Bertrand, Y., Patte, C., Pacquement, H., Vérité, C., Robert, A., Michel, G., Margueritte, G., Gandemer, V., Hémon, D., & Clavel, J. (2007). Household exposure to pesticides and risk of childhood hematopoietic malignancies: The ESCALE Study (SFCE). Environmental Health Perspectives, 115(12), 1787–1793. https://doi.org/10.1289/ehp.10596

Salam, M. T., Li, Y. F., Langholz, B., & Gilliland, F. D. (2004). Early-life environmental risk factors for asthma: findings from the Children's Health Study. Environmental Health Perspectives, 112(6), 760–765. https://doi.org/10.1289/ehp.6662

Saldana, T. M., Basso, O., Hoppin, J. A., Baird, D. D., Knott, C., Blair, A., Alavanja, M. C., & Sandler, D. P. (2007). Pesticide Exposure and Self-Reported Gestational Diabetes Mellitus in the Agricultural Health Study. Diabetes Care, 30(3), 529–534. https://doi.org/10.2337/dc06-1832

Shim, Y. K., Mlynarek, S. P., & van Wijngaarden, E. (2009). Parental exposure to pesticides and childhood brain cancer: U.S. Atlantic Coast Childhood Brain Cancer Study. Environmental Health Perspectives, 117(6), 1002–1006. https://doi.org/10.1289/ehp.0800209

Tang, J. X., & Siegfried, B. D. (1996). Bioconcentration and Uptake of a Pyrethroid and Organophosphate Insecticide by Selected Aquatic Insects. Bulletin of Environmental Contamination and Toxicology, 57(6), 993–998. https://doi.org/10.1007/s001289900288

Thomas, R. D. (1995). Age-specific carcinogenesis: environmental exposure and susceptibility. Environmental Health Perspectives, 103(suppl 6), 45–48. https://doi.org/10.1289/ehp.95103s645

Torres-Sánchez, L., Rothenberg, S. J., Schnaas, L., Cebrián, M. E., Osorio, E., del Carmen Hernández, M., García-Hernández, R. M., del Rio-Garcia, C., Wolff, M. S., & López-

Carrillo, L. (2007). In Utero p , p '-DDE Exposure and Infant Neurodevelopment: A Perinatal Cohort in Mexico. *Environmental Health Perspectives, 115*(3), 435–439. https://doi.org/10.1289/ehp.9566

Tulve, N. S., Suggs, J. C., Mccurdy, T., Cohen Hubal, E. A., & Moya, J. (2002). Frequency of mouthing behavior in young children. *Journal of Exposure Science & Environmental Epidemiology, 12*(4), 259–264. https://doi.org/10.1038/sj.jea.7500225

US Environmental Protection Agency. (2018). *What is a pesticide.* https://www.epa.gov/ingredients-used-pesticide-products/basic-information-about-pesticide-ingredients

Van Maele-Fabry, G., Gamet-Payrastre, L., & Lison, D. (2017). Residential exposure to pesticides as risk factor for childhood and young adult brain tumors: A systematic review and meta-analysis. *Environment International, 106,* 69–90. https://doi.org/10.1016/j.envint.2017.05.018

Virtanen, H. E., & Adamsson, A. (2012). Cryptorchidism and endocrine disrupting chemicals. *Molecular and Cellular Endocrinology, 355*(2), 208–220. https://doi.org/10.1016/j.mce.2011.11.015

Vrijheid, M., Casas, M., Gascon, M., Valvi, D., & Nieuwenhuijsen, M. (2016). Environmental pollutants and child health—A review of recent concerns. *International Journal of Hygiene and Environmental Health, 219*(4–5), 331–342. https://doi.org/10.1016/j.ijheh.2016.05.001

Wang, A., Padula, A., Sirota, M., & Woodruff, T. J. (2016). Environmental influences on reproductive health: the importance of chemical exposures. *Fertility and Sterility, 106*(4), 905–929. https://doi.org/10.1016/j.fertnstert.2016.07.1076

Whyatt, R. M., Rauh, V., Barr, D. B., Camann, D. E., Andrews, H. F., Garfinkel, R., Hoepner, L. A., Diaz, D., Dietrich, J., Reyes, A., Tang, D., Kinney, P. L., & Perera, F. P. (2004). Prenatal insecticide exposures and birth weight and length among an urban minority cohort. *Environmental Health Perspectives, 112*(10), 1125–1132. https://doi.org/10.1289/ehp.6641

Whyatt, R. M., Garfinkel, R., Hoepner, L. A., Holmes, D., Borjas, M., Williams, M. K., Reyes, A., Rauh, V., Perera, F. P., & Camann, D. E. (2007). Within- and between-home variability in indoor-air insecticide levels during pregnancy among an inner-city cohort from New York City. *Environmental Health Perspectives, 115*(3), 383–389. https://doi.org/10.1289/ehp.9546

Whyatt, R. M., Garfinkel, R., Hoepner, L. A., Andrews, H., Holmes, D., Williams, M. K., Reyes, A., Diaz, D., Perera, F. P., Camann, D. E., & Barr, D. B. (2009). A biomarker validation study of prenatal chlorpyrifos exposure within an inner-city cohort during pregnancy. *Environmental Health Perspectives, 117*(4), 559–567. https://doi.org/10.1289/ehp.0800041

Yolton, K., Xu, Y., Sucharew, H., Succop, P., Altaye, M., Popelar, A., Montesano, M. A., Calafat, A. M., & Khoury, J. C. (2013). Impact of low-level gestational exposure to organophosphate pesticides on neurobehavior in early infancy: a prospective study. *Environmental Health, 12*(1). https://doi.org/10.1186/1476-069x-12-79

Yolton, K., Cornelius, M., Ornoy, A., McGough, J., Makris, S., & Schantz, S. (2014). Exposure to neurotoxicants and the development of attention deficit hyperactivity disorder and its related behaviors in childhood. *Neurotoxicology and Teratology, 44,* 30–45. https://doi.org/10.1016/j.ntt.2014.05.003

Zahm, S. H., & Ward, M. H. (1998). Pesticides and childhood cancer. *Environmental Health Perspectives, 106*(suppl 3), 893–908. https://doi.org/10.1289/ehp.98106893

IMMIGRANTS AND REFUGEES AS A VULNERABLE POPULATION

Ruth McDermott Levy, PhD, MPH, RN
Professor
Co-Director, Mid-Atlantic Center for Children's Health and the Environment
Villanova University
M. Louise Fitzpatrick College of Nursing

INTRODUCTION

Currently, there are 44 million people who were born in another country and have made the United States their home. They represent every country in the world; thus the United States has the largest and most diverse immigrant population (Radford, 2019). Although immigrants to the U.S. represent many nations, the foreign-born U.S. residents who immigrated to the U.S. and comprise the largest segment of the immigrant population were born in Mexico (25 %), China (6%), India (6%), Philippines (4%), and El Salvador (3%) (Pew Research Center, 2020). Climate change is influencing migration and it is expected to be a driver of rising rates of refugees and asylum seekers in the future (see climate change section on Migration in this e-text).

Those immigrating to and seeking refuge in the U.S. have primarily resided in California, Florida, Illinois, New York and Texas. There has been a recent trend, however, in which immigrants and refugees are settling throughout the country (U.S. Census Bureau, n.d.). This trend leads to greater diversity within our communities and requires the nurse to have an understanding of the needs of foreign-born populations related to their past environmental exposures and their unique environmental risks with resettlement in the U.S.

ENVIRONMENTAL EXPOSURES FROM COUNTRY OF ORIGIN

Like everyone else, we are influenced by our environments. Body burden studies have found that people living in industrialized countries, such as the U.S., have a legacy of chemical exposures (Gennings et al, 2012). Immigrants and refugees arrive in the U.S. with past environmental exposures from their native land. Depending on the circumstances of the immigrating person those environmental exposures can place an immigrant or refugee at greater health risk.

OCCUPATIONAL EXPOSURES

Workplace environmental exposures in the country of origin influence the health of people immigrating to the U.S. The World Health Organization (n.d.) has identified that people from developing countries are more likely to be exposed airborne particulates, carcinogens, and risks of workplace injury. Those employed in agricultural jobs are at risk for pesticide exposures and depending on the climate of the country of origin, heat related illnesses such as skin cancer and renal disease (Wesseling, Crowe, Hogstedt, Jakobsson, Lucas & Wegman, 2013). Outdoor workers are particularly vulnerable to greater risk of heat related illnesses as a result of climate change. Climate change is also expected to exacerbate existing chronic diseases such as pulmonary and cardiac disease (Intergovernmental Panel on Climate Change, 2014).

It is helpful to remember that not all resettled immigrants and refugees were employed in countries with strict occupational health requirements for worker protections. Assessment of past employment activities and exposures is an important first step to determine environmental risks. In addition to the risk described for agricultural workers in the previous paragraph, workers in manufacturing may be at risk for musculoskeletal injury from repetitive activities or chemical and noise exposures from working with industrial equipment and lubricants. Those who were employed in the health care sector may have risk of biological exposures, while the extraction (mining) industry presents the risk of radiation, poor air quality, and chemical exposures (Frumkin, 2016). For more information regarding global occupational health risk see WHO Occupational Health web site.

The role of many women from developing countries remains traditional and their work is in the home. This makes immigrating women from some developing countries vulnerable to household indoor smoke from indoor cook stoves that use wood or other biomass fuel. Poor indoor air quality is associated with pulmonary conditions such as acute respiratory infections, tuberculosis, and lung cancer, as well as heart disease and poor pregnancy outcomes such as low birth weight (World Health Organization, 2006). Nursing assessments should include identifying chronic diseases and previous exposures in the immigrating person's country of origin.

CULTURAL & FOLK PRACTICES

Cultural practices can put immigrants and refugees at risk for environmental hazards. For example, women from some parts of Africa, South Asia, and the Middle East may use traditional eye cosmetics known as kolh (Arabic: kuhl; Punjabi: sirma; Hindi: kajal; Telegu: katuka from: https://theurbanmuslimwomen.wordpress.com/2008/09/22/kohl-for-the-eyes/). Kohl can also be applied to infants' eyes at birth as it is believed to strengthen the eyes and protect the child from the evil eye. Kolh preparations may contain lead and this practice can put women and infants at risk of lead toxicity. change (See lead section in this e-text).

Furthermore, some traditional medicines that are used as part of Hispanic, Chinese, Middle Eastern, Indian and other Asian folk health practices have been noted to contain heavy metals including lead. The U.S. Center for Disease Control and Prevention (n.d.) offers detailed information about folk medications that may place immigrant and refugee families at risk for lead and other heavy metal exposures. The nurse should assess past use of traditional medicines and determine if the immigrating family continues to rely on these traditional medicines.

DISASTERS

Natural and manmade disasters have the capacity to disrupt the infrastructure that provides clean water and air as well as safe food and medicines. Consequently, immigrant and refugee families may present with health problems related to exposure to poor air and water quality as a result of disruptions of utilities. These disasters could be the reason for immigration to the U.S. Natural disasters such as volcanoes, earthquakes, tornadoes and hurricanes can create health problems for the people in the surrounding communities. For example, volcanic activity generates gasses such as sulfur dioxide, carbon dioxide and hydrogen chloride as well as particulate matter that can affect human health. The U.S. Geological Survey website describes air pollution related to volcanic activity.

With increasing development, natural disasters can influence the built environment and lead to a manmade disaster. This was the case with the 2011 earthquake and subsequent tsunami near Fukushima, Japan that ultimately led to the release of radiation from the nearby nuclear power plant. Following the Fukushima nuclear disaster, WHO (2013) conducted a health risk assessment and identified that those people living closest to the nuclear reactors at the time of the accident had an increased risk of solid cancers (4%), breast cancer (6% increase for infant females), leukemia (7% increase for infant males) and thyroid cancer (70% increase for infant females). It is important that the nurse takes the time to learn the history of the country of origin and reason for immigration so that health screening can be targeted to the patient's environmental health risks. For more information regarding environmental health impacts of disasters, please go to the Natural Disasters, Climate Change, & Preparedness section in Unit 6.

WAR AND AREAS OF CONFLICT

Disputes of our world's limited natural resources such as water rights can be an antecedent to war. War itself, a manmade disaster, presents additional environmental risks to immigrant and refugee families. Psychological trauma and physical disability as consequence of military conflict can be complicated by environmental exposures of warfare including chemical weapons that affect military and civilian populations (Dworkin, Prescott, Jamal, Hardawan, Aras, & Sandro, 2008). Iraqi refugee families attributed congenital anomalies of children that were born following maternal exposure to chemicals used during the Iraqi war (McDermott-Levy & Al Balushi, 2015).

IMMIGRANTS & REFUGEES LIVING IN THE U.S.

Immigrants to the U.S. are less likely to have health insurance and are less likely to seek care from a health care professional. Furthermore, citizenship influences access to U.S. sponsored health insurance programs such as Medicaid and Medicare. Consequently, in 2018, 24% of lawfully present, nonelderly and 45% of undocummented immigrants were not insured (Kaiser Family Foundation, 2020).

Access to health care is further limited by language barriers, cultural differences, perception of health needs, and immigrant status (Ku & Jewers, 2013). These factors influence how an immigrant patient or family would respond to or understand the risks or impacts of environmental exposures.

LANGUAGE

Language and access to interpreters also creates barriers to health information for refugees (Morris et al., 2009) who may come to the U.S. with a variety of physical and mental health problems (Jamil, Farrag, Hakim-Larson, Kafaji, Adbulkhaleqm & Hammad, 2007; Ramos, Orozovich, Moser, Phares, Stauffer, & Mitchell, 2010). One problem for those new to the country is the ability to access environmental health information related to the area of resettlement and to read instructions on chemical labels such as pesticides and cleaning agents. The National Service Center for Environmental Publications of the EPA has environmental health resources in 23 languages and dialects to support the immigrant and refugee family. Safe and proper use of household pesticides and cleaning agents can be a problem for recent immigrants who may not be able to read instructions in English. One thing that may assist those new to the U.S. is that in 2003 the member countries of the United Nations published a harmonized chemical hazard communication system called the "Globally Harmonized System of Classification and

Labeling of Chemicals" (OSHA, n.d.). As a result of harmonization, most countries rely on standardized warning symbols and standardized safety data sheets (formally MDS). While this will not completely overcome some language barriers for recent immigrant or refugee families, standardization does provide common warning pictographs from country to country. For more information regarding international chemical labeling standardization see Occupational Safety & Health Administration web site regarding global harmonization.

CULTURAL IMPLICATIONS IN THE U.S.

Adding to barriers of access to a health professional regarding environmental health information is the perceptions of the role of the nurse. In some cultures it is not acceptable to ask questions of the providers and nurses do not have a role other than following the physician's orders. Also the U.S. healthcare system is very complex and can be confusing to a newly arriving immigrant; therefore, someone with an environmentally related problem may not know how to access a health care provider for assistance. Nurses need to make themselves available to immigrant and refugee communities in order to educate those new to the U.S. in the role of the nurse and environmental risks and safe practices. Social organizations and the faith community are groups in which the nurse can access immigrant and refugee communities. For example, Villanova University nursing students partnered with a senior center that serviced elderly Asian immigrants to teach healthy gardening practices that did not rely on pesticides. See How does your garden grow?

ECONOMICS & HOUSING

Many immigrants and refugees arrive in the U.S. and find themselves living at a lower standard of living than they had in their home country (Morris et al., 2009). In the U.S. they may find themselves living in substandard housing, older homes in disrepair, or be victims of unscrupulous landlords. Home environmental risks that may be a problem for this population is lead based paint, carbon dioxide from poorly maintained furnaces, or pests such as roaches or rodents. The nurse should assess the age of homes, the availability and policies related to carbon monoxide detectors, and if pests are a problem for the immigrating family. If an environmental risk is identified the nurse should make appropriate referrals and educate the family in mitigation methods.

CONCLUSIONS

Immigrants and refugees may come to the U.S. with previous environmental health exposures that require assessment and management if there are health consequences. Additionally, once in the U.S., immigrants and refugees are at risk as a result of language and cultural barriers as well as potential challenges accessing the health care system. Nursing assessments should focus on the unique previous exposures and potential risks for the resettled immigrant. Once risks and health problems are identified the nurse can make appropriate referrals and participate in interventions that promote the health of this vulnerable population.

REFERENCES

Centers for Disease Control (n.d.) *Complementary and alternative medicine.* https://www.cdc.gov/cancer/survivors/patients/complementary-alternative-medicine.htm

Dworkin, J., Prescott, M., Jamal, R., Hardawan, S. A., Abdullah, A., & Galea, S. (2008). The Long-Term Psychosocial Impact of a Surprise Chemical Weapons Attack on Civilians in Halabja, Iraqi Kurdistan. *Journal of Nervous & Mental Disease, 196* (10), 772-775. doi: 10.1097/NMD.0b013e3181878b69.

Frumkin, H. (Ed). (2016). *Environmental health: From global to local (3rd ed.).* Jossey-Bass.

Gennings, C., Ellis, R., & Ritter, J. K. (2012). Linking empirical estimates of body burden of environmental chemicals and wellness using NHANES data. *Environment International, 39*(1), 56–65. https://doi.org/10.1016/j.envint.2011.09.002

George Washington University, Department of Health Policy (2012). Analysis of data from the US Current Population Survey. *March Annual Social and Economic Supplement.*

Intergovernmental Panel on Climate Change. (2014). *Climate change 2014: Impacts, adaptation, and vulnerability.* http://www.ipcc.ch/report/ar5/wg2/.

Jamil, H., Farrag, M., Hakim-Larson, J., Kafaji, T., Adbulkhaleqm, H., & Hammad, A. (2007). Mental health symptoms in Iraqi refugees: Post traumatic stress disorder, anxiety, and depression. *Journal of Cultural Diversity, 14* (1), 19-25.

Kaiser Family Foundation. (2020). *Health coverage of immigrants.* https://www.kff.org/racial-equity-and-health-policy/fact-sheet/health-coverage-of-immigrants/

Ku, L. & Jewers, M. (2013). *Health care for immigrant families: Current policies and issues.* Migration Policy Institute. http://www.migrationpolicy.org/pubs/COI-HealthCare.pdf.

Martin, P. & Midgley, E. (2006). Immigration: Shaping and reshaping America. *Population Bulletin, 61.*

McDermott-Levy, R. & N. Al Balushi (2015). Philadelphia Arab immigrant health needs assessment. *Research & Reviews: Journal of Nursing and Health Sciences, 1*(3), 4-13.

Morris, M.D., Popper, S.T., Rodwell, T.C., Brodine, S.K., & Brouwer, K.C. (2009). Healthcare barriers of refugees post-resettlement. *Journal of Community Health, 34,* 529-538. doi:10.1007/s10900-009-9175-3.

Occupational Safety & Health Administration (OSHA) (n.d.). *Modification of the hazard communication standard(HCS) to conform with the United Nations' (UN) Globally Harmonized System of Classification and Labeling of Chemicals (GHS).* https://www.osha.gov/dsg/hazcom/hazcom-faq.html.

Pew Research Center. (2020). *Key Findings About U.S. Immigrants: Mexico, China and India are among top birthplaces for immigrants in the U.S.* https://www.pewresearch.org/fact-tank/2020/08/20/key-findings-about-u-s-immigrants/ft_2020-08-20_immigrants_03b/.

Radford, J. & Noe-Bustamante, L. (2019). *Facts on U.S. Immigrants, 2017: Statistical portrait of the foreign-born population in the United States.* Pew Research Center.https://www.pewresearch.org/hispanic/2019/06/03/facts-on-u-s-immigrants-2017-data/.

Ramos, M., Orozovich, P., Moser, K., Phares, R., Stauffer, W., & Mitchell, T. (2010). Health of resettled Iraqi refugees San Diego County, California, October 2007-September 2009. *Morbidity and Mortality Weekly Report, 59*(49), 1614-1618.

Wesseling, C., Crowe, J., Hogstedt, C., Jakobsson, K., Lucas, R., & Wegman, D. (2013). The epidemic of chronic kidney disease of unknown etiology in Mesoamerica: A call for interdisciplinary research and action. *American Journal of Public Health, 13*(11), 1927-1929.

World Health Organization (WHO) (2006). *Fuel for life: Household energy and health.* http://www.who.int/indoorair/publications/fuelforlife.pdf.

World Health Organization (2013). *Global report on Fukushima nuclear accident details health risks.* http://www.who.int/mediacentre/news/releases/2013/fukushima_report_20130228/en/.

World Health Organization (n.d.). *Global estimates of occupational burden of disease.* http://www.who.int/quantifying_ehimpacts/global/occrf2004/en/.

DENTAL AMALGAM AND VULNERABLE POPULATIONS

Linda Cifelli, BA, RN
Co-owner of Innovative Pain Release
Williamsburg, VA
Member of Dental Amalgam Mercury Solutions

Jeanne Leffers, PhD, RN, FAAN
Professor Emeritus
University of Massachusetts Dartmouth
College of Nursing and Health Sciences

INTRODUCTION

This chapter examines several vulnerable populations for whom mercury used in dental amalgams poses risk to health. The first three groups are pregnant and breastfeeding people, and children, and the fourth is the occupational setting that includes dentists, dental assistants and dental hygienists as a vulnerable group due to their occupational exposure to mercury in dental office settings. Mercury is a heavy metal that is a neurotoxin. It can affect the brain and nervous system leading to neuromuscular effects and function. People can present with headaches and tremors, to more serious effects such as disturbances in mental function or neuromuscular changes. Additional adverse health effects include difficulties with coordination, changes in vision or hearing, memory disorders (including possible links to Alzheimer's Disease), mood disorders (anxiety, depression), sleep disturbances, and fatigue (Haley & Mutter, 2013), as well as cardiac disease and hypertension in older adults (HCWH, 2018). Human exposure to mercury occurs most commonly through ingestion of seafood contaminated with mercury, dental amalgams, some vaccines that contain thimerosal such as multi-dose flu (CDC, n.d.)), and air and water contaminated by mercury chloride. Fish highest in mercury levels are bluefish, grouper, marlin, salmon (farmed Atlantic), Chilean Sea Bass, swordfish, and all types of tuna (NRDC, 2021). (This textbook offers additional information in the chapter on heavy metals located in the Environmental Health Sciences Unit). Studies indicate that pregnant and breastfeeding people are at risk for mercury exposure. However, workers, such as dentists and dental hygienists, can be exposed to mercury in their occupational settings. For those working in the dental field their exposure comes from dental amalgam. Dental amalgam is composed of mercury, copper, silver and tin, often referred to as "silver" fillings. These fillings have been used for more than 180 years (FDA, 2020). Although composite resin fillings are used more frequently today for filling decayed areas of teeth, amalgam fillings are still in use and are also replaced as the tooth and filling age, such as amalgam restoration, decay under a filing and fractures of teeth among others occur (Warwick, Young, Palmer & Ermel, 2019).

Mercury is released during dental restorations through volatilization of mercury vapor and is absorbed into the body through inhalation. (FDA, 2020, Warwick, Young, Palmer & Ermel,2019). In the USA there are more than 400, 000 (USBLS 2019) dentists and dental hygienists employed in dental offices who come in direct contact with dental amalgam (Tibau &Grube, 2019; Tucek, Busova, Cejchanova, Schlenker & Kapitan, 2020). Dental workers have be found to have increased levels of mercury and more health issues associated with mercury exposure than the general public (Warwick, Young, Palmer & Ermel, 2019). However, the Food and Drug Administration (FDA, 2020) notes that factors such as other dietary or environmental exposures to mercury, limitations in study design and execution and conflicting study findings result in contradictory data; thus, limiting the establishment of safe levels of exposure, and conclusive evidence for health recommendations (FDA, 2020).

Testing for the presence of mercury in the body can be done by testing urine, blood, or hair; however, this is not widely available, is generally not covered by insurance and can be costly. Testing can indicate toxic levels of mercury in the body but that does not lead to the cause of exposure. Additionally, dental fillings are likely to remain in the body for many years beyond the time of testing, resulting in further mercury exposure.

EVIDENCE OF RISK

Although the issue of human health risk from dental amalgam has been controversial, most studies confirm that microleakage of mercury does occur. Thus, mercury from dental amalgam can enter the body at low levels (Yip, Li & Yau, 2003). For example, studies of amalgam use for tooth decay in children followed for 5-7 years reviewed by the National Institutes of Health (NIH) (2006) reported that no detectable loss of memory, coordination, concentration or other symptoms of severe mercury exposure were noted, that children in studies in both the United States and Europe who have amalgam fillings did show elevated levels of mercury in their urine. It should be noted that no level of mercury in the human body is considered normal. Studies of dentists and dental assistants show that they are more likely to have elevated blood levels of mercury than the control group (Jamil et al, 2016; Jonidi Jafari, Esrafili, Moradi & Mahmoudi, 2020).

VULNERABLE POPULATIONS

The FDA recommends that resin-based composites be considered for populations who can be more sensitive to the adverse effects of mercury vapor exposure. (FDA, 2020). Groups that are at higher risk include: pregnant people, those who are breastfeeding, children (particularly those under age 6), people planning to become pregnant, persons with chronic diseases such as kidney dysfunction, neurologic impairment, and those people who have a known allergy to mercury (Napierska, 2018).

Scholars claim that studies of differential treatment based upon race or socioeconomic factors in dentistry is not well established (Sabbah, Tsakos, Chandola, Sheiham & Watt, 2007; Bastos, Celeste, & Paradies, 2018) that disparities in dental care exist. Disparities in treatment options exist with studies that show differential treatment decisions based upon the person's skin color (Chisini et al, 2019, Sabbah, Tsakos, Chandola, Sheiham & Watt). Health disparities persist among those who face financial barriers for dental care than for any other form of health care (Vujicic, Buchmueller & Klein, 2016). More research into racial and ethic disparities in treatment options related to dental amalgams and risk reduction.

REGULATION OF DENTAL AMALGAM

In the United States, the regulatory agency for health and safety for chemical safety is the Environmental Protection Agency (EPA). They regulate the safety of mercury overall but make brief reference to dental amalgam as a source of mercury exposure (EPA, 2020). However the EPA regulates mercury waste for all sources and is discussed later in this chapter. Because dental amalgam is considered a medical device it is regulated by the Food and Drug Administration (FDA). The FDA offers a recent literature review for Epidemiologic Evidence on the Adverse Health Effects Reported in Relation to Mercury from Dental Amalgams (2019). They note that the 30 studies reviewed fail to provide consistent evidence between detectable adverse clinical outcomes and dental amalgams however they recommend methodological approaches that can differentiate between exposures from diet (generally methyl mercury) and other sources of elemental mercury from occupational and other such as dental amalgams (FDA, 2019). Recommendations from the FDA (2009) indicate the need for more study about the effects of dental amalgam and due to the potential adverse impacts upon vulnerable groups that the Precautionary Principle be followed. The European Union (EU) has taken steps to phase out dental amalgam for human health safety as well as environmental health of all species and the planet (Napierska, 2018). In July 2018 a EU dental amalgam phase-out program for vulnerable populations was put into effect. This phase-out focuses upon pregnant and breastfeeding women, children, and, (not specifically upon dental professionals) it includes vulnerability into the 2017 Regulation on Mercury (Regulation (EU) 2017/852. This regulation dictates methods for amalgam waste, requires amalgam separators, and prohibits bulk forms of amalgam in dental offices (Napierska, 2018).

AMALGAM WASTE

Common to many medical procedures, waste results in potential exposures to materials used for treatment. Dental clinics have been shown to be a point source for mercury pollution as well as silver, tin, copper, and zinc found in amalgam fillings (Shraim, Alsuhaimi, & Al-Thakafy,2011). Organizations such as Practice Greenhealth and Healthcare Without Harm were developed to address safe disposal of medical waste. The American Dental Association's publication Best Management Practices for Amalgam Waste (ADA, 2007) provides guidance for the use of amalgam separators, amalgam capture devices, and recycling to protect the environment and to reduce exposures. Dental waste management is also addressed in the European Union's 2017 Regulation (Napierska, 2018).

CONCLUSION

Advocates for safer products for use in dental restorations continue to press for research, regulation and practice changes. Advocacy groups such as the International Academy of Oral Medicine and Toxicology continue to advocate for change in policy the use of composite materials to replace amalgams as well as restrictions on the use of fluoride in public water supplies. Other organizations advocate for a precautionary approach until safe levels of exposure can be determined and for phase-out of dental amalgam over time to protect health and the environment. Nursing research can add to this discussion to investigate the influence of dental amalgam on human health.

RESOURCES:

- Food and Drug Administration Adverse reactions to dental amalgam filling http://www.fda.gov/Safety/MedWatch/HowToReport/default.htm.

- Health Care Without Harm Moving towards a Phase-Out of Dental Amalgam in Europe: What Dental Practitioners Need to Know.

- International Academy of Oral Medicine and Toxicology https://iaomt.org/resources/dental-mercury-facts/understanding-risk-assessment-mercury-dental-amalgam/

REFERENCES

American Dental Association (ADA). (2007). *Best management practices for amalgam waste.* https://www.ada.org/~/media/ADA/Member%20Center/Files/topics_amalgamwaste_brochure.ashxx

Bastos J. L, Celeste R. K, Paradies Y. C. (2018). Racial inequalities in oral health. *Journal of Dental Research,* 97(8), 878-886. doi: 10.1177/0022034518768536.

Brownawell, A. M., Berent, S., Brent, R. L. Burckner, J. V., Doull, J., Gershwin, E. M., Hood, R. D., Matanoski, G. M., Rubin, R. Weiss, B. & Karol, M. H. (2012) Potential adverse health effects of dental amalgam. *Toxiological Reviews, 24,* 1-10 https://doi.org/10.2165/00139709-200524010-00001

Center for Disease Control and Prevention (CDC) (n.d.) *Understanding thimerosal, mercury, and vaccine safety.* https://www.cdc.gov/vaccines/hcp/patiented/conversations/downloads/vacsafe-thimerosal-color-office.pdf

Chisini, L. A., Noronha, T. G., Ramos, E. C., Baptisa dos Santos, R., Sampaio, K. H., Faria-e-Silva, A. L., & Correa, M. B. (2019). Does the skin color of patients influence the treatment decision-making of dentists? A randomized questionnaire-based study. *Clinical Oral Investigations 23,* 1023–1030. https://doi.org/10.1007/s00784-018-2526-7

Haley, B. E., & Mutter, J. (2013) Mercury and Alzheimer's Disease. In Kretsinger, R. H., Ulversky, V. N., Permyakov, E. A. (Eds). *Encyclopedia of Mettaloproteins,* Springer. doi.org/10.1007/978-1-4514-1533-6_317

Jamil, N., Baqar, M., Ilyas, S., Qadir, A., Arslan, M., Salman, M., Ahsan, N., & Zahid, H. (2016). Use of mercury in dental silver amalgam: An occupational and environmental assessment. BioMed *Research International, 2016,* 6126385. https://doi.org/10.1155/2016/6126385

Jonidi Jafari, A., Esrafili, A., Moradi, Y., & Mahmoudi, N. (2020). Mercury level in biological samples of dentists in Iran: a systematic review and meta-analysis. *Journal of Environmental Health Science & Engineering, 18*(2), 1655–1669. https://doi.org/10.1007/s40201-020-00558-w

Napierska, D. (2018). *Moving towards a phase-out of dental amalgam in Europe: What dental practitioners need to know.* Health Care Without Harm Europe. (HCWH Europe). https://noharm-uscanada.org/sites/default/files/documents-files/5740/2018-12_Moving_towards_a_phase-out_of_dental_amalgam_in_Europe_WEB.pdf

National Institutes of Health (2006). *Studies evaluate health effects of dental amalgam fillings in children.* https://www.nih.gov/news-events/news-releases/studies-evaluate-health-effects-dental-amalgam-fillings-children

Natural Resources Defense Council (NRDC). *Mercury in fish.* https://www.nrdc.org/sites/default/files/walletcard.pdf

Sabbah, W., Tsakos, G., Chandola, T., Sheiham, A., & Watt, R. G. (2007). Social gradients in oral and general health. *Journal of Dental Research, 86*(10), 992–996. https://doi.org/10.1177/154405910708601014

Shraim, A., Alsuhaimi, A. & Al-Thakafy, J.T. (2011) Dental clinics" A point pollution source, not only of mercury but also of other amalgam constituents. *Chemosphere, 84* (8), 1133-1139.

Tibau, A. V., & Grube, B.D., (2019) Mercury contamination from dental amalgam. *Journal of Health and Pollution, 9*(22): 190612. https://doi.org/10.5696/2156-9614-9.22.190612

Tucek, M., Bosova, M., Cejchanova, M, Schlenker, A, & Kapita, M. (2020). Exposure to mercury from dental amalgam: Actual contribution for risk assessment. *Central European Journal of Public Health, 28*(1), 40-43.

USBLS: United States Bureau of Labor Statistics. (2019) *Occupational employment statistics.* https://www.bls.gov/oes/current/oes_nat.htm#29-0000

Vujicic, M., Buchmueller, T., & Klein, R. (2016). Dental care presents the highest level of financial barriers, compared to other types of health care services. *Health Affairs, 35* (12), 2176-2182.

Warwick, D. Young, M., Palmer, P., & Ermel, R.W. (2019) Mercury vapor volatilization from particulate generated from dental amalgam removal with a high-speed dental drill-a significant source of exposure. *Journal of Occupational and Medical Toxicolicology,* 14, 22. https://www.ncbi.nlm.nih.gov/pmc/articles/PMC6637613/

Yip, H. K., Li, D. K., & Yau, D.C. (2003). Dental amalgam and human health. *International Dental Journal, 53*(6), 464-8. doi: 10.1002/j.1875-595x.2003.tb00888.x

Unit III:
Environmental Health Sciences

INTRODUCTION

Nursing history includes nurses who have identified environmental dimensions that could promote health or be a risk factor in illness and disease development. Florence Nightingale identified the role of hygiene and fresh air in improved patient outcomes. Lillian Wald addressed poor housing, close living situations, and social environments in the health of immigrants. Nurses have continued to use the evidence of environmental exposures to reduce health risks to patients, families, and communities.

In our first edition of this e-textbook in 2016, the Environmental Health Sciences section spanned 25 pages with eight subsections. The first edition included the current knowledge of environmental exposures that influence human health. Now, five years later with the second edition of Environmental Health in Nursing, environmental health science and knowledge continues to grow, and nurses have played an important role in generating environmental health science, interpreting the science, and educating the public and other nurses in the application of environmental health science to protect health and reduce exposure risks.

This revised Environmental Health Science section includes 17 new or revised sections written by nurse scientists and environmental health nursing experts. The sections of epidemiology, exposure routes, biomonitoring, toxicology, and epigenetics provide a foundation in understanding the science of environmental health. In this edition, we have added environmental health toxicants of electromagnetic fields, noise, and per- and polyfluoroalkyl substances (PFAS) to the revised content of air quality, water, endocrine disruptors, and lead. The information contained in this section provides the building blocks to identify environmental health vulnerabilities and to develop interventions to reduce the risks. We encourage you to use the materials in this section to expand your own knowledge and include your understanding of environmental health science in your nursing practice.

INTRODUCTION TO EPIDEMIOLOGY AND THE RELATIONSHIP TO ENVIRONMENTAL HEALTH

Azita Amiri, PhD, RN
Associate Professor
University of Alabama Huntsville
College of Nursing

Epidemiology is the study of disease distribution and its underlying factors in populations (Celentano & Szklo, 2019), which is an essential discipline for public health and environmental health. Today, epidemiology is used to establish distribution and prevention of disease, determine causal relationships, compare different intervention outcomes, and evaluate and propose primary and secondary prevention programs and public health policies.

Epidemiology and environmental heath are related. The basic principle of epidemiology is to clarify the relationship between environmental agents and human health. Epidemiology can help with validating models that are used in predicting hazards and their potential health outcomes. Human acute or chronic health problems arise from the interaction between humans as the host and an agent (e.g, virus) and/or the environment (e.g., lead in contaminated water). However, not everyone is vulnerable to a particular disease, vulnerability is determined by many factors such as genetic background, immunological characteristics, and nutritional status (Gordis, 2013). Some of the most studied environmental exposures are toxic air pollutants such as particulate matter (PM), pesticides such as organophosphates, personal care products such as phthalates and triclosan, plastics such as Bisphenol A (BPA), flame retardants such as Polybrominated Diphenyl Ethers (PBDEs), and water pollutants such as lead and Per- and polyfluoroalkyl substances (PFAS).

Nurses' knowledge for diagnosis, prognosis, and treatment of diseases and even patient education are based on epidemiologic data and heavily rely on population concepts. For instance, encouraging patients to quit smoking or to vaccinate their children are based on previous epidemiologic and population based studies. Furthermore, in everyday practice, nurses use the basic epidemiologic approach, to determine possible etiologies of poor clinical outcomes and to evaluate the existing preventive policies and protocols. For instance, a public health nurse uses the epidemiologic approach when conducting home visits to gather information about possible environmental risks that may lead to children's low IQ in the specific community. Another example is when nurses use the epidemiologic approach to prevent in-hospital elderly fall incidence and its related injuries by studying characteristics of the unit and patients to determine whether there are any relationships between characteristics of the unit or patients with fall incidence.

REFERENCES

Celentano, D., & Szklo, M. (2019). *Gordis epidemiology (6th ed.)*. Elsevier.

Gordis, L. (2013). The epidemiologic approach to disease and intervention. In *Epidemiology*. (5th ed.). Elsevier.

CONTAMINATION PATHWAYS

Azita Amiri, PhD, RN
Associate Professor
University of Alabama Huntsville
College of Nursing

A contamination pathway describes a mechanism that occurs when a substance contaminates a person from an environmental source (National Research Council Commission on Engineering Technical, 2000). The Agency for Toxic Substances and Disease Registry (ATSDR) identifies the following five elements of a contamination pathway (ATSDR, 2005):

11. **source of contaminant or release**, such as chemical container drums and landfills;

12. **environmental fate and transport** after being released, in other words how contaminants move or degrade through and across different media;

13. **exposure point or specific locations** where people encounter an existing contaminated medium;

14. **exposure route,** which means how people contact contaminants at the exposure point, such as inhalation, ingestion, or dermal contact;

15. **current or future exposed populations** and their characteristics, if any.

In environmental health, the concept of exposure "can be applied to the primary explanatory variable of interest and to other variables that may be associated with the outcome, such as confounders or effect modifiers..." (Velentgas, Dreyer, Nourjah, Smith, & Torchia, 2013, p. 45). The exposure event is characterized by the following factors: substance physicochemical properties and concentration, route of exposure, time/space scale of substance concentration, duration of exposure, time scale of potential health effects, exposure medium, and of course demographic characteristics of the exposed individual, such as age and gender (National Research Council Commission on Engineering Technical, 2000).

Developing a site conceptual model early in the environmental assessment is very helpful in evaluating a contamination pathway and putting together all of the above elements for a better understanding of what is going on in a community (ATSDR, 2005). In constructing a conceptual model, consider including links to an individual or a population group with a series of time-specific activities and with geographic locations. Figure I is an example of a site conceptual model in a community that is exposed to a coal ash landfill and a cheese plant. Also,

Figure I An example of a contamination pathway conceptual model

consider completing an exposure evaluation form (Figure 2), which applies to sites that have one or multiple contamination sources. Figure 3 is an example of a site with multiple contamination sources.

Nurses can communicate with public health specialists about environmental exposures in their state to familiarize themselves with the common environmental hazards. Also, nurses should work with patients' primary care providers, and the local epidemiologists and public health researchers to optimize patient care and community engagement. For the unknown and questionable exposures and symptoms, nurses are encouraged to search the literature and contact well-known researchers in the field. Also, the Alliance of Nurses for Healthy Environments is a great resource for connecting with nurse specialists in environmental health.

CONTAMINATION SOURCE(S)

A contamination source indicates the location of the contamination; in other words, a contamination pathway starts with a source of contamination. Contamination sources can be from a variety of sites, including drums (or containers), incinerators, landfills (e.g., coal ash landfill), buried waste, impoundments, spills, open burning areas, industry, power plants, lagoons, sewage spray fields, and transportation. It is also necessary to study the location of contamination sources, operating periods, remedial actions (e.g., landfill liners, scrubbers, wastewater treatment system, plans), characteristics, history, and types and amount of substances that are released to the media. Sometimes the details about contamination are not clear and conclusive, which makes it difficult for assessors to take appropriate action (ATSDR, 2005). Identifying contamination sources helps assessors to identify possible hazardous substances, types of media that might be contaminated by these substances, and how they may reach a population. For example, if the source of contamination is a coal ash landfill, reviewing levels of contamination in soil, soil gas, groundwater, and air are necessary to determine if people are being exposed.

For nurses to identify possible contamination sources, it is necessary to collect some background information about the proposed site, e.g. regulatory actions, site operation and history, physical hazards, and demographics. This information can be found using NEPAssits (https://nepassisttool.epa.gov/nepassist/entry.html) and EJscreen (https://ejscreen.epa.gov/mapper/) tools and by contacting the state's environmental department (Amiri & Zhao,

2019; Environmental Protection Agency, 2018; EPA, 2018). Reviewing the location of the site and its proximity to residential areas, schools, and places of worship is also necessary. This information can be obtained using Google maps or NEPAssits and EJScreen tools.

TRANSPORT AND FATE OF CONTAMINANTS

Transport and fate of contaminants indicate how contaminants travel or are transformed in the environment. Contaminants can accumulate in a local area or be transported by cross-media to a different location or another medium. Besides, contaminants can be biologically transformed to a new agent or chemically broken down and deteriorated. Therefore, for a meaningful description of a contaminant, nurses should look at the environment as a series of interacting compartments. Estimating transport and fate of contaminants helps nurses to understand better the contaminants of interest, exposure points, and a population that is exposed to contaminants.

Reviewing possible transport processes and physical, chemical, and biological factors that can affect travel and transformation of contaminants in media is important. Assessors may refer to local topographic characteristics to understand the relative steepness of slopes and elevation of site and rate of soil erosion. Studying soil type also will help identify groundwater recharge, contaminant release, and transport rate. Other factors include the rate of rainwater infiltration, evaporation, and soil erosion that influences the direction of contaminant transport. In addition, climatic and meteorological factors, such as temperature and precipitation, can affect contamination transport and fate; for instance, warmer temperature increases the volatilization of contaminants, and more rain escalates the chance of flooding and groundwater recharge rate. Furthermore, wind speed and direction influence contaminant transportation (ATSDR, 2005).

POINTS OF EXPOSURE

The point of exposure refers to the points or places in which someone can encounter environmental contaminants. Points of exposures should be identified for each medium. The most common points of exposures are ambient air, a residential yard, surface water, on-site, private well, drinking water, food, indoor air, public water supply, surface and subsurface soil, and sediment (ATSDR, 2005; The Texas Risk Reduction Program (TRRP), 2009). Information about the points of exposure can be obtained by reviewing site information and conducting a public health assessment. Patterns of land use may change over time; therefore, assessment of current, past, and future exposure points are important during the point exposure

evaluation. Moreover, it is necessary to collect and compare available environmental contamination records, exposure pathway information, substance-specific information, and health-related data in different periods. To make a proper assessment, the nurse must also do a site visit and interview residents and other stakeholders about their health and environmental concerns.

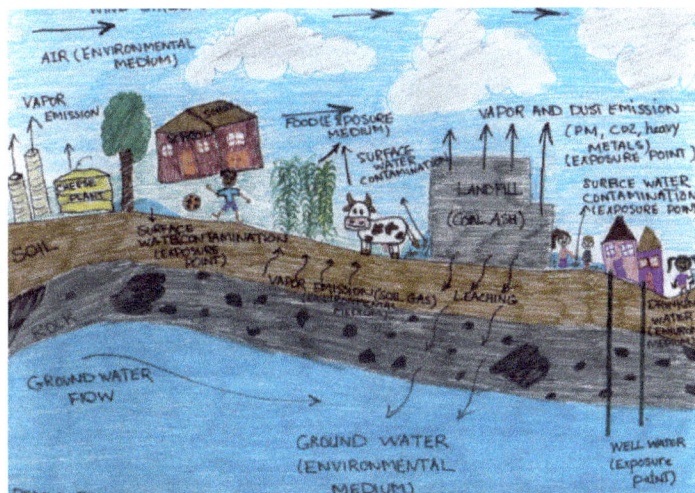

ENVIRONMENTAL MEDIUM

The media that can be affected by contamination sources are air, soil gas, food chain, groundwater, surface water, surface and subsurface soil, sediment, sludge, leachate, and waste materials. When investigating groundwater, as a medium for possible contamination, assessors should consider investigating the location and possibility of any groundwater or well water contamination, location and depth of potentially contaminated wells, and location of liners or slurry walls for landfills (ATSDR, 2005). In the case of potential drinking water contamination, reviewing the source of drinking water (e.g., utility) and existing reports are helpful. It is necessary to study boundaries and controls such as physical barriers and institutional controls, which are in place by the government, regulatory committee, or industry to prevent contamination of the media; however, be aware that sometimes the boundaries are not effective and can contaminate the media.

The next step is to confirm the possible contaminations by determining the concentration of the contaminants in the media and comparing them with the baseline data and data from other non-contaminated sites, if available. Information on air permits and reports of the amount of substances that are released to the environment are helpful and can be obtained from the NEPAssist (Amiri & Zhao, 2019; Environmental Protection Agency, 2018). If the adequacy and quality of available data are not acceptable, then samples of media should be taken and sent to a

Figure 2. Contamination pathway evaluation form (a modified version from ATSDR, 2005)

Contamination Source 1				
Source	Environmental medium	Exposure point	Exposure route	Potentially exposed population
Drums	air	Ambient air	inhalation	Family members in source proximity
Incinerator	soil	Residential yard	Digestion	Nearby residents
Landfill	drinking water	Surface water	Dermal	City residents
Industry	ground water	On site		State residents
Power plant	Biota	Well water		School children
Lagoon	Physical hazards	Public drinking water		workers
Sewage spray field	Radiological parameters	Indoor air		Minority and low socioeconomic
Transportation		Public water supply		Live stock
Impoundments		Surface and subsurface soil		Birds and fish
Other (Add)		Sediment		

Contamination Source 2				
Source	Environmental medium	Exposure point	Exposure route	Potentially exposed population
Drums	air	Ambient air	inhalation	Family members in source proximity
Incinerator	soil	Residential yard	Digestion	Nearby residents
Landfill	drinking water	Surface water	Dermal	City residents
Industry	ground water	On site		State residents
Power plant	Biota	Well water		School children
Lagoon	Physical hazards	Public drinking water		workers
Sewage spray field	Radiological parameters	Indoor air		Minority and low socioeconomic
Transportation		Public water supply		Live stock
Impoundments		Surface and subsurface soil		Birds and fish
Other (Add)		Sediment		

Contamination Source 3				
Source	Environmental medium	Exposure point	Exposure route	Potentially exposed population
Drums	air	Ambient air	inhalation	Family members in source proximity
Incinerator	soil	Residential yard	Digestion	Nearby residents
Landfill	drinking water	Surface water	Dermal	City residents
Industry	ground water	On site		State residents
Power plant	Biota	Well water		School children
Lagoon	Physical hazards	Public drinking water		workers
Sewage spray field	Radiological parameters	Indoor air		Minority and low socioeconomic
Transportation		Public water supply		Live stock
Impoundments		Surface and subsurface soil		Birds and fish
Other (Add)		Sediment		

Figure 3. Contamination pathway evaluation form: Example of a community with a coal ash landfill, spray field, and cheese plant

Contamination Source 1

Source	Environmental medium	Exposure point	Exposure route	Potentially exposed population
Drums	air	Ambient air	inhalation	Family members in source proximity
Incinerator	soil	Residential yard	Digestion	Nearby residents
Landfill, Coal Ash	drinking water	Surface water	Dermal	City residents
Industry	ground water	On site		State residents
Power plant	Biota	Well water		School children
Lagoon	Physical hazards	Public drinking water		workers
Sewage spray field	Radiological parameters	Indoor air		Minority and low socioeconomic
Transportation		Public water supply		Live stock
		Surface and subsurface soil		Birds and fish
Other (Add)		Sediment		

Contamination Source 2

Source	Environmental medium	Exposure point	Exposure route	Potentially exposed population
Drums	air	Ambient air	inhalation	Family members in source proximity
Incinerator	soil	Residential yard	Digestion	Nearby residents
Landfill	drinking water	Surface water	Dermal	City residents
Industry	ground water	On site		State residents
Power plant	Biota	Well water		School children
Lagoon	Physical hazards	Public drinking water		workers
Sewage spray field	Radiological parameters	Indoor air		Minority and low socioeconomic
Transportation		Public water supply		Live stock
		Surface and subsurface soil		Birds and fish
Other (Add)		Sediment		

Contamination Source 3

Source	Environmental medium	Exposure point	Exposure route	Potentially exposed population
Drums	air	Ambient air	inhalation	Family members in source proximity
Incinerator	soil	Residential yard	Digestion	Nearby residents
Landfill	drinking water	Surface water	Dermal	City residents
Industry	ground water	On site		State residents
Power plant	Biota	Well water		School children
Lagoon	Physical hazards	Public drinking water		workers
Sewage spray field	Radiological parameters	Indoor air		Minority and low socioeconomic
Transportation		Public water supply		Live stock
Impoundments		Surface and subsurface soil		Birds and fish
CHEESE PLANT(Add)		Sediment		

laboratory for analysis. In some instances, e.g., when it is expected for contaminants to migrate, serial media sampling over time in different locations or depths is required. The goal of exposure assessment is to combine data on the current and past exposures to any contaminants with activities and lifestyle of the individuals. Therefore, environmental contamination data on different media and different times is necessary to identify potential exposure points. Keep in mind that in the case of multiple contaminants, assessment of all contaminants at any given time is impossible; therefore, assessments should be prioritized (ATSDR, 2005).

When media sampling from the source and exposure point is necessary, assessors should consider taking samples from upstream and downstream of the proposed site, and impoundments and drainage ditches in case of surface water and sediment sampling. When soil is the potential contaminated medium, sampling from surface soil (0-12 inches) and subsurface soil (below the surface soil, depending on the depth of surface soil) is required (ATSDR, 2005). The concentration of potential contaminants in the air should be studied on-site (e.g., stack emission, soil gas, buries liners) and off-site (e.g., indoor and outdoor air in residential areas or schools). In addition, home visits might be necessary for learning about potential indoor contaminants (e.g., lead paint, lead in dust, and drinking water). Furthermore, the potential contaminated foods and livestock can be tested for the existence of substances. Finally, physical hazards and radiologic parameters can be identified by inspection of the site for any missing fences, gates, and warning signs close to the sources of hazard, e.g., electric boxes, industrial equipment, polluted impoundment or drainage ditches. Radiologic parameters can be measured using appropriate testing kits (e.g., radon) (ATSDR, 2005). Different techniques are used for the collection of samples from different media, for example, groundwater (EPA: Region 4, 2017); however, discussing techniques is not in the scope of this chapter. Assessors can consult with their region's EPA office or the state's environmental department to learn about the specific techniques.

EXPOSURE ROUTES

The exposure route refers to the way a substance enters the body via environmental media. Environmental pollutants may contaminate humans through multiple routes. The common exposure routes are inhalation of polluted indoor air and outdoor air (e.g., particulate matter, volatile organic compounds, and radon gas), ingestion (e.g., water, food, soil contents, medication), dermal contact (e.g., water, soil, food, other media such as personal products or contaminated waste), and internal/

external exposure to radiation. The external radiation exposure can come from various resources such as sun, x-ray, radiation generators, buildings, or the ground. The internal radiation may happen when the radiation is emitted within the body due to inhalation or ingestion of radioactive materials (e.g., radon, radiopharmaceuticals), radioactive iodine (e.g., in the Chernobyl nuclear accident) and contaminated foods and drinks (ATSDR, 2005; Ministry of the Environment Government of Japan, 2013). The injection is another exposure route, but it is not the case in an environmental exposure event.

Another classification of exposure routes is direct or indirect exposure. A direct exposure route is when someone is exposed to a substance that directly comes from the source, for instance, inhalation of ambient air with a high level of ultrafine particulate matter in coal power plant proximity. However, the indirect route is when a person is exposed to a contaminant from a secondary source, for example when a chemical agent is transferred from air to soil and then deposited onto vegetation and transferred to food (Bachmann, 2006; National Research Council Commission on Engineering Technical, 2000). In the event of acute exposure to a contaminant, inhalation, and to a lesser extent, dermal is the most common exposure route. However, when assessing chronic exposures to a contaminant, persistent and indirect routes must also be taken into account (Bachmann, 2006; National Research Council Commission on Engineering Technical, 2000).

POTENTIAL EXPOSED POPULATIONS

When assessing human exposure, it is useful to focus on contact media, which includes the air surrounding a community; the water and food ingested; the layer of soil, water, surface water or other substances that contact skin surface (National Research Council Commission on Engineering Technical, 2000). Identifying the characteristics and size of the potentially contaminated population is necessary. The demographic information can be obtained using the EJSCREEN tool (EPA, 2018). The conceptual model (Figure 1) helps determine the potential exposed populations. To develop an exposure model, an individual or a population group is linked with a series of time-specific activities and with the geographic locations and macro and microenvironments associated with those activities (National Research Council Commission on Engineering Technical, 2000). For instance, when characterizing exposed populations, the assessors should find answers to the following questions (ATSDR, 2005).:

1. Who is exposed? Residential population, worker populations, vulnerable populations (children, elderly, disabled)

2. What is the estimated number of potentially exposed people?

3. What activities are occurring and where? Local fish consumption, locally grown food consumption, groundwater use, well water use, surface water contamination

4. What is the history of exposure (past, current, and future)?

5. How long has the exposure occurred?

16. What are the exposure points? Is there any site accessibility?

17. What is the climate condition?

18. Is there any institutional control?

CONCLUSION

Evaluating source, environmental medium, exposure point, exposure route, and potentially exposed populations are five main elements of contamination pathway. The exposure process can be short term (over hours or days) or long term (over months or years). Reviewing available information on emission factors, transport and transformation processes, exposure scenarios and pathways, and routes of intake or uptake are important components of a contamination pathway. The critical step is combining the collected information. When the quality or quantity of available data is not acceptable, collecting additional information by sampling the media and interviewing the potentially exposed populations is required.

REFERENCES

Amiri, A., & Zhao, S. (2019). Environmental justice screening tools: Implications for nursing. *Public Health Nursing, 36*(3), 411-421. doi:10.1111/phn.12593

ATSDR. (2005). *Public health assessment guideline manual (update)*. https://www.atsdr.cdc.gov/hac/phamanual/pdfs/phagm_final11-27-05.pdf

Bachmann, T. M. (2006). 2 - assessment of human health impacts and the approach followed. In T. M. Bachmann (Ed.), *Trace metals and other contaminants in the environment* (Vol. 8, pp. 5-31). Elsevier.

Ministry of the Environment Government of Japan. (2013). *Radiation exposure. BOOKLET to Provide Basic Information Regarding Health Effects of Radiation. 1st.* https://www.env.go.jp/en/chemi/rhm/basic-info/1st/02.html

National Research Council Commission on Engineering Technical. (2000). In T. E. McKone, B. M. Huey, E. Downing, & L. M. Duffy (Eds.), *Strategies to protect the health of deployed U.S. Forces: Detecting, characterizing, and documenting exposures.* National Academies Press.

The Texas Risk Reduction Program (TRRP). (2009). *Human health points of exposure.* https://www.tceq.texas.gov/assets/public/comm_exec/pubs/rg/rg-366-trrp-21.pdf

US Environmental Protection Agency (EPA). (2018). *Nepassist.* https://www.epa.gov/nepa/nepassist

US Environmental Protection Agency (EPA). (2018). *EJScreen: Environmental justice screening and mapping tool.* https://www.epa.gov/ejscreen

US Environmental Protection Agency (EPA): Region 4 (2017). *Groundwater sampling.* https://www.epa.gov/sites/production/files/2017-07/documents/groundwater_sampling301_af.r4.pdf

Velentgas, P., Dreyer, N. A., Nourjah, P., Smith, S. R., & Torchia, M. M. (2013). *Exposure definition and measurement. In Developing a protocol for observational comparative effectiveness research: A user's guide* (pp. 45). Agency for Healthcare Research and Quality.

INTRODUCTION TO TOXICOLOGY IN ENVIRONMENTAL HEALTH NURSING

Ruth McDermott-Levy, PhD, MPH, RN, FAAN
Professor
Co-Director, Mid-Atlantic Center for Children's Health and the Environment
Villanova University
M. Louise Fitzpatrick College of Nursing

Nurses must have a broad understanding of environmental health that relies on knowledge of social, biological, chemical, and physical sciences. A clear understanding of basic toxicology is the foundation for nurses to understand and communicate environmental risk and exposures. According to the National Institute of Environmental Health Sciences (NIEHS, n.d.) of the National Institutes of Health, "toxicology is a field of science that helps us understand the harmful effects that chemicals, substances, or situations, can have on people, animals, and the environment." This includes the source and route of exposure of the chemicals, substances, or situations.

PHARMACOLOGY AND TOXICOLOGY

Many nurses have not studied toxicology and the idea of addressing chemical or other environmental exposures can be overwhelming. However, nurses have the knowledge and skill of monitoring patients when they take medications. How a medication is taken (the route), the amount of medication (the dose), the length of time that a patient takes a medication (the treatment plan), how the medication is absorbed, distributed, metabolized, and excreted (pharmacokinetics) and the patient's response whether it be therapeutic or with side effects are all skills that support nurses to better understand environmental exposures and human health.

There is different terminology for toxicology when compared pharmacology. A chemical substance that can cause an adverse health problem that occurs naturally is called a toxin and one that is made synthetically is called a toxicant (American Academy of Pediatrics, 2019; Miller, 2016). For example, methane (natural gas) is a toxin and human made per- and polyfluoroalkyl substances (PFAS) are toxicants. Unlike the expectation of improving health with medications, in toxicology there is an assumption that substances have the potential to be harmful to humans (Miller, 2016). Therefore, it is important to understand that the investigation of toxicant exposure has a unique difference between toxicology and pharmacology. This makes the study of toxicology and the determination of toxic exposures more challenging than the study of pharmacology.

In the field of pharmacology, drugs have been tested in human populations and are given in prescribed dosages — We know how much medication and the route that the medication is being administered. When giving medications, for the most part, conditions are controlled; vital signs and therapeutic levels are monitored. Whereas, in the case of a toxicant often we have no control of the route of exposure and we may not have knowledge of the exact amount of exposure (how much was ingested or breathed in). Also, for ethical reasons, toxic chemicals or other toxicants have not been tested on human beings. Therefore, when we examine toxicological data, we frequently rely on animal studies and accidental human exposures where we are approximating the amount of exposure to make an informed decision regarding human health (Richards & Bourgeois, 2013). Consequently, many times we make the best decision we can with the available scientific evidence while recognizing that there may be limitations in the data. For example, in animal studies we are asked to make inferences to humans when the study was conducted on a different species and we may not know threshold level of toxic human exposure. Pharmacology and toxicology share some similar concepts; but toxicology is much more complex and frequently toxicologist must make inferences from the data to determine human toxicity of a particular chemical.

HUMAN RESPONSES TO TOXICANTS

Environmental exposures can occur at every level of human development and can have a single effect or cumulative effects across the lifespan. Health impacts can be mild such as nasal irritation, to more severe such as birth defects, cancer, or death. Exposures to toxicants can influence an entire population, a family, a specific body organ (such as the brain or reproductive organs), the body's cells, or influence genetic response (Richards & Bourgeois, 2013; Miller, 2016). For example, the lead chapter in this section describes the impact of physiological impact of lead within the human body.

Like medications, the toxicant's chemical properties determine how the human body absorbs, distributes, metabolizes, and excretes the chemical. The movement of a toxicant from the environment through the human body is called toxicokinetics (Miller, 2016). It is important to understand this so that one can determine the risk to human health of a specific toxicant. At the end of this chapter there are resources to learn about the toxicological effects of specific toxicants. There are also, specific chapters within this e-textbook regarding toxicants such as lead, PFAS, and radiation.

DOSE-RESPONSE

When medications are studied, they are examined to determine the appropriate dose to be administered without causing untoward and unacceptable effects for the person taking the medication. This is referred to as the dose-response. This is the amount of medication or exposure to an environmental toxicant in which there are effects on the human body (DNA, cells, organs). The threshold response is the point at which there is a response to the lowest dose of exposure. The human response can be immediate, occur over time, be cumulative, or have a latency period as seen with radiation or exposure to asbestos.

Humans and animals respond to various toxicants in different ways. Most of us think it is a linear response. With a small exposure of a toxicant there is a mild response, and as the exposure increases, there is a greater response leading to toxicity and possible death. In this case one would see a standard dose response curve (Figure 1). However, depending on the toxicant, the amount or concentration of exposure, the length of exposure, and the route of exposure the curve can look very different. Additionally, there are many factors that can influence a biological response such as genetics, previous exposures, concurrent exposures to other substances, and existing morbidities within a population (Aleksunes & Eaton, 2019). In this case the dose response may appear as an inverted U-shaped curve, where there is initially an increase in response, but as the dose increases there is a lower response (Figure 2). The dose response curve can have a variety of slopes and curves depending on multiple factors.

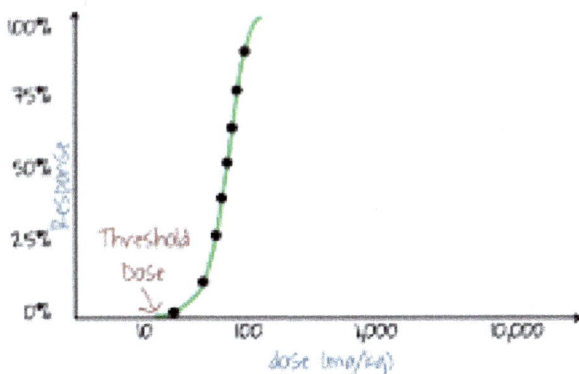

Figure 1: Standard Dose Response Curve: as the dose increases, the response increases. (National Institutes of Health, ToxTutor), reproduced as part of the public domain.

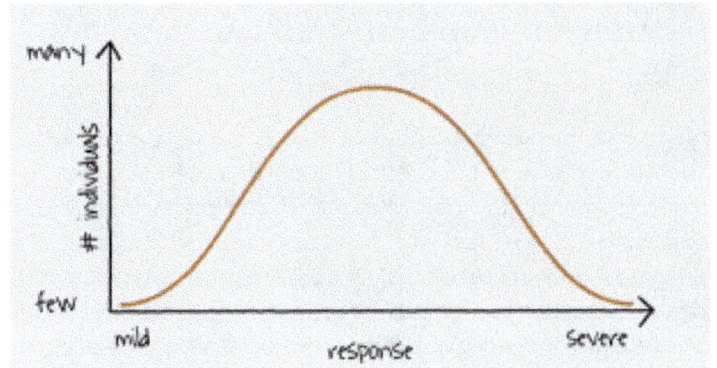

Figure 2: An Inverted U-shaped Curve: there is initially an increase in response, but as the dose increases there is a lower response. (National Institutes of Health, ToxTutor), reproduced as part of the public domain.

According to Richards and Bourgeois (2014) understanding the dose-response relationship can used to:

- Establish the threshold of the exposure.

- Quantitatively determine the relationship between exposure to a toxicant and the response.

- Provide basic evidence of a causal relationship.

- Compare relative toxicity to other toxicants tested under similar exposure conditions.

TOXICANT CLASSIFICATION

Like medications, toxicants or toxins are classified. There are three general classifications of toxins/toxicants: biological, chemical, and physical. Biological toxins are disease causing pathogens such as viruses, microorganisms, and parasites. This category also includes animals such as toxic shellfish, venomous snakes, and spiders. Toxic plants are also in the biological category (Richards & Bourgeois, 2013).

The chemical category includes solid, liquid, or gas toxicants. These poisons can be found in household items such as personal care products or cleaning agents. Other common examples of chemical toxicants are pesticides, painting products, gasoline, and carbon monoxide (Richards & Bourgeois, 2013).

Physical toxicants are found in the built environment, in nature, and from industry. Physical toxicants are toxicants such as radiation, lead, or asbestos. Radon, a colorless, odorless gas from the breakdown of uranium is a residential risk in some regions of the United States and globally. Radiation risks are also found in our electronics (see chapter Wireless Smog). Health care facilities where radiation is used for therapeutic and diagnostic procedures are another area where there is risk of radiation exposure and toxicity. Lead and asbestos can be found in homes, schools, and workplaces.

NURSE'S ROLE IN TOXICOLOGY

Much like monitoring a patient who is taking a medication, the nurse's environmental health role related to toxicology includes risk prevention and managing a toxic exposure. Regardless of practice setting, nurses are educated and prepared to address health promotion and disease prevention. An important part of promoting health is educating individuals, families, and populations related to potential environmental exposures in their homes, schools, places of employment and worship, and communities. Nurses must be aware of the toxicological risks within their practice setting and monitor for risk, educate those in the setting to reduce risk, and advocate for safe policies and practice. This may also include collaborating with facilities management and purchasing within an organization to ensure proper ventilation and that products are stored safely and marked appropriately. Safety Data Sheets must be available for all chemicals that are used within an organization. If standards are not being met, the nurse's role of advocacy for clients, fellow-employees, and self is important to reduce toxic exposures and health risks. Additionally, nurses must advocate for the least toxic materials and safe chemical policies. The policy section of this text has examples of nurses' advocacy for policies that protect our health.

If the nurse is caring for an individual, toxic risk reduction and management would follow the nursing process as described below:

- Observe the environment and determine risks and the routes of exposures. When possible, attempt to reduce risk.

- Assess the patient's physical status, health history including exposure history and risk.

- Plan methods to safely remove the patient from the toxicant (some exposures can present risk for the health provider and personal protective equipment may be required). Identify referrals and resources. Educate for prevention of future risk and management of exposure.

- Intervention: If a patient is demonstrating symptoms, refer to primary provider, contact poison control, or if symptoms are severe call 911 for transport to emergency services.

- Evaluate: continue to monitor patient status, effects of interventions, collaboration of health care team, and methods to reduce risk in the future.

Nurses have excellent observation and assessment skills, as well as the scientific knowledge to support patients, families, and communities in addressing environmental exposures. Collaborating with experts in toxicology to address exposures can assure the health of those in the care of the nurse. Please find more detailed information about specific toxicants throughout this e-textbook and from the electronic resources listed below.

ELECTRONIC TOXICOLOGY RESOURCES

- Chemical IDPlus has links to scientific information about specific toxicants. https://chem.nlm.nih.gov/chemidplus/chemidlite.jsp

- Consumer Product Safety this website contains information about automobile, lawn, cleaning, and other products that are used in homes and workplace. https://www.whatsinproducts.com/

- Haz-map provides information regarding hazardous chemicals and occupational diseases: https://haz-map.com/

- Pediatric Environmental Health Specialty Units. Provides education and consultation related to reproductive and children's exposures. Regional environmental health experts can answer your questions: https://www.pehsu.net/

- ToxTutor from the National Library of Medicine. Basic toxicology information for further understanding of the topic: https://toxtutor.nlm.nih.gov/01-002.html

REFERENCES

Aleksunes, L.M. & Eaton, D.L. (2019) Principles of Toxicology. In Casarett & Doull's Toxicology: The Basic Science of Poisons, 9th edition, Klaasen, E.D. (Ed) (2019).

American Academy of Pediatrics, Council on Environmental Health. (2019). *Pediatric Environmental Health, 4th ed.* American Academy of Pediatrics.

Miller, G. (2016). Toxicology. In Frumkin, H. (Ed.). *Environmental health from global to local*, (3rd ed., pp. 123-152).

National Institute of Environmental Health Sciences (n.d.). *Toxicology: Introduction. What is toxicology.* https://www.niehs.nih.gov/health/topics/science/toxicology/index.cfm

Richards, I.S. & Bourgeois, M. (2013). *Principles and practice of toxicology in public health* (2nd ed). Jones and Bartlett Publishers.

BIOMONITORING IN ENVIRONMENTAL HEALTH: IMPLICATIONS FOR NURSES

Katie McElroy, PhD, RN
Assistant Professor
University of Maryland
School of Nursing

Biomonitoring is the assessment of individual or population exposure to environmental contaminants, by measuring the concentration of chemicals or their metabolites in human specimens (Association of Public Health Laboratories [APHL], 2013, pg. 1). It is beneficial to measure the contaminants that have been absorbed into the body because those findings reflect the multiple sources and routes of contamination. Therefore biomonitoring, as compared to self-reported history or environmental measures (i.e. air quality), provides nurses with a more comprehensive assessment of overall, cumulative exposure to specific toxins.

Biomonitoring has many applications in the study and practice of environmental health, including (APHL, 2013; Council of State and Territorial Epidemiologists [CSTE], 2012):

- General surveillance of exposures

- Comparison of exposure levels in various populations

- Targeted investigations of specific exposures (see Success Story: New York)

- Rapid response activities during actual or potential threats

- Planning and evaluation of new policies

- Evaluation of policy change or elimination

Most importantly, results from biomonitoring offer a critical link between the presence of contaminants in the environment and observed adverse health effects in humans. Biomonitoring has the potential to become an integral aspect of environmental health nursing. For this reason, nurses with an interest in environmental health must have a basic understanding of biomonitoring concepts. This chapter provides background information on biomonitoring, including common methods, past and current efforts, and existing challenges related to biomonitoring in the United States. Implications for nurses in the areas of practice, education and research are discussed. Finally, success stories, resources and references for further reading are provided.

WHAT DOES BIOMONITORING HAVE TO DO WITH NURSING?

Practicing nurses often unknowingly participate in biomonitoring activities while delivering routine care. For example, pediatric nurses that conduct lead screenings on their young patients are directly measuring the level of a contaminant (lead) in a human specimen (blood). However, the topic of biomonitoring is rarely introduced in the undergraduate nursing curriculum, leaving many practicing nurses without the necessary background knowledge of basic definitions (Table 1) and methods.

Table 1: Biomonitoring definitions

Absorption	The process by which a toxin enters the body via the skin, gastrointestinal tract, lungs or eyes
Biomarker	The contaminant or its metabolite that is measured during biomonitoring
Body burden	Overall amount of a contaminant in all parts of the body
Distribution	The process by which a toxin moves within the body to various organs
Lipophilic	Describes a compound that dissolves in fat instead of water
Metabolite	Substance produced by the breakdown of a chemical in the body, can be more or less harmful than the parent chemical
Reference range	Lowest and highest values that will be used for comparison with another value, helpful for identifying levels that may be unexpected
Reference value	Single value used for comparison with another value, helpful for identifying levels that may be unexpected
Sensitivity	How low of a level of a contaminant can the biomonitoring test detect?
Specificity	Can the biomonitoring test detect a particular contaminant or just the class of chemical?

Currently, methods for most biomonitoring activities involve the collection of blood and/or urine specimens. However, some chemicals and metabolites quickly exit the circulatory system to be stored in various parts of the body prior to being excreted, making blood and urine testing inaccurate measures of the body burden of many contaminants. Therefore, researchers continue to explore other types of specimens to be used in biomonitoring, including saliva, expired breath, hair, fingernails, teeth, stool, and breast milk. Table 2 has a list of potential specimens with advantages and disadvantages of each. Although smaller studies have investigated the feasibility of using other types of specimens, to date, large biomonitoring programs still rely on blood and urine.

Table 2: Types of specimens used in biomonitoring

Specimen	Examples of contaminants detected	Advantages	Disadvantages
Adipose Tissue	Dioxin	Can be used for lipophilic contaminants	Invasive
Blood	POPs, lead, mercury (recent exposure only)	Good for contaminants with very long half-lives; in contact with entire body; familiar to people	Invasive
Bone Marrow	Benzene, Lead	Can represent long-term exposures	Invasive
Breast Milk	Persistent bioaccumulative substances (POPs, PCBs, dioxin, perflourinated compounds, bromated flame retardants)	Noninvasive; can be used for lipophilic contaminants	Limited population
Expired Air	Benzene, VOCs	Noninvasive; can link directly to exposure from air	Difficulty storing and transporting
Fingernails	Trace elements (cobalt, copper, nickel)	Noninvasive; can represent long-term exposure	Easily contaminated
Hair	Trace elements, mercury, organic pollutants	Noninvasive; can represent long-term exposure	Easily contaminated; volume of specimen needed can be difficult to collect
Saliva	Cotinine, organic solvents, some pesticides	Noninvasive	
Stool	Flame retardants	Noninvasive	Unpleasant for people to collect
Teeth	Lead, trace elements	Noninvasive	Difficult to obtain
Urine	Phthalates, arsenic, lead (only reflects recently absorbed lead); non-persistent pesticides, BPA, VOCs, some metals	Noninvasive; good for contaminants that are excreted quickly	Wide variety of excretion rates among individuals

Source: Centers for Disease Control & Prevention, 2016; World Health Organization, 2015.
Notes: POP= persistent organic pollutants; PCB= polychlorinated biphenyl; VOC= volatile organic compounds; BPA=bisphenol A

PAST AND CURRENT BIOMONITORING EFFORTS

Biomonitoring has been used for over 100 years as a tool for assessing toxic exposures. One of the first examples in the 1890s involved testing the blood and urine of factory workers for elevated levels of lead (Sexton, Needham &

Table 3: Websites and resources on biomonitoring for the practicing nurse

Pirkle, 2004). Figure I outlines the history of formal biomonitoring programs in various US agencies (Committee on Human Biomonitoring for Environmental Toxicants, 2006). Of particular interest, the Nurses' Health Study (NHS) collected toenail, blood and urine samples from tens of thousands of nurses between 1982 and 2012. These specimens have been used to examine exposure to heavy metals and chemicals. To date, the NHS and the National Health and Nutrition Examination Survey (NHANES) remain the only national surveys that include biomonitoring.

The Centers for Disease Prevention and Control's (CDC) National Center for Environmental Health houses the National Biomonitoring Program (NBP), which reports on NHANES biomonitoring data via the National Report on Human Exposure to Environmental Chemicals. In the National Report, the CDC publishes reference values for certain contaminants based on the NHANES data. These values can be used by researchers and providers to determine if the exposure level of an individual or a population is elevated and possibly requires action. The most recently published tables reflect population-level exposure to over 300 toxins. The NBP also works to disseminate best practices and methodology for laboratories, and to fund state-level biomonitoring programs (CDC, 2016).

BIOMONITORING IN NURSING PRACTICE

Practicing nurses already routinely participate in biomonitoring activities in acute care, primary care, and in the community setting, but many may be unaware of the implications that exist. For example, nurses may not know that public health labs often perform the analyses on specimens. Public health labs are government laboratories that function as a network at the local, state and federal level. Public health labs serve many purposes in the testing of environmental and human specimens for contaminants, including newborn screening, food safety and emergency response (APHL, n.d.).

A central public health lab is present in each state and territory, and some states have more than one lab. The necessary tests that are involved in biomonitoring can be too complicated, sophisticated or costly for commercial labs, but public health labs work closely with the federal government and the national network of labs to share knowledge, resources and methodology. Every nurse that participates in biomonitoring should know the location of their appropriate public health lab.

Nurses that conduct biomonitoring activities as part of practice have critical factors to consider, particularly around planning for the interpretation and communication of findings. Possible questions to contemplate include (CSTE, 2012):

- Will you be testing for a single contaminant or multiple?

- What are the requirements for obtaining, storing and transporting the specimen (consider cost, stability of specimen, timing factors)?

- Is there a reputable lab that can run the analysis?

- How invasive and time-consuming will it be to obtain the specimen?

- How much of the specimen is needed?

- Do reference values exist for the contaminant?

- How long will the analysis take?

- How will you communicate findings to the public?

- How will you follow-up with those who were tested?

Results from biomonitoring tests are often complex and nurses may be responsible for communicating the results to individuals or groups. Interpretation can be complicated by individual variability and a lack of reference values for certain populations. Additionally, most contaminant reference values do not correspond to the presence of disease or symptoms, they strictly serve to allow comparisons among people. Only a small number of contaminants have clinically relevant reference values (CSTE, 2012). Therefore, when communicating results, the nurse must consider the relevance of the information to the health of the individual or population. However, if evidence does exist that links specific levels of a contaminant with adverse health effects, nurses should include information on ways to decrease exposure to and absorption of the contaminant.

BIOMONITORING IN NURSING EDUCATION

Biomonitoring activities are becoming more prevalent, therefore education on biomonitoring principles and practice must be incorporated into nursing education. Introductory content can be introduced in a variety of classes at the undergraduate level, including pediatrics, obstetrics and acute care courses. As diseases linked to environmental exposures are discussed in those classes, a definition of biomonitoring can be presented accompanied by simple examples of current strategies (i.e.

lead testing in pediatrics). More extensive coverage can occur in formal environmental health education that is part of undergraduate or graduate nursing programs. Biomonitoring concepts can be explored within a toxicology course or module. Nursing students can examine emerging trends in biomonitoring, best practice related to methods, and existing or proposed policies. As students transition into the workplace, a basic understanding of biomonitoring will serve to inform nursing care, advance nursing practice, and could improve patient outcomes.

Practicing nurses can take advantage of online training and education. In the past, Coursera has offered a course developed by the Johns Hopkins University called Chemicals and Health that purports to examine both toxicology and biomonitoring. Additionally, the Environmental Protection Agency (EPA) has online tutorials on exposure assessment, one of which covers biomonitoring. Please note that this author has neither taken nor reviewed these online offerings. Additional

Success Story: New York

Routine surveillance revealed that immigrants from the Dominican Republic had much higher levels of mercury in their urine specimens than native-born New Yorkers. Public health officials conducted follow-up interviews and discovered that a popular imported personal care product used in the Dominican population contained very high levels of mercury. An educational campaign for store owners and consumers ensued, followed by an eventual embargo of the dangerous product.

Source: CSTE, 2012

websites and resources for practicing nurses can be found in Table 3. Armed with fundamental knowledge about biomonitoring, nurses will be equipped to more fully protect the health of individuals and populations.

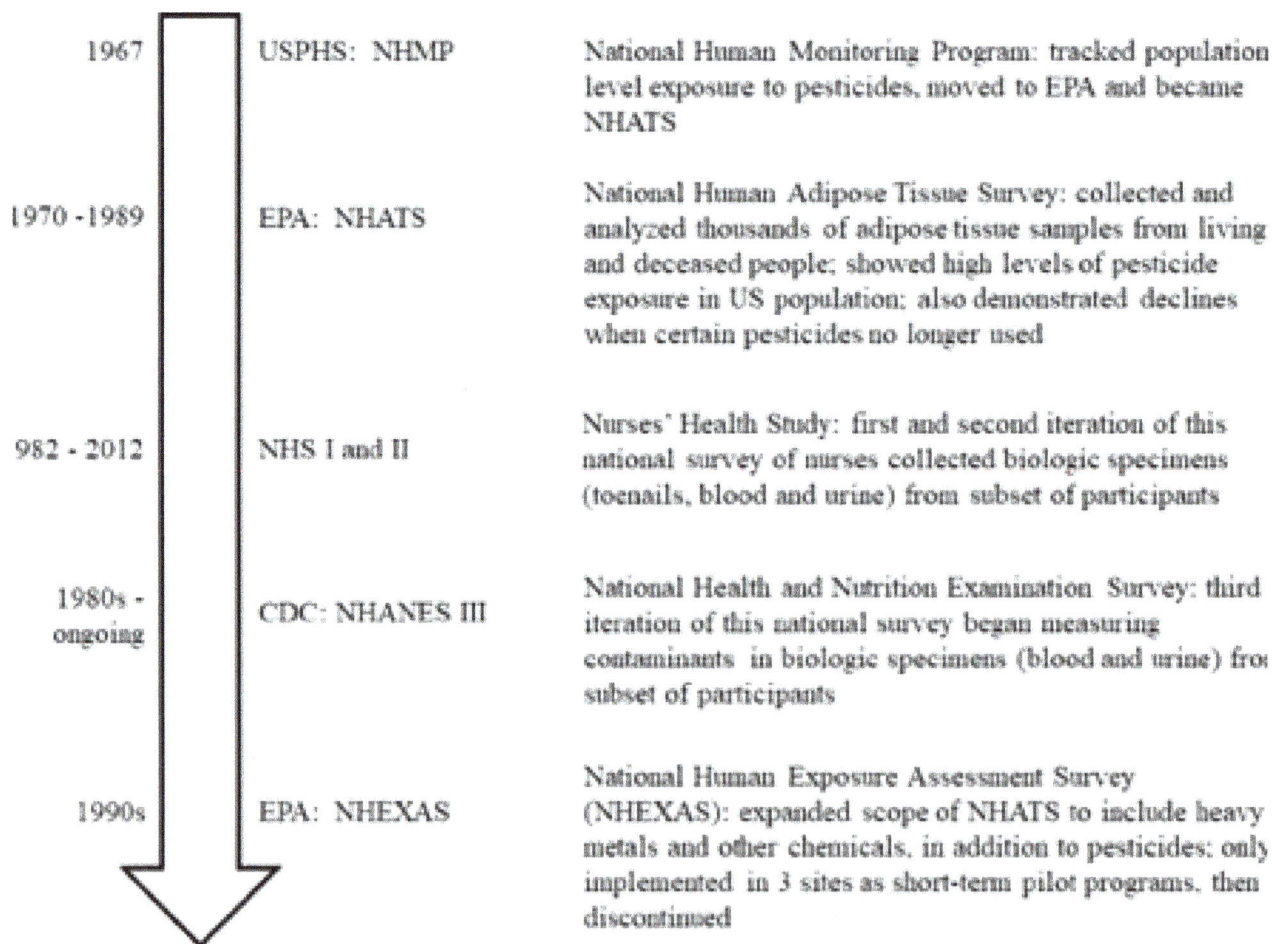

Date	Agency	Description
1967	USPHS: NHMP	National Human Monitoring Program: tracked population level exposure to pesticides, moved to EPA and became NHATS
1970-1989	EPA: NHATS	National Human Adipose Tissue Survey: collected and analyzed thousands of adipose tissue samples from living and deceased people; showed high levels of pesticide exposure in US population; also demonstrated declines when certain pesticides no longer used
982-2012	NHS I and II	Nurses' Health Study: first and second iteration of this national survey of nurses collected biologic specimens (toenails, blood and urine) from subset of participants
1980s-ongoing	CDC: NHANES III	National Health and Nutrition Examination Survey: third iteration of this national survey began measuring contaminants in biologic specimens (blood and urine) from subset of participants
1990s	EPA: NHEXAS	National Human Exposure Assessment Survey (NHEXAS): expanded scope of NHATS to include heavy metals and other chemicals, in addition to pesticides; only implemented in 3 sites as short-term pilot programs, then discontinued

Figure 1. Timeline of formal biomonitoring programs in US agencies. USPHS= United States Public Health Service; EPA= Environmental Protection Agency; CDC= Centers for Disease Prevention and Control.

BIOMONITORING IN NURSING RESEARCH

Nurses that conduct environmental health research should consider building biomonitoring activities into the research study design. The linkage of metadata with data from environmental samples and human specimens can be a powerful tool to investigate research questions. Connecting an exposure or a health issue to a particular source remains a major challenge in biomonitoring and environmental health research. Currently, our ability to detect low levels of contaminants far surpasses our ability to link the contaminant with a specific exposure or with a disease (Committee on Human Biomonitoring for Environmental Toxicants, 2006). This is an area of research that needs further exploration.

APHL	www.aphl.org/Pages/default.aspx	Provides information and resources on biomonitoring. Note: some areas of the website are for members only.
CDC	www.cdc.gov/biomonitoring/	National Biomonitoring Program
CDC	www.cdc.gov/exposurereport/	National Report on Human Exposure to Environmental Chemicals
CDC	www.cdc.gov/nchs/nhanes/index.htm	NHANES – reports, information and data
COPHES	www.eu-hbm.info/cophes/human-biomonitoring	Consortium to Perform Human Biomonitoring on a European Scale: take a look at what's happening internationally
EPA	www.epa.gov/ace	America's Children and the Environment
EPA	www.epa.gov/expobox	Toolbox for assessing exposures
EPA	https://ephtracking.cdc.gov/showHome	View data in maps, tables and charts, connect to state data
OSHA	www.osha.gov/	Provides information regarding worker protection and employer responsibilities for biomonitoring
PSR	www.psr.org/resources/hazardous-chemicals-in-health.html	Physicians for Social Responsibility's report on Hazardous Chemicals in Health Care

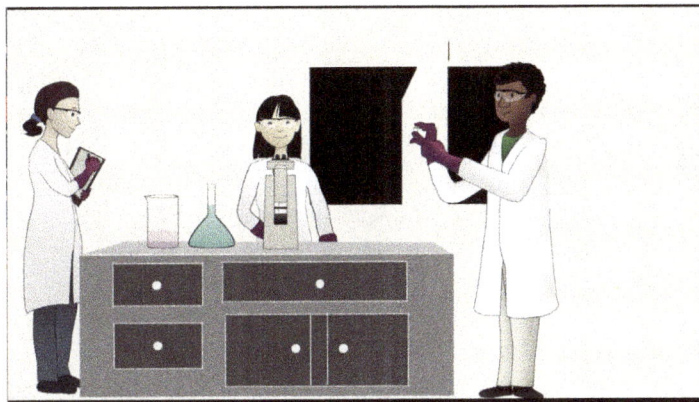

Ethical considerations are amplified when including biomonitoring activities in research. Participants must be fully informed of all procedures involved in the collection of specimens. They will also want reassurance that confidentiality will be maintained at all times, and that their specimens will not be used for purposes other than what has been described. Research nurses will need to make decisions about specimen banking if there will be any substance left over after the analyses are completed. Specimen banking typically involves additional costs and may require specific storage conditions, with no guarantee that specimens will remain useful over time. Finally,

---

Success Story: 4CSBC

The Four Corners States Biomonitoring Consortium (4CSBC), a collaboration between Arizona, Colorado, New Mexico and Utah, helped to address public concern after an accidental mining waste release. The spill impacted a major waterway that flows through all four states and led to increased levels of metals in the water, including lead, mercury, arsenic, and cadmium. As a result, the Consortium increased biomonitoring efforts in the immediate area and assisted in the development of educational materials to provide to affected communities.

Source: Chaudhuri et al., 2017

participants may want to know the results for their individual specimens. Researchers are ethically bound to maximize benefits and minimize harm to participants, but must also consider the reliability and validity of the test and the usefulness of the information to the participant. Although the incorporation of biomonitoring into research studies presents challenges, potential benefits from the findings are important.

Nurses that want to conduct population-level biomonitoring research without collecting their own specimens can leverage existing NHS and NHANES data to investigate novel research questions. Data and resources may also be available from other large biomonitoring programs or federally-funded studies that have been completed. For example, the Four Corners States Biomonitoring Consortium (see Success Story: 4CSBC) offers information on lessons learned related to many aspects of the biomonitoring studies conducted, including participant recruitment and reporting results. Finally, nurses can be encouraged that individual biomonitoring studies do help to inform action and policy on a national level, as evidenced by the removal of lead from gasoline and paint (see Success Story: Leaded Gasoline), and the removal of bisphenol A from many plastic products (APHL, 2015).

CHALLENGES IN BIOMONITORING

Despite decades of collecting NHANES biomonitoring data, limitations in our ability to effectively and efficiently use the data exist. Because of the survey design, NHANES biomonitoring data can only be used for national level estimates; there is no way to use the data to drill down to state or local level estimations (Latshaw et al., 2017). Therefore, a national environmental health surveillance system that provides granular biomonitoring data to states and localities remains unavailable in the United States. Additionally, linkages between large-scale exposure data and data on health outcomes are lacking. For instance, the EPA's report entitled America's Children and the Environment collates NHANES biomonitoring data with environmental and health data, but offers no linkage between indicators. As an example, the report details the percentage of children with asthma and the percentage of children with elevated lead levels, but not the combination of asthma and elevated lead levels.

A small number of states have attempted to address these limitations by using NBP funds to increase biomonitoring capacity. Some have even collaborated with neighboring states to leverage regional-level data. Additionally, the CDC developed the Environmental Public Health Tracking Network (EPHT) to connect population-level biomonitoring data with data from environmental sources

and human exposures. These collaborations and efforts aim to provide extensive biomonitoring data at state and local levels, but fall short of delivering a robust monitoring system capable of covering much of the country (Latshaw et al., 2017).

To tackle this problem, the APHL and the CDC recently launched the National Biomonitoring Network that integrates existing labs and biomonitoring programs into a cohesive, comprehensive network (Latshaw et al., 2017). Once the framework is built, additional partners and stakeholders can be added, with a goal of providing a formal system that can be used for routine surveillance and emergency response (Latshaw et al., 2017). In the meantime some organizations, including the CSTE and APHL, are providing resources and guidance for thoughtful, effective policy development at local and state levels.

NEXT STEPS

The direct measurement of contaminants in humans is a critical part of advancing the field of environmental health. However, biomonitoring is currently used primarily as a research tool as opposed to an integral component of public health practice. To date, the topic is not included in formal nursing education, and many nurses lack basic biomonitoring knowledge. Additionally, the US lags far behind other countries in developing a large-scale integrated repository for biomonitoring data. Despite these limitations and challenges, opportunities exist for environmental health nurses to be involved in planning, implementing and evaluating biomonitoring programs. Practicing nurses that already participate in biomonitoring activities are well-suited to contribute to policy development and evaluation, as well. Nurses are encouraged to critically appraise findings from biomonitoring studies and to conduct their own biomonitoring research. By incorporating biomonitoring practice, education and research into environmental

---

Success Story: Leaded Gasoline

Prior to the ban of leaded gasoline, mathematical and statistical modeling suggested that removing lead from gasoline would not significantly lower blood levels in people. However, measurements of the actual lead levels in human specimens obtained after unleaded gasoline was introduced demonstrated a much more dramatic decrease than the models predicted. In this case, biomonitoring was a critical tool that aided in the evaluation and validation of a policy change.

Source: CSTE, 2012

health nursing, we can begin to bridge the evidence gap between harmful levels of contaminants that we know exist in our environments and adverse health effects that we see daily in our patients.

REFERENCES

Association of Public Health Laboratories. (n.d.). *About public health laboratories.* https://www.aphl.org/aboutAPHL/pages/aboutphls.aspx.

Association of Public Health Laboratories (APHL). (2013). *Biomonitoring: An integral component of public health practice. Issues in Brief: Biomonitoring.* APHL.

Association of Public Health Laboratories. (2015). *APHL position statement: Biomonitoring.* APHL. https://www.aphl.org/policy/Position_Documents/EH_2015_Biomonitoring.pdf.

Centers for Disease Control and Prevention. (2017). *National Environmental Public Health Tracking Network.* https://ephtracking.cdc.gov/showHome.action.

Centers for Disease Control and Prevention. (2016). *National Biomonitoring Program.* https://www.cdc.gov/biomonitoring/about.html

Chaudhuri, S. Broekemeier, M., Butler, C., Coyle, A., Iuliano, K., James, K. & LeFevre, S. (2017). Four Corners States Biomonitoring Consortium: Lessons learned during implementation. *Journal of Public Health Management and Practice, 23*(5 supp), S93-6. DOI: 10.1097/PHH.0000000000000602

Committee on Human Biomonitoring for Environmental Toxicants. (2006). *Human biomonitoring for environmental chemicals.* National Academies Press.

Council of State and Territorial Epidemiologists (CSTE). (2012). *Biomonitoring in public health: Epidemiologic guidance for state, local and tribal public health agencies.* CSTE.

Latshaw, M., Degeberg, R., Patel, S., Rhodes, B., King, E., Chaudhuri, S. & Nassif, J. (2017). Advancing environmental health surveillance in the US through a national human biomonitoring network. *International Journal of Hygiene and Environmental Health, 220*, 98-102. doi.org/10.1016/j.ijheh.2016.09.010

Sexton, K., Needham, L.L. & Pirkle, J.L. (2004). Human biomonitoring of environmental chemicals. *American Scientist, 92*, 38-45.

World Health Organization. (2015). *Human biomonitoring: Facts and figures.* World Health Organization.

INTRODUCTION TO RISK ASSESSMENT IN ENVIRONMENTAL HEALTH

Poonam Sandhu, RN, BSN, BGS, MPH
Nurse Manager
Stanford Health Care
Palo Alto, CA

WHAT IS RISK?

The Environmental Protection Agency defines risk as "the chance of harmful effects to human health or to ecological systems resulting from exposure to an environmental stressor" (EPA, 2012a).

The EPA defines a stressor as "any physical, chemical, or biological entity that can induce an adverse response. Stressors may adversely affect specific natural resources or entire ecosystems, including plants and animals, as well as the environment with which they interact" (EPA, 2012a).

It is important to keep in mind that risk can be actual (based on empirical data) or perceived (based on cultural and/or personal beliefs). For a noteworthy view on the difference between the two read Perceived vs. Actual Risk (Schneier, 2006).

Remember, risk is also a matter of perception. For example, every time you work with paper, you are at risk of getting a paper cut. One could say that the risk of a paper cut has minimal perceived risks to human health and therefore people continue to work with this material without warning labels.

Changing perception is a matter of gathering relevant and accurate data and balancing this against beliefs and values.

If the negative outcomes of a paper cut were perceived as significant, one could demand that all reams of paper include a warning label informing the end user of the impending dangers. Sound a little extreme? That's because we don't perceive paper cuts as a major threat to human health. On the other hand, warning labels are found on cigarette packages, medication bottles, household cleaning agents, plastic bags and thousands of other products that are perceived and proven to negatively impact health.

WHY IS RISK ASSESSMENT IMPORTANT TO NURSES?

Nurses perform risk assessments on a daily basis. For example, an acute care nurse must assess a patient's risk of developing pressure ulcers in the hospital. Alternatively, a discharge coordinator will assess a client's risk of falls based on their home environment. In doing so, nurses seek to reduce and prevent harmful effects to human health, including disease, disability, and premature death. One way of achieving this is to limit human exposure to environmental stressors and promote healthy, sustainable environments. Nurses need to know how to identify environmental hazards and assess human risk related to these hazards. Thus, risk assessments can be done for individuals, families, communities or larger cohorts.

HOW DOES ONE ASSESS A RISK?

The first step in risk assessment is to define a problem. What is the problem, how big is it, how does it impact humans or the environment and which stakeholders are salient enough to help solve the problem? The methodology used in this section combines two excellent risk assessment frameworks:

1. Health Canada's Decision-Making Framework for Identifying, Assessing and Managing Health Risks (Health Canada, 2000)

2. EPA's Human Health Risk Assessment (EPA, 2012b).

Problem solvers beware! New risk managers make the mistake of skipping over risk assessment and jumping straight to a solution. Do not make this mistake. The assessment process is what tells you whether or not you even have a risk.

Step One: Identify and Characterize a Problem

For all things risk related, identifying a problem is the starting point. A problem could be a hunch, an observation, or the product of existing information. Below is a list of questions to ask in order to fully understand the problem.

Who is impacted by the problem?

Whenever possible provide a quantitative value.

- Individual/ group

- General population

- Life stages such as children, teenagers, pregnant/ breastfeeding people

- Population subgroups - highly susceptible (for example, due to asthma, genetics, etc.) and/or highly exposed (for example, based on geographic area, gender, racial or ethnic group, or economic status) (EPA, 2012b)

Example: "75% of South Asian men and women aged 45 and up, living in Surrey, have diabetes."

What type of problem/hazard is in question?

- Chemicals (single or multiple/cumulative risk)

- Radiation

- Physical (dust, heat)

- Microbiological or biological

- Nutritional (for example, diet, fitness, or metabolic state)

- Socio-Economic (for example, access to health care) (EPA, 2012b).

Example: "Children aged 0-10 are experiencing increased heat exhaustion due to the recent record breaking temperatures."

How is the problem reaching humans?

- Point sources (for example, smoke or water discharge from a factory; contamination from a Superfund site)

- Non-point sources (for example, automobile exhaust; agricultural runoff)

- Natural sources (EPA, 2012b).

Example: "There is an increase in reports of asthma attacks downwind of the power plant."

How does this problem enter the human body?

- Pathways (recognizing that one or more may be involved)

  - Air

  - Surface Water

  - Groundwater

  - Soil

  - Solid Waste

  - Food

  - Non-food consumer products, pharmaceuticals

- Routes (and related human activities that lead to exposure)

  - Ingestion (both food and water)

  - Contact with skin

  - Inhalation

  - Non-dietary ingestion (for example, "hand-to-mouth" behavior)

Example: "Residents of the Kingston neighborhood are complaining of a change in the taste of their water and an increase in unusual skin rashes."

Lastly, it is important to define whether the problem is acute or chronic; what the severity of the adverse effects are; what time frame the problem occurs in; and if the risk is only to humans or to other species as well (EPA, 2012c).

Health Canada (2000) suggests drawing from one or more of the following sources to characterize a risk:

- Toxicology studies (e.g. on laboratory animals, cultured cells, or tissues);

- Epidemiology studies (e.g. of occupationally exposed workers);

- Environmental monitoring (e.g. levels of chemical contaminants in air);

- Biological monitoring (e.g. lead levels in blood);

- Product surveillance (e.g. adverse reactions to specific therapeutic products);

- Disease surveillance (e.g. distribution of cases of a disease over time);

- Investigations of disease outbreaks;

- Targeted risk assessment programs;

- Targeted public health research;

- Information supplied by industry as required by legislation;

- Lack of compliance with legislative requirements;

- Consultation with experts (e.g. advisory committees);

- Literature review;

- Monitoring of the news media;

- Communications from interested and affected parties (e.g. health care professionals, consumers, industry);

- Focus groups

- Examination of public perceptions and concerns.

Step Two: Identify and Characterize the Salient Stakeholders

In this step, identify and characterize the key stakeholders. You will discover that certain stakeholders exhibit power, urgency and/or legitimacy or a combination thereof. Mitchel et al. (1997) categorized stakeholders using these

Figure I

Stakeholder Typology:
One, Two, or Three Attribute Present

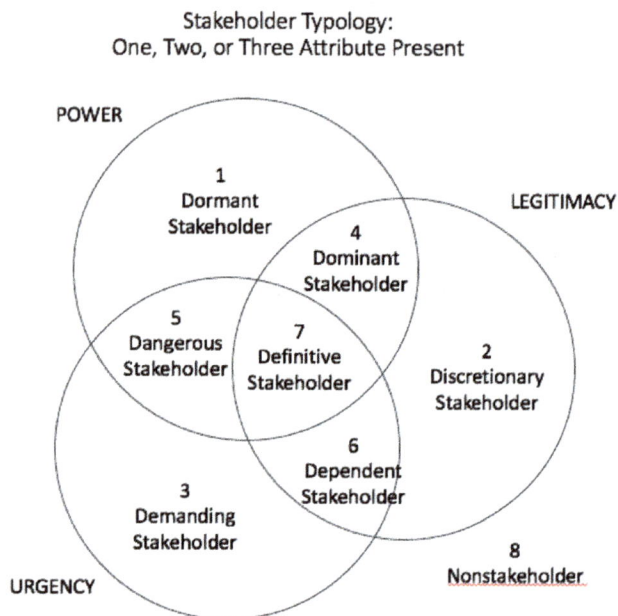

three main attributes as depicted in the Venn diagram below (Figure I). For more information on how to characterize stakeholders read Mitchel et al. (1997).

Step Three: Formulate a Problem Statement

If the nurse has done a good job collecting the data above, then this step will be easy. Take your "hunch" from step one and make it more specific.

For example, the problem, "Sudden Infant Death Syndrome occurs more often in babies than before" can be transformed to a thorough problem statement.

Problem Statement: (data is fictitious) "Sudden Infant Death Syndrome (SIDS) impacts 1 in 10 infants aged 0-5 months old in North America. This number is equitably distributed across socioeconomic status, ethnicity and geographic regions. Sleeping position is a strong precursor of SIDS; infants sleeping prone (face down) have a 30% increased risk of SIDS as compared to infants that sleep face up."

Resources about Risk Assessment

- EPA Risk Assessment

- Healthy People 2020. Environmental Health

- National Research Defense Council. (2012). Strengthening Toxic Chemical Risk Assessments to Protect Human Health

- World Health Organization. Children's Environmental Health: Environmental Risks

CONCLUSION

This section presented the steps of identifying a problem and gathering pertinent information to assess whether or not a problem poses a health risk. In addition to assessing actual risks it is important to identify the perceived risks through your most salient stakeholders. Selected resources about risk assessment are provided. Finally, this is an iterative process which allows one to truly assess, is this problem really putting the target population at risk?

REFERENCES

EPA. (2012a, July 31). *Risk assessment - Basic information.* http://epa.gov/riskassessment/basicinformation.htm#risk

EPA. (2012b, July 31). *Human health risk assessment.* http://epa.gov/riskassessment/health-risk.htm

EPA. (2012c, July 31). *Risk characterization.* http://www.epa.gov/risk_assessment/eco-risk-characterization.htm

Health Canada. (2000, August 1).*Health Canada Decision-Making Framework for Identifying, Assessing, and Managing Health Risks.* http://www.hc-sc.gc.ca/ahc-asc/pubs/hpfb-dgpsa/risk-risques_tc-tm-eng.php

Mitchell, R. K., Agle, B. R., & Wood, D. J. (1997). Toward a theory of stakeholder identification and salience: Defining the principle of who and what really counts. *Academy of Management Review, 22*(4), 853-886.

Schneier, B. (2006, November). *Perceived risk vs. actual risk.* https://www.schneier.com/blog/archives/2006/11/perceived_risk_2.html

EPIGENETICS

Emily E. Hopkins, PhD, RN, WHNP, FNP-BC
Associate Professor of Nursing
Chatham University
School of Health Sciences

Nicole Zangrilli Hoh, PhD, RN
Assistant Professor of Nursing
Chatham University
School of Health Sciences

The concept of epigenetics has been in existence since the 1940s. First recognized by developmental biologist Conrad Waddington, epigenetics provided a way to describe gene environment interactions (Van Speybroeck, 2002). When defined by its Greek origin, epi translates to on top of, outside of, or around and genetics becomes genesis or origin. Epigenetics itself is a simple term. However, when looking at the overall concept it becomes rather involved. To fully understand the process of epigenetics, some basic genetic concepts and knowledge are needed. This conceptual foundation provides recognition of the complexity associated with epigenetic change. Additionally, this information will assist in appreciation for the role of gene and environment interactions.

"The behavior of a person's genes doesn't just depend on the genes' DNA sequence - it's also affected by so-called epigenetic factors. Changes in these factors can play a critical role in disease" (Simmons, 2008, p.6)

GENETIC UNDERPINNINGS FOR EPIGENETICS

Epigenetics are biochemical alterations that do not affect the sequence of DNA but influence gene expression or the way in which proteins are formed. Although this definition is easily comprehended, it is of the utmost importance to note that these biochemical alterations are not always easily identified nor readily understood. To explain this further, there are some genetic underpinnings that must be reviewed to understand how epigenetics affects health and how it is related to the environment. This includes some basic genetic principles, the genetic code, and the genomic era of healthcare.

Basic Genetic Principles

Deoxyribonucleic acid (DNA) is the blueprint of the cell. "DNA" has become such a common term that it is used to sell televisions, facial cream, and chips. But what does it really mean to say that it is in our DNA? Humans start as a single cell organism when the haploid (23 chromosomes) sperm fertilizes a haploid egg (23 chromosomes) and creates a diploid zygote cell (46 chromosomes) with all of the genetic "blueprint" the human will ever need. Through the process of replications and cell division the single cell becomes a trillion-cell organism. Cells as they divide through embryonic development contain the same exact DNA sequence. However, cells will become specialized and as a result will perform different functions. This allows the human body to function and is why a cardiac cell can behave differently than a nerve cell.

The Genetic Code

The central dogma of genetics is that DNA provides instructions to make a functional product for the body. This is done by a two-step process. First, DNA synthesizes or transcribes a ribonucleic acid (RNA) copy of its sequence. Second, the RNA leaves the nucleus of the cell and carries this sequence or code of information into the cytoplasm where it is translated into amino acids that produce proteins (National Institute of Health [NIH], 2020a). As such, human bodies function based on enzymatic processes that stem from a DNA sequence converting to an RNA sequence which is then converted to proteins. This is known as gene expression and conveys how the cell gets from a DNA double helix of base sequences containing nucleic acids (adenines (A), thymines (T), cytosines (C), and guanines (G)) and then interprets this "genetic code" to making protein. So, while every cell contains the "genetic code" to behave like every other cell and has the information to make any protein, certain genes are turned on or off by design otherwise known as differentiation. This results in a gene expression that has been modified and therefore, only makes the necessary proteins for their cell specific function.

Genomic Era of Healthcare

The Human Genome Project (1990-2003) sought to identify the genetic code for human species. This task was accomplished through a collaboration of international researchers, permitting the world for the first time ever to see nature's blueprint (NIH, 2020b). Prior to this endeavor, healthcare focused on gene-disease models. This would be the classic Mendelian Genetics where patterns of inheritance are basic autosomal dominant (AD) and autosomal recessive (AR) disorders. These genetics forms of transmission are well known and understood with use of the traditional Punnett square that determines probability or likelihood of an offspring acquiring a disorder. For people with an AD disorder, only one copy of the variant gene is needed to have the disease process or phenotype. A prime example of an AD inheritance pattern is achondroplasia dwarfism. However, for individuals with AR disorders two copies of a variant gene are required to have the phenotype. For example, cystic fibrosis or sickle cell anemia are common disorders passed through AR inheritance. Both AD and AR inheritance patterns are clear and predictable. Their associated genes are easily identified because there is a variant in the DNA sequence that differs from people who do not display the phenotype—or atypical congenital/disease process. Simply presence of the gene (genotype), whether one copy or two is required, equals phenotypic expression (disease state).

However, healthcare has evolved, and the genetic knowledge provided through the Human Genome Project has demonstrated that many of the complex disorders common in healthcare today do not follow simple Mendelian genetic inheritance patterns. The role of the environment in combination with genetic vulnerabilities play a role in phenotypic expression of the disorder. A patient may have a genetic vulnerability, but if they were never exposed to environmental triggers that turned that gene on or off, they may never present with the disease phenotype. For example, a patient may have a genetic vulnerability to high cholesterol, but if they were never exposed to a diet that was high in cholesterol, they may never develop the disease process of hyperlipidemia. Or, an environmental exposure may trigger an epigenetic change, creating a disease process that was not originally in the individual's genetic blueprint. Subsequently, it is the environmental exposures that are thought to be the basis of epigenetic change. This is exemplified among identical twins who share the same DNA, yet exhibit different characteristics and have varying disease history making epigenetic changes resultant of dissimilar environments the most likely contributing factor.

EPIGENETICS AND THE ENVIRONMENT

Epigenetics provides a causal link between the environment and chemical changes to DNA that can result in disease. Environmental triggers that can be related to disease processes are numerous and heterogenous and can occur through a variety of mechanisms such as nutrition, chemical, and physical exposures (Jirtle &, Skinner, 2007). Although epigenetic changes can occur throughout the lifespan, the most susceptible period is from prenatal development when rapid cellular growth occurs to two years of age (Braid & Zelac, 2019). In fact, it is during prenatal development that research findings indicate certain threats such as lack of nutrition or exposure to chemicals can lead to the development of disease later in adulthood known as the "fetal basis of adult disease" (Perera & Herbstman, 2011). For example, poor maternal nutrition resulting in low birth weight infants and subsequent rapid postnatal infant

growth, can increase risk for adult obesity, hypertension, heart disease, and type 2 diabetes (Alfaradhi & Ozanne, 2011). Additionally, prenatal exposures to arsenic, tobacco smoke, polycyclic aromatic hydrocarbon air pollutants, phthalates, and bisphenol A have been indicated with a greater risk for cancers, asthma, obesity, type 2 diabetes, low birth weight, and problems with cognitive development or behavioral disorders (Perera & Herbstman, 2011).

There is also evidence to suggest that epigenetic changes may be involved with nonsyndromic birth defects. Many birth defects do not have a single genetic mutation as their cause; rather, it is an unknown interaction of genes, environment, and lifestyle. (Hobbs et al., 2014). For instance, cleft lip and palate are among the most common birth defects in the world. Although genes and inheritance patterns have been identified with its development, many other environmental factors such as smoking, diabetes, and use of anticonvulsants during pregnancy are known to contribute to its occurrence (Center for Disease Control [CDC], 2019).

Moreover, there are many other known postnatal environmental factors resulting in a disease state. Evidence suggests that certain viral exposures may trigger onset of type 1 diabetes (Filippie & von Herrath, 2008). Ionizing radiation has been a known causative agent of leukemia and lymphoma (Leuraud et al., 2015). Furthermore, an association has been identified with night shift work and subsequent development of breast cancer (Szkiela, 2020). These few examples are not exhaustive as there are countless other causal relationships between the environment and disease processes.

EPIGENETICS

Epigenetics is the changes that affect how genes work. Epigenetic changes do not change the DNA sequence or code. These changes are best thought of as a separate cover or the outermost layer from an individual's DNA structure. If this DNA were sequenced, results would indicate that the actual "genetic code" has not been altered. The additional epigenetic alteration on top of the DNA sequence is responsible for changes in actual expression of the "genetic code". Pathway modification, or a change in the process of transcription and translation, for gene expression may occur as the result of epigenetic enhancers or silencers, that turn on or turn off the ability for DNA to make RNA which in turn alters specific proteins for cell function. Therefore, gene expression is changed even though the gene sequence is unchanged. As previously mentioned, these changes are related to different environmental exposures. And although genes are reset during the process of conception or ovum fertilization, some of the epigenetic changes can still be passed onto offspring. Currently, the three main ways identified for epigenetics to make its mark on DNA are: 1) histone modification, 2) DNA methylation, and 3) noncoding RNA (Wei et al., 2017).

Histone Modification

Histones are an integral part of DNA structure. The double helix model which to many looks like a spiral staircase is the known structure of DNA. Given the length of the model or staircase, it needs additional packaging to fit within the cell nucleus. Histones are responsible for aiding with this task. Histones are essentially little proteins that allow the DNA to wind up tightly around them forming chromatin and condensing their size to one suited for housing in the nucleus of the cell. As such, they play a significant role in gene regulation by affecting accessibility of the gene for transcription and DNA repair from cell damage. However, histones can be modified through the process of acetylation, phosphorylation, or methylation (Fessele & Wright, 2018). This modification does not affect the sequence of the DNA but creates a chemical tag on the histone that can be detected by other cell proteins to determine if a particular region of the DNA should be recognized or overlooked within that cell (NIH, 2016a). By modifying the histones with acetyl groups (acetylation) or with phosphate groups (phosphorylation) the gene turns transcription on. This is also known as the process of synthesizing RNA to make a protein. Likewise, if you remove methyl groups from histones (demethylation) the gene turns transcription, or the process of synthesizing RNA to make a protein, off (Fessele & Wright, 2018).

DNA Methylation

Perhaps the most well-known mechanism of epigenetic changes is DNA methylation. The DNA methylation mark or alteration occurs when chemical tags, otherwise known as methyl groups, are attached to specific DNA nucleic acid bases. These DNA nucleic acid bases are the steps of the double helix model's spiral staircase. As DNA is transcribed into RNA and RNA translated into a protein the pattern of methylation can alter protein function resulting in different cell behaviors depending on the type of body tissue. Essentially, these methyl groups patterns can interact between other proteins and DNA and affect their communication process. This results in turning genes on or off altering their expression (Fessele & Wright, 2018).

DNA methylation can be a normal process for cells to ensure proper functioning with gene expression. For example, genomic imprinting is a normal biological pattern of DNA methylation based upon maternal and paternal inheritance. Remember offspring receive two copies of every gene. One copy comes from the mother and the other from the father. For some genes only the copy from the mother is turned on: for others, only the copy of their father is turned on. This pattern of imprinting is determined by methylation (NIH, 2016a).

Unfortunately, abnormal imprinting can occur. Prader-Willi and Angelman syndrome are two notable syndromes related to abnormal imprinting (NIH, 2016a). Prader-Willi syndrome is often noted in infancy due to poor muscle tone, feeding abilities, and growth. Individuals with Prader-Willi are likely to have developmental delays, cognitive disabilities, and behavioral problems. During childhood, they will exhibit excessive hunger resulting in obesity (NIH, 2016b). Angelman syndrome mainly affects the nervous system resulting in a small head size, seizures, developmental impairment, intellectual and speech disabilities, and difficulties with movement or balance. Those affected tend to display excessively happy emotions with frequent laughter, smiling, and hand-flapping motions (NIH, 2015). Although characteristics of these two syndromes are very different, both originate with abnormal imprinting or abnormal methylation on chromosome 15.

In addition to abnormalities with imprinting, humans can accumulate abnormal DNA methylation patterns that can disrupt gene expression associated with other disease processes. These processes include cancer, neurological disorders, autoimmune diseases, neuropsychiatric disorders, and genetic syndromes (Rodenhiser & Mann, 2006). Research indicates that cancer can be a direct cause of methylation turning tumor genes on or off. Neurological disorders may also arise from the aging process and this epigenetic mechanism contributing to development of Alzhiemer's disease. In addition, autoimmune diseases such as systemic lupus erythematosus (Patel & Richardson, 2010) and neuropsychiatric disorders such as schizophrenia, mood disorders, and autism have also been associated with DNA methylation. Lastly, some genetic syndromes, such as Rett syndrome which results in a small brain and developmental delays, have been identified as a result of a gene mutation that interacts with the epigenetic pathway through binding of an abnormal protein to methylated DNA (Rodenhiser & Mann, 2006).

Non-coding RNA

RNA plays a significant role in the transcription and translation of DNA to make proteins for cell function. However, modifications can occur to RNA prior to translation and subsequent production of a protein. One key modification is "splicing" where a portion of RNA is not coded for making a protein and therefore, is cut out of the sequence. The short non-coding RNA (20-25 nucleotide bases) that become spliced out, are called microRNA. MicroRNA can bind to other functioning RNA and DNA sequencing limiting or preventing gene expression. Long non-coding RNA (greater than 25 nucleotide bases) can recruit transcription factors and increase gene expression. They can also condense the chromatin of the chromosomes and decrease access to transcription. This results in decreased gene expression (Fessele & Wright, 2018).

Of the epigenetic mechanisms, non-coding RNA's role in disease processes is the least understood. Nevertheless, research has linked non-coding RNA to several ailments. Among these associated non-coding RNA conditions are prostate cancer, melanoma, colorectal cancer, and leukemia as well as neurodegenerative disorders such as Huntington's disease. Furthermore, there is evidence that Fragile X syndrome which is a known cause of autism may result from non-coding RNA's (Fessele & Wright, 2018).

EPIGENETICS AND CLINICAL APPLICATION

Epigenetic changes occur throughout the human lifespan. For example, research indicates that as individuals age the amount of DNA methylation decreases. Meaning that newborns will have a greater amount of DNA methylation than older adults. Evidence further suggests that epigenetic changes such as DNA methylation can both occur and resolve based on behaviors and environmental changes. Smoking cigarettes, for instance, can impact rates of DNA methylation which resolve with smoking cessation (CDC, 2020). In addition, different nutrients and vitamins. such as tea polyphenols (Hardy & Tollefsbol, 2011) and folic acid (Crider, et al., 2012), have been explored in relation to epigenetic changes associated with cancer prevention. It is important to note that these behavioral and dietary changes are just a few of the many being explored. As for epigenetic testing, clinical screening for illnesses is limited to DNA methylation analysis. This analysis can be performed for diagnosis of some cancers as well as Prader Willi and Angelman Syndromes. While we are gaining knowledge on epigenetics and the intersection with human diseases much of the treatment and testing are still in the research arena.

EPIGENETIC RESEARCH

To better understand the role of epigenetics in the human disease process the National Institute of Health formed the Roadmap Epigenomics Project. The purpose of this project was to provide a resource for epigenomic data which is data on epigenetic changes of all cells. This store of information was then made available to the public for research. Much like the human genome project, this project used sequencing technologies to map histone modifications, DNA methylation, and small non-coding RNA in stem cells and tissues. The resulting roadmap presents normal tissues and organ systems epigenomes for comparison of epigenomes in human disease processes. By February 2015, over 100 cell and tissue types had been mapped. These data have enabled valuable insights to the genetic information used for the development of different cell types (Roadmap Epigenomics Project, 2010).

CONCLUSION

Epigenetics is a remarkable genetic concept uniting the science between gene-environment interactions. The nature of epigenetic mechanisms covering DNA without altering its structure and sequence, is truly a unique albeit challenging design. With resources such as the Roadmap Epigenomics Project, research progress can be made to grow the current body of epigenetic knowledge. This research will assist in unveiling healthy behaviors and other environmental factors that promote or impede personal wellness. Truly, we are only beginning to understand the full epigenetic impact on disease processes and management.

REFERENCES

Alfaradhi M, & Ozanne, S. (2011). Developmental programming in response to maternal overnutrition. *Frontiers in Genetics, 2*, 27. https://doi.org/10.3389/fgene.2011.00027

Braid, S., & Zelac, D.E. (2019). Epigenetic mechanisms: An introduction for the NICU nurse. *Neonatal Network, 38*(5), 278-284, http://dx.doi.org/10.1891/0730-0832.38.5.278

Center for Disease Control and Prevention. (2019, December 5). *Facts about cleft lip and cleft palate.* https://www.cdc.gov/ncbddd/birthdefects/cleftlip.html

Center for Disease Control and Prevention. (2020, August 3). *Genomics & precision health.* https://www.cdc.gov/genomics/disease/epigenetics.htm#ref2

Crider, K. S., Yang, T. P., Berry, R. J., & Baily, L. B. (2012). Folate and DNA methylation: a review of molecular mechanisms and the evidence for folate's role. *Advanced Nutrition, 3*(1), 21-38. https://doi.org/10.3945/an.111.000992

Filippie, C. M., & von Herrath, M. G. (2008). Viral trigger for type 1 diabetes. *Diabetes, 57*(11), 2863-2871. https://doi.org/10.2337/db07-1023

Hobbs, C. A., Chowdhury, S., Cleves, M. A., Erickson, S., MacLeod, S. L., Shaw, G. M., Shete, S., Witte, J. S., & Tycko, B. (2014). Genetic epidemiology and nonsyndromic structural birth defects: from candidate genes to epigenetics. *Journal of the American Medical Association Pediatrics, 168*(4), 371–377. https://doi.org/10.1001/jamapediatrics.2013.4858

Jirtle, R. L., & Skinner, M. K. (2007). Environmental epigenomics and disease susceptibility. *Nature Reviews Genetics, 8*(4), 253-262, https://doi.org/10.1038/nrg2045

Leuraud, K., Richardson, D. B., Cardis, E., Daniels, R. D., Gillies, M., O'Hagan, J. A., Hamra, G. B., Haylock, R., Laurier, D., Moissonnier, M., Schubauer-Berigan, M. K., Thierry-Chef, I., & Kesminiene, A. (2015). Ionising radiation and risk of death from leukaemia and lymphomona in radiation-monitored workers (INWORKS): an international cohort study. *The Lancet Haematology, 2*(7), e271-e281, https://doi.org/10.1016/S2352-3026(15)00094-0

Fessele, K. S., & Wright, F. (2018). Primer in genetics and genomics, article 6: basics of epigenetic control. *Biological Research for Nursing, 20*(1), 103-110. https://doi.org/10.1177/1099800417742967

Hardy, T. M., & Tollefsbol, T. O. (2011). Epigenetic diet: impact on the epigenome and cancer. *Epigenomics, 3*(4), 503-518. https://doi.org/10.2217/epi.11.71

National Institute of Health Genetic and Rare Diseases Information Center. (2015, December 31). *Angelman syndrome.* https://rarediseases.info.nih.gov/diseases/5575/prader-willi-syndrome

National Institute of Health National Human Genome Research Institute. (2016a, April 1). *Epigenomics fact sheet.* https://www.genome.gov/about-genomics/fact-sheets/Epigenomics-Fact-Sheet

National Institute of Health Genetic and Rare Diseases Information Center. (2016b, July 7). *Prader-willi syndrome.* https://rarediseases.info.nih.gov/diseases/5575/prader-willi-syndrome

National Institute of Health National Human Genome Research Institute. (2020a, August 24). *Deoxyribonucleic acid (DNA) fact sheet.* https://www.genome.gov/about-genomics/fact-sheets/Deoxyribonucleic-Acid-Fact-Sheet

National Institute of Health National Human Genome Research Institute (2020b). *The human genome project.* https://www.genome.gov/human-genome-project

Patel, D. R., & Richardson, B. C. (2010). Epigenetic mechanisms in lupus. *Current Opinion in Rheumatology, 22,* 478-482, https://doi.org/10.1097/BOR.0b013e32833ae915

Perera, R., & Herbstman, J. (2011). Prenatal environmental exposures, epigenetics, and disease. *Reproductive Toxicology, 31*(3), 363-373, https://doi.org/10.1016/j.reprotox.2010.12.055

Roadmap Epigenomics Project. (2010). *NIH roadmap epigenomics mapping consortium.* http://www.roadmapepigenomics.org/

Rodenhiser, D., & Mann, M. (2006). Epigenetics and human disease: translating basic biology into clinical applications. Canadian *Medical Association Journal, 174*(3), 341-348, https://doi.org/10.1503/cmaj.050774

Simmons, D. (2008) Epigenetic influence and disease. *Nature Education, 1*(1), 6. https://www.nature.com/scitable/topicpage/epigenetic-influences-and-disease-895/

Szkiela, M., Kusidel, E., Mkowiec-Dabrowska, T., & Kaleta, D. (2020). Night shift work—a risk factor for breast cancer. *International Journal of Environmental Research and Public Health, 17*(2), 659, https://doi.org/10.3390/ijerph17020659

Van Speybroeck, L. (2002). From epigenesis to epigenetics: the case of CH Waddington. *Annals New York Academy of Sciences, 981*(1), 61–81, https://doi.org/10.1111/j.1749-6632.2002.tb04912.x

Wei, J. W., Huang, K., Yang, C., & Kang, C. S. (2017). Non-coding RNAs as regulators in epigenetics. *Oncology Reports, 37*(1), 3-9. https://doi.org/10.3892/or.2016.5236

AIR QUALITY AND AIR POLLUTION

Jessica Castner, PhD, RN-BC, FAEN, FAAN
President and Principal Investigator
Castner Incorporated

INTRODUCTION

Air pollution is the largest environmental risk to human health (World Health Organization, 2016). Globally, outdoor air pollution contributes to an estimated 4.2 million annual deaths and is among the top nine risk factors for lost years of health (Lim et al., 2012; World Health Organization, 2016). High levels of outdoor air pollution have been classified as a human carcinogen, with an estimated 15% of lung cancer deaths attributable to outdoor air pollution (International Agency for Research on Cancer, 2016). Other major health conditions impacted by outdoor air pollution include acute lower respiratory disease, obstructive lung diseases, ischemic heart disease and conductive disorders, and stroke (Lim et al., 2012; World Health Organization, 2016). These are all health conditions commonly seen by nurses in a wide variety of clinical practice settings. The major sources of outdoor air pollution are combustion from energy, industry, transportation, and household energy practices; agricultural practices; waste management, and dust (World Health Organization, 2020a).

Indoor household air pollution is also a major determinant of health, with substantial regional variations in specific exposures and burden of disease. For example, the health effects in regions with high levels of lead from old paint sources in the household dust, compared to global regions where solid fuels are routinely used for cooking, present vastly different exposure types, intensity, duration, and health effects. Household pollution from polluting cooking fuels is estimated to lead to 3.8 million annual deaths, which is a problem that tends to be seen more often in low and middle income countries, compared to in the United States (World Health Organization, 2020a). In the future, the average person's exposure to harmful indoor air pollution may worsen, without intervention, due to the ongoing effects of climate change (Institute of Medicine, 2011). In particular, climate change may lead to more air pollution that penetrates the indoor environment; increased mold, moisture, and flooding conditions; increased risks of thermal (heat and cold) extremes in both the indoor and outdoor environment; more hospitable conditions for rodent or insect disease vectors or infectious agents that intrude into the indoor environment; and increased likelihood the household resident uses mitigation strategies, like pesticides, that worsen hazardous exposures indoors (Institute of Medicine, 2011).

PEOPLE AT RISK FROM AIR POLLUTION EXPOSURE

Globally, only 1 in 10 people live in an area where the air is clean enough outdoors to meet the World Health Organization's air quality guidelines (World Health Organization, 2020a). In the United States, outdoor air quality has steadily improved for decades. Unfortunately, over 122 million Americans still live in counties that do not meet federal air quality standards (Office of Disease Prevention and Health Promotion, 2014). Black/African American and Latino communities are disproportionately exposed to higher levels of air pollution compared to predominantly Caucasian/White communities (Amiri & Zhao, 2019a, 2019b; Castner, 2020b). The Environmental Protection Agency calls those at high risk for health effects from poor outdoor air quality "sensitive groups." These sensitive groups include individuals with pre-existing heart disease, respiratory disease, diabetes, older adults, children, and people with low income (Environmental Protection Agency, 2017b). Those at highest risk for poor indoor air quality include those from low and middle income countries that cook with solid fuels, homes where cigarette smoking or vaping is allowed indoors, those in poverty or who reside in low income housing in the United States, those who live in homes built before 1978 from before lead paint was banned in the United States, and individuals who live in flood plains or regions with high levels of radon (Castner, Barnett, Moskos, Folz, & Polivka, 2020; Centers for Disease Control and Prevention, 2017; Hahn et al., 2019; World Health Organization, 2020a).

CRITERIA AIR POLLUTANTS

In the United States, the Environmental Protection Agency regulates 187 hazardous air pollutants outdoors. The most common and pervasive harmful outdoor air pollutants are called "criteria" air pollutants (Castner, Gittere, & Seo, 2015; Environmental Protection Agency, 2015). These six criteria air pollutants are particulate matter (PM), ozone (O_3), sulfur oxides, nitrogen oxides, carbon monoxide (CO), and lead (Pb). PM is further defined by size, with mean diameter of less than 10 µg (PM10), less than 2.5 µg (PM2.5), or ultrafine (UFP). The regulatory standards for these pollutants are called the National Ambient Air Quality Standards (NAAQS), based on the Clean Air Act of 1970, which was amended in 1990.

Regulatory science is the technical and scientific foundation for environmental protection policies and standards. There is a difference in the ethical considerations between research studies that test therapeutic interventions for clinical practice, compared to exposing human participants to harmful pollutants and toxicants in regulatory science. The clinical sciences that inform evidence-based nursing practice are based on a hierarchy of scientific designs from meta-analysis of randomized controlled trials as the highest level to expert consensus. In contrast, regulatory science is generally based on different research evidence evaluations that comprehensively integrate results from a range of epidemiology, exposure and atmospheric science, animal model toxicology, ecological, and controlled human exposure research study designs (Environmental Protection Agency, 2015).

Periodically, the Environmental Protection Agency conducts and extensive literature review and quality appraisal of the research evidence, called an Integrated Science Assessment (ISA) (Environmental Protection Agency, 2015). This culminates in a causality determination. The causality determination for each pollutant-health effect relationship relays the EPA's confidence in the strength, consistency, coherence, and biological plausibility of the research evidence. Table 1 lists the most recent causality determination by health effect for PM2.5, PM2.5-10, UFP, O3, SOx, and NO2 (Environmental Protection Agency, 2016a, 2017a, 2019, 2020b). CO and Pb have not been evaluated in an ISA since 2010 and 2013, respectively, and are not included in the table (Environmental Protection Agency, 2010, 2013). The evidence from the ISAs causality determination inform policy recommendations, and ultimately the EPA Administrator's decision to set and update the standards on what levels of pollution are considered harmful to public health and the environment. Where is the evidence the strongest? The strongest evidence supports that cardiovascular disease and mortality are caused by both short- and long-term exposure to PM2.5, and

respiratory effects are caused by short-term increases in O3, SOX, and NO2. Research evidence also indicates that Pb causes decreased cognitive function and behavioral disorders in children, reproductive, hematologic, coronary artery disease, and hypertension in adults (Environmental Protection Agency, 2013). While high levels of carbon monoxide are known to cause acute poisoning that can lead to death, the strength of evidence for health effects

Table 1: Strength of evidence that the criteria pollutant causes health problem

	$PM_{2.5}$	$PM_{2.5-10}$	UFP	Ozone	SO_X	NO_2
Date of ISA (MM/YY)	12/19	12/19	12/19	04/20	12/17	01/16
Short Term Effects						
Respiratory effects	L	S	S	C	C	C
Cardiovascular effects	C	S	S	S	I	S
Metabolic effects	S	I	I	L		
Total mortality	C	S	S	S	S	S
Nervous system effects	S	I	S	S		
Long Term Effects						
Respiratory effects	L	I	I	L	S	L
Cardiovascular effects	C	S	I	S	I	S
Metabolic effects	S	S	I	S		
Total mortality	C	S	S	S	I	S
Reproductive effects	S	I	I	S	I	S
Nervous system effects	L	S	S	S		
Cancer	L	S	S	I	I	S

C=Causal relationship
L=Likely to be a causal relationship
S=Suggestive of, but not sufficient to infer, a causal relationship
I=Inadequate to infer a causal relationship

of outdoor pollution levels of CO is less conclusive. The strongest link between outdoor CO levels and health problems is a 'likely to be causal' relationship between short-term exposure and cardiovascular disease outcomes (Environmental Protection Agency, 2010).

How does the pollutant cause the health problem? For each relationship in Table 1, the Environmental Protection Agency's ISA summarizes the research evidence on the causal mechanisms, often called the pathophysiology in nursing or the potential biological pathway in regulatory science. The pathways begin with the specific pollutant exposure and initial effect. Generally, the initial effects include inflammation and oxidative stress of barrier tissue in direct contact with the pollutant (mucus membrane and epithelium of the skin, eyes, nose, throat, and lungs), acid-base changes in barrier tissue fluid, activation of sensory nerves, and direct mechanical irritation (Kousha & Castner, 2016). In some instances, the initial effect is a systemic penetration of soluble or ultrafine particle pollutants from the alveoli of the lungs into the bloodstream, surrounding lung tissue, or lymphatic system. Next, a series of intermediate effects are depicted, such as how the immediate effect is linked to altered homeostasis in the body, temporary increases in blood pressure, blood clot formation, or other evidence of endocrine, immune, and nervous system responses. The clinical and population effects as endpoints of the pathways are depicted last, generally measured as emergency department visits, hospital admissions, mortality, or long-term disease morbidity diagnosis.

While the Environmental Protection Agency's ISAs provide comprehensive and substantial synthesis of the state of the scientific evidence on criteria air pollutants, they are far from complete to inform the full practice of nursing. For example, pollution from agricultural sources, rural areas, and large-scale fire disasters (often called wildfires regardless of the human or geologic cause) are not adequately represented in the measurement, scientific evaluation, and regulation of air pollutants. In real life, human beings are exposed to a mixture of harmful pollutants, and rarely to a single pollutant alone. Further, symptom and syndromic health effects that may have a substantial impact on an individual patient's quality of life are not conceptually well defined in the review process and final documents. Symptom science and emerging evidence on pollutant exposure impacts on headache, general irritation of the eyes, nose, and throat, chemical or environmental sensitivity, fatigue, depression, abdominal pain, skin and mucus membrane irritation, renal insufficiency, and interaction with allergy and infection require further attention in the regulatory sciences (Castner, Amiri, & Huntington-Moskos, 2020; Castner et

al., 2019; Kousha & Castner, 2016; Szyszkowicz, Kousha, & Castner, 2016). Thus, the need for the ongoing leadership, influence, and work of clinical nurses, nurse policymakers and administrators, and nurse scientists in the environmental and regulatory sciences is evident.

INDOOR AIR QUALITY

The qualities of a healthy home, from the physical environment perspective, can be summarized in the following eight ways: 1) dry, 2) clean, 3) safe, 4) well-ventilated, 5) pest free, 6) contaminant free, 7) well-maintained, and 8) energy efficient (Brand, Caine, Rhodes, & Ravenscroft, 2016; Green & Healthy Homes Initiative, 2020). Three major health outcomes in the United States linked to poor indoor air quality include neurological and developmental delays from lead exposure, asthma development and exacerbation from multiple triggers, and lung cancer from radon (Butz et al., 2019; Reddy, Gomez, & Dixon, 2017).

The dust in homes built before 1978 in the United States can contain lead (Pb) from peeling or cracking paint on windows or walls that leach into the dust coating household items (Centers for Disease Control and Prevention, 2020). Children are susceptible to neurological developmental delays from lead poisoning when they breathe or swallow this dust. Lead exposure can also occur from pipes that carry water to the home, certain homeopathic remedies, or from high risk hobbies or occupations. Nurses often contribute to lead poisoning prevention through home assessment and education, routine screening and case finding, and treatment of acute lead poisoning (Spanier, McLaine, & Gilden, 2019). Nursing educational interventions include sharing information on routine cleaning practices to limit dust contamination, water testing, referral to home maintenance programs for resources for window replacements, and home maintenance education to safely eliminate areas of peeling or cracked paint.

Common home exposures that can cause and exacerbate asthma, and other allergic or chronic respiratory disorders include pets (more specifically, proteins from their dander, saliva, or other fluids), cockroaches, dust mites and other pests, mice or rats, mold, pollen, tobacco smoke exposure, and other chemical irritants (Castner, Barnett, et al., 2020; Institute of Medicine, 2011). The sources for these indoor pollutants can come from cooking (including gas and solid fuel burning), heating, smoking or vaping, any type of combustion (including scented candles), cleaning or pesticide sprays, and off-gassing from new furnishing or construction materials. There are several integrated pest management, home environment modification, and trigger reduction programs and interventions the clinical nurse can learn more about and provide to patients. These programs often focus on (Green & Healthy Homes Initiative, 2020; Reddy et al., 2017):

- Reducing and eliminating cigarette and vape smoke exposure

- Improved ventilation, including use of working bathroom and cooking fan

- Safe cleaning practices, including use of high-efficiency particulate air (HEPA) filter vacuums

- Integrated pest management

- Removing, washing, or covering reservoirs for dust mites and allergens

- Mold and moisture remediation

- Alternating to less polluting heating and cooking sources

- Caretaking practices for pets

EXAMPLE PATHOPHYSIOLOGY PATHWAY FOR SHORT-TERM PM2.5 EXPOSURE AND CARDIOVASCULAR EFFECTS

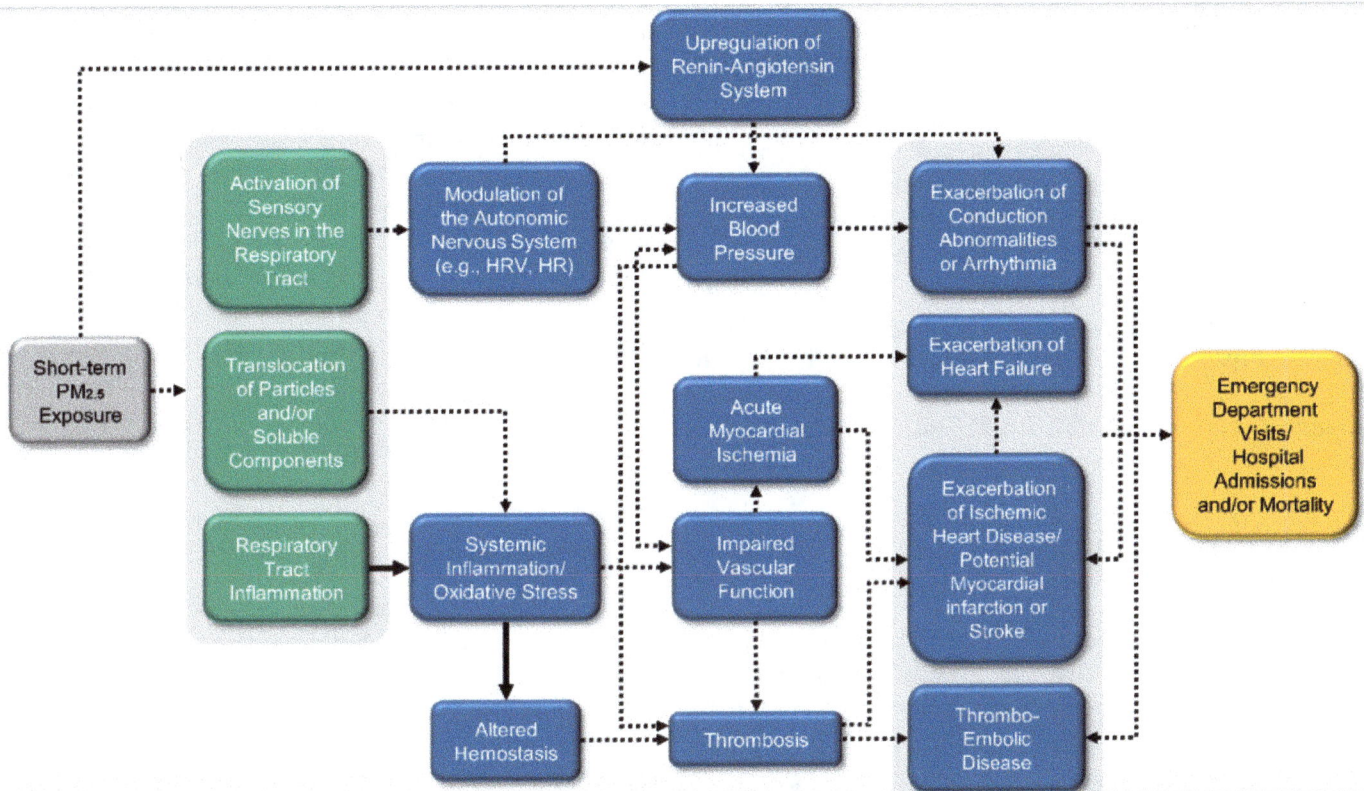

Reprint of Figure 6-1 (Environmental Protection Agency, 2019), reproduced as part of the public domain. Potential biological pathways for cardiovascular effects following short-term exposure to PM2.5.

"HR = heart rate; HRV = heart rate variability; PM2.5 = particulate matter with a nominal mean aerodynamic diameter less than or equal to 2.5 μm.

Note: The boxes above represent the effects for which there is experimental or epidemiologic evidence related to short-term PM2.5 exposure, and the arrows indicate a proposed relationship between those effects. Solid arrows denote evidence of essentiality as provided, for example, by an inhibitor of the pathway or a genetic knockout model used in an experimental study involving PM2.5 exposure. Shading around multiple boxes is used to denote a grouping of these effects. Arrows may connect individual boxes, groupings of boxes, and individual boxes within groupings of boxes. Progression of effects is generally depicted from left to right and color coded (gray = exposure; green = initial effect; blue = intermediate effect; orange = effect at the population level or a key clinical effect). Here, population-level effects generally reflect results of epidemiologic studies. When there are gaps in the evidence, there are complementary gaps in the figure."

Indoor, household radon is a leading risk factor for developing lung cancer (Hahn et al., 2019; Huntington-Moskos, Rayens, Wiggins, & Hahn, 2016). Radon generally enters household air from the soil or rocks that surround a house's foundations through cracks and gaps. Some regions of the United States have higher levels of radon compared to others, and a map can be found at the Environmental Protection Agency's Radon website (Environmental Protection Agency, 2020c). As inhaled radon decays, it creates a risk for cancer by irradiating surrounding lung tissue (Institute of Medicine, 2011). The human senses cannot detect radon because it is odorless, tasteless, and colorless. The only way to detect radon is through testing. Each state has a radon program to contact for information about obtaining a test kit, and many home improvement stores carry radon testing kit supplies (Environmental Protection Agency, 2020c). In homes where radon levels are high, solutions focus on new or improved ventilation systems.

There are several other important topics and exposures to consider in regards to patients' home indoor air quality, such as asbestos, carbon monoxide, formaldehyde, flood cleanup, volatile organic compounds, semi-volatile organic compounds, and endocrine disrupting chemicals, nurses can find more exposure specific information at the Environmental Protection Agency, World Health Organization, Centers for Disease Control and Prevention, National Institute of Environmental Health Sciences, and Agency for Toxic Substances and Disease Registry websites.

NURSES' ROLE IN REDUCING EXPOSURE TO HARMFUL AIR POLLUTANTS AND HAZARDS

The nurses' role in protecting and promoting health from harmful environmental exposures can occur on the individual, family, organizational, community, regional, state, national, and/or international level (Campbell & Anderko, 2020). Nurses equipped with knowledge about common indoor and outdoor air pollutants are in key positions to apply the nursing process to assess, diagnose, plan, intervene, and evaluate the provided care. In particular, nurses, including advanced practice nurses, are in key positions to educate patients and families on strategies to reduce exposures and risks. Clinical nurses can lead and inform ongoing organizational quality improvement projects or policy by sharing their clinical experiences about the human suffering and health consequences in caring for affected patients, families, and communities (Association, 2007; Castner et al., 2015; Castner & Polivka, 2018; Johnson & Schenk, 2019). At the organizational level, nurses are crucial to implementing assessments, interventions, and programs to improve air quality in

schools, clinical practice sites, and other organizational settings (Environmental Protection Agency, 2020a; Johnson & Schenk, 2019). Nurses in formal higher education, leadership or administration, research, and policymaking roles are tasked with advancing environmental health knowledge, policy, and curricula through the nursing and interdisciplinary lens (Castner, 2020b; Castner, Amiri, et al., 2020; Castner et al., 2019; Dodd-Butera, Beaman, & Brash, 2019; Leffers et al., 2015; McDermott-Levy, Jackman-Murphy, Leffers, & Jordan, 2019).

PATIENT EDUCATION AND SELF-MANAGEMENT

Nursing interventions to reduce the health effects of air pollution include patient education and self-management recommendations that individuals can take to reduce their personal exposures (Castner & Polivka, 2018). While the most effective and impactful interventions take place at the broader public health level aimed at changing public policy and regulation that reduces emissions, these individual interventions are a particularly relevant priority to prevention and chronic disease management among high risk groups (World Health Organization, 2020b). There are several resources for clinical nurses to obtain evidence-based professional development, patient education videos, handouts, and posters about air quality for use in their practice settings. In addition to full reports, the World Health Organization's website on Air Pollution includes links to short videos, fact sheets, and infographics about ambient and household air pollution as a resource for individual clinical nurses to learn more about the topic, as well as to drive quality improvement projects at their clinical site (World Health Organization, 2020a).

Here are several resources to locate evidence-based patient education material ready for use in clinical nursing practice, with internet links that can be accessed from the reference list. The American Thoracic Society's Information Series includes 2-page, ready to use, Patient Education handouts focused on patients with, or at risk for, respiratory disease (American Thoracic Society, 2020). Topics for these patient education handouts include outdoor air pollution (Rice, Balmes, & Malhotra, 2016), indoor air quality problems (Mainardi & Redlich, 2018), mold exposure after water damage (Graham Carlos et al., 2017), work exacerbated asthma (Harber, Redlich, & Henneberger, 2018), military burn pit exposure (Sotolongo et al., 2020), burning indoor fuels (Sood, Kapoor, Doo, & Blount, 2018), among many others. The National Institute of Environmental Health Sciences (NIEHS) also publishes brochures and fact sheets for the layperson audience that the clinical nurse might consider using as patient education handouts (National Institute of Environmental Health Sciences, 2020). These NIEHS brochures tend to be lengthier than the American Thoracic Society's patient education handouts, and include toxin specific content (e.g. arsenic, asbestos, bisphenol A), disease specific topics (e.g. asthma, autism, breast cancer), general topics (e.g. climate change, air pollutants), and information about ongoing NIEHS supported studies and initiatives. For summaries about specific hazardous pollutants and toxins, the Agency for Toxic Substances and Disease Registry hosts ToxFAQs™ which are written at an appropriate level to be included in patient and public education (Agency for Toxic Substances & Disease Registry, 2014). Last, the Environmental Protection Agency (EPA) provides open access links to posters on the health effects of common air pollutants; fact sheets about air pollution and diseases like stroke, heart disease, and asthma; and health behavior education about how to limit exposure to large scale fire disaster smoke and receiving notifications about air quality alerts (Environmental Protection Agency, 2016b, 2017b). Despite the widespread and open access availability of these patient education tools on air quality and health, little is known from an implementation science perspective about the overall reach, effectiveness, adoption, implementation, or sustainability of these patient education interventions into clinical nursing practice and individual patient care (Castner, 2020a).

Specific areas for the clinical nurse to consider focusing on when providing patient education and self-management coaching include: 1) "Know your Numbers," 2) avoiding exposure by place and time, 3) air filters, and 4) respirator use. First, the goals of "Know your Numbers" interventions are to improve patient knowledge, skill, and attitudes about air quality alerts or indices with subsequent government-recommended health protective behaviors (World Health Organization, 2020b). Nurses can assist patients on ways to receive and understand air quality index, air quality health index, or air quality alerts through media, emergency management, and personal communication systems. For example, the nurse can assist patients to access, download, and practice using freely available smartphone compatible software applications, such as the Environmental Protection Agency's AirNow app (available in the Apple App Store or the Google Play Store) in order to receive an email or cell phone alert notifications and follow behavior recommendations when air quality presents a health risk in the patient's community, while tailoring the education and behavior change recommendation to the patients' personalized risks and preferences. Research evidence demonstrates the need for additional nursing intervention, as most patients currently do not follow recommended guidance from air quality alerts (D'Antoni, Smith, Auyeung, &

Weinman, 2017). There are several additional experimental self-management software apps in various stages of research and development, such as measuring the level of indoor formaldehyde exposure (Castner, Gehrke, Shapiro, & Dannemiller, 2018).

Clinical nurses are in an important position to individualize patient education and self-management coaching to avoid air pollution by specific place and time (World Health Organization, 2020b). It is important to support and encourage outdoor physical activity for overall health and wellbeing. However, it is also important that patients avoid, if possible, major roadways during heavy traffic times or late afternoon on ozone action days. Discussing the specific routes patients may use for outdoor exercise, with considerations for industrial corridors or other pollution sources can aide in reducing the patient's short- and long-term exposures to pollutants. The overall research evidence on the use of small area or home air filtration on health is mixed, and caution should be followed when recommending any particular filtration device or product to patients. For patients with high risk for allergies, asthma, or other cardio-respiratory diseases, attention to routine home maintenance that includes following manufacturer instructions for the frequency of furnace/air conditioner filter cleaning or change is needed. Additional air purifiers or cleaners, particularly those using High Efficiency Particulate Air (HEPA) filtration systems may be promising to reduce symptoms and exposures, especially in high pollution areas or during high pollution times or disasters. While the priority is to eliminate exposure to second and third hand smoke from cigarette, or other smoking, in the home, air filtration may help mitigate exposures where second or third hand exposures indoor still do occur (Schuers, Chapron, Guihard, Bouchez, & Darmon, 2019). Last, clinical nurses can provide evidence-based information on face masks and respirators for patients. There is little evidence to support the use of face masks or respirators to reduce exposure to general outdoor air pollution. However, there are specific occupational job exposures, geological disasters (volcanic eruption, desert dust storm), disaster clean up (mold-related water damage in homes), or specific immunocompromised populations (patient with HIV/AIDs at risk for aspergillosis) where face coverings and masks are recommended. In these instances, specialty consults and training for the care of immunocompromised patients, specialty training to provide occupational health nursing or fit testing and occupational wear (Occupational Safety and Health Administration, nd), and Centers for Disease Control and Prevention disaster guidance on respirator use in disasters (Centers for Disease Control and Prevention, 2017, 2018) offer key evidence-based recommendations and material to inform patient education interventions.

REFERENCES

Agency for Toxic Substances & Disease Registry. (2014). *Toxic Substances Portal.* https://www.atsdr.cdc.gov/toxfaqs/index.asp

American Thoracic Society. (2020). *Fact sheets: A-Z. Patient education handouts.* https://www.thoracic.org/patients/patient-resources/fact-sheets-az.php

Amiri, A., & Zhao, S. (2019a). Environmental justice screening tools: Implications for nursing. *Public Health Nurs, 36*(3), 411-421. doi:10.1111/phn.12593

Amiri, A., & Zhao, S. (2019b). Working with an environmental justice community: Nurse observation, assessment, and intervention. *Nursing Forum, 54*(2), 270-279. doi:10.1111/nuf.12327

Association, A. N. (2007). *ANA's principles of environmental health for nursing practice with implementation strategies.* http://www.nursingworld.org/MainMenuCategories/WorkplaceSafety/Healthy-Nurse/ANAsPrinciplesofEnvironmentalHealthforNursingPractice.pdf

Brand, J. E., Caine, V. A., Rhodes, J., & Ravenscroft, J. (2016). Rewards and Lessons Learned From Implementation of a Healthy Homes Research Project in a Midwestern Public Health Department. *Journal of Environmental Health, 79*(1), 20-23.

Butz, A. M., Bollinger, M. E., Ogborn, J., Morphew, T., Mudd, S. S., Kub, J. E., . . . Tsoukleris, M. (2019). Children with poorly controlled asthma: Randomized controlled trial of a home-based environmental control intervention. *Pediatric Pulmonology, 54*(3), 245-256. doi:10.1002/ppul.24239

Campbell, L. A., & Anderko, L. (2020). Moving upstream from the Individual to the community: Addressing social determinants of health. *NASN School Nurse, 35*(3), 152-157. doi:10.1177/1942602x20902462

Castner, J. (2020a). Knowledge translation of science advances into emergency nursing practice with the Reach, Effectiveness, Adoption, Implementation, and Maintenance Framework. *Journal of Emergency Nursing, 46*(2), 141-146.e142. doi:10.1016/j.jen.2020.01.006

Castner, J. (2020b). Ozone alerts and respiratory emergencies: The Environmental Protection Agency's Potential Biological Pathways for Respiratory Effects. *Journal of Emergency Nursing, 46*(4), 413-419.e412. doi:10.1016/j.jen.2020.05.008

Castner, J., Amiri, A., & Huntington-Moskos, L. (2020). Applying the NIEHS translational research framework (NIEHS-TRF) to map clinical environmental health research trajectories. *Nursing Outlook, 68*(3), 301-312. doi:10.1016/j.outlook.2020.01.005

Castner, J., Amiri, A., Rodriguez, J., Huntington-Moskos, L., Thompson, L. M., Zhao, S., & Polivka, B. (2019). Advancing the symptom science model with environmental health. *Public Health Nursing, 36*(5), 716-725. doi:10.1111/phn.12641

Castner, J., Barnett, R., Moskos, L. H., Folz, R. J., & Polivka, B. (2020). Home environment allergen exposure scale in older adult cohort with asthma. *Canadian Journal of Public Health.* doi:10.17269/s41997-020-00335-0

Castner, J., Gehrke, G. E., Shapiro, N., & Dannemiller, K. C. (2018). Community interest and feasibility of using a novel smartphone-based formaldehyde exposure detection technology. *Public Health Nursing, 35*(4), 261-272. doi:10.1111/phn.12384

Castner, J., Gittere, S., & Seo, J. Y. (2015). Criteria air pollutants and emergency nursing. *Journal of Emergency Nursing, 41*(3), 186-192. doi:10.1016/j.jen.2014.08.011

Castner, J., & Polivka, B. J. (2018). Nursing practice and particulate matter exposure. *American Journal of Nursing, 118*(8), 52-56. doi:10.1097/01.NAJ.0000544166.59939.5f

Centers for Disease Control and Prevention. (2017). *Mold cleanup & remediation.* https://www.cdc.gov/mold/cleanup.htm

Centers for Disease Control and Prevention. (2018). *During an eruption. Natural disasters and severe weather.* https://www.cdc.gov/disasters/volcanoes/during.html

Centers for Disease Control and Prevention. (2020). *Childhood lead poisoning prevention.* https://www.cdc.gov/nceh/lead/prevention/sources.htm

D'Antoni, D., Smith, L., Auyeung, V., & Weinman, J. (2017). Psychosocial and demographic predictors of adherence and non-adherence to health advice accompanying air quality warning systems: a systematic review. *Environmental Health, 16*(1), 100. doi:10.1186/s12940-017-0307-4

Dodd-Butera, T., Beaman, M., & Brash, M. (2019). Environmental Health Equity: A Concept Analysis. *Annual Reviews in Nursing Research, 38*(1), 183-202. doi:10.1891/0739-6686.38.183

Environmental Protection Agency. (2010). *Integrated science assessment for carbon monoxide (EPA/600/R-09/019F)*. www.epa.gov/isa

Environmental Protection Agency. (2013). *Integrated science assessment for lead (EPA/600/R-10/075F)*. www.epa.gov/isa

Environmental Protection Agency. (2015). *Preamble to the integrated science assessments (EPA/600/R-15/067)*. www.epa.gov/isa

Environmental Protection Agency. (2016a). *Integrated science assessment for oxides of nitrogen - health criteria (EPA/600/R-15/068)*. www.epa.gov/isa

Environmental Protection Agency. (2016b). *Patient education tools. Ozone and your patients' health*. https://www3.epa.gov/ttn/ozonehealth/tools.html

Environmental Protection Agency. (2017a). *Integrated science assessment for sulfur oxides - health criteria (EPA/600/R-17/451)*. www.epa.gov/isa

Environmental Protection Agency. (2017b). *Patient education tools for particle pollution. Particle pollution and your patients' health*. https://www.epa.gov/particle-pollution-and-your-patients-health/patient-education-tools

Environmental Protection Agency. (2019). *Integrated science assessment for particulate matter (EPA/600/R-19/188)*. www.epa.gov/isa

Environmental Protection Agency. (2020a). *Creating healthy indoor air quality in schools*. https://www.epa.gov/iaq-schools

Environmental Protection Agency. (2020b). *Integrated science assessment for ozone and related photochemical oxidants (EPA/600/R-20/012)*. www.epa.gov/isa

Environmental Protection Agency. (2020c). *Radon. Environmental Topics*. https://www.epa.gov/radon

Graham Carlos, W., Dela Cruz, C., Jamil, S., Kipen, H., & Rose, C. (2017). Mold-specific concerns associated with water damage for those with allergies, asthma, and other lung diseases. *American Journal of Respiratory Critical Care Medicine, 196*(7), P13-p14. doi:10.1164/rccm.1967P13

Green & Healthy Homes Initiative. (2020). *8 elements of a green and healthy home. Healthy Homes*. https://www.greenandhealthyhomes.org/home-and-health/elements-green-healthy-home/

Hahn, E. J., Huntington-Moskos, L., Mundy, M., Rademacher, K., Wiggins, A. T., Rayens, M. K., . . . Butler, K. M. (2019). A Randomized Trial to Test Personalized Environmental Report Back to Reduce Lung Cancer Risk. *Health Education and Behavior, 46*(1), 165-175. doi:10.1177/1090198118788602

Harber, P., Redlich, C. A., & Henneberger, P. (2018). Work-exacerbated asthma. *American Journal of Respiratory Crit ical Care Medicine, 197*(2), P1-p2. doi:10.1164/rccm.1972P1

Huntington-Moskos, L., Rayens, M. K., Wiggins, A., & Hahn, E. J. (2016). Radon, secondhand smoke, and shildren in the home: Creating a teachable moment for lung cancer prevention. *Public Health Nursing, 33*(6), 529-538. doi:10.1111/phn.12283

Institute of Medicine. (2011). *Climate change, the indoor environment, and health*. National Academies Press.

International Agency for Research on Cancer. (2016). *Outdoor air pollution*. IARC Monographs on the Evaluation of Carcinogenic Risks to Humans, 109. https://publications.iarc.fr/538.

Johnson, S., & Schenk, E. (2019). A Proposal: Nurse-Sensitive Environmental Indicators. *Annual Reviews of Nursing Research, 38*(1), 265-274. doi:10.1891/0739-6686.38.265

Kousha, T., & Castner, J. (2016). The Air Quality Health Index and Emergency Department Visits for Otitis Media. *Journal of Nursing Scholarship, 48*(2), 163-171. doi:10.1111/jnu.12195

Leffers, J. M., Smith, C. M., McDermott-Levy, R., Resick, L. K., Hanson, M. J., Jordan, L. C., . . . Huffling, K. (2015). Developing curriculum recommendations for environmental health in nursing. *Nurse Educator, 40*(3), 139-143. doi:10.1097/nne.0000000000000133

Lim, S. S., Vos, T., Flaxman, A. D., Danaei, G., Shibuya, K., Adair-Rohani, H., . . . Memish, Z. A. (2012). A comparative risk assessment of burden of disease and injury attributable to 67 risk factors and risk factor clusters in 21 regions, 1990-2010: a systematic analysis for the Global Burden of Disease Study 2010. *Lancet, 380*(9859), 2224-2260. doi:10.1016/s0140-6736(12)61766-8

Mainardi, A. S., & Redlich, C. A. (2018). Indoor air quality problems at home, school, and work. *American Journal of Respiratory Critical Care Medicine, 198*(1), P1-p2. doi:10.1164/rccm.1981P1

McDermott-Levy, R., Jackman-Murphy, K. P., Leffers, J. M., & Jordan, L. (2019). Integrating climate change into nursing curricula. *Nurse Educator, 44*(1), 43-47. doi:10.1097/nne.0000000000000525

National Institute of Environmental Health Sciences. (2020). *Brochures and fact sheets. Health Education*. https://www.niehs.nih.gov/health/materials/index.cfm

Occupational Safety and Health Administration. (nd). *Respiratory protection. Safety and health topics.* https://www.osha.gov/respiratory-protection

Office of Disease Prevention and Health Promotion. (2014, September 16, 2020). *Environmental quality. Leading Health Indicators Healthy People 2020.* https://www.healthypeople.gov/2020/leading-health-indicators/2020-lhi-topics/Environmental-Quality

Reddy, A. L., Gomez, M., & Dixon, S. L. (2017). The New York State Healthy Neighborhoods Program: Findings from an evaluation of a large-scale, multisite, state-funded healthy homes program. *Journal of Public Health Management Practice, 23*(2), 210-218. doi:10.1097/phh.0000000000000529

Rice, M., Balmes, J., & Malhotra, A. (2016). Outdoor air pollution and your health. *American Journal of Respiratory Critical Care Medicine, 194*(10), P17-p18. doi:10.1164/rccm.19410P17

Schuers, M., Chapron, A., Guihard, H., Bouchez, T., & Darmon, D. (2019). Impact of non-drug therapies on asthma control: A systematic review of the literature. *European Journal of General Practice, 25*(2), 65-76. doi:10.1080/13814788.2019.1574742

Sood, A., Kapoor, V., Doo, K., & Blount, R. (2018). Health problems and burning indoor fuels. *American Journal of Respiratory Critical Care Medicine, 198*(5), P9-p10. doi:10.1164/rccm.1985P9

Sotolongo, A., Falvo, M., Santos, S., Johnson, I., Arjomandi, M., Hines, S., . . . Osterholzer, J. (2020). Military burn pits. *American Journal of Respiratory Critical Care Medicine, 201*(7), P13-p14. doi:10.1164/rccm.2017P13

Spanier, A. J., McLaine, P., & Gilden, R. C. (2019). Screening for Elevated Blood Lead Levels in Children and Pregnant Women. *JAMA, 321*(15), 1464-1465. doi:10.1001/jama.2019.2594

Szyszkowicz, M., Kousha, T., & Castner, J. (2016). Air pollution and emergency department visits for conjunctivitis: A case-crossover study. *International Journal of Occupational and Medical Environmental Health, 29*(3), 381-393. doi:10.13075/ijomeh.1896.00442

World Health Organization. (2016). *Ambient air pollution: A global assessment of exposure and burden of disease.* https://www.who.int/phe/publications/air-pollution-global-assessment/en/

World Health Organization. (2020a). *Air pollution.* Health topics. https://www.who.int/health-topics/air-pollution#tab=tab_1

World Health Organization. (2020b). *Personal interventions and risk communication on air pollution.* https://www.who.int/publications/i/item/9789240000278

WHERE DOES OUR DRINKING WATER COME FROM?
Anne Huilck, RN, MSN, JD
Clean Water Action
State Director, Connecticut

Many Americans don't think too much about where drinking water comes from or the infrastructure and processes that enable us to get safe, clean water from our faucets. The United States is fortunate to have one of the most reliable and safest systems for drinking water in the world (United States Environmental Protection Agency [US EPA], 2018). Yet, aging infrastructure, gaps in federal and state law, climate change, land use practices and pollution pose significant threats to drinking water sources.

The majority of Americans get their drinking water from public water utilities that pump and treat groundwater from aquifers and surface water from reservoirs, rivers, lakes and streams, before pumping it to our faucets. There are more than 170,000 public water systems in the United States, both publicly or privately owned, all required to meet federal and state standards for safety (US EPA, 2020h).

Recent crises of public drinking water like in Flint, Michigan, heighten awareness of the critical importance of assuring safe drinking water. As the most trusted profession, it is important for nurses to have an understanding of not only where local water supplies come from but potential sources of risk to drinking water. A very helpful report from ANHE is here: ([United States Environmental Protection Agency, 2018](#))

Protecting drinking water sources, also referred to as source waters, requires a variety of pollution prevention methods including protecting the source itself and assuring the infrastructure and processes to deliver the water are safe. Both are required to protect public health.

PROTECTING WATER SOURCES

- Protect watershed land: A watershed encompasses the land that drains rainwater or snow into a water body used for drinking water, agricultural and industrial processes and for plants and wildlife. The land around the water body, including the small streams, helps filter water going into the waterbody. Protecting this land from environmental impacts and pollution protects these vital water sources for millions of Americans.

- Stormwater runoff: Stormwater runoff is the rain or snowmelt that flows over land and impervious surfaces, such as paved streets, parking lots, and building rooftops,

that does not soak into the ground. The runoff picks up pollutants like trash, chemicals, oils, and dirt/sediment that can harm our rivers, streams, lakes, and coastal waters. Preventing or minimizing runoff is critical to protecting watersheds. Under federal law, municipal separate storm sewer systems (MS4s), construction activities, and industrial activities may be required to implement stormwater runoff practices (US EPA, 2020c). Despite this, stormwater runoff continues to be a significant source of pollution flowing into waterways (US EPA, 2020e). Protecting land around a drinking water source from stormwater runoff is critical.

- Agriculture: Manure and wastewater from farms, particularly large-scale confined animal feeding operations (CAFOs) are often significant sources of nitrogen and phosphorus, organic matter, sediments, pathogens, hormones, and antibiotics to the environment (US EPA, 2020b).

- Nutrients: Nutrients, like nitrogen and phosphorus found in fertilizers and in pet and animal waste can be harmful to water bodies. When excessive amounts of nutrients run off into water bodies, they can cause excessive growth of algae and algal blooms which significantly impair water quality. Some algae blooms contain cyanobacteria which can harm the health of humans, pets and other wildlife (Centers for Disease Control and Prevention, n.d.). Excessive nutrients and algae growth can also lead to areas of low or no oxygen, known as dead zones. Severe algal growth blocks light that is needed for aquatic plants. As the plants die and decay, they take up more dissolved oxygen in the water which can kill aquatic life (US NOAA, 2020).

- Pesticides: Pesticides are toxic chemicals designed to kill pests. They contain a variety of chemicals, many of which are carcinogenic, neurotoxic and hormone-disruptors. Pesticides are applied to farmlands, gardens and lawns and can make their way into groundwater or surface water systems that feed drinking water supplies. According to the U.S. EPA, the question of whether these contaminants pose a health risk depends on how toxic the pesticides are, how much is in the water, and how much exposure occurs on a daily basis. Numerous other studies show that many of these chemicals are present in umbilical cord blood and have health concerns at low levels (Earth Justice, 2014; Formuzis, 2020).

- Climate change: Changing weather patterns and warming temperatures affect drinking water sources in a variety of ways. Frequent, intense storms contribute to erosion and stormwater runoff and potentially more nutrient pollution. Longer periods of warm temperatures and lack of rain impact water supply. Warmer temperatures can lead to algal blooms, cyanobacteria growth and low levels of dissolved oxygen all of which impair water quality (Union of Concerned Scientists, 2010).

PROTECT AND UPGRADE INFRASTRUCTURE

Aging infrastructure

Much of the water infrastructure in the United States is aging and in need of repair or replacement (Sedlack, 2019). There are approximately one million miles of underground pipes, laid in the early to mid-19th century. These pipes generally have an estimated lifespan of 75-100 years. According to a 2017 report, there are approximately 240,000 leaks from water infrastructure each year, wasting over two trillion gallons of treated drinking water (Infrastructure Report Card, n.d.). Overall, according to the American Society of Civil Engineers Infrastructure 2017 Report card, the U.S. drinking water infrastructure system scored a grade of D and approximately $105 billion dollars in funding is needed to address the country's aging infrastructure. You can learn more about conditions in your state here: Water Infrastructure | ASCE's 2017 Infrastructure Report Card.

Water utilities are responsible to maintain, monitor, repair and upgrade infrastructure to assure safe drinking water (US EPA, 2020a). They must also comply with the federal Safe Drinking Water Act (SDWA) and regulations to meet drinking water standards. The U.S. Environmental Protection Agency set limits for ninety contaminants in drinking water, under SDWA authority. The Safe Drinking Water Act also enables states to adopt their own drinking water standards that at least meet or are more protective than the EPA (US EPA, 2017).

Lead Service Lines

Congress banned lead pipes in 1986 but the problem of lead service lines is extensive. Lead service lines are the portion of pipe that connects the main water line under the street to the building or home and most are made of lead. Lead can enter drinking water when this portion of the pipe corrodes-usually from acidic water or water with low levels of minerals. Corrosion of lead into drinking water is also impacted by other factors including water temperature and the age and status of the pipes. Sources of lead may also include the solder and fixtures (US EPA, 2020f).

In most communities, the water utility is responsible for the water main and the portion of the lead service line up to the property line. The property owner is responsible for the portion from the property line to the building or home. It is impractical, expensive and unsafe to replace only a portion of the lead service line as disconnecting the line can cause lead and other contaminants to get into the pipe. The dual responsibility for the lead service line replacement poses many legal challenges as states and municipalities often have different requirements and funding streams for service line replacement. These barriers, along with other challenges, have hindered robust progress in replacing all lead service lines in the U.S. More information on legal aspects of LSL replacement is here: Legal Factors - LSLR Collaborative (lslr-collaborative.org).

Water utilities are required to monitor lead levels in drinking water supplies and submit a Consumer Confidence Report annually by July 1 to all residents. Residents that have small community or private wells should contact their local health department about testing their water.

Nurses know there is no safe level of lead. Lead is a heavy metal that is persistent and bioaccumulative. The federal Safe Drinking Water Act set the maximum contaminant level (MCL) for lead at zero due to serious health impacts including premature birth, lowered IQ, behavioral disorders, hyperactivity, delayed growth and hearing disorders. Fetuses, infants and young children are particularly vulnerable to extremely low levels of lead. Understanding sources of lead in drinking water, local issues and what is being done to address lead exposure is a critical role for nurses.

THE CRISIS IN FLINT: CAN IT HAPPEN AGAIN?

The public health crisis that occurred in Flint Michigan was an enormous tragedy, the result of cost-cutting decisions that exposed approximately 99,000 residents to high levels of lead in their drinking water and caused 12,000 cases of lead poisoning and many others to Legionnaires disease. In 2014, Flint, Michigan officials switched the city's water supply from the Detroit Water and Sewage Department to the Karegnondi Water Authority to save money. In the interim before the connection was built, the city used water from the Flint River. The acidity of the water from the river corroded pipes, leaching lead into the drinking water supplies for Flint residents. Despite complaints from residents about foul smelling, brown water that caused rashes and other health concerns, city officials failed to take rapid action, often denying that there was a problem. In August 2020 after five years of litigation, the state of Michigan and other defendants agreed to pay $600 million that will go to a victims' compensation fund to support residents. Despite the settlement, more than five years later, not all pipes have been replaced and residents remain fearful that the drinking water is still unsafe (Smith et al., 2019). The magnitude of this tragedy, the slow response and blatant failures on the part of city and government officials are rooted in systemic racism and caused one of the biggest man-made public health crises in the U.S, highlighting potential gaps in how we assure safe drinking water for all.

WATER PROTECTION LAWS---AND GAPS

Despite strong laws protecting drinking water in the U.S., the tragedy in Flint Michigan pointed to the serious consequences that occur when laws are violated, not enforced or accountability is lacking. The federal Safe Drinking Water Act (SDWA), passed in 1974, protects drinking water sources in the U.S, authorizes the Environmental Protection Agency (EPA) to establish minimum standards to protect tap water and requires all owners or operators of public water systems to comply with these primary (health-related) standards (US EPA, 2020d). The EPA has set health-based standards for ninety contaminants that all public utilities must monitor and comply with. The SDWA also allows states to set their own health protective standards that at a minimum, meet the federal standard or are more health protective.

Although most Americans receive their drinking water from public utilities, there are gaps. EPA estimates that approximately 8,000 schools and child care facilities maintain their own water supply and are regulated under the Safe Drinking Water Act (SDWA).

There are approximately 98,000 public schools and 500,000 child care facilities not regulated under the SDWA. These unregulated schools and child care facilities may or may not be conducting voluntary drinking water quality testing (US EPA, 2019). Prior to the passage of the revised Lead and Copper Rule (December 2020), only twenty-four states and the District of Columbia required testing water in schools (Vock, 2019).

In 2015, the National Resources Defense Council (NRDC) analyzed reports from public water systems regulated under the SDWA. They found "more than 80,000 reported violations of the Safe Drinking Water Act by community water systems. Nearly 77 million people were served by more than 18,000 of these systems with violations in 2015. These violations included exceeding health-based standards, failing to properly test water for contaminants, and failing to report contamination to state authorities or the public. What's worse, 2015 saw more than 12,000 health-based violations in some 5,000 community water systems serving more than 27 million people" (Fedinick et al., 2017).

The report clearly shows that despite laws, concerns about safe drinking water exist in Flint and across the country.

LEAD AND COPPER RULE

In 1991, the EPA published the Lead and Copper Rule. This regulation requires public water utilities to monitor drinking water at customer taps and implement a treatment technique if levels of lead are above 15ppb or if copper concentrations exceed an action level of 1.3 ppm in more than 10% of customer taps sampled. If either occur, the system must undertake a number of additional actions to control corrosion. If the action level for lead is exceeded, the utility must also inform the public about steps they should take to protect their health and may have to replace lead service lines under their control (US EPA, 2021). The rule was revised in December 2020 and has better protections for children in schools and childcare facilities. The rule includes:

- Using science-based testing protocols to find more sources of lead in drinking water.

- Establishing a trigger level to jumpstart mitigation earlier and in more communities.

- Driving more and complete lead service line replacements.

- For the first time, requiring testing in schools and child care facilities.

- Requiring water systems to identify and make public the locations of lead service lines (US EPA, 2020g).

Unfortunately, while the inventory of lead service lines is helpful, the rule does not require all water utilities to fund and replace this portion of the pipes, leaving residents at risk. The failure will continue to disproportionately affect low-income communities as they cannot bear the burden of paying for partial replacement of these lines. The gap in the revised rule prolongs the potential of lead exposure for all Americans and perpetuates the inequities faced by vulnerable communities. Environmental advocacy organizations will continue to press for fully funded and complete lead service line replacement.

WHAT NURSES CAN DO

As the most trusted profession, nurses can play an important role in educating patients about safe drinking water issues in their community. Nurses can take steps to understand local drinking water sources, any local or state laws regarding testing drinking water in schools, any inventory on lead service lines in the community and drinking water issues raised by local health departments or water utilities. Nurses can also share steps on what individuals can do:

Important Steps Individuals Can Take to Reduce Lead in Drinking Water

- Have your water tested. Contact your water utility to have your water tested and to learn more about the lead levels in your drinking water.

- Learn if you have a lead service line. Contact your water utility or a licensed plumber to determine if the pipe that connects your home to the water main (called a service line) is made from lead.

- Run your water. Before drinking, flush your home's pipes by running the tap, taking a shower, doing laundry, or doing a load of dishes. The amount of time to run the water will depend on whether your home has a lead service line or not, and the length of the lead service line. Residents should contact their water utility for recommendations about flushing times in their community.

- Learn about construction in your neighborhood. Be aware of any construction or maintenance work that could disturb your lead service line. Construction may cause more lead to be released from a lead service line.

- Use cold water. Use only cold water for drinking, cooking and making baby formula. Remember, boiling water does not remove lead from water.

- Clean your aerator. Regularly clean your faucet's screen (also known as an aerator). Sediment, debris, and lead particles can collect in your aerator. If lead particles are caught in the aerator, lead can get into your water.

- Use your filter properly. If you use a filter, make sure you use a filter certified to remove lead. Read the directions to learn how to properly install and use your cartridge and when to replace it. Using the cartridge after it has expired can make it less effective at removing lead. Do not run hot water through the filter. (see more here: Basic Information about Lead in Drinking Water | Ground Water and Drinking Water | US EPA)

REFERENCES

Centers for Disease Control and Prevention. (n.d.). *Cyanobacteria blooms FAW*. https://www.cdc.gov/habs/pdf/cyanobacteria_faq.pdf

Earth Justice. (2014, January 31). *Targeting the most dangerous chemicals*. Earthjustice. https://earthjustice.org/healthy-communities/toxic-chemicals/most-dangerous

Fedinick, K. P., Wu, M., & Olson, E. D. (2017, May 2). *Threats on tap: Widespread violations highlight need for investment in water infrastructure and protections*. NRDC. https://www.nrdc.org/resources/threats-tap-widespread-violations-water-infrastructure

Formuzis, A. (2020, February 12). *EWG study: EPA fails to follow landmark law to protect children from pesticides in food*. https://www.ewg.org/release/ewg-study-epa-fails-follow-landmark-law-protect-children-pesticides-food

Infrastructure Report Card. (n.d.). *Drinking water*. ASCE's 2017 Infrastructure Report Card. https://www.infrastructurereportcard.org/cat-item/drinking_water/

Sedlack, D. (2019, March 3). *How development of America's water infrastructure has lurched through history*. Pew. https://pew.org/35mMYCF

Smith, M., Bosman, J., & Davey, M. (2019, April 25). *Flint's water crisis started 5 years ago. It's not over*. The New York Times. https://www.nytimes.com/2019/04/25/us/flint-water-crisis.html

Union of Concerned Scientists. (2010, January 24). *Water and climate change*. https://www.ucsusa.org/resources/water-and-climate-change

United States Environmental Protection Agency. (2018, December 19). *Basic information about your drinking water*. US EPA. https://www.epa.gov/ground-water-and-drinking-water/basic-information-about-your-drinking-water

United States Environmental Protection Agency. (2017, September 1). *Drinking water regulations*. US EPA. https://www.epa.gov/dwreginfo/drinking-water-regulations

United States Environmental Protection Agency. (2019, March 15). *Lead in drinking water in schools and childcare facilities*. US EPA. https://www.epa.gov/node/116045_

United States Environmental Protection Agency. (2020a, July 2). *Asset management for water and wastewater utilities*. US EPA. https://www.epa.gov/sustainable-water-infrastructure/asset-management-water-and-wastewater-utilities

United States Environmental Protection Agency. (2020b, August 3). *Animal feeding operations (AFOs)*. US EPA. https://www.epa.gov/npdes/animal-feeding-operations-afos

United States Environmental Protection Agency. (2020c, August 6). *NPDES stormwater program*. US EPA. https://www.epa.gov/npdes/npdes-stormwater-program

United States Environmental Protection Agency. (2020d, October 6). *Safe drinking water act (SDWA)*. US EPA. https://www.epa.gov/sdwa

United States Environmental Protection Agency. (2020e, November 24). *Soak up the rain: What's the problem?*. US EPA. https://www.epa.gov/soakuptherain/soak-rain-whats-problem

United States Environmental Protection Agency. (2020f, December 9). *Basic information about lead in drinking water*. US EPA. https://www.epa.gov/ground-water-and-drinking-water/basic-information-about-lead-drinking-water

United States Environmental Protection Agency. (2020g, December 22). *Lead and copper rule long-term revisions*. US EPA. https://www.epa.gov/sdwa/lead-and-copper-rule-long-term-revisions

United States Environmental Protection Agency. (2021, February 10). *Lead and copper rule*. US EPA. https://www.epa.gov/dwreginfo/lead-and-copper-rule

United States Environmental Protection Agency. (2020h, January 14). *Overview of the Safe Drinking Water Act*. US EPA. https://www.epa.gov/sdwa/overview-safe-drinking-water-act

United States National Oceanic and Atmospheric Administration. (2020, December 4). *What is nutrient pollution?* https://oceanservice.noaa.gov/facts/nutpollution.html

Vock, D. (2019, January 9). *For most U.S. students, lead testing isn't required for their school's water*. Governing the Future of States and Localities. https://www.governing.com/archive/gov-lead-water-schools-testing-flint.html

CARCINOGENS AND ENVIRONMENTAL HEALTH

Jeanne Leffers, PhD, RN, FAAN
Professor Emeritus
University of Massachusetts Dartmouth
College of Nursing and Health Sciences

Liz Clark, BSN, RN
Staff Nurse
Wills Eye Hospital
Philadelphia, PA

INTRODUCTION

What are carcinogens?

Carcinogens are commonly known as cancer causing substances. These substances have been shown to cause carcinogenesis or the process whereby normal cells are transformed. Carcinogens are commonly known as cancer causing substances. These substances have been shown to cause carcinogenesis or the process whereby normal cells are transformed into cancer cells. Carcinogens can either be physical, biological or chemical. Physical carcinogens include ultraviolet light and ionizing radiation. A biological example would be the Human Papillomavirus (HPV) which is known to cause cervical cancer in women. Carcinogens can also come from chemicals that we use daily in our personal and professional lives.

Carcinogenesis

In simple terms, carcinogenesis is a complex process that involves gene interaction with a carcinogen through 3 distinct phases of carcinogenesis: initiation, promotion and progression. During initiation there is an irreversible alteration in cellular genes or mutation. In the promotion stage, these abnormal cells self-proliferate and the final stage is progression where the cancer cells transform and grow and can lead to malignant proliferations and further mutations. (Baba & Catoi, 2007). Cancers generally come from genetic, environmental, and lifestyle factors and scientific investigators work to identify how these processes intersect in order to learn more about etiology and more effective treatments. Health professionals and the lay public are well aware of some of the risks from lifestyle such as tobacco use and some workplace exposures such as asbestos and radiation as well as more recent publicity about viral carcinogens such as Human Papilloma Virus (HPV). However, there is mounting concern about the 80,000 chemicals in our environment of which only about 7% have been tested for safety. This chapter looks at those chemicals that are known carcinogens or are considered as potentially hazardous.

WHAT NURSES HAVE LEARNED IN THEIR BASIC EDUCATION

Nurses first learn about carcinogens in their pre-licensure education, particularly in their pathophysiology course. During their medical-surgical courses they are likely to revisit the topic but very briefly as those courses focus upon the care and management of patients with acute and chronic diseases, with limited discussion of prevention. In courses such as community/public health, there is a strong emphasis upon health promotion and disease prevention but extensive content about carcinogens again is limited. Commonly used pathophysiology textbooks are more likely to include information about cancer epidemiology and identify risk factors than other course textbooks. For example, in one popular textbook, there is a chapter on cancer epidemiology with discussion and graphics to guide the learner in understanding epigenetics, DNA methylation, methylation of a gene region and gene transcription, free radical formation and modeling for radiation exposure (Huether & McCance, 2012). Huether & McCance (2012) include a table of environmental and occupational links to cancer citing the category (e.g. aromatic amines, metals, chlorination by-products, environmental tobacco smoke [ETS], natural fibers, pesticides, petrochemicals, radiation, and solvents), carcinogenic agents (e.g. arsenic, lead, benzidine, asbestos, herbicides, polycyclic aromatic hydrocarbons, ionizing radiation, formaldehyde, vinyl chloride and benzene), strong association for cancer (e.g. aromatic amines and bladder cancer; ETS and lung cancer; asbestos and mesothelioma; ionizing radiation and leukemia, brain, thyroid, and sarcoma cancers; benzene and leukemia) as well as suspected link for cancer (2012). If nurses enter the profession with a strong background in carcinogenesis, it should be clear that knowledge of carcinogens must become integral to their nursing practice.

GENE-ENVIRONMENT INTERACTION

In the prior discussion of carcinogenesis, genetic sequences in the cell interface with environmental factors to begin the process of carcinogenesis known as initiation. Epigenetics is that branch of science that examines heritable changes in gene expression or more simply mechanisms that will switch genes. Genes are composed on DNA sequencing but epigenetics is the field that looks at epigenetic processes that influence genetic functioning. In simpler terms, epigenetics looks at gene activity that occurs without changing DNA sequencing. These are generally natural and essential to the function of the organism but can occur improperly resulting in many illnesses and adverse health events. The etiology of cancer is one of the most studied areas of epigenetic research leading to greater knowledge of how epigenetic processes influence cancer. (Weinhold, 2006). (For more information about epigenetics, please see the chapter on epigenetics.)

UPSTREAM APPROACH

Nurses have long understood the importance of an upstream approach to health. Initially introduced into nursing literature in 1990 by Dr. Patricia Butterfield (2018) the roots extend to sociologists Dr. Irving Zola and John McKinley in the late 1970s. The concept is explained by the analogy of a bystander seeing someone being swept downstream in a river and struggling with the current. The bystander quickly jumps into the river and pulls the person to shore only to see a second, then third being swept downstream. He was asked later what was pushing the victims into the river and his response was that he was so busy rescuing victims that he had not had time to look or focus upstream (Butterfield, 2017). This approach has become part of nursing discourse particularly when examining social determinants of health, contextual factors in disease etiology, system level influences on health and illness and environmental health (Butterfield, 2018). For our understanding of carcinogens this approach is very important. Many of the chemicals commonly used in our daily lives are known or suspected carcinogens. Using an upstream approach to safer choices for chemical use in health care settings as well as personal choices can promote health and can likely reduce the prevalence of cancer.

PRECAUTIONARY PRINCIPLE

Related to an upstream approach is the concept of precaution. In 1998, a group of scientists, environmental activists, lawyers and philosophers convened at the Johnson Foundation Wingspread Conference Center in Wisconsin where they developed the Wingspread Statement. The significant result of that statement is the Precautionary Principle that is stated as, "When an activity raises threats of harm to human health or the environment, precautionary measures should be taken even if some cause-and-effect relationships are not fully established scientifically. In this context the proponent of an activity, rather than the public, should bear the burden of proof. The process of applying the precautionary principle must be open, informed, and democratic and must include potentially affected parties. It must also involve an examination of the full range of alternatives, including no action." – Wingspread Statement on the Precautionary Principle, Jan. 1998

NURSING AND THE ENVIRONMENT

The landmark book, Nursing, Health and the Environment (Pope, Snyder & Mood, 1995), recommends that environmental health content be integrated into nursing education, practice, research and policy/advocacy. At the time of publication there was reference to human exposures to toxicants in occupational settings that had high risk for the development of cancers such as liver (vinyl chloride), lung /mesothelioma (asbestos), and blood dyscrasias (benzene). In the intervening 26 years since its publication, the nursing profession has built a stronger body of work in the four key areas outlined by the IOM report. In particular, the work includes the publication of the original e-text, Environmental Health in Nursing (2016), manuscripts with recommendations for how to integrate environmental health content into nursing education, webinars with essential content to advance knowledge, journal clubs, publications that highlight nursing research about toxic chemicals (Pak & McCauley, 2007) or make recommendations for practice (Rafferty & Limonik, 2013) or advocacy (Ballard, 2008)

WHY IS THIS IMPORTANT?

The group of diseases known as cancer can result in death if the growth of the abnormal cells is not controlled. Nurses work in many settings where people who have developed cancer are being treated. According to the American Cancer Society, as many as 1 in 3 Americans are likely to develop cancer in their lifetime. Data shows that 7.6 million women and 6.9 million men had a cancer diagnosis during 2014. Cancer costs are high for both individuals and for society as well with estimates of direct medical costs for cancer in the US in 2015 totaling $80.2 billion (American Cancer Society, 2018). Globally, the numbers of those diagnosed with cancer is higher with people living in low-income countries and people of color in the US more likely to die from the effects of cancer. Efforts to inform health professionals and the public about carcinogens to reduce risk can have benefits to the health of populations as well as reduction in health care expenditures (Department of Health and Human Services, 2016).

HOW IS DETERMINATION MADE TO CLASSIFY AS A CARCINOGEN?

National and international agencies select the chemicals of concern to be studied based upon the likelihood of risk to human health. Scientific research is conducted using laboratory animal studies as well as human epidemiologic studies. Environmental epidemiologic studies include surveillance systems, ecologic studies, cluster studies, case control studies, cohort studies and cross-sectional designs.

Comparison of data from a body of research on a particular chemical can lead to conclusive evidence that a substance can be designated as a carcinogen or has a high probability of causing the mutations in DNA that lead to carcinogenesis (National Research Council, 1997).

Three agencies, the International Agency for Research on Cancer (IARC), part of the World Health Organization, the US National Toxicology Program (NTP) and the EPA are the major agencies that make classifications about substances that are then labeled as carcinogens. Each has its own standards and reporting mechanism as identified below:

International Agency for Research on Cancer (IARC)

The IARC has evaluated more than 900 likely carcinogens in order to develop their classifications.

Group 1: Carcinogenic to Humans

Group 2A: Probably Carcinogenic to Humans

Group 2B: Possibly Carcinogenic to Humans

Group 3 Unclassifiable as to Carcinogenicity to Humans

Group 4 Probably NOT Carcinogenic to Humans

National Toxicology Program (NTP)

The second agency, the National Toxicology Program was formed from the National Institutes of Health, the Centers for Disease Control and Prevention, and the Food and Drug Administration. They compile a report on carcinogens with the belief that the identification of carcinogens is a key step in prevention (Department of Health and Human Services, 2016).

Report on Carcinogens, 14th Report

The Report on Carcinogens is designed to be a public health and scientific document, and includes a list of substances that pose a potential hazard. Placement on that list does not mean that the substance will cause cancer in any individual. Cancer etiology is dependent upon many factors such as susceptibility on the part of the individual, the amount of exposure and the duration of the exposure. Classifications of potential carcinogens on the Report of Carcinogens are:

- "Known to be human carcinogens": There is sufficient evidence of carcinogenicity from studies in humans, which indicates a causal relationship between exposure to the agent, substance, or mixture, and human cancer.

- "Reasonably anticipated to be human carcinogens": There is limited evidence of carcinogenicity from

studies in humans, which indicates that causal interpretation is credible, but that alternative explanations, such as chance, bias, or confounding factors, could not adequately be excluded, or there is sufficient evidence of carcinogenicity from studies in experimental animals, which indicates there is an increased incidence of malignant and/or a combination of malignant and benign tumors (1) in multiple species or at multiple tissue sites, or (2) by multiple routes of exposure, or (3) to an unusual degree with regard to incidence, site, or type of tumor, or age at onset, or there is less than sufficient evidence of carcinogenicity in humans or laboratory animals; however, the agent, substance, or mixture belongs to a well defined, structurally related class of substances whose members are listed in a previous Report on Carcinogens as either known to be a human carcinogen or reasonably anticipated to be a human carcinogen, or there is convincing relevant information that the agent acts through mechanisms indicating it would likely cause cancer in humans. From US Department of Health and Human Services, Report of Carcinogens, 14th edition (2016)

Additionally, the EPA maintains the Integrated Risk Information System (IRIS) that is an electronic database containing information on human health effects from substances in the environment. Their rating system is:

- Group A: Carcinogenic to humans

- Group B: Likely to be carcinogenic to humans

- Group C: Suggestive evidence of carcinogenic potential

- Group D: Inadequate information to assess carcinogenic potential

- Group E: Not likely to be carcinogenic to humans

There are other federal agencies, such as the National Cancer Institute , CDC's National Institute for Occupational Safety and Health (NIOSH),and the Food and Drug Administration (FDA) that do not maintain listings but may comment on whether a substance or exposure may cause cancer.

WHAT SHOULD NURSES DO?

According to the ANA Scope and Standards (2015) for nursing practice, nurses must incorporate environmental health knowledge into professional practice. Nurses can learn essential knowledge about environmental health risks not only through formal educational offerings in academic and professional settings but also through independent learning. This e-text is one effective way but there are also webinars, journal articles, and many other resources available. Many of these can be accessed on the Alliance of Nurses for Healthy Environments website. For our focus here on carcinogens and risk reduction we can examine three ways this is important to nursing practice. First, inclusion of knowledge about carcinogens will improve nurse's ability to conduct nursing health assessments that include hazardous chemical risks and exposures. Second, nurses can use that knowledge gained to educate patients and community members about hazardous chemicals and carcinogens. Increased knowledge about carcinogens can lead to greater engagement for nurses in nursing research and finally, nurses can include an exposure history into nursing assessments. This allows nurses to identify areas for patient or community education. Nurses should educate patients about exposure risks for chemicals in their workplace, schools, or homes. Exposure routes for chemicals into the body include absorption through the skin, ingestion of food and water, injection, and inhalation. A discussion of exposures from chemicals through absorption must include those used in household cleaning, personal care, and cosmetic use. Excellent sources of information for the lay population include the Environmental Working Group's Home Guide, Skin Deep, Healthy Cleaning and Consumer Products databases. Further, the National Library of Medicine offers a Household Products Database that includes sections for inside the home, landscape/yard, home maintenance, personal care, pet care, arts and crafts, auto products, home office, and commercial/institutional products commonly used in homes. The databases examine the products, the manufacturers, the ingredients, and health effects. The user can either search for the products they commonly use or locate those products rated as safest through the chemical testing results. Resources for education about food and water, the most common ingestion routes of exposure, include the Environmental Working Group's Tap Water Database, Shopper's Guide to Pesticides in Produce, and Food Scores. The Environmental Working Group also sponsors a Healthy Living App that can be used on a mobile telephone for use when shopping. Additionally, for specific source and exposure risk to carcinogens see the chapters about air, PFAS, and wireless technology in this e-textbook.

The ANHE site offers a menu of many tools including a Home Environmental Health and Safety Tool. Planned Parenthood offers an Environmental Health Assessment Form, and assessments for pesticides, personal care products, and cleaning products.

Many nurses practice in acute care settings where there is increasing emphasis upon sustainability. These initiatives which have been steadily increasing over the past 20 years include efforts to create healthier environments, eliminate mercury, establish green purchasing policies, reduce energy and water use, reduce and recycle solid waste and reduce chemical waste by phasing out toxic substances (Practice Greenhealth, 2018). Initiatives are driven by concerns for healthier environments for patients and staff, climate change and the significant contribution made by healthcare facilities to greenhouse gas emissions, and financial incentives to reduce expenditures for waste removal, energy consumption and water use. Many of the toxic substances include carcinogens. Nurses have been leaders as sustainability coordinators for health care facilities as well as participants on Green teams. Dr. Beth Schenk is one of those leaders.

Research

Nurses are actively involved in research that looks at environmental health risks. What is most foremost in the public's view is nurse participation in the Nurses Health Study that began in 1976 and has followed more than 275,000 nurses longitudinally. Key findings have made contributions to scientific knowledge related to lifestyle

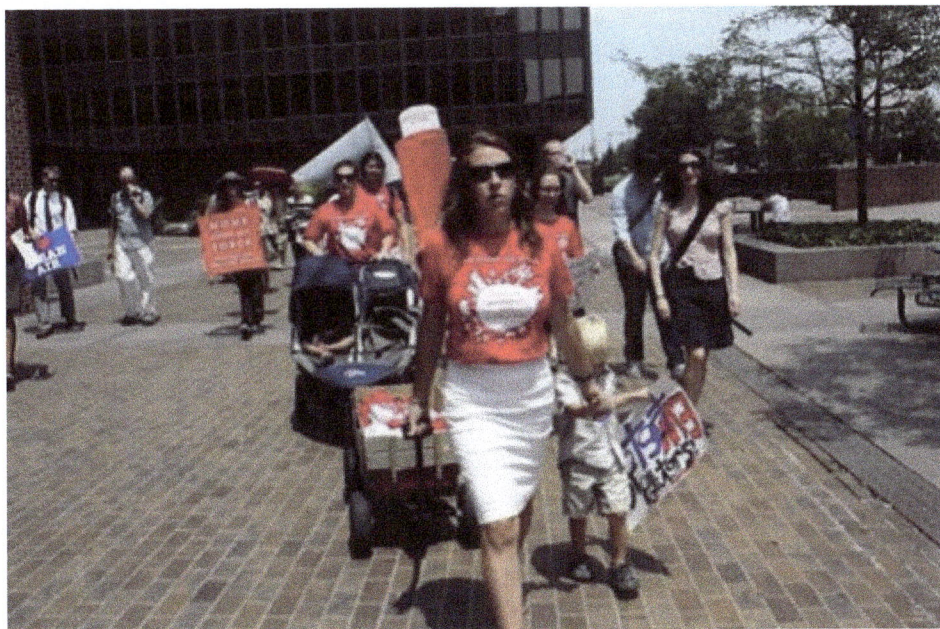

Mom's Clean Air Force advocating for stronger clean air policy with a stroller brigade. This photo by an unknown author is licensed under CC BY-SA-NC.

factors such as cigarette smoking, alcohol use, physical activity and diet, and biomarkers (exposures to heavy metals, cancer risks, role of Vitamin D in disease prevention). Increased risks associated with breast and colon cancer was determined through this longitudinal study. Further nurses conduct research in many areas of environmental health. Some of this research directly relates to exposure to carcinogens such as hydraulic fracturing (McDermott-Levy et al, 2016), pesticides (Runkle et al, 2013) and water (ONeal et al, 2013).

Advocacy and Policy

A final area where nursing practice can advance risk reduction for carcinogens is through policy and advocacy work. First, nurses must be knowledgeable about regulations, policies and legislation that relates to toxic chemical exposures. Advocacy can occur in the workplace setting where nurses advocate for the use of safer products. Advocacy can occur at the local level in their own communities to reduce risk in areas such as the elimination of crumb rubber and pesticide application to playing fields where children can be exposure to carcinogens. This can occur at the federal level to identify areas where public comment can be made or by participation with alliances, coalitions and advocacy groups that target hazardous chemicals such as Safer Chemicals, Healthy Families, Clean and Healthy New York, Connecticut Clean Water Action, Children's Environmental Health Network, and Health Care without Harm. These and many other organizations dedicated to reducing toxic exposures have nurses as directors or in leadership positions. In particular the Cancer Free Economy (CFE) part of the Garfield Foundation promotes networks and funds programs to specifically address the carcinogens prevalent in our everyday lives. Their work to build networks includes nurses and funds initiatives to engage the public for advocacy. The CFE goal is to create a cancer free economy or one that is healthy by shifting the current culture based upon risk reduction to that of an upstream preventive approach.

TOXIC SUBSTANCES CONTROL ACT (TSCA)

Beginning in 1970 with the establishment of the Environmental Protection Agency (EPA), the US government began taking steps to control sources of hazardous exposures in the environment through the Clean Air Act, the Clean Water Act and the Toxic Substances Control Act. (TSCA). In 1976 Congress approved TSCA to evaluate chemicals for their safety for human health. At that time, all existing chemicals were not required to be evaluated and were considered to be safe. That allowed those chemicals to have a "grandfather clause" to consider their safe use. All new chemicals were

MY PERSONAL ACCOUNT OF CANCER AS A PRACTICING BEDSIDE NURSE

By Liz Clark:

I graduated from nursing school in 1997 and worked at an emergency department. Initially, I had limited exposure and experience with the oncology patients because there were always rooms available on the oncology floor for them to be directly admitted. The ED was just considered "too dirty" of a place for immunocompromised oncology patients. As my career and time progressed, I have found oncology patients sitting in waiting rooms for hours waiting to get a gurney in the emergency department. Now, there are times when there is a whole section with active oncology patients or patients with a history of cancer in the ED. My journey to environmental nursing started when I started to get "burnt out" and realized I suffered from moral distress. To witness the physical decline and pain and emotional upheaval cancer has on a patient and family made me question my role as a nurse. I realized that I needed to get more involved in advocacy, working up stream, and having the moral courage to speak out on behalf of my patients. I needed to become more active in reducing the likelihood of cancer. That meant that I needed to understand the environmental risks of cancer and teach patients ways to avoid those risks and advocate to policies that reduced exposures to carcinogens.

then subject to regulation by the Environmental Protection Agency (EPA). For almost 40 years EPA was unable to enact strong regulatory action on chemical hazards due to the limitations of the 1976 ruling. Building upon work began in 2004 by those concerned about the need to improve TSCA, Senators Frank Lautenberg and David Vitter introduced the Chemical Safety Improvement Act in 2013. During the time that the bill faced challenges until 2015 when in December 2015 a revised version garnered 60 co-sponsors and was passed in the Senate by an unanimous vote. Prior to that, the House of Representatives had passed a similar bill that was less comprehensive. While the two bills had to be reconciled to enact the legislation that was passed and signed into law in June 2016, it greatly improves TSCA of 40 years earlier. Despite the death of Senator Lautenberg in 2013 his work was recognized through the naming the legislation Frank R. Lautenberg Chemical Safety for the 21st Century Act. This act mandates stronger reviews of chemicals, strengthens the protection of vulnerable populations such as pregnant people and children and requires EPA to prioritize persistent and bioaccumulative chemicals while enhancing the agency's authority to test new and existing chemicals. Safer Chemicals, Healthy Families provides a readable summary of the law on their website.

CONCLUSION

If nurses are to practice to meet the standards put forth in the ANA Scope and Standards of Practice (2015) they must be knowledgeable about carcinogens and incorporate that knowledge into their professional practice. Further, to fulfill that professional role, nurses should use evidence from research and advance nursing knowledge of hazardous carcinogenic chemicals. They must also become advocates to reduce and eliminate carcinogens for cancer prevention and a healthier world.

REFERENCES

American Cancer Society (2018). *Cancer prevalence.* https://www.cancer.org/cancer/cancer-basics/lifetime-probability-of-developing-or-dying-from-cancer.html

Baba A. I. & Câtoi, C. (2007). Carcinogenesis. In *Comparative Oncology.* The Publishing House of the Romanian Academy. https://www.ncbi.nlm.nih.gov/books/NBK9552/

Department of Health and Human Services. *Report on Carcinogens, 14th Edition.* https://ntp.niehs.nih.gov/ntp/roc/content/introduction_508.pdf

Department of Veterans Affairs. (2017). *VA's rule establishes a presumption of service connection for diseases associated with exposure to contaminants in the water supply at Camp Legeune.* https://www.blogs.va.gov/VAntage/35977/vas-rule-establishes-presumption-service-connection-diseases-associated-exposure-contaminants-water-supply-camp-lejeune/

Despommier, D. (n.d.) *The vertical farm.* http://www.verticalfarm.com/

Environmental Protection Agency (EPA). (2020). *Pesticides.* https://www.epa.gov/pesticides.

Etzl, R. A. (2012). *Pediatric environmental health, (3rd Ed.).* American Academy of Pediatrics.

Gilden, R., Huffling, K., & Sattler, B. (2010) Pesticides and health risks. *JOGNN, 39* (1), 103-110

Huether, S. E. & McCance, K. L. (2012). *Understanding physiology (5th Ed.).* Mosby.

Imai, N., Imai, Y., Kido, Y. (2008). Psychosocial factors that aggravate the symptoms of sick house syndrome in Japan. *Nursing and Health Sciences, 10* (2), 101-109

International Agency for Research on Cancer (IARC). (n.d.). *IARC Carcinogen Monographs.* www.monographs.iarc.fr/

Larsson, L. S. (2014). Risk-Reduction strategies to expand radon care planning with vulnerable groups. *Public Health Nursing, 31*(6), 526-536. https://doi.org/10.1111/phn.12111

McBride, D. (2015). Residential exposure to pesticides tied to childhood cancers. *ONS Connect, 30*(4), 86.

McDermott-Levy, R. & Garcia, V. (2016). Health concerns of Northeastern Pennsylvania residents living in an unconventional oil and gas development county. *Public Health Nursing, 33* (6), 502-510. Doi:10.1111/phn.12265

National Research Council (US) Committee on Environmental Epidemiology; National Research Council (US) Commission on Life Sciences. (1997). Environmental-Epidemiology Studies: Their Design and Conduct. In *Environmental epidemiology: Volume 2: Use of the gray literature and other data in environmental epidemiology.* National Academies Press. https://www.ncbi.nlm.nih.gov/books/NBK233644/

National Cancer Institute. www.cancer.gov

National Institute of Environmental Health Sciences (2020). *Bisphenol A.* https://www.niehs.nih.gov/health/topics/agents/sya-bpa/index.cfm

National Toxicology Program. https://www.epa.gov/tsca-inventory

National Toxicology Program (NTP). https://ntp.niehs.nih.gov/

O'Neal, G., Odom-Maryon, T., Postma, J., Hill, W., & Butterfield, P. (2013). The Household Risk Perception instrument and the Self-Efficacy in Environmental Risk Reduction instrument: psychometric testing using principal component analysis. *Journal of Advanced Nursing, 69*(9), 2107-2115.

Pak, V. M. & McCauley, L. A. (2007). Risks of phthalate exposure among the general population. *AOHONN, 55*(1).

Pollitt, P., Sattler, B., Butterfield, P. G., Anderko, L., Brody, C., Mood, L., ... & Cook, K. (2020). Environmental nursing: Leaders reflect on the 50th anniversary of Earth Day. *Public Health Nursing, 37*(4), 614-625. https://doi-org.libproxy.umassd.edu/10.1111/phn.12703

Pope, A.M., Snyder, M.A. & Mood, L. H. (1995). *Nursing, health, and the environment.* National Academies Press.

Practice Greenhealth. *About.* https://practicegreenhealth.org/about.

Rafferty, M. A. & Limonik, E. (2013). Is shale gas drilling an energy solution or public health crisis? *Public Health Nursing, 30*(5), 454-462. https://doi.org/10.1111/phn.12036

Runcle, J. D., Tovar-Aguilar, J. A., Economos, E., Flocks, J., Williams, B., Muniz, J. F. & McCauley, L. (2013). Pesticide Risk Perception and biomarkers of exposure in Florida female farmworkers. *Journal of Occupational and Environmental Medicine, 55*(11), 1286-1292. Doi:10:1097/IOM.ObO 13e3182973396

US Department of Health and Human Services. Public Health Service, National Toxicology Program. (2016). *Report on Carcinogens (14th ed.).* https://ntp.niehs.nih.gov/whatwestudy/assessments/cancer/roc/index.html

Valentine-Maher, S. K., Butterfield, P. G., & Laustsen, G. (2018). Environmental health: Advancing emancipatory policies for the common good. *Advances in Nursing Science, 41*, 57-69. https://doi.org/10.1097/ANS.0000000000000194

Weinhold, B. (2006). Epigenetics: The science of change. *Environmental Health Perspectives, 114*(3), A160–A167.

PHARMACEUTICAL WASTE

Kathryn P. Jackman-Murphy EdD, MSN, RN
Director, RN/BSN Program
Charter Oak State College

Ruth McDermott-Levy, PhD, MPH, RN, FAAN
Professor
Co-Director, Mid-Atlantic Center for Children's Health and the Environment
Villanova University
M. Louise Fitzpatrick College of Nursing

Jeanne Leffers, PhD, RN, FAAN
Professor Emeritus
University of Massachusetts Dartmouth
College of Nursing and Health Sciences

As the most trusted profession, nurses have a responsibility to instruct and advocate for not only proper medication use but also for proper disposal to keep our families, children, and communities safe. Nurses have opportunities daily to educate patients and their families about the medications they are taking including proper dosage, timing, effect(s), side effects, and interactions. These instructions must also include proper disposal of each medication as a part of their interactions with patients and their families. Every professional in the healthcare continuum should include this information, including the prescriber, pharmacists, and nurses. Despite this, researchers found that only 67.9% of pharmacists provided education only once a month to their customers and less than 16% of the pharmacists were able to select all the appropriate medication disposal recommendations (Tai, Hata, Wu, Frausto, and Law, 2016). A review of the literature did not reveal any research regarding nurses and providing appropriate disposal recommendations or patient education.

In 2002, the U.S. Geological Survey published a study of the ground and surface waters tested from 30 U.S. states. The findings revealed that there were low levels of pharmaceuticals such as antibiotics, contraceptives, hormones, and steroids in 80% of the water samples (Earth Talk, n.d). In 2009 waterways in rural Central Pennsylvania were found to be contaminated with caffeine, antibiotics, ibuprofen, and diphenhydramine. These findings were attributed to run off from municipal effluents and animal feeding operations (Loper, Crawford, Otto, Manning, Meyer, & Furlong, (2007). The concentrations of pharmaceuticals in the water remains low; however, there is no evidence to identify the human health impacts of long-term exposure of the pharmaceutical agents, their metabolites, and the health impacts of combined exposures to contaminated water and other contaminants.

Pharmaceuticals enter the environment in several ways. First, human consumption of medications leads to excretion of pharmaceutical waste and metabolites into sewage that can be released into aquifers or surface water. In fact, 30-90% of medication is excreted unchanged after ingestion (Pharmaceutical Technology, 2017). While this is unintentional contamination, there is also the purposeful flushing of unused or expired medications. Contamination also occurs as part of pharmaceutical manufacturing and waste disposal. There is also the excretion of pharmaceuticals by animal sources, due to use of medications (generally steroids and antibiotics) in livestock production (Becker, Mendez-Quigley, & Phillips, 2010).

As our population ages there are increases in chronic illnesses with subsequent increases in prescription medication use that leads to a greater likelihood of pharmaceutical waste in the environment. It is estimated that hospitals and long-term care facilities contribute up to 65% of the unused pharmaceuticals into wastewater facilities (Becker, Mendez-Quigley & Phillips, 2010). The article Managing Pharmaceutical Waste: What Pharmacists Should Know (Smith, 2002) is very helpful to understand federal regulations related to waste management; the definition of pharmaceutical waste; who is generating it; common waste streams and characterization of hazardous waste streams; and how pharmaceutical waste should be managed. In addition, Figure 1 in this chapter provides a visual description of how pharmaceutical waste enters the environment.

In the third edition of Nursing: Scope and Standards of Practice (2015), the American Nurses Association (ANA), Standard 17: Environmental Health specifically states that the registered nurse "advocates for the safe, judicious, and appropriate use, and disposal of products used in health care (p. 84)." This standard of nursing practice is related to medication use and proper disposal. In other words, our code of nursing practice acknowledges the nurse's professional responsibility to the environment by assuring our knowledge of these issues and proper management and disposal of medications to assure the health of everyone.

Medications that are unwanted, expired, or unused collect in our homes. Patients may have excess medications, including over the counter and prescription drugs, in their homes due to a change in dosage or medication, intolerance, or over-purchasing such as buying medications in bulk at a big box store or ordering long term supplies from their pharmacy as a means to save money on insurance co-pays. There are significant concerns regarding these excess stores of medications including accidental ingestion, poisoning of children and pets, accidentally taking the wrong medication, illness from taking expired medications, and diversion. The opioid crisis has placed a greater focus on eliminating excess medications from homes to protect from diversion and accidental ingestion, but additional conversations about minimizing excess medications in homes due to environmental concerns are needed. Despite the concerns of excess medications in our homes, they are rarely disposed of properly (Daughton, 2014).

Healthcare facilities have guidelines and resources for disposal of medications, but nurses in all practice settings, must educate the public about how to properly dispose of unneeded medications to protect the environment, and safety from diversion and accidental ingestion. Often in the community medications are discarded in the trash, in the toilet, or down the drain (Tong, Peake, & Braund, 2011). These disposal methods can contribute to water contamination and cause health issues for humans and animals alike. For example, in homes with septic tanks and wells as a water source, medications flushed down the drain can leach into the ground, seep into groundwater, and ultimately come out of their tap. Those with private wells are vulnerable of not only what they may be flushing down the drain but also the actions of others in their surrounding area.

Homes that obtain their water from a municipal water source can also be at risk for water contaminated from medications and other chemicals of concern. The municipality may not be equipped or able to test for pharmaceuticals in the water supply (EPA, 2018), and may not have the means to remediate the water if medications are detected and remain in sewage even with water treatment (Daughton, 2014). Low-income, rural, and communities of color may be more likely to have poor infrastructure, or the resources to manage contaminants including discarded pharmaceuticals (Cook, Curtis, & Huffling, 2017). Education for all community members regarding pharmaceutical disposal and other means for protecting water quality is vital to ensure optimal water quality for all. Hospital nurses should include proper medication disposal in the discharge plans. School nurses should talk to students (depending on child's age) and parents about proper storage and disposal of medications. Nurses working in the community should make medication storage and disposal part of the care that is provided to the individual, family, or community. (See the end of this chapter for resources to support the nurse in medication disposal information.)

Proper prescribing, purchasing, and disposal of medications helps to protect our water supply, protects from accidental ingestion and misuse, removes potentially harmful expired medications, and protects pets and wildlife. Daughton (2014) calls for changes to the current practice of prescribing medications by avoiding imprudent, unnecessary, excessive prescribing, misuse and overconsumption as effective "upstream" measures to protect our water supply. Other suggestions are to consider the excretion profile of the medication and prescribing the lowest dose necessary. It is noted that some medications can even be ordered at a lower "off-label" dose but still be effective (Daughton, 2014). Additionally, proper prescribing and administration of antibiotics may help to prevent antibiotic resistance.

The Environmental Protection Agency (EPA) and the Food and Drug Administration (FDA) specifically instructs citizens not to flush medications down the drain or toilet unless the label or patient instructions specifically tell the patient to do so. Medications such as controlled substances and narcotics have specific instructions to discard via flushing down the drain to reduce the danger of overdose stemming from unintentional or illegal use (EPA (a), 2018). An example of this is a fentanyl patch, which after use may still have medication remaining in the patch and the FDA recommends the patch be discarded by flushing. The FDA recognizes there are concerns with medications being disposed of this method, but states "there has been no sign of environmental effects caused by flushing recommended drugs" (2018). For aerosol medications and inhalers, instructions include following local regulations and contacting the local trash and recycling facility (FDA, n.d.).

Proper disposal of medications is not always available due to high costs and knowing the appropriate method. The FDA and EPA recommend citizens dispose of excess medications at community take-back programs in which they will be disposed of in a "safe and environmentally-conscious way" (EPA (a), 2018, FDA, 2018). Community take-back programs may be combined with a hazardous waste collection event but may also require a pharmacist for identifying medications and security for controlled substances that may be submitted. In 2018, over 6,000 sites participated in the bi-annual National Prescription Drug Take Back Days and collected nearly one million pounds of unwanted drugs. Click here for more information on National Prescription Drug Take Back Days.

Other sources for community disposal of medications include drug disposal kiosks at pharmacies or secure drop-off containers in police departments. Click here to

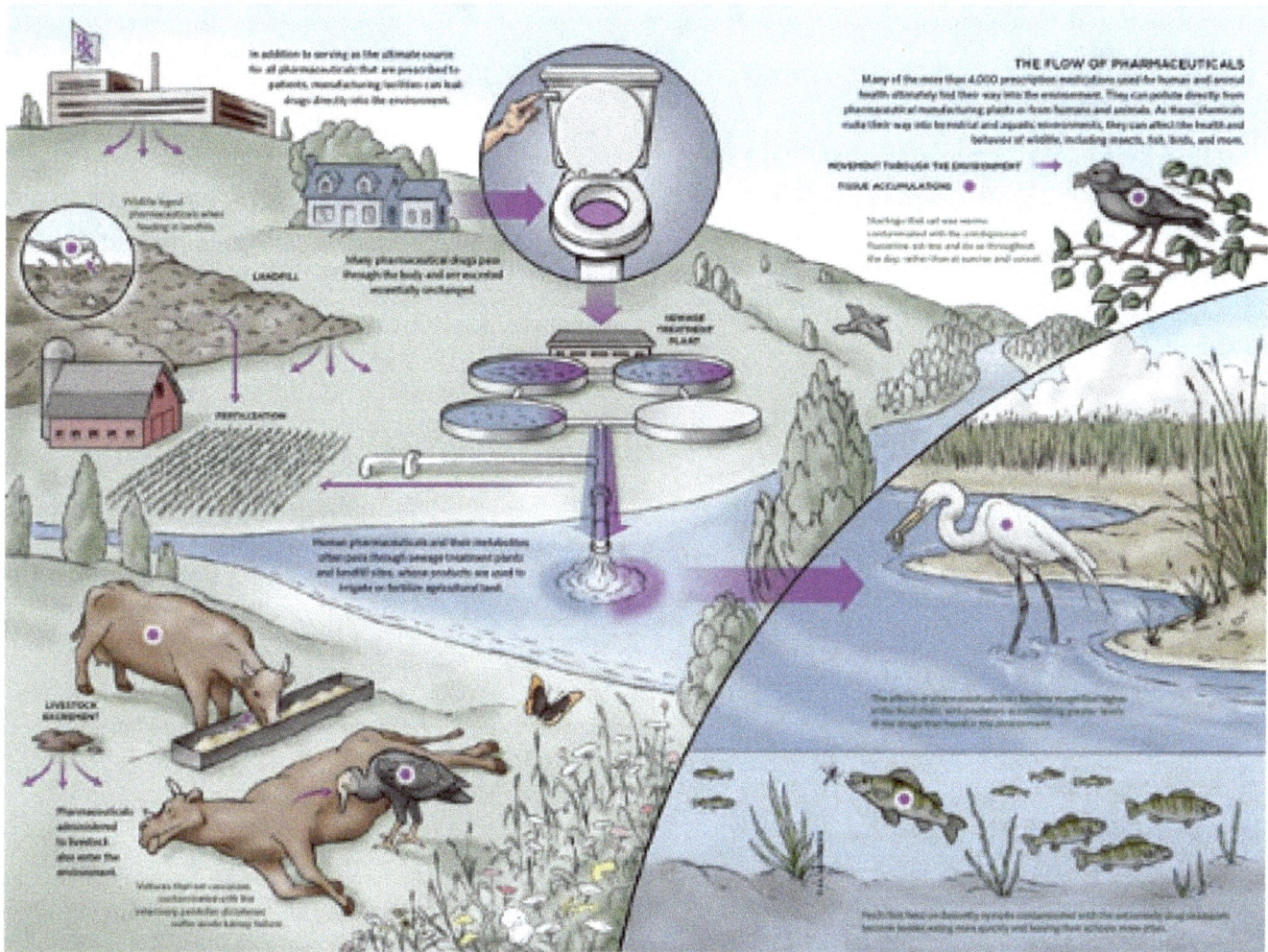

Figure 1: Pharmaceuticals found in our waterways come from human or animal use, or from the pharmaceutical industry. Image from U.S. Geological Survey web site, public domain

find a Controlled Substance Public Disposal Location by using your zip code. An informal survey of a few towns with these collection containers found the police bring the medications to an incineration company. The EPA describes the disposal of medications via incineration as a "environmentally responsible" and "safe and environmentally-conscious" (EPA (b), 2018). There are significant concerns with this method of disposal on the contributions to particulate air pollution not only from the incinerated medications but also for the containers that hold the medication, which are often plastic. Plastic when burned releases dioxin, a known carcinogen and hormone disruptor, which can enter the air and waterways. Some in the pharmaceutical industry recognize the problem of inadvertent pharmaceuticals in the environment and are working on "Green Pharma", an initiative that addressed more environmentally safe drug discovery, development, and medication products (Pharmaceutical Technology, 2017).

If a community take-back program is not available, the EPA recommends the following for disposal: remove the medication from the original container, making sure to remove any identifying information from the medication label, mix the medication with an inedible substance such as kitty litter, place the medication in a disposable container with a lid (i.e. margarine container, plastic laundry detergent container), and place the sealed container with your trash. While this may make the medication safer from diversion or accidental ingestion there are still concerns with this method of disposal contributing to water contamination, as the container may leak if it becomes torn or crushed and its contents may leach into the water supply. Click here for the EPA's How to Properly Dispose of Medications.

Nurses must take every opportunity to teach our patients, families, and communities the importance of proper medication administration, storage, and disposal to not only protect from accidental ingestion, poisoning of children and pets, and diversion, but also to protect our water supply.

RESOURCES FOR NURSES:

DEA: Controlled Substances https://www.deadiversion.usdoj.gov/schedules/orangebook/c_cs_alpha.pdf

EPA: Collecting and Disposing of Unwanted Medications: https://www.epa.gov/hwgenerators/collecting-and-disposing-unwanted-medicines

EPA: Resource Conservation and Recovery Act (RCRA) https://www.epa.gov/rcra

FDA: Disposal of unused medicines: What you should know. https://www.fda.gov/drugs/safe-disposal-medicines/disposal-unused-medicines-what-you-should-know

Health Care Without Harm: https://noharm-uscanada.org/

Practice Greenhealth: Pharmaceutical Waste: https://practicegreenhealth.org/topics/waste/pharmaceutical-waste

U.S. Geological Survey Podcast: Pharmaceuticals in the Nation's Water https://www.usgs.gov/media/audio/pharmaceuticals-nations-water

REFERENCES

American Nurses Association (ANA) (2010). *Nursing: Scope and standards of practice.* American Nurses Association.

American Nurses Association (ANA) (2015). *Nursing: Scope and standards of practice (2nd ed.).* American Nurses Association.

Becker, J., Mendez-Quigley, T., & Phillips, M. (2010). Nursing role in the pharmaceutical life cycle. *Nursing Administration Quarterly, 34*(4), 297-305.

Cook, C., & Curtis, K. Huffling, K. (2017). *Water and health: Opportunities for nursing action.* Alliance of Nurses for Healthy Environments

Daughton, C.G. (2014). Eco-directed sustainable prescribing: feasibility for reducing water contamination by drugs. *Science of the Total Environment, 493,* 392-404. doi: 10.1016/j.scitotenv.2014.06.013

Earth Talk. (n.d.). *External medicine: Discarded drugs may contaminate 40 million Americans' drinking water.* Scientific American. https://www.scientificamerican.com/article/pharmaceuticals-in-the-water/

Environmental Protection Agency. (n.d.). *Pharmaceuticals collected by law enforcement during take-back events and programs memo.* https://www.epa.gov/sites/production/files/2018-09/documents/signedwheeler_barnes_pharmaceuticaltakebacks.pdf

Environmental Protection Agency (a). (2018, September 12). *Collecting and disposing of unwanted medicines.* https://www.epa.gov/hwgenerators/collecting-and-disposing-unwanted-medicines

Loper, C. A., Crawford, J. K., Otto, K. L., Manning, R. L., Meyer, M. T., & Furlong, E. T. (2007). Concentrations of selected pharmaceuticals and antibiotics in south-central Pennsylvania waters, March through September 2006. In *U.S. Geological Survey Data Series 300* (p. 101).

Pharmaceutical Technology (2017). *Green pharma: The growing demand of environmentally friendly drugs.* https://www.pharmaceutical-technology.com/comment/commentgreen-pharma-the-growing-demand-for-environmentally-friendly-drugs-5937344/

Smith, C.A. (2002). Managing pharmaceutical waste: What pharmacists should know. *Journal of the Pharmacy Society of Wisconsin, Nov/Dec,* 17-22. https://gecap.org/pdf/managing_pharmaceutical_waste.pdf

Tai, B., Hata, M., Wu, S., Frausto, S. & Law, A. (2016). Prediction of pharmacist intention to provide medication disposal education using the theory of planned behaviour. *Journal of Evaluation in Clinical Practice, 22,* 653-661.

Tong, A., Peaks, B., & Braund, R. (2011). Disposal practices for unused medications around the world. *Environmental International, 37*(1), 292-298. doi:10.1016/j.envint.2010.10.002

U. S. Department of Health and Human Services. (2018, Sept 10). *Where and how to dispose of unused medicines.* U.S. Food and Drug Administration. https://www.fda.gov/ForConsumers/ConsumerUpdates/ucm101653.htm

PERFLUOROALKYL AND POLYFLUOROALKYL SUBSTANCES (PFAS): FOREVER CHEMICALS AND HEALTH EFFECTS

Dr. Laura Anderko, PhD, RN
Co-Director, Mid-Atlantic Center for Children's Health and the Environment
Villanova University
M. Louise Fitzpatrick College of Nursing

Emma Pennea, BA, MSGH
The Mid-Atlantic Center for Children's Health and the Environment
Villanova University
M. Louise Fitzpatrick College of Nursing

BACKGROUND

Perfluoroalkyl and polyfluoroalkyl substances (PFAS) refer to a family of synthetic chemicals used for over 70 years to make products that resist heat, oil, stains, grease, and water.

Most people in the United States and other industrialized countries have measurable amounts of PFAS in their blood (Agency for Toxic Substances and Disease Registry (ATSDR), 2023a). Thousands of chemicals that are designated as PFAS are commonly found in drinking water, food, and a wide range of consumer products (see Figure 1). For example, PFAS may be used to keep food from sticking to cookware, sofas and carpets more resistant to stains, packaging more resistant to grease, clothes and mattresses more waterproof, and as a component of some firefighting foams. PFAS can also be found in medical equipment, such as stents and commonly used pharmaceuticals (e.g., Lipitor) (Hammel et al., 2022). Because PFAS are chemically stable, they are unaffected by typical environmental degradation processes, and are persistent in the environment (ATSDR, 2023).

PFAS remain in the human body for long periods of time, and data from human studies suggest that some PFAS can take many years to be cleared from the body. Certain PFAS have estimated half-lives that can be as long as 35 years (ATSDR, 2020). These long half-lives result in body burdens that persist for years through bioaccumulation, even after identified exposure sources have been reduced (ATSDR, 2020; Bartell et al., 2010). Bioaccumulation is the buildup of toxicants, such as PFAS, in the body from various exposures such a water and food sources.

In August 2022, the National Academies of Sciences, Engineering and Medicine (NASEM) published a report, *Guidance on PFAS Exposure, Testing, and Clinical Follow-Up*, that examined the current evidence regarding human health effects of the most widely studied PFAS, and developed recommendations for risk reduction, lab testing, and clinical management (NASEM, 2022).

HEALTH IMPACTS

A large number of studies have examined possible relationships between levels of PFAS in blood and the associated harmful health effects. There is evidence that exposure to PFAS can lead to a variety of adverse health outcomes. If humans ingest contaminated food, water, and/or dust, the PFAS are absorbed and can accumulate in the body. There are many negative health outcomes associated with PFAS exposure. Health outcomes with sufficient evidence of increased health risks associated with PFAS exposure include: 1. Decreased antibody response (adults and children), 2. Dyslipidemia (adults and children), 3. Decreased infant and fetal growth, 4. Increased risk of kidney cancer (adults). The NASEM (2022) report outlines

Figure1: PFAS Exposure Sources

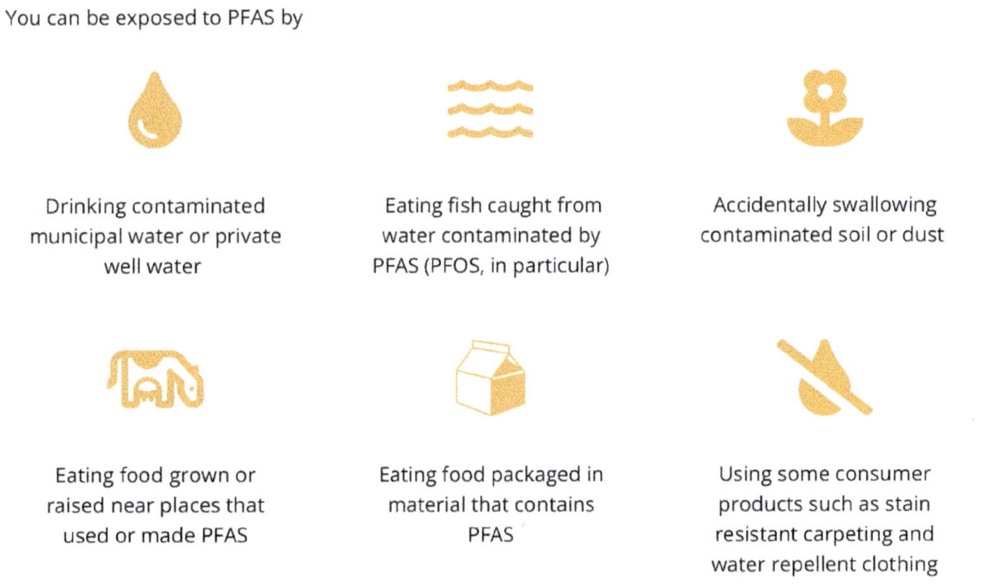

You can be exposed to PFAS by

Drinking contaminated municipal water or private well water

Eating fish caught from water contaminated by PFAS (PFOS, in particular)

Accidentally swallowing contaminated soil or dust

Eating food grown or raised near places that used or made PFAS

Eating food packaged in material that contains PFAS

Using some consumer products such as stain resistant carpeting and water repellent clothing

(ATSDR, 2023) https://www.atsdr.cdc.gov/pfas/health-effects/exposure.html
Reproduced as part of public domain

Table 1: Evidence of Health Outcomes Associated with PFAS Exposure

CATEGORY OF ASSOCIATION	HEALTH OUTCOMES WITH INCREASED RISK ASSOCIATE WITH PFAS EXPOSURE
Sufficient evidence of an association Based on strong evidence, there is high confidence that there is an association between exposure to PFAS and the health outcome. It is unlikely that the association is due to chance or bias.	• Decreased antibody response (in adults and children) • Dyslipidemia (in adults and children) • Decreased infant and fetal growth • Increased risk of kidney cancer (in adults)
Limited suggestive evidence of an association Based on limited evidence, there is moderate confidence that there is an association between exposure to PFAS and the health outcome. It is possible that the association is due to chance or bias.	• Increased risk of breast cancer (in adults) • Liver enzyme alterations (in adults and children) • Increased risk of pregnancy-induced hypertension (gestational hypertension and preeclampsia) • Increased risk of testicular cancer (in adults) • Thyroid disease and dysfunction (in adults) • Increased risk of ulcerative colitis (in adults)
Inadequate or Insufficient Evidence to Determine an Association Based on inconsistent evidence, a lack of evidence, or evidence of insufficient quality, there is moderate confidence that there is an association between exposure to PFAS and the health outcome. No conclusion can be made about a potential association.	• Immune effects other than reduced antibody response, and ulcerative colitis; Cardiovascular outcomes other than dyslipidemia; • Developmental outcomes other than small reductions in birthweight • Cancers other than kidney, breast, and testicular; Reproductive effects other than hypertensive disorders of pregnancy; Endocrine disorders other than thyroid hormone levels; Hepatic effects other than liver enzyme levels; Respiratory effects; Hematological effects • Musculoskeletal effects, such as effects on bone mineral density; Renal effects, such as renal disease; Neurological effects
Limited Suggestive Evidence of No Association Based on at least limited evidence, there is at least moderate confidence that there is NO association between PFAS and the health outcome.	• No outcomes were identified.

(NASEM, 2022) Reproduced as part of public domain.

additional health outcomes and the category of association (e.g., limited suggestive evidence of an association) in Table 1.

The widespread and ubiquitous nature of PFAS exposures from everyday consumer products and drinking water, coupled with the potential for long-term health impacts has raised community concerns about health impacts from exposure. There is a critical need to reduce and eliminate these exposures to improve community health over a lifetime.

Since 1999, the National Health and Nutrition Examination Survey (NHANES) has measured blood PFAS in the U.S. population. Most recent estimates report that 97% of the US population has been exposed. A 2006 agreement by eight major companies in the PFAS industry to voluntarily phase out perfluorooctane sulfonic acid (PFOA) and perfluorooctanoic acid (PFOS), two compounds that are part of the PFAS family, by 2015 has resulted in blood levels of PFOS and PFOA to decline (see Figure 2) (ATSDR, 2023b). This underscores the need to reduce the production and use of PFAS to protect the public's health.

A major source of PFAS is drinking water and the appropriate level that can be in drinking water is currently not federally regulated in the U.S. The U.S. Environmental Protection Agency (EPA) has not yet issued an enforceable standard called a Maximum Contaminant Level (MCL). In 2016, the EPA established a lifetime Health Advisory Level (HAL), which was set at 70 parts per trillion (ppt) for the combined concentrations of PFOS and PFOA. HALs are not legally enforceable and are not designed to be a definitive health-effect level but rather, provide a margin of protection over a lifetime. In June 2022, EPA revised its level from 70 ppt. to 4 ppt. for two of the most common PFAS (PFOS and PFOA) (EPA, 2023). Table 2 offers a summary of health advisories, for a complete list of PFAS health advisories go to: https://www.epa.gov/sdwa/questions-and-answers-drinking-water-health-advisories-pfoa-pfos-genx-chemicals-and-pfbs.

finalizes a national primary drinking water regulation for those contaminants (EPA, 2023). Clinical Implications

In addition to the absence of a drinking water regulation, there are no established clinical reference levels for PFAS in the blood. This absence provides uncertainty by healthcare providers looking to manage cases, especially of mothers exposed to PFAS and their children. The NASEM report developed a set of clinical management recommendations for healthcare providers based on PFAS blood levels (see Table 3). In general, when health concerns arise that might be associated with PFAS, it is important to conduct an environmental exposure history and physical exam relative to any symptom(s) reported and manage the issue with established evidence-based guidelines (e.g., routine cholesterol screening; thyroid function tests if a patient has symptoms consistent with thyroid dysfunction) (Anderko & Pennea, 2020; Anderko, Pennea, & Chalupka, 2020).

Since at this time there is no consensus related to long-term medical management for those exposed to levels higher than the background, reducing and preventing exposure is a critical intervention. This can be accomplished by offering guidance to families about how to identify and reduce current sources of PFAS exposure, including drinking water and consumer products (Anderko & Pennea, 2020; Anderko, Pennea, & Chalupka, 2020).

Health providers should determine the need for long-term monitoring based on risk factors such as age, source of drinking water, consumer products used, and occupational exposures. If there are concerns about PFAS exposure, a blood sample can test for the level of PFAS in

Figure 2: Blood Levels of the Most Common PFAS Found in Humans in the US
*Average = geometric mean

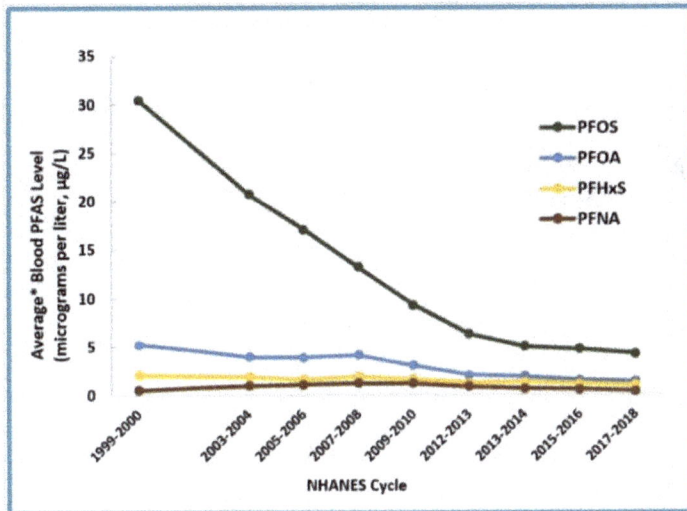

Blood Levels of the Most Common PFAS in People in the United States Over Time

(ATSDR, 2023b). Reproduced as part of the public domain

Above these levels, EPA recommends that public drinking water systems take steps to assess contamination, inform consumers, and limit exposure. Because of the lack of federal regulation, some states are beginning to establish their own guidelines. The Association of State Drinking Water Administrators (2019) provides information on states with proposed or established standards.

In the spring of 2023, EPA proposed a National Primary Drinking Water Regulation (NPDWR) to establish legally enforceable Maximum Contaminant Levels (MCLs), for six PFAS in drinking water. These include PFOA and PFOS as individual contaminants, and PFHxS, PFNA, PFBS, and HFPO-DA as a PFAS. The 2022 interim Health Advisories for PFOA and PFOS will continue to remain available as EPA

Table 2: Summary of Four PFAS Health Advisories

Summary of Four PFAS Health Advisories

- **Interim Health Advisories**:
  - Perfluorooctanoic acid (PFOA)
  - Perfluorooctane sulfonate (PFOS)
- **Final Health Advisories**:
  - GenX chemicals (PFOA replacement)
  - Perfluorobutane sulfonic acid (PFBS) (PFOS replacement)
- For PFOA and PFOS, some negative health effects may occur at concentrations that are near zero and below our ability to detect at this time.
- The lower the level of these chemicals in drinking water, the lower the risk to public health.

Chemical	Health Advisory Value (ppt)	Minimum Reporting Level (ppt)
PFOA	0.004 (Interim)	4
PFOS	0.02 (Interim)	4
GenX Chemicals	10 (Final)	5
PFBS	2,000 (Final)	3

EPA United States Environmental Protection Agency   Office of Water

(EPA,   2023).

Table 3: PFAS Clinical Management Recommendations

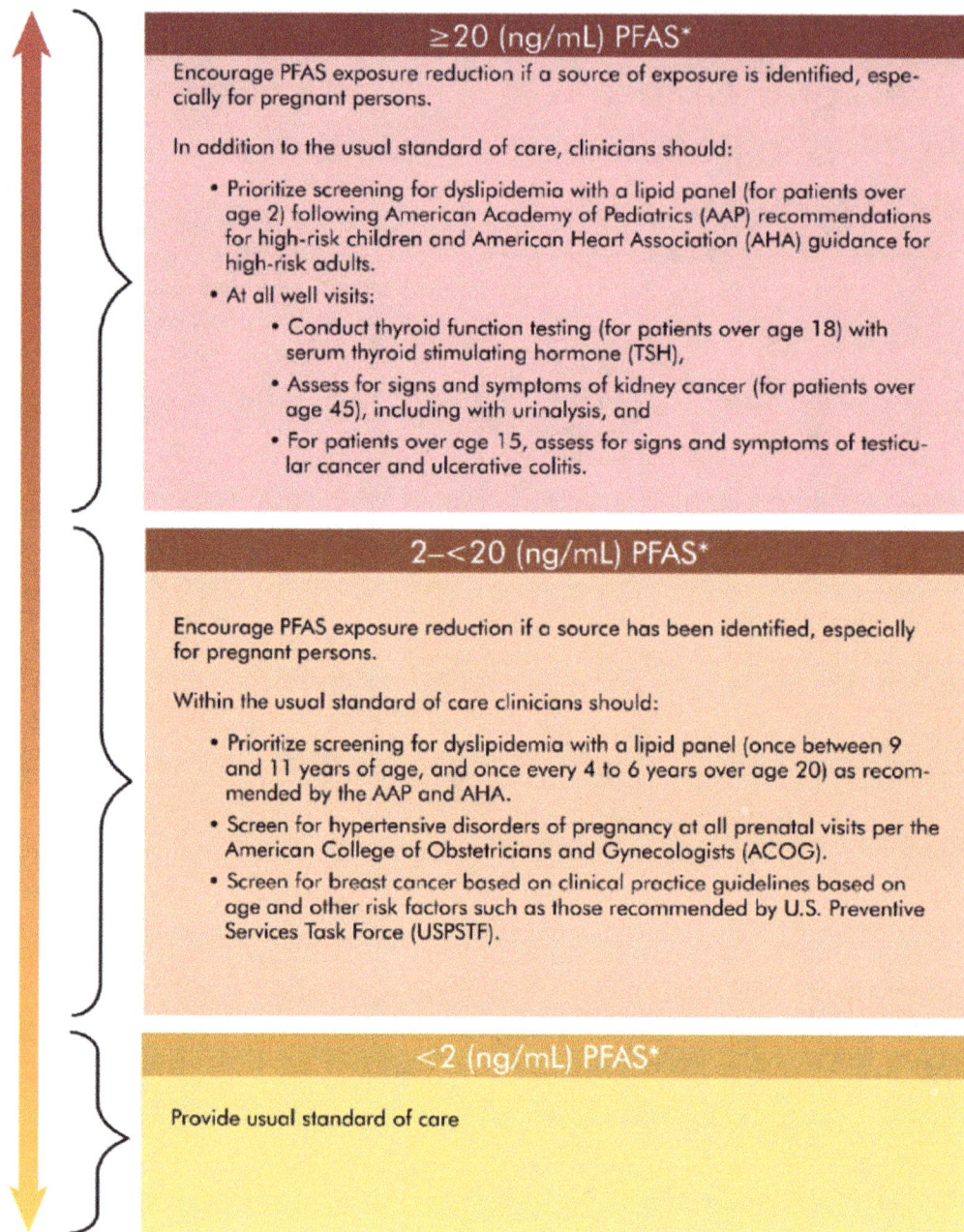

≥20 (ng/mL) PFAS*

Encourage PFAS exposure reduction if a source of exposure is identified, especially for pregnant persons.

In addition to the usual standard of care, clinicians should:

- Prioritize screening for dyslipidemia with a lipid panel (for patients over age 2) following American Academy of Pediatrics (AAP) recommendations for high-risk children and American Heart Association (AHA) guidance for high-risk adults.
- At all well visits:
  - Conduct thyroid function testing (for patients over age 18) with serum thyroid stimulating hormone (TSH),
  - Assess for signs and symptoms of kidney cancer (for patients over age 45), including with urinalysis, and
  - For patients over age 15, assess for signs and symptoms of testicular cancer and ulcerative colitis.

2–<20 (ng/mL) PFAS*

Encourage PFAS exposure reduction if a source has been identified, especially for pregnant persons.

Within the usual standard of care clinicians should:

- Prioritize screening for dyslipidemia with a lipid panel (once between 9 and 11 years of age, and once every 4 to 6 years over age 20) as recommended by the AAP and AHA.
- Screen for hypertensive disorders of pregnancy at all prenatal visits per the American College of Obstetricians and Gynecologists (ACOG).
- Screen for breast cancer based on clinical practice guidelines based on age and other risk factors such as those recommended by U.S. Preventive Services Task Force (USPSTF).

<2 (ng/mL) PFAS*

Provide usual standard of care

* Simple additive sum of MeFOSAA, PFHxS, PFOA (linear and branched isomers), PFDA, PFUnDA, PFOS (linear and branched isomers), and PFNA in serum or plasma

(NASEM, 2022) Reproduced as part of the public domain.

the body. Since there currently is no established blood level range of PFAS, the tests cannot predict past or future health problems. Most laboratories do not have testing methods for PFAS, however, a growing number of laboratories can offer these tests (See Appendix A).

Another option is an online tool offered by CDC/ATSDR that estimates blood PFAS levels. It requires information such as current levels of PFAS in drinking water, which can be obtained from the annual drinking water report for public drinking water systems. Citizens with well water can contact their local public health department for information on how to get their water tested available at:

https://www.atsdr.cdc.gov/pfas/bloodlevelestimator/index.html

Additional PFAS information can be found by contacting your local Pediatric Environmental Health Specialty Unit (PEHSU). Dedicated to educating health professionals and the general public about reproductive and children's environmental health issues, the federally funded PEHSU national network offers fact sheets, webinars, and lectures to discuss emerging research and assist in translating findings to clinical practice and public health protections (www.pehsu.net).

PREVENTING EXPOSURES

Since there is no known treatment once exposure occurs, prevention of exposures is critical. In the absence of federal regulation, clinicians can provide pregnant people and families with resources and several strategies for reducing exposures including:

- Water filtration of contaminated water sources by using granulated activated carbon (GAC) and/or reverse osmosis (RO). NSF updates a list of home water filtration systems that will remove some PFAS chemicals available at: https://www.nsf.org/consumer-resources/articles/home-water-treatment.

- Dust control in the home (including wet mopping, wet dusting, and vacuuming) to reduce exposure from PFAS-contaminated dust.

- Avoid purchasing and using products with PFAS such as non-stick pans, waterproof garments, and stain-resistant carpet.

- Check local fish and wildlife advisories in your community.

LOOKING FORWARD

The CDC/ATSDR measures PFAS as part of its national biomonitoring program. They also launched a nationwide multi-site risk assessment to expand the science about the relationships between PFAS exposure near current or former military installations (CDC, 2023a) and conducted a multi-site study on the human health effects of exposures to PFAS through drinking water (CDC, 2023b). See Appendix B for information about the Exposure Assessments. Findings from the exposure assessment can be found at: https://www.atsdr.cdc.gov/pfas/activities/assessments/final-report.html.

The goal of the Multi-Site Study project (MSS) conducted by CDC/ATSDR is to learn more about the relationship between PFAS exposure and health outcomes among differing populations (See Appendix C). These findings can be used to advance the science and help health professionals to address health issues in individuals, families, and communities impacted by PFAS. At this time, the MSS is still in progress and results have not been published.

While research continues to emerge on health outcomes associated with PFAS exposure, the PEHSU national network is working closely with CDC/ATSDR to provide the most up-to-date information to guide clinicians' practice and protect the public's health (www.pehsu.net). Ultimately, a healthy public policy that regulates PFAS is needed to reduce exposures and health impacts negatively impacting children, families, and communities.

APPENDIX A

Laboratories capable of processing individual clinical serum samples collected by health care providers include:

- Eurofins

  https://www.eurofinsus.com/environment-testing/pfas-testing/services/blood-and-serum/

- AXYS Analytical

  https://www.sgsaxys.com/sampling-analysis/pfas/

- Quest Diagnostics

  https://testdirectory.questdiagnostics.com/test/test-detail/39307/perfluoroalkyl-substances-pfas-serumplasma?cc=SEA&q=PFAS

- Vista Analytical www.vistaanalytical.com

- NMS www.nmslabs.com

Note: Billing code for blood draw is 83921; CPT code 82542

APPENDIX B

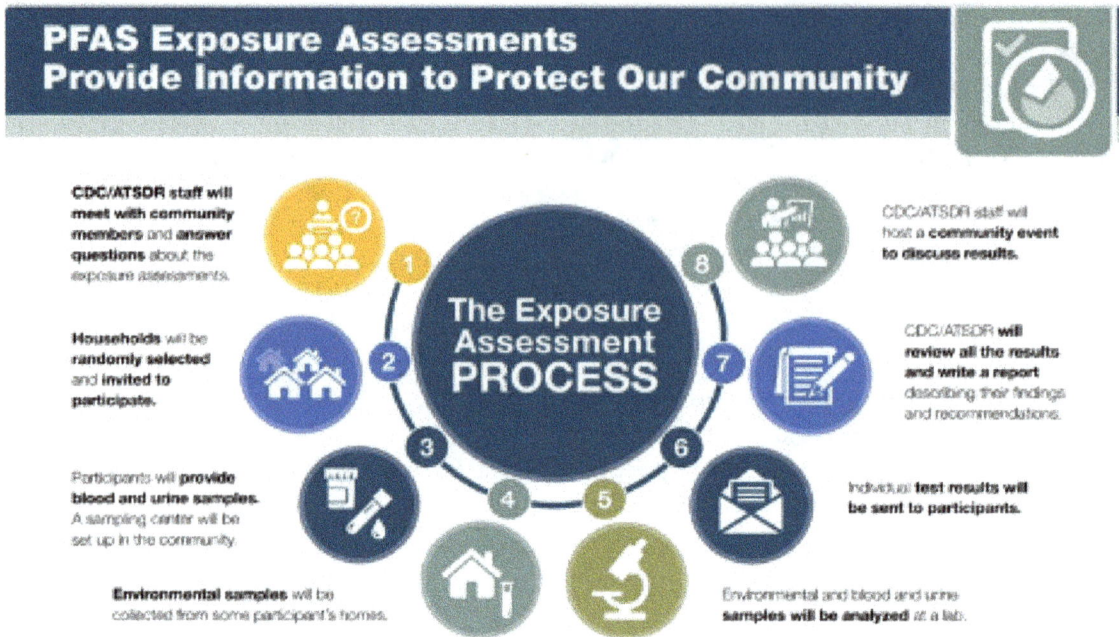

(ATSDR, 2023) https://www.atsdr.cdc.gov/pfas/docs/PFAS-EA-Factsheet-508.pdf Reproduced as part of the public domain.

APPENDIX C

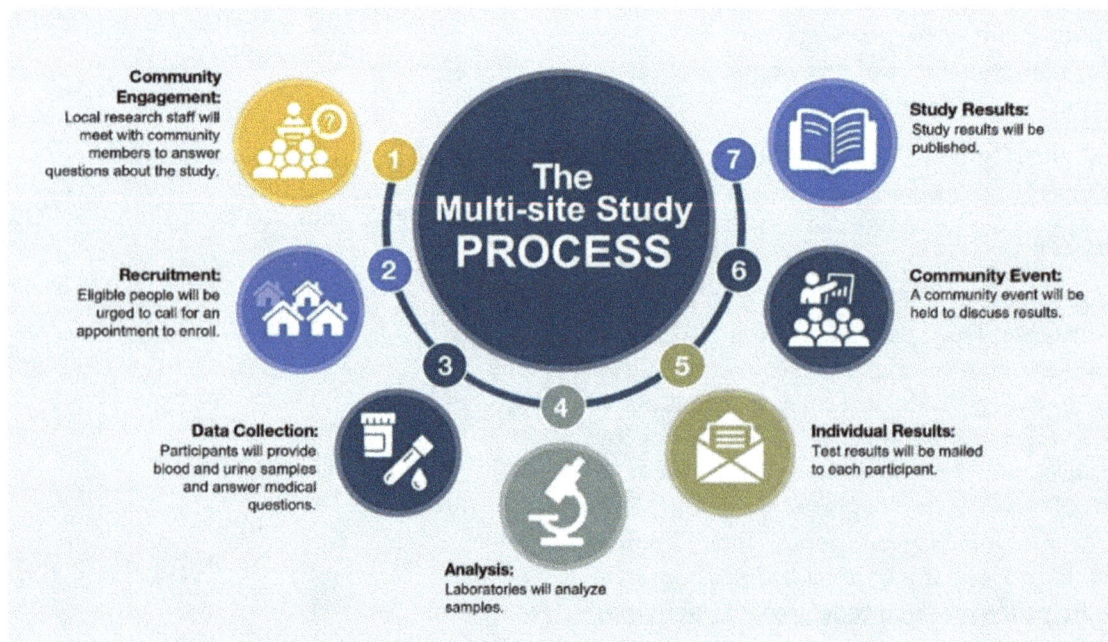

(ATSDR, 2023) https://www.atsdr.cdc.gov/pfas/activities/studies/multi-site.html#about Rreproduced as part of the public domain.

REFERENCES

Agency for Toxic Substances and Disease Registry (ATSDR). (2020). *ToxGuide for Perfluoroalkyls*. U.S. Department of Health and Human Services, Public Health Service. https://www.atsdr.cdc.gov/toxguides/toxguide-200.pdf

Agency for Toxic Substances and Disease Registry (ATSDR) (2023a). *PFAS and your health*. https://www.atsdr.cdc.gov/pfas/health-effects/exposure.html

Agency for Toxic Substances and Disease Registry (ATSDR). (2023b). *PFAS in the US population*. U.S. Department of Health and Human Services, Public Health Service. https://www.atsdr.cdc.gov/pfas/health-effects/us-population.html

Anderko, L. & Pennea, E. (2020). Exposures to per-and polyfluoroalkyl substances (PFAS): Potential risks to reproductive and children's health, *Current Problems in Pediatric and Adolescent Health Care*, 100760.

Anderko, L., Pennea, E., & Chalupka, S. (2020). Per-and polyfluoroalkyl substances: An emerging contaminant of concern. *Annual Review of Nursing Research*, 38(1), 159-182.

Association of State and Drinking Water Association. (2019). *Per- and polyfluoroalkyl substances (PFAS) and State Drinking Water Program challenges*. www.asdwa.org/wp-content/uploads/2019/04/ASDWA-PFAS-2-Pager-March-2019.pdf

Bartell, S. M., Calafat, A. M., Lyu, C., Kato, K., Ryan, P. B., & Steenland, K. (2010). Rate of decline in serum PFOA concentrations after granular activated carbon filtration at two public water systems in Ohio and West Virginia. *Environmental Health Perspectives*, 118(2), 222–8.

Centers for Disease Control and Prevention (CDC). (2023a). *PFAS exposure assessments*. US Department of Health and Human Services. https://www.atsdr.cdc.gov/pfas/PFAS-Exposure-Assessments.html

Centers for Disease Control and Prevention (CDC). (2023b). *CDC/ATSDR PFAS related activities*. US Department of Health and Human Services. https://www.atsdr.cdc.gov/pfas/related_activities.html#Multi-Site-Health-Study

Environmental Protection Agency (EPA). (2023). *Per- and polyfluoroalkyl substances (PFAS) proposed PFAS National Primary Drinking Water Regulation*. https://www.epa.gov/sdwa/and-polyfluoroalkyl-substances-pfas

Hammel, E., Webster, T. F., Gurney, R., & Heiger-Bernays, W. (2022). Implications of PFAS definitions using fluorinated pharmaceuticals. *iScience*, *25*(4), 104020. https://doi.org/10.1016/j.isci.2022.104020

National Academies of Sciences, Engineering, and Medicine (NASEM). 2022. *Guidance on PFAS exposure, testing, and clinical follow-up*. The National Academies Press. https://doi.org/10.17226/26156

LEAD RISK AND PREVENTION
Lois Wessel, RN, FNP, MS
Instructor
Georgetown University
School of Nursing & Health Studies

Lead, a toxic metal, is found in air, soil, dust, water and consumer products. For many years, its uses in household plumbing, and paint, as well as gasoline, were sources of human exposure. The declining lead levels in children since the 1970s, resulting from the use of unleaded gasoline and lead-free paint, form an important public health progress over the last several decades. Ingestion and inhalation form the two primary modes of entry into the body.

Lead exposure can lead to adverse cognitive problems, neurobehavioral issues, poor test scores and Attention Deficit Disorder. In the 1970s, the Surgeon General deemed a serum level of 40 µg/dL as safe (Wessel & Dominski, 1977). As science advanced, blood levels of less than or equal 10 µg/dL was considered an acceptable level. However, in 2012, the Centers for Disease Control and Prevention (CDC) dropped the standard blood level to 5 µg/dL (Raymond, Wheeler, & Brown, 2014). As more evidence becomes available, it is clear that small amounts of lead still pose harm.

Even low lead levels affect IQ, academic achievement and mental and behavioral problems (Hauptman, Bruccoleri & Woof, 2017). While decreases in the acceptable lead level reflect an improved understanding of the consequences of lead exposure, the United States Environmental Protection Agency (EPA) states that there is no safe level of lead exposure. Numerous factors increase a child's likelihood of lead poisoning including normal hand-to-mouth behaviors and an immature blood brain barrier during a period of rapid brain development (Schnur & John, 2014).

While prevalence data by exposure type remains scarce, nursing advocates continue to stress the need to educate consumers and patients regarding unusual sources which plague low income, ethnic minorities, and immigrants disproportionately (Hauptman, Bruccoleri & Woof, 2017). Children of low socioeconomic means may have increased risks of lead poisoning due to poor housing and nutritional deficits, as iron deficiency anemia increases lead absorption through the gastrointestinal track. The New York City Department of Health provides outreach to clinicians and patient education materials regarding common potential lead sources in the ethnically diverse city, including spices, candies, nuts brought from abroad, health remedies, cosmetics, jewelry, and toys (Hore,

Ahmed, Nagin & Clark, 2014). A convenience sample in the United States of Afghani eye liner products (also called Surma or Kohl), used on children to ward off evil, showed that 70% of the samples contained lead (McMichael & Stoff, 2018). Researchers in India found out of 97 random toys selected to assess for lead, 22 samples showed levels above the permissible rate (Dutta, et al., 2016). Forbes magazine investigated the lack of regulations on permissible lead levels in shooting ranges and military facilities where lead bullet dust on clothing led to cases of elevated levels in adults and subsequently in their infant children inhaling the dust from the parents' clothing (MacBride, 2018). The concept of take-home lead, a term from the National Institute for Occupational Safety and Health (NIOSH), includes lead brought into the home from building renovations, scrap metal work, recycling, and shooting range work (Hauptman, Bruccoleri, & Woof, 2017). Researchers in China identified numerous folk and herbal medications as a source of childhood lead poisoning (Ying, Markowitz & Yan, 2018).

Lead also produces long-term social and economic costs to society. A study by Columbia University's Mailman School of Public Health on the lead crisis in Flint, Michigan, reported that the social cost of lead poisoning is valued over $400 million (Muennig, 2016) and that high lead levels costs to society include lower economic productivity, dependence on welfare programs and costs to the criminal justice system due to neurological problems leading to aggression and violence that can occur as poisoned children mature into adulthood. Additionally, young men jailed for juvenile delinquency issues show higher lead levels than other men in their same neighborhoods (Landrigan & Landrigan, 2018). Lead-exposed children require an estimated $5600 in medical and special health services (Hauptman, Bruccoleri & Woolf, 2017)

Therefore, recognizing potential sources of lead risk allows for interventions to prevent lead exposure before they occur as a primary prevention strategy, as well as potentially making an impact on disparities in lead poisoning cases. Lead risk assessment screening questionnaires help nurses identify potential lead sources in a patient's environment and most state health departments can provide them to nurses. Increasingly, electronic health records (EHRs) are adopting these screening questions as part of routine history and physicals for children.

EXPOSURE SOURCES: THE ROLE OF NURSES

Lead screening tests focus on secondary prevention in that they identify lead exposure hopefully before it manifests to a problem. However, given that there is no known safe level and the risk of extreme toxicity of lead exposure, nurses can reframe the issue with a primary prevention approach. This focus should be on regulation and legislation to prevent lead in the environment, as well as patient education on potential exposure sources. The most common source of lead exposure in the US is attributed to paint exposure, but numerous other sources exist and should be part of preventive education.

Household exposures: Windows, walls and door frames, as well as old painted furniture, are potential exposure sites for children in the home setting. Additionally, remodeling and home construction can stir up lead in the home. Most homes built prior to 1978 contain lead paint and nurses should discuss this with patients and offer prevention methods for families at risk of lead exposure. Flaking and peeling paint are potential exposure sources for children and if noted, should be addressed by homeowners and landlords.

Water Systems: Lead in water systems is most likely caused by lead service lines or lead solder, both banned in 1986. Many communities coat lead pipes with biofilms to keep the lead pipes from contact with the water and sometimes additional chemicals need to be added to protect this film. This important step was missing in Flint, Michigan, thus causing numerous cases of lead poisoning in 2014. Local and state health and water officials must inform consumers about lead issues in public water sources. Nationally, lead in public drinking water is regulated under the Clean Drinking Water Act. Lead can be eliminated in water by running cold water to flush the lines when it has been sitting in the pipes all day.

Cosmetics: Traditional eye make-up and other cosmetics manufactured in Asia, the Middle East, and Africa have been reported to contain lead. Known as khol, kajal, tiro or surma in different countries, the practice of putting on eyeliner is thought to protect the eyes and ward off evil in several countries (McMichael & Stoff, 2018). Yet, this practice can result in lead absorption through the conjunctiva. In the US, this problem shows up mostly in newly arrived refugee children and thus, the CDC recommends that all refugee children in the US ages 6 months-16 years be screened upon arrival and six months later, as outlined in a tool kit focusing on lead poisoning prevention for newly arrived refugee children. Nurses can raise awareness about this potential source of

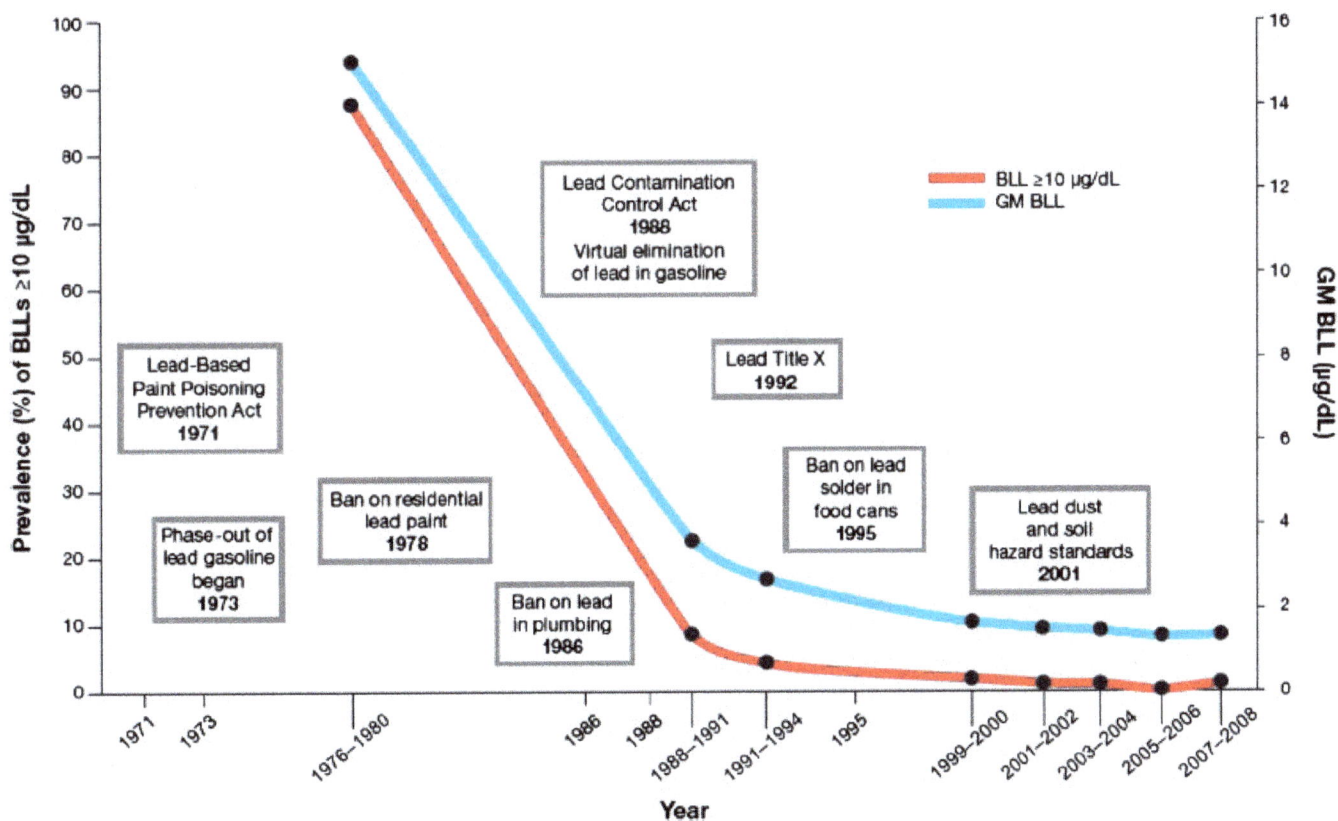

Table I: Lead Levels and Legislation to Reduce Lead in the Environment

lead exposure and discuss lead-free alternative products to families engaging in this cultural practice.

Occupational/Recreational exposures: Lead ammunition continues to be used for hunting and shooting. Lead poisoning from game hunted with lead ammunition posed a threat to those eating the meat (Arnemo, et al, 2016). Nontoxic shot has been required nationally in the US, though it is rarely enforced. Furthermore, military and police personnel as well as staff in shooting ranges, may be exposed to lead dust through their activities involving lead bullets. Lead dust on their clothing has been shown to lead to elevated lead levels in their children, due to inhalation (Gorospe& Gerstenberger, 2008). In a study of lead contamination among construction workers, researchers found that children of lead-exposed construction workers were six times more likely to have blood lead levels over the recommended limit than children whose parents did not work in lead-related industries (Whelan, 1997). This study indicates the importance of conducting an occupational history with the parents of pediatric patients and providing appropriate education on prevention of childhood exposure from parents. The Minnesota Department of Health offers guidance on what types of occupations may lead workers to carry lead home with them including battery manufacturing, radiator repair, and home remodeling.

Gardening: Urban soils may be contaminated with lead particles from old homes, proximity to highways, and previous industrial sites. Nurses should encourage that urban gardeners learn the previous use of the site, place garden plots far from wooden homes with peeling paint built prior to 1940 and test the soil for lead and other toxicants before planting. Food should not be grown in soil over 400 ppm. Lead is more likely to be found in leafy green vegetables and root vegetables. Plants in potted receptacles or raised beds with fresh soil are safer options.

Children's Toys, Jewelry, other household items: Imported toys and jewelry made in China and older toys painted with lead paint can contain lead. Children putting toys and other objects in their mouths increases the risk of lead ingestion. Some mini-blinds contain lead, as well. Ceramic and pottery with lead-based glazes can leach into food. Glassware with painted surfaces or leaded crystal are other sources. Families should be counseled to check all dishes, especially those from abroad and antiques, with lead testing kits that are easily available from local hardware stores. A thorough environmental assessment by the nurse can address these potential lead exposures.

Consumables: Candies, spices and herbs from abroad have been associated with high levels of lead. Both the packaging and the product could contain lead particles. Families should be asked about the country of origin of their food sources, as well as the folk remedies used. Local alternatives should be suggested in exchange for goods brought into the country or purchased in local ethnic stores.

Perinatal Exposure: Lead crosses the placenta and has been detected in the fetal brain as early as the first trimester (ACOG, 2012). Elevated lead levels during pregnancy have been associated with preeclampsia, spontaneous abortion, low birthweight, and impaired neurological functioning. Not all pregnant people should be tested for lead exposure, however, risk assessments, such as the one utilized in Illinois provide nurses with an overview of potential exposure sources and blood testing should be performed if a single risk is identified. The lead exposures sources discussed here should all be discussed with the pregnant or preconceptual patients.

According to the CDC, homes with pregnant people where water lead levels exceed 15 ppb should use water filters or bottled water for cooking, drinking, and baby formula. Breast milk is a potential source of lead exposure. Lead is found in breast milk as the result of a current exposure or a past exposure where lead is stored in the bones and leaches out during the breast-feeding process. Mothers with elevated risks should be screened and counseled appropriately if maternal lead levels are high. The CDC offers Guidelines for the Identification and Management of Lead Exposure in Pregnant and Lactating Women. If someone in the home has been identified as having an elevated lead level, the pregnant person should be tested.

LEAD TESTING

The only way to know if a child has been exposed to lead is through blood testing. This is particularly important for children ages 1 to 3 both because of brain development and normal hand-to-mouth developmental processes occurring at that age. Universal lead screening guidelines recommend testing all children twice before the age of two, generally at 9-12 months and again at 2 years. Previous best practices focus on targeted screening based on year of housing, foreign-born status or Medicaid recipient. Lead screening laws vary by state, but most focus on the idea of "2 by 2" or two screenings by age 2.

Venous lead testing is more accurate than capitally testing, due to potential for contamination from the skin's surface. Elevated capillary blood lead levels are confirmed with follow up venous samples.

NATIONAL SURVEILLANCE

The CDC collects data to understand what areas of the country face continued high exposures to lead. Financial support to states and local governments vary, but nurses should advocate for appropriate lead poisoning data collection, surveillance, case coordination, and remediation in their community.

ASSESSMENT AND MANAGEMENT OF CHILDHOOD LEAD EXPOSURES

Once screening tests indicate an elevated lead level from capillary testing, venous blood samples are used to confirm. Treatment options include identifying lead sources through home assessments and continued testing to assure lead levels are decreasing, notification of the local or state health department, nutritional counseling to treat potential iron deficiency, development and psychological evaluations and interventions, and consultation with specialists if chelation therapy indicated. The state of Maryland has a simple set of guidelines for the assessment and management of childhood lead exposure. The Pediatric Environmental Health Specialty Unit and the American Academy of Clinical Toxicology have a chelation therapy guide for the general public.

PREVENTION STRATEGIES FOR PATIENT EDUCATION

Children with mildly elevated lead levels typically are asymptomatic. Conducting risk assessments regarding potential exposures through screening forms is part of the nursing role. Nutritional assessments are important, as good nutrition can minimize lead absorption. Children with iron and calcium deficiencies are at increased risk for lead poisoning. Nurses working with the childbearing population should assess the country of origin of recent arrivals, due to industrial, and automobile emissions. The location and year of construction of housing should be assessed, as homes near lead mines, and battery recycling plants can put the pregnant person at risk. Pregnant people should avoid living in an older home during renovation or remodeling. Water systems should be checked for lead. Any pregnant person with pica during pregnancy requires testing for lead exposure. Occupational exposure from factory work or exposure to lead bullets should be discussed, as well as potential exposure from hobbies including stained glass work and lead fishing lures. Complementary and alternative medications and herbs pose a risk for lead exposure as well. There is a greater risk of lead exposure from alternative medications and herbs if the product comes from India, Africa, Asia or Latin America.

In addition to the resources listed here, videos in office waiting rooms can provide patients with education on lead poisoning prevention. Be Proactive-Lead Poisoning Prevention PSA is one such resource. Nurses must inform themselves and their communities of the hazards of lead poisoning and ways communities are affected by it through the Public Broadcasting System's Poisoned Water show, focusing on the situation in Flint, Michigan leading up to the recent lead crisis there.

Table 2: Lead Resources

Pediatric Health Specialty Unit (PEHSU) Interpreting and Managing Low Blood Lead Levels	https://envirn.org/documents/PEHSU-interpreting-and-managing-lead-levels.pdf
Agency for Toxic Substances and Disease Registry (ATSDR)	https://www.atsdr.cdc.gov/substances/toxsubstance.asp?toxid=22
Environmental Protection Agency (EPA): Lead	https://www.epa.gov/lead
American Academy of Pediatrics: Lead Exposure and Lead Poisoning	https://www.aap.org/en-us/advocacy-and-policy/aap-health-initiatives/lead-exposure/Pages/default.aspx
Environmental Working Group (EWG): Lead	https://www.ewg.org/key-issues/toxics/lead#.W7ZC_FJRdBw
Centers for Disease Control and Prevention (CDC): Lead	https://www.cdc.gov/nceh/lead/toolstraining.htm

REFERENCES

American College of Obstetricians and Gynecologists (2012). *Lead screening during pregnancy and lactation.* https://www.acog.org/Clinical-Guidance-and-Publications/Committee-Opinions/Committee-on-Obstetric-Practice/Lead-Screening-During-Pregnancy-and-Lactation

Arnemo, J. M., Andersen, O., Stokke, S., Thomas, V. G., Krone, O., Pain, D. J., & Mateo, R. (2016). Health and environmental risks from lead-based ammunition: science versus socio-politics. *EcoHealth, 13*(4), 618-622.

Brown, M. J., Margolis, S., & Centers for Disease Control and Prevention. (2012). *Lead in drinking water and human blood lead levels in the United States.* US Department of Health and Human Services, Centers for Disease Control and Prevention.

Dutta, S., Srivastava, S., Panda, S., Thakur, D., Pokhrel, D., & Venkatesh, T. (2016). Estimation of lead (Pb) in toys using x-ray fluorescence technology. *Journal of Krishna Institute of Medical Sciences (JKIMSU), 5*(1).

Gorospe, E. C., & Gerstenberger, S. L. (2008). Atypical sources of childhood lead poisoning in the United States: a systematic review from 1966–2006. *Clinical Toxicology, 46*(8), 728-737.

Hauptman, M., Bruccoleri, R., & Woolf, A. D. (2017). An update on childhood lead poisoning. *Clinical Pediatric Emergency Medicine, 18*(3), 181-192. doi:10.1016/j.cpem.2017.07.010 [doi]

Hore, P., Ahmed, M., Nagin, D., & Clark, N. (2014). Intervention model for contaminated consumer products: A multifaceted tool for protecting public health. *American Journal of Public Health, 104*(8), 1377-1383. doi:10.2105/AJPH.2014.301912 [doi]

Landrigan, P. J., & Landrigan, M. M. (2018). *Children and Environmental Toxins: What Everyone Needs to Know®.* Oxford University Press.

MacBride, E. (2018, April 26). *Despite evidence, lead standards in shooting ranges haven't been updated since 1978.* Forbes. https://www.forbes.com/sites/elizabethmacbride/2018/04/26/lead-exposure-rules-would-protect-more-than-1m-americans-they-havent-been-updated-since-1978/#5c21b53f6770

McMichael, J. R., & Stoff, B. K. (2018). Surma eye cosmetic in Afghanistan: A potential source of lead toxicity in children. *European Journal of Pediatrics, 177*(2), 265-268. doi:10.1007/s00431-017-3056-z

Muennig, P. (2016). The social costs of lead poisonings. *Health Affairs (Project Hope), 35*(8), 1545. doi:10.1377/hlthaff.2016.0661

Raymond, J., Wheeler, W., & Brown, M. (September 12, 2014). Lead screening and prevalence of blood lead levels in children aged 1–2 years — child blood lead surveillance system, United States, 2002–2010 and National Health and Nutrition Examination Survey, United States, 1999–2010. *Morbidity and Mortality Weekly Report (MMWR), 63*(2), 36-42. doi:https://www.cdc.gov/mmwr/preview/mmwrhtml/su6302a6.htm

Schnur, J., & John, R. M. (2014). Childhood lead poisoning and the new Centers for Disease Control and Prevention guidelines for lead exposure. *Journal of the American Association of Nurse Practitioners, 26*(5), 238-247.

Wessel, M. A., & Dominski, A. (1977). Our children's daily lead: Lead poisoning is a continuing, underestimated, and preventable danger. *Scientific America, 65,* 294-298. doi:http://www.jstor.org/stable/27847839

Whelan, E. A., Piacitelli, G. M., Gerwel, B., Schnorr, T. M., Mueller, C. A., Gittleman, J., & Matte, T. D. (1997). Elevated blood lead levels in children of construction workers. *American Journal of Public Health, 87*(8), 1352-1355.

Ying, X. L., Markowitz, M., & Yan, C. H. (2018). Folk prescription for treating rhinitis as a rare cause of childhood lead poisoning: A case series. *BMC Pediatrics, 18*(1), 219-018-1193-9. doi:10.1186/s12887-018-1193-9

ENVIRONMENTAL NOISE IMPACTS HEALTH AND WELL-BEING

Marjorie McCullagh, PhD, RN, COHN-S, PHNA-BC, FAAOHN, FAAN,
Professor
University of Michigan
School of Nursing

Sally L. Lusk
Collegiate Professor of Nursing
University of Michigan
School of Nursing

Sally Lechlitner Lusk, PhD, RN, FAAOHN, FAAN
Professor Emerita
University of Michigan
School of Nursing

OVERVIEW

Hearing loss is the third most common chronic physical condition in the United States and is twice as prevalent as diabetes or cancer (Blackwell et al., 2014). Although noise is one of the leading causes of hearing loss (Center for Hearing and Communication, n.d.), the debilitating and potentially life-altering effects of environmental noise on health are not limited to hearing loss. They extend to virtually every system of the human body, affecting millions of people annually. Nurses, healthcare workers, and others will recognize the problem of noise as a cause of hearing loss (Humes et al., 2006). Although the relationship between noise and hearing loss is well-recognized, far fewer are aware of the non-auditory effects of noise on health that place a high economic burden on our society, comparable to the economic impact of passive smoking (Basner et al., 2014). On a global level, the World Health Organization conservatively estimates that at least one million healthy years of life are lost every year in western Europe because of traffic-related noise alone (WHO, 2015) (Figure 1).

Similar to other environmental hazards, such as air pollution and hazardous waste, the problem of environmental noise is not evenly distributed across different groups. There is evidence that socially disadvantaged groups such as racial minorities, the poor, and those with lower levels of educational attainment experience the highest levels of exposure. The dual stresses of noise and low socio-economic status represent a double jeopardy for marginalized populations, contributing to observed health disparities across diverse groups in the United States and elsewhere (Casey et al., 2017; Dale et al., 2015; Dreger et al., 2019; Park et al., 2018).

NOISE AND OTOTOXINS: A DANGEROUS COMBINATION

A number of environmental chemicals have toxic effects on the cochlea, vestibula, or auditory nerve, with related negative effects on hearing and balance. These include exposure to tobacco smoke, many industrial solvents, and some medicinal drugs. In a meta-analysis involving 27 studies and 30,000 participants, there was a direct relationship between smoking and hearing loss (Li et al., 2020). Furthermore, smoking is believed to have a synergistic effect on noise and hearing loss (Wang et al., 2017). Drugs that are associated with auditory nerve damage include aspirin (in large doses), nonsteroidal anti-inflammatory drugs (NSAIDS), aminoglycosides (such as gentamicin, streptomycin, and neomycin), diuretics (including furosemide), and cancer chemotherapeutic agents (cyclophosphamide, cisplatin, and bleomycin) (Ganesan et al., 2018). Industrial solvents that are known to have ototoxic effects include toluene, styrene, carbon disulfide, trichloroethylene, and xylene (Hodgkinson & Prasher, 2006). Persons exposed to these chemicals are more likely to experience hearing loss, particularly if they are exposed to hazardous noise.

WHAT IS NOISE?

We commonly refer to any unwanted sound as noise. Noise volume is measured in decibels (dB) and can be determined using a noise level meter or (somewhat less accurately) a smartphone app, such as the NIOSH sound level meter for iPhone (EA LAB, 2016) and the Sound Meter for android, both free. Some common noise levels are illustrated in Figure 2 Noise Thermometer. A person's noise exposure is a function of both noise level (volume) and duration (time exposed). However, a commonly used way to estimate hazardous noise is to apply the following standard: if you need to raise your voice to be heard by a person standing at arm's length from you, then you are in hazardous noise and should use hearing protection or other noise control strategy, such as removing yourself from the source.

Occupational Noise

Occupational sources of noise vary by economic sector and job type, but are particularly problematic in manufacturing, construction, agriculture, and mining. Common noise sources include machinery such as air jets, exhaust fans, compressors, motors, woodworking machines, pneumatic tools (Gerges et al., 2020).

In the US, the National Institute for Occupational Safety and Health has determined that workplace noise exposure at or above 85 decibels is hazardous and should be limited. The US Occupational Safety and Health Administration (OSHA) sets legal limits for workers' exposure to noise and has set a permissible exposure limit (PEL) at 90 decibels for an eight-hour day, while acknowledging that implementation of that standard does not protect 25% of the workers from hearing loss (NIOSH, 1998).

Occupational hearing loss is one of the most prevalent work-related illnesses in the United States. In the US alone, about 22 million workers are exposed to hazardous noise levels at work. Over 30 million US workers are exposed to chemicals, some of which are harmful to the ear (ototoxic) and hazardous to hearing. In addition to damaging workers' quality of life, occupational hearing loss carries a high economic price to society, including lost productivity, medical costs, social isolation, communication difficulties, and stigma (NIOSH, 2018).

Environmental Noise

In contrast with occupational noise exposures, environmental ones are more difficult to measure and quantify due to their multiple sources and variable exposures. These sources include noise from aircraft, road traffic, trains, construction machinery, lawn maintenance equipment, and windmills, as well as from entertainment (concerts and movie theaters) and recreational equipment (motorboats, power water skis, motorcycles, and off-road vehicles). Further, unlike the work setting, there are no standards for acceptable levels of environmental noise exposure, or science-based knowledge regarding the effects of noise on human health at various decibel levels. Little attention has been devoted in the US to attempting to quantify the effects on human health, but with leadership from the World Health Organization, more studies are currently being conducted in Europe. Much more data will be needed to determine "safe" levels of noise exposure.

Although OSHA published a graphic in 1980 depicting the non-auditory stress response effects on the body due to worksite exposure to noise, research was primarily conducted on its effects on hearing (Figure 3). Around the turn of the last century, studies around the world expanded to focus on the non-auditory effects of noise, and on environmental noise sources. These studies found significant effects on body systems, contributing to multiple negative effects on health (Figure 4). There are several reasons why these effects are relatively unknown: (a) the effects slowly build over time; (b) health professionals are not aware of all of these effects so fail to

assess for noise as a contributor to health problems; and (c) while most persons are aware of the effect on hearing, they are not well informed that noise also causes tinnitus, or contributes to many other health problems.

WHAT ARE THE EFFECTS OF NOISE ON HEALTH?

Many of the negative effects of noise on health are believed to be related to stimulation of the human stress response and interference with sleep. Noise initiates a cascade of events that includes the release of stress hormones, which in turn, trigger inflammatory and oxidative stress pathways (Hahad et al., 2019).

In the following pages, selected research studies reporting the adverse effects of noise on health are described (Figure 4). Although many of the effects of noise on health are interrelated, for simplicity, they are discussed separately. For example, the physiological stress response effects, as well as the noise itself, contribute to sleep problems which in turn, contribute to many of the other health problems and diseases.

Cognition/Learning/Memory

Effects of noise on cognition, learning, and memory have primarily been studied in children in school settings, finding learning difficulties, decreased reading skills, and memory for children in noisier environments while controlling for other factors such as intelligence and socioeconomic status. As reported in the analysis by WHO, this results in 45,000 healthy years of life due to the cognitive impairment of children (Figure 1).

Behavior/Performance

As noted above, noise decreases children's school performance, but it also impacts adults' performance and interpersonal behaviors (WHO, 2015). WHO (2015) has documented its effect on negative emotions including anger, dissatisfaction, withdrawal, disappointment, helplessness, depression, anxiety, distraction, agitation, and exhaustion; all of which would affect behavior and performance.

Sleep/Fatigue

Acute and chronic sleep disorders can lead to fatigue, and obvious effects on quality of life. Additionally, sleep problems can lead to changes in insulin and appetite-regulating hormones which in turn contribute to metabolic syndrome and Type 2 diabetes (Hume, 2010; Münzel et al., 2014). As noted in Figure 1, studies by WHO indicated that 903,000 healthy years of life were lost due to sleep disturbance from noise.

Cardiovascular

Noise exposure is linked to multiple diseases that are among the top causes of death (e.g., heart disease, heart attacks, and strokes) in the US and the world. Elevated blood pressure is a well-known contributor to heart disease and stroke (Subramaniam & Lip, 2009). Lusk, et al. (2002 & 2004) reported both a chronic effect and an acute effect of noise exposure on blood pressure as noise levels increased. In meta-analyses of studies, both Babisch (2014) and Vienneau, et al. (2015) found a relationship between road noise and heart disease. Novel experimental studies have revealed oxidative stress-related vascular damage and changes in the genes responsible for vascular function, vascular remodeling and cell death due to noise exposure providing a physiological explanation for increased cardiovascular disease due to noise (Münzel, Schmidt, Steven, Herzog, Daiber, Sørensen, 2018). WHO estimates that 61,000 years of healthy life are lost annually due to ischemic heart disease related to noise (Figure 1). Important to note is a projected reduction in health care costs of 3.9 billion dollars per year in the USA alone with a small reduction on decibel levels! (Swinburn, et al, 2015).

Mental Health/Depression

It should come as no surprise that environmental noise has an effect on mental health and depression, and several studies have found relationships. A very large case-control study involving 77,295 persons with new depression diagnoses over a 5-year period, found increased risk for depression related to aircraft, road traffic, and railway noise. All three sources of noise, and the combined sources, contributed to increasing the odds for a depression diagnosis, with traffic noise the greatest contributor (Seidler et al., 2017).

Figure 1 Noise and Health: By the Numbers

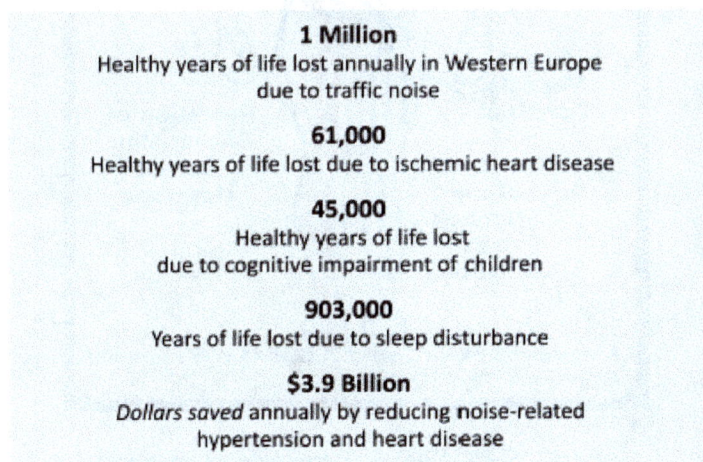

1 Million
Healthy years of life lost annually in Western Europe due to traffic noise

61,000
Healthy years of life lost due to ischemic heart disease

45,000
Healthy years of life lost
due to cognitive impairment of children

903,000
Years of life lost due to sleep disturbance

$3.9 Billion
Dollars saved annually by reducing noise-related hypertension and heart disease

Source: WHO, 2015

Low Birth Weight

An infant weighing less than 2500 g. is considered to be low birth weight (LBW), regardless of gestational age. LBW is the leading cause of infant mortality and contributes to serious morbidity problems such as ophthalmologic, neurologic, cognitive, and pulmonary disorders. This is a major public health problem and care of these infants is very costly. Ristovska, Lazlo, and Hansell (2014) reviewed 23 studies of reproductive outcomes associated with noise exposure. Their conclusions were: (a) although the evidence is sparse, it supports interactions between noise exposure and reproductive outcomes (LBW, preterm birth, spontaneous abortion, and gestation length); (b) of these reproductive outcomes, epidemiological studies have shown very high noise exposure was associated only with LBW; and (c) a hierarchy of biological mediators may create a pregnancy stress syndrome that leads to increased susceptibility for problems in the mother and fetus.

Body Weight

Because obesity contributes to a multitude of health problems, it is a serious public health problem. In a 2015 Swedish study of over 50,000 persons, Pyko et al. (2015) found a significant rise in both waist circumference and waist/hip ratio as decibel levels of noise exposure from road, railway, and aircraft noise increased, with the largest effect from a combination of these sources of noise. These effects remained, even after controlling for the numerous confounders of obesity, such as age, gender, socioeconomic status, and dietary habits. It is of less concern that these changes were not seen for body mass index (BMI), because more recent research has identified problems in using BMI as a measure of obesity, as it is not accurate due to differences in musculature, body type, age, gender, and ethnicity (O'Sullivan, 2020).

Hearing and Tinnitus

Tinnitus may be experienced as ringing, chirping, or other sounds in one or both ears (or in the head) when there is no source of sound in the environment. It often accompanies hearing loss. Tinnitus and hearing loss are prevalent in the U.S., but especially among noise-exposed workers. Particularly affected are workers in agriculture, manufacturing, and construction. Tinnitus can disrupt sleep and concentration, increase fatigue, decrease alertness, erode performance, and potentially increase risks for injuries at work, while driving, and at home. Although many work settings offer programs to reduce noise exposure and associated development of tinnitus, the prevalence of this problem demonstrates the need for increased awareness, and improvised programs and

Figure 2 Noise Thermometer

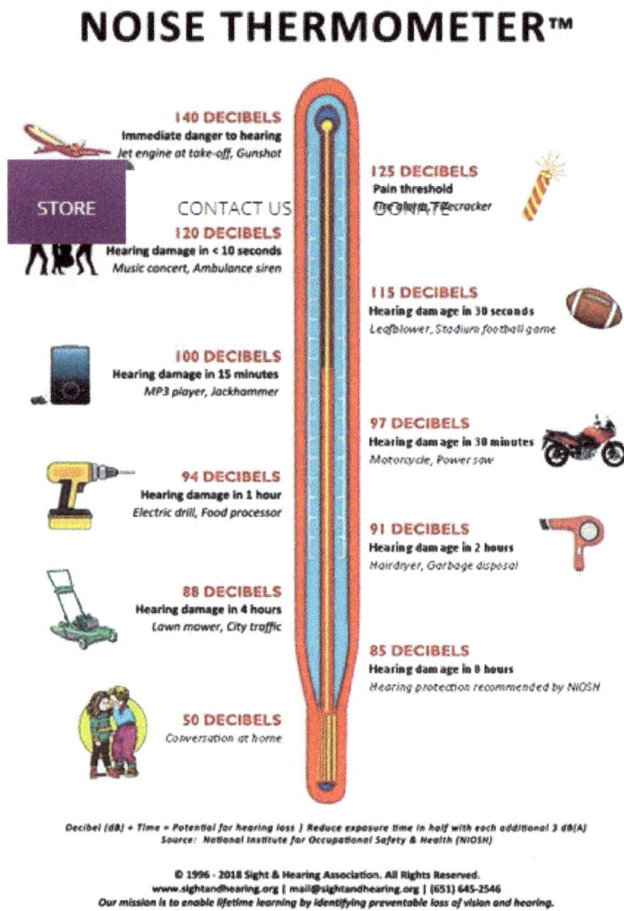

NOISE THERMOMETER™

140 DECIBELS
Immediate danger to hearing
Jet engine at take-off, Gunshot

STORE

CONTACT US

125 DECIBELS
Pain threshold
Fire alarm, Firecracker

120 DECIBELS
Hearing damage in < 10 seconds
Music concert, Ambulance siren

115 DECIBELS
Hearing damage in 30 seconds
Leafblower, Stadium football game

100 DECIBELS
Hearing damage in 15 minutes
MP3 player, Jackhammer

97 DECIBELS
Hearing damage in 30 minutes
Motorcycle, Power saw

94 DECIBELS
Hearing damage in 1 hour
Electric drill, Food processor

91 DECIBELS
Hearing damage in 2 hours
Hairdryer, Garbage disposal

88 DECIBELS
Hearing damage in 4 hours
Lawn mower, City traffic

85 DECIBELS
Hearing damage in 8 hours
Hearing protection recommended by NIOSH

50 DECIBELS
Conversation at home

Decibel (dB) + Time = Potential for hearing loss | Reduce exposure time in half with each additional 3 dB(A)
Source: National Institute for Occupational Safety & Health (NIOSH)

© 1996 - 2018 Sight & Hearing Association. All Rights Reserved.
www.sightandhearing.org | mail@sightandhearing.org | (651) 645-2546
Our mission is to enable lifetime learning by identifying preventable loss of vision and hearing.

Image reproduced with permission.

policies to promote personal and public safety, and quality of life.

More recently, studies have focused not on just the level of environmental noise, but on noise annoyance as a factor influencing health, finding that individuals vary in their response to noise and their level of response affects health issues. For example, Hammersen, et al. (2016), used data obtained from a German national health interview survey of adults (n= 19,294) to measure associations between individual levels of noise annoyance due to noise (road traffic, neighbors, and air traffic) and mental health. While controlling for covariates, they found a more than doubled odds of impaired mental health among those annoyed. This, of course, does not prove causation, but suggests the need for further study.

Other European research has focused on the relationship between well-being and noise exposure. Braubach et al. (2015) studied the effect of traffic noise reduction projects in three cities on perceived well-being. The noise reduction projects in the three cities used different methods to mitigate noise and resulted in marginal, but positive effects on population well-being. While noting the inadequacies of the measures of both noise and well-being, researchers reported that survey data showed that perceptions of high noise levels were associated with lower reported levels of well-being.

Lawton & Fujiwara (2016) obtained records of 24-hour decibel levels of noise at the 17 main airports in England, and using mail codes, correlated the noise data with five subjective measures of well-being collected by the Office of National Statistics. They found that daytime noise, but not nighttime noise, consistently negatively impacted wellbeing, and there was also a marginal effect with each additional decibel of noise. They concluded that the negative effect of living in airport flight paths on overall and momentary wellbeing was equivalent to one-half the negative effect of smoking (Lawton & Fujiwara, 2016).

SUMMARY

Environmental noise is a public health hazard, not merely an annoyance. The impact of noise on health is universal and widespread, and this impact increases health care costs, creating an additional burden on society. As noted

Figure 3 Non-auditory effects of noise

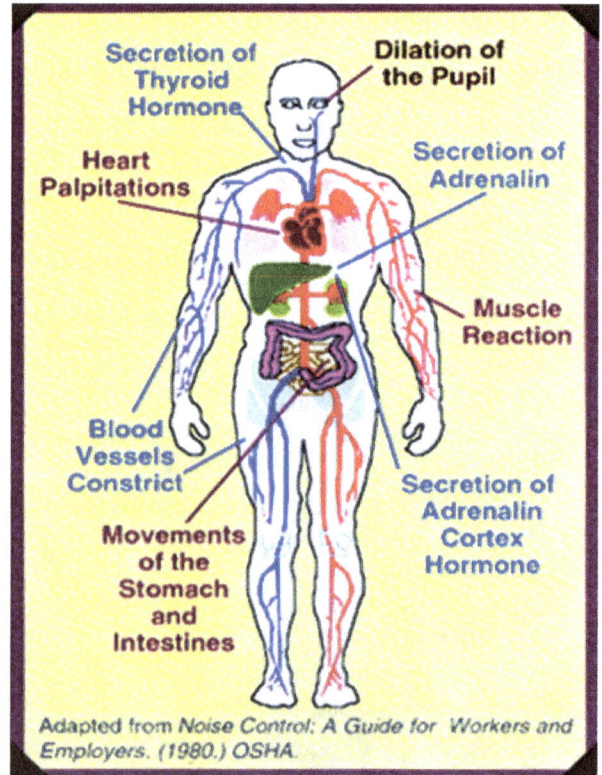

Secretion of Thyroid Hormone

Dilation of the Pupil

Heart Palpitations

Secretion of Adrenalin

Muscle Reaction

Blood Vessels Constrict

Movements of the Stomach and Intestines

Secretion of Adrenalin Cortex Hormone

Adapted from Noise Control: A Guide for Workers and Employers. (1980.) OSHA.

Source: OSHA, 1980. Reproduced as part of the public domain.

above, WHO has supported many studies documenting the effect on healthy life years, validating this impact by association. The seriousness of these associations is well accepted; however, for a number of reasons, it has not been possible to prove causation. These reasons include (a) inadequacies of surveillance and measurement of noise levels and sources; (b) inconsistencies in the measurement of noise exposure (both objective and subjective measures have been recommended by Ristovska et al. (2014); (c) lack of knowledge regarding "safe" levels of noise for the human body; and (d) inability to conduct controlled experimental studies to document causation.

Of critical importance are environmental justice issues when assessing the impact of all these negative health effects noise and the burden of health care costs. Although the authors of the previously described study on depression, Seidler et al. (2017) did not address the issue of socioeconomic status as a factor, their study may well represent an example of environmental justice concerns. Areas of the community where lower income and underrepresented persons reside are also more likely to be those with greater environmental noise. Thus, it is reasonable to assume that this noise exposure contributes to the higher rates of mortality and morbidity in disadvantaged populations. There is a growing body of literature that supports the concept of environmental racism. For example, both polluters and pollution are often disproportionately located in communities of color (Miranda, 2016). Environmental racism can be readily applied to noise pollution of neighborhoods. To achieve health equity, promote health, and prevent disease, environmental noise must be reduced.

CAN NOISE EXPOSURE BE CONTROLLED?

Many people think of using hearing protection as a primary method of protecting themselves from hazardous noise exposure. Actually, the use of hearing protection is the least desirable approach to the problem. Using the NIOSH hierarchy of controls (Figure 5), the most preferred approach is to eliminate the noise source. If elimination is not possible (for occupational or environmental noise), then it may be possible to use engineering controls to isolate people from the noise. Engineering controls might include sound insulation, lubrication, securing loose parts, and other mechanical means of reducing the noise generated or peoples' exposure to it in the occupational setting. Engineering controls for controlling environmental noise exposure may include erecting sound barriers (around highways and airports), adjusting flight patterns (for airport noise), and using electric-powered vehicles (rather than internal combustion engines). Another approach would be to use

Figure 4 Selected Effects of Noise on Auditory and Somatic Health

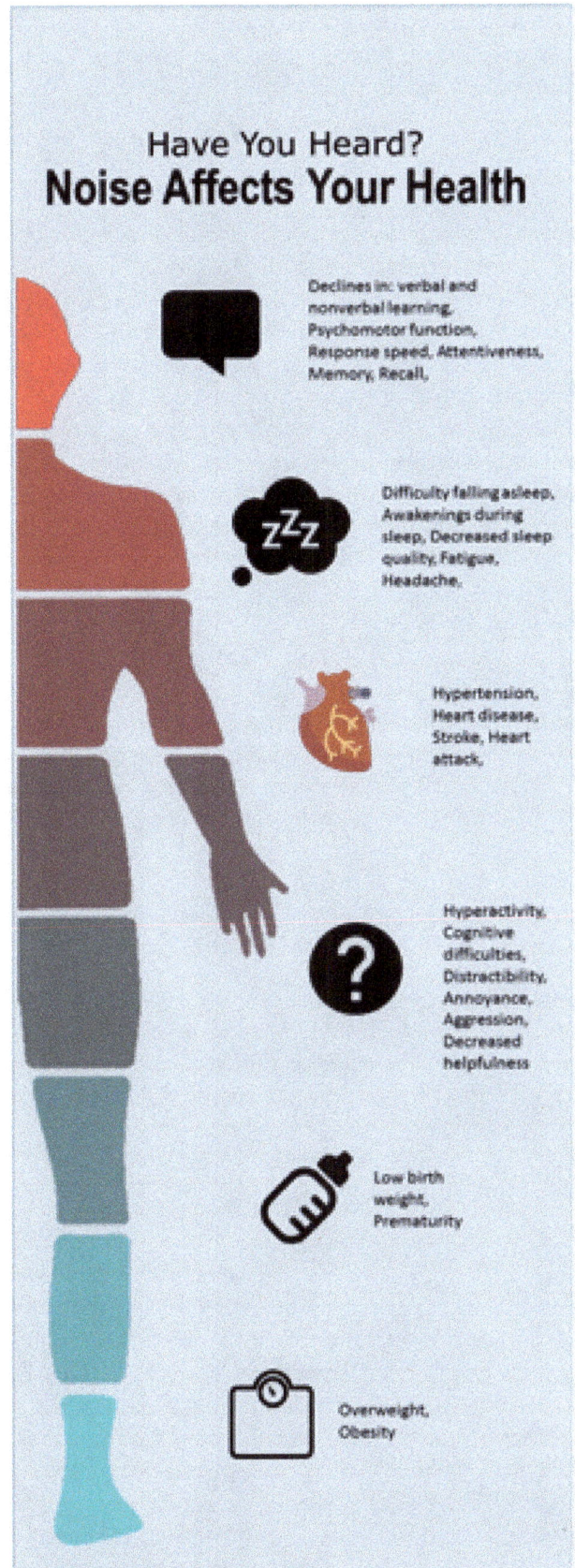

administrative controls, such as relocating workers to a location remote from the hazardous noise. Administrative controls for environmental noise include policy changes (e.g., limiting the use of train horns). Only after these alternative approaches are exhausted is it appropriate to recommend use of personal protective devices to reduce exposures to hazardous noise.

Personal protective devices for noise exposure control are called hearing protection devices (HPDs). Several types are available: roll-down (foam) ear plugs, pre-molded ear plugs, semi-aurals (or canal caps), and muffs. All of these choices are available for purchase in stores and online. Purchase in bulk is more cost-effective. (Some people may also use custom-molded ear plugs.) Selection of hearing protection is highly individual; the best hearing protector is the one that the noise-exposed person will use. Many factors influence personal preference of type of protector, including noise intensity, duration, weather, personal anatomy, exposure to harmful chemicals or animal waste, and type of work. Each type of HPD has its own benefits and drawbacks. For example, some users will find earmuffs easy to apply, and cleaner to use around chemicals, but uncomfortable in warm environments. With the large number of variables, many experts recommend that users purchase a sample package of hearing protection devices and use several types on a trial basis before investing in a larger supply. Since convenience is highly associated with level of use, hearing protectors should be strategically placed near common noise sources and in settings where hearing protectors are supplied by one other than the user, more than one type should be available to enable each worker to select what works best (Lusk et al., 1995).

The effectiveness of ear plugs is highly dependent on their proper insertion. Short videos are available online to guide clinicians in developing this skill and training their clients (3M, 2015). A properly inserted ("fitted") ear plug should be barely visible beyond the tragus of the ear, should offer some resistance to being removed, and should result in the user's voice sounding lower, or more resonant.

Hearing protection devices are labeled for the level of noise that they reduce in a laboratory setting; this rating is called the noise reduction rating (NRR). Although this rating indicates that the device may reduce noise by 20 or more decibels, in field use, users should expect the level of protection to be far less, perhaps as much as 50 percent less. Although some shoppers select HPDs with larger NRR levels, the best hearing protector simply lowers the hazardous noise level down to a safe level (e.g., 84 dB or less), and allows the user to benefit from hearing

desirable sounds, such as voices, warning sounds, and unusual equipment noises. Use of hearing protection is usually not practicable for most environmental noise but is useful when homeowners are exposed to more time-limited sources, such as gas-powered leaf blowers, mowers, and heavy equipment.

HOW CAN HEALTHCARE WORKERS DISPEL MYTHS ABOUT NOISE AND HEARING?

Some people may attribute their hearing loss to age, rather than noise exposure. However, for most people, age-related hearing loss is usually not detectable until after age 60. So most healthy people can expect to keep their good hearing for much of their lives, as long they protect themselves from noise. However, we know that noise-exposed people who do not protect their hearing begin to lose their hearing at an early age (CDC, 2018; McAdams et al., 2011; NIOSH, 2018). For example, farm youth are known to have noise-induced hearing loss by the time they are in high school (Marlenga, 2012).

One factor that sometimes is a barrier to people wearing hearing protection is fear of not hearing warning sounds, like sirens. Failure to react to warning sounds is more often the result of high background noise or severe hearing loss; rarely because of wearing hearing protectors. Most hearing protectors will reduce both the background noise and the warning sound, so the person will hear both sounds (NIOSH, 2018).

Some people are reluctant to wear hearing protection because they fear that it will make hearing equipment noises, warning sounds, and co-workers' voices difficult or impossible to hear. One's hearing protection should lower environmental noise levels, but not eliminate them. However, for workers in settings where hearing certain sounds is particularly important, workers can seek the assistance of an audiologist or safety specialist, who can help select a hearing protection device that will reduce the unwanted frequencies more than the frequencies one needs to hear. Another option is to consider a noise-activated hearing protector that allows normal sounds to pass through the device, and block only the hazardous noise. Musicians can select devices that lower the sound volume, while retaining sound fidelity (NIOSH, 2018).

Some people mistakenly think that if they already have hearing loss, then protecting their hearing is not necessary. However, exposure to loud noise can continue to damage a person's hearing, making communication and other hearing functions even more difficult. Also, the exposure to noise will continue to contribute to the non-auditory (somatic) effects of noise, such as cardiovascular disease (NIOSH, 2018). Reducing noise and the health problems it causes will result in a reduction in disease and health care costs (Swinburn et al., 2015), and improve public health.

WHAT HEALTH POLICIES CAN REDUCE NOISE EXPOSURES?

In recognition of the importance of noise reduction, the federal government enacted two landmark legislations: The Noise Control Act of 1972 and the 1978 Quiet Communities Act. The Office of Noise Abatement and Control (ONAC) in the Environmental Protection Agency was created and charged with coordinating federal noise reduction programs, promoting noise education and research, and assisting state and local noise abatement (Shapiro, 1992). For the first time, this legislation established the primary responsibility for control of noise at the state and local levels. Today, state and local regulations vary widely (FindLaw Attorney Writers, 2018). Additionally, ONAC funding was terminated in 1982, and today there is little action in noise abatement and control (Shapiro, 1992).

Consistent with the WHO guidelines, the United Kingdom and other European countries previously established legislation that requires quieter industrial and household equipment, product labeling for noise levels, and incentives for manufacturers to develop quieter products. In comparison, the US National Institute for Occupational Safety and Health promotes the implementation of Buy Quiet programs that encourage companies to use quieter machinery to reduce worker exposure to noise (CDC, 2014). Although well-intended, these US noise reduction programs are not required by law, creating a need for additional legislation to reduce environmental noise and enhance enforcement in workplaces, the community, and at all levels: local, state, and national. Examples include, but are not limited to, noise surveillance, and development and testing of programs to reduce noise exposure.

As noted in the reports of research regarding the effects of environmental noise exposures, few studies have addressed the differential effects of varying levels of noise and length of the exposures. Although there is debate about whether the standards for occupational noise exposures are stringent enough, some standards do exist. This is not the case for environmental noise. Surveillance to determine the actual level of noise is almost nonexistent, and thus far scientific studies can only report associations between noise of varying levels and health problems. For, example, while multiple studies support the negative health effects of traffic noise, they do not provide enough consistency in types, levels, and duration of the noise to develop specific guidelines. Therefore, even though there is agreement about the deleterious effect of

noise on health, it is not possible to set permissible levels of exposure to prevent health problems.

The WHO is providing direction and leadership in identifying the harmful effects of environmental noise and promoting programs to mitigate its effects. However, in the US, with the defunding of the Office of Noise Abatement and Control (ONAC) at the EPA, there is no organization to lead efforts to reduce environmental noise and its harmful effects on health. In addition to supporting the reestablishment of ONAC, the American Academy of Nursing has indicated its support for:

1. "requiring production and use of quieter equipment and appliances;

2. "implementing measures to reduce airport, railway, and road noise;

3. "enacting legislative restrictions at state and local levels to reduce environmental noise levels, including those at public events" (Lusk et al., 2017, pp. 655).

Further, the Academy has committed to collaborate "with federal agencies, state and federal legislators, and nursing and non-nursing organizations to support the reduction of environmental noise.

Actions that individual nurses can take to influence policy should include:

1. Become an advocate for reducing noise by informing state and local governments about the hazards of noise;

2. Promote local ordinances and their enforcement to reduce noise;

3. Promote state efforts to enact legislation to assist with surveillance of noise sources and remediation programs to reduce it;

4. Inform legislators at all levels of government, and the public, of environmental justice and environmental racism issues associated with environmental noise and its effects on health and disease disparities.

5. Be a resource to US congressional members in promoting federal legislation to address the problems of environmental noise and environmental justice; and

6. Collaborate with relevant groups, for example health professional organizations and societies, National Hearing Conservation Association, American Speech-Language-Hearing Association, and Noisefree America: A Coalition for Quiet.

Figure 5 Hierarchy of Controls

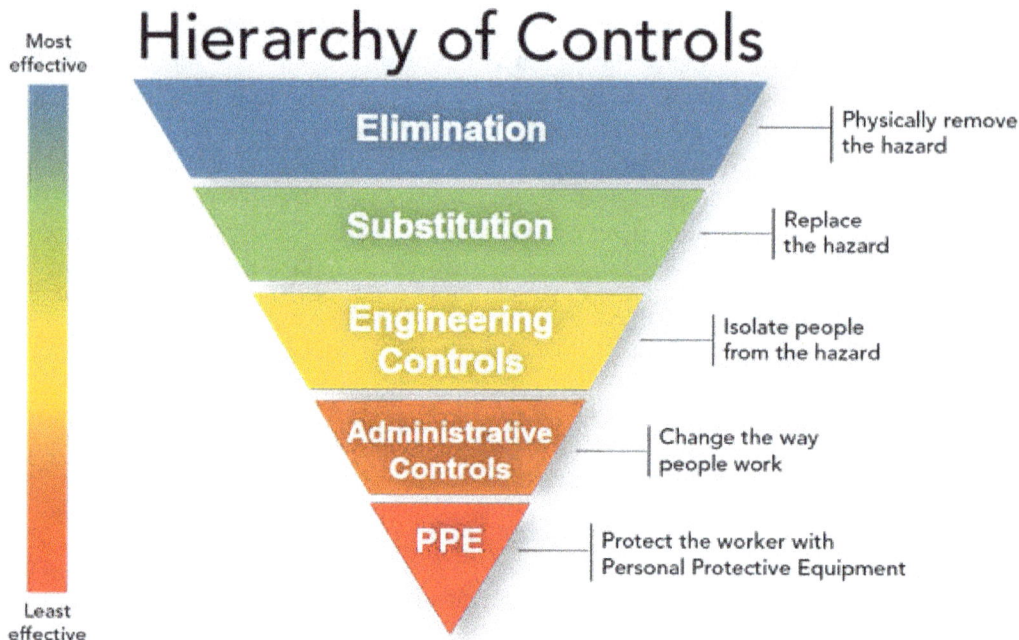

Source: NIOSH, 2018. Reproduced as part of the public domain.

WHAT EDUCATION MEASURES OF HEALTH PROFESSIONALS AND THE PUBLIC CAN REDUCE NOISE EXPOSURES?

Persons who are well-informed about their noise exposures at work, home, school, and in the community are more prepared to protect themselves from the adverse health effects of noise. A few suggestions for health professionals and the public are listed here.

1. Develop and distribute worker and employer education materials specific to the use of engineering controls to reduce noise exposure;

2. Disseminate information regarding risk factors for noise exposure, hearing loss, and other adverse effects of noise exposure to workers, employers, and students;

3. Prepare and distribute resource materials to aid in educating health professionals and the public about the harmful effects of noise exposure, using existing web and other media;

4. Seek opportunities to provide education, guidance, and advice regarding how workers, employers, and students can protect themselves from noise exposure;

5. Collaborate with other professionals, and organizations with common interests to assist in dissemination of information, and promotion of strategies to mitigate noise, e.g., Alliance of Nurses for a Healthy Environment, American Public Health Association, and American Association of Nurse Practitioners; and

6. Ensure that curricula in health professional schools include content on the effects of noise on health and environmental justice issues associated with noise.

HOW CAN CLINICIANS IN PRACTICE REDUCE NOISE EXPOSURES?

Nurses and others can implement evidence-based practice to promote hearing health and prevent the adverse effects of noise on health. Much can be done to help workers, employers, students, and others increase their awareness of hazardous noise in their work and home environments, and in the community. In addition, they can help their clients understand the hazards to their hearing and non-auditory health that noise presents, and promote measures to protect oneself, such as reducing the volume, distancing themselves from noise, and using hearing protection. Nurses in clinical practice can include an assessment of noise exposure and use of protective measures in their routine health assessment procedures. Based on assessment data, nurses can tailor information to clients in meeting their needs to acknowledge their hazardous noise exposures, and implement strategies to reduce noise exposures. One of the most impactful messages that nurses can offer persons exposed to noise is to store hearing protection near commonly-used noise sources, where they can be conveniently accessed when needed (McCullagh & Robertson, 2009). Nurses can work with employers and government agencies to reduce noise exposure and implement effective noise control measures. Nurses and other healthcare workers can contribute to the development of business cases to justify adopting noise control interventions. Furthermore, nurses can work with interdisciplinary teams to develop, test, and promote programs to reduce noise exposures among workers and in communities.

HOW CAN RESEARCH REDUCE NOISE EXPOSURES?

There are many opportunities to develop our understanding of noise and prevention of its negative effects on health. For many workers, industries, and communities, there is a need to identify and inventory sources of noise and ototoxic chemical exposures putting populations at risk for noise-related health problems. Because development of hearing loss and other noise-related health problems have multiple causative and risk factors, there is a need to determine the contribution of individual, behavioral, and exposure factors on the development of these health problems. Employers and communities need to know how to develop and maintain cost-effective interventions (such as engineering controls) to reduce noise exposure, or mitigate its effects. Finally, policy makers and others need information about the effectiveness of individual-, family-, and population-based interventions.

As previously described, researchers have typically used cross-sectional studies and correlational methods to find associations between noise and several health conditions. However, these types of studies are not robust enough to establish a causal relationship between noise and disease. While the associations found in multiple and repeated studies clearly indicate negative effects of noise exposures, more specific information about the types of noise and its sources, as well as the levels at which it causes problems would be useful in designing prevention programs. Knowledge of levels of noise which may be acceptable from a health standpoint, and evaluation of the cost-effectiveness of various mitigation programs will inform the development of related policies and services.

HOW CAN COMMUNITY ACTIONS REDUCE NOISE EXPOSURES?

As concerned citizens and informed health professionals, nurses have a role in influencing noise issues in their communities. Actions include ensuring that local ordinances are promulgated and enforced to reduce environmental noise which may require meeting with city and county officials, police, and legislative bodies. Health professionals have a responsibility to call attention to health disparities and work to alleviate them. Therefore, it is critical to address environmental justice and environmental racism issues in relation to noise exposures.

REFERENCES

3M. (2015). *How to fit your 3M roll down earplugs* [Video]. YouTube. https://www.youtube.com/watch?v=kMMHudYoQ40

Babisch, W. (2014). Updated exposure-response relationship between road traffic noise and coronary heart diseases: A meta-analysis. *Noise and Health, 16*(68), 1-9.

Basner, M., Babisch, W., Davis, A., Brink, M., Clark, C., Janssen, S., & Stansfeld, S. (2014). Auditory and non-auditory effects of noise on health. *Lancet, 383*(9925), 1325–1332. https://doi.org/10.1016/S0140-6736(13)61613-X

Blackwell, D. L., Lucas, J. W., & Clarke, T. C. (2014). *Summary health statistics for US adults: National Health Interview Survey, 2012. (Issue Vital health statistics series 10, 260).* Centers for Disease Control. http://www.cdc.gov/nchs/data/series/sr_10/sr10_260.pdf

Braubach, M., Tobolik, M., Mudu, P., Hiscock, R., Chapizanis, D., Sarigiannis, D. A., Keuken, M., Perez, L., & Martuzzi, M. (2015). Development of a quantitative methodology to assess the impacts of urban transport interventions and related noise on well-being. *International Journal of Environmental Research and Public Health, 12*(6), 5792-5814. doi: 10.3390/ijerph120605792

Bravo, M. A., Anthopolos, R., Bell, M. L., & Miranda, M. L. (2016). Racial isolation and exposure to airborne particulate matter and ozone in understudied US populations: Environmental justice applications of downscaled numerical model output. *Environmental International, 92-93,* 247-255. https://doi.org/10.1016/j.envint.2016.04.008

Casey, J. A., Morello-Frosch, R., Mennitt, D. J., Fristrup, K., Ogburn, E. L., & James, P. (2017). Race/ethnicity, socioeconomic status, residential segregation, and spatial variation in noise exposure in the contiguous United States. *Environmental Health Perspectives, 125.* https://doi.org/doi.org/10.1289/EHP898

CDC. (2014). *Buy Quiet. CDC/NIOSH Buy Quiet.* https://www.cdc.gov/niosh/topics/buyquiet/default.html#:~:text=Buy

CDC. (2018). *Noise and hearing loss prevention.* https://www.cdc.gov/niosh/topics/noise/reducenoiseexposure/noisecontrols.html

Center for Hearing and Communication, (n.d.). *Statistics and facts about hearing loss.* https://chchearing.org/facts-about-hearing-loss/

Dale, L. M., Goudreau, S., Perron, S., Ragettli, M. S., Hatzopoulou, M., & Smargiassi, A. (2015). Socioeconomic status and environmental noise exposure in Montreal, Canada. *BMC Public Health, 15,* 205. https://doi.org/10.1186/s12889-015-1571-2

Dreger, S., Schule, S. A., Hilz, L. K., & Bolt, G. (2019). Social inequalities in environmental noise exposure: A review of evidence in the WHO European region. *International Journal of Environmental Research and Public Health, 16,* 1011.

EA LAB. (2016). *NIOSH Sound Level Meter (Version 1.2.1)* [Mobile App]. Apple Store. https://apps.apple.com/us/app/niosh-sound-level-meter/id1096545820

FindLaw Attorney Writers. (2018, Jan 30). *Guidelines for Drafting Municipal Noise Control Ordinances. FindLaw for Legal Professionals.* https://corporate.findlaw.com/law-library/guidelines-for-drafting-municipal-noise-control-ordinances.html

Ganesan, P., Schmiedge, J., Manchaiah, V., Swapna, S., Dhandayutham, S., & Kothandaraman, P. P. (2018). Ototoxicity: A challenge in diagnosis and treatment. *Journal of Audiology & Otology, 22*(2), 59–68. https://www.ncbi.nlm.nih.gov/pmc/articles/PMC5894487/pdf/jao-2017-00360.pdf

Gerges, S., Sehrndt, G. A., & Parthey, W. (2020). Noise Sources. In Goelzer, B., Hansen, C. H., & Sehrndt, G. A. (Eds.), *Occupational exposure to noise: evaluation, prevention and control (pp. 103–124).* https://www.who.int/occupational_health/publications/noise5.pdf?ua=1

Hahad, O., Prochaska, J. H., Daiber, A., & Münzel, T. (2019). Environmental noise-induced effects on stress hormones, oxidative stress, and vascular dysfunction: Key factors in the relationship between cerebrocardiovascular and psychological disorders. *Oxidative Medicine and Cellular Longevity.* https://doi.org/10.1155/2019/4623109

Hammersen, F., Niemann, H., & Hoebel, J. (2016). Environmental noise annoyance and mental health in adults: Findings from the Cross-Sectional German Health Update (GEDA) *Study. International Journal of Environmental Research and Public Health, 13,* 954. doi: 10.3390/ijerph13100954

Hodgkinson, L., & Prasher, D. (2006). Effects of industrial solvents on hearing and balance: A review. *Noise and Health, 8,* 114–133.

Hume, K. (2010). Sleep disturbance due to noise: Current issues and future research. *Noise and Health, 12*(47), 70–76.

Humes, L. E., Joellenbeck, L. M., & Durch, J. S. (2006). *Noise and Military Service: Implications for Hearing Loss and Tinnitus.* https://doi.org/https://doi.org/10.17226/11443

Lawton, R. N., & Fujiwara, D. (2016). Living with aircraft noise: Airport proximity, aviation noise and subjective wellbeing in England. *Transportation Research, 42,* 104–118.

LeBron, A. M. W., Torres, I. R., Valencia, E., Dominguez, M. L., Garcia-Sanchez, D. G., Logue, M.D., & Wu. J. (2019). The state of public health lead policies: Implications for urban health inequities and recommendations for health equity. *International Journal of Environmental Research and Public Health, 16*(6), 1604. doi: 10.3390/ijerph16061064

Li, X., Rong, X., & Lin, A. (2020). Association between smoking and noise-induced hearing loss: A meta-analysis of observational studies. *Journal of Environmental Research and Public Health, 17*(4), 1201. https://doi.org/10.3390/ijerph17041201

Lusk, S. L., Eakin, B. L., Kazanis, A. S., McCullagh, M. C. (2004). Effects of booster interventions on factory workers' use of hearing protection. *Nursing Research, 53*(1), 53-58.

Lusk, S. L., Hagerty, B., Gillespie, B., & Caruso, C. C. (2002). Chronic effects of workplace noise on blood pressure and heart rate. *Archives of Environmental Health, 57*(4), 273-281.

Lusk, S. L., McCullagh, M. C., Dickson, V. V, & Xu, J. (2017). Reduce noise: Improve the Nation's health. *Nursing Outlook, 65*(5), 652–656. https://doi.org/org/10.1016/j.outlook.2017.08.001

Lusk, S. L., Ronis, D. L., & Kerr, M. J. (1995). Predictors of hearing protection use among workers: Implications for training programs. *Human Factors, 37*(3), 635–640.

Marlenga, B., Berg, R. L., Linneman, J. G., Wood, D. J., Kirkhorn, S. R., Pickett, W. (2012). Determinants of early-stage hearing loss among a cohort of young workers with 16-year follow-up. *Occupational and Environmental Medicine, 69,* 479-484. doi:10.1136/oemed-2011-100464

McAdams, M. T., Kerwin, J. J., Olivo, V., & Goksel, H. A. (2011). *National Assessment of the Occupational Safety and Health Workforce (Issues 200-2000–08017, Task Order 18).* http://www.cdc.gov/niosh/oshworkforce/pdfs/NASHW_Final_Report.pdf

McCullagh, M., & Robertson, C. (2009). Too late smart: Farmers' adoption of self-protective behaviors in response to exposure to hazardous noise. AAOHN Journal: Official *Journal of the American Association of Occupational Nurses, 57*(3), 99-105. https://doi.org/10.1177/216507990905700304

Münzel, T., Schmidt, F.P., Steven, S., Herzog, J., Daiber, A.,& Sørensen, M. (2018). Environmental noise and the cardiovascular system. *Journal of American College of Cardiology, 71*(6):688–697.

Münzel, T., Gori, T., Babisch, W., & Basner, M. (2014). Cardiovascular effects of environmental noise exposure. *European Heart Journal, 35*(13), 829–836. https://doi.org/ http://dx.doi.org/10.1093/eurheartj/ehu030

NIOSH. (1998). *Criteria for a Recommended Standard: Occupational Noise Exposure (NIOSH Publication No. 98-126).*

NIOSH. (2018). *Noise and Hearing Loss Prevention.* https:// www.cdc.gov/niosh/topics/noise/faq.html

O'Sullivan, S. (2020). *BMI Can't Tell The Full Story Of A Person's Health, So Why Are We Still Using It?* Refinery 21. https://www.refinery29.com/en-gb/problem-with-bmi

Park, C., Sim, C. S., Sung, J. H., Lee, J., Ahn, J. H., Choe, Y. M., & Park, J. (2018). Low income as a vulnerable factor to the effect of noise on insomnia. *Psychiatry Investigations, 15*(6), 602–612. https://doi.org/10.30773/pi.2018.01.14

Ristovska, G., Laszlo, H. E., & Hansell, A. L. (2014). Reproductive outcomes associated with noise exposure - A systematic review of the literature. *International Journal of Environmental Research and Public Health, 11*(8), 7931-7952.

Seidler, A., Hegewalda, J., Seidlera, A. L., Schuberta, M., Wagnera, M., Drögea, P., Haufea, E., Schmitta, J., Swartc, E., & Zeebd, H. (2017). Association between aircraft, road and railway traffic noise and depression in a large case-control study based on secondary data. *Environmental Research, 152,* 263–271. https://doi.org/https://doi.org/10.1016/ j.envres.2016.10.017

Shapiro, S. A. (1992). Lessons from a public policy failure: EPA and noise abatement. *Ecology Law Quarterly, 19*(1), 1–61. https://doi.org/10.15779/Z384N9B

Subramaniam, V., & Lip, G. Y. (2009). Hypertension to heart failure: A pathophysiological spectrum relating blood pressure, drug treatments and stroke. *Expert Review of Cardiovascular Therapy, 7*(6), 703–713. https://doi.org/ doi:10.1586/erc.09.43

Swinburn, T. K., Hammer, M. S., & Neitzel, R. L. (2015). Valuing quiet: An economic assessment of US environmental noise as a cardiovascular health hazard. *American Journal of Preventive Medicine, 49*(3), 345–353. https://doi.org/10.1016/j.amepre.2015.02.016

Vienneau, D., Schindler, C,; Perez, L., Probst-Hensch, N., Röösli, M. (2015). The relationship between transportation noise exposure and ischemic heart disease: A meta- analysis. *Environmental Research, 10*(138), 372-380. doi:10.1016/j.envres.2015.02.023

Villarosa, L. (2020). *Pollution is killing Black Americans: This community fought back.* New York Times Magazine.

Wang, D., Wang, Z., Zhou, M., & Al, E. (2017). The combined effect of cigarette smoking and occupational noise exposure on hearing loss: Evidence from the Dongfeng-Tongji Cohort Study. *Scientific Reports, 7*(1), 11142. https:// doi.org/10.1038/s41598-017-11556-8

World Health Organization (WHO). (2015). *Burden of disease from environmental noise: Quantification of healthy life years lost in Europe.* http://www.who.int/ quantifying_ehimpacts/publications/e94888.pdf?ua=1

INTRODUCTION TO FRACKING AND RENEWABLE ENERGY

Katie Du
Major: Cell Biology Class of 2021
University of Alberta
ANHE Intern

While renewable energy accounted for only 11% of total U.S. primary energy consumption in 2019 by source, petroleum and natural gas has dominated U.S. energy consumption and represents 69% of total primary energy use (U.S. Energy Information Administration, 2020). This is problematic because a widespread method to obtain unconventional natural gas and oil trapped underneath shale rock layers, known as hydraulic fracturing or fracking, is deeply harmful to both the local environment and communities.

Given the numerous health effects with hydraulic fracturing and the influence of fossil fuels on climate change (which is outlined in this chapter), it is important to consider alternative energy sources such as renewable energy. There are many different types of renewable energy, such as wind, solar, geothermal, and hydroelectric. Each of these energy sources has its own advantages and disadvantages.

Wind turbines, which are powered by wind, can generate substantial amounts of electricity without contaminating the air or water, unlike hydraulic fracturing (Office of Energy Efficiency and Renewable Energy, n.d.). Furthermore, since wind is a form of solar energy, evoked by uneven heating across Earth's surface, it is sustainable. Recently, the Biden Administration has supported the development of offshore wind energy off the East Coast (Massachusetts, Rhode Island, New York, and New Jersey) and the Gulf Coast.

Solar energy can also be converted to electricity through technology such as photovoltaic panels. The generated electricity can be stored in batteries which would allow for later use, even in the absence of sunlight. According to the Office of Energy Efficiency and Renewable Energy, if all the sunlight that reached the Earth's surface in an hour and a half could be captured, converted, and stored as useful forms of energy, that would be enough to satisfy the total energy demand across the entire globe for a year (Office of Energy and Efficiency and Renewable Energy, n.d.).

Geothermal energy is another form of clean energy, meaning its extraction does not rely upon the burning of fossil fuels and lead to the emission of greenhouse gases

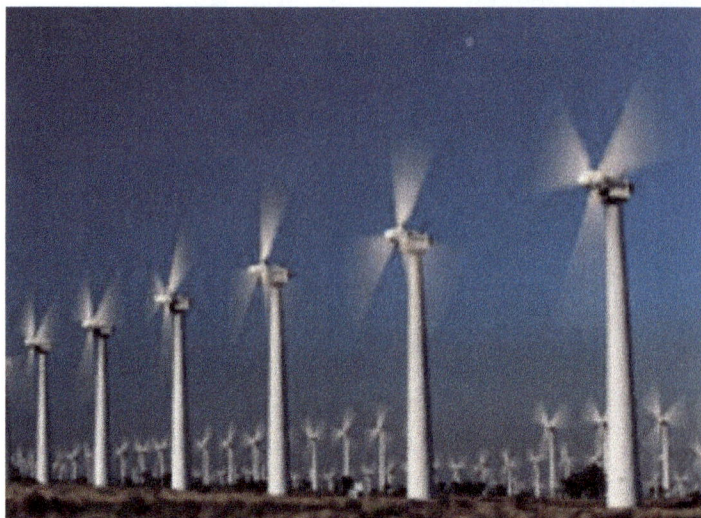

Reprint (Environmental Protection Agency, 2016), reproduced as part of the public domain.

(Office of Energy and Efficiency and Renewable Energy, n.d.). The source of geothermal energy is heat harnessed from natural processes that occur at Earth's core, such as the decay of radioactive isotopes. Hydraulic turbines convert the potential energy of water in motion into mechanical energy, much like wind turbines with moving air.

Overall, renewable energy produces minimal greenhouse gas emissions, and is an avenue that has the potential to diversify energy stores as well as the economy (Environmental Protection Agency, n.d.). For the consumer, renewable energy may also be a cheaper means to achieve household energy demands. According to a New York Times article, solar panels deliver power to homes at $31 to $111 a megawatt-hour compared to natural gas plants which deliver power at $122 to $162 a megawatt-hour (Penn, 2020). There are concerns, however, that renewable energy alone cannot meet the demands due to the current storage issues of renewable energy. This is an area that will require greater investment in renewable energy technology.

Despite the environmental and other benefits associated with transitioning to renewable energy, it is important to acknowledge that there are still environmental concerns. For example, although hydropower does not directly produce carbon emissions, manufacturing the dams required for the process does depend upon machinery which emit pollutants similar to those that are required to maintain a natural gas well. Furthermore, diverting water to a dam may be harmful to local ecosystems. Some have also pointed out that biomass burning plants produce 300% to 400% the carbon dioxide emissions as natural gas plants (Partnership for Policy Integrity, n.d.). Although it is important to note here that approximately equivalent amounts of plant used for fuel would be able to sequester the carbon dioxide they release while burning (U.S. Energy Information Administration, 2020).

This section addresses the fracking process and the associated health risks. Nurses have been involved in educating, researching, and advocating for fracking communities. Additionally, nurses have also advocated for cleaner renewable energy to protect the health of communities and mitigate climate change risks. As more renewable sources are used, studying the impacts of renewable energy on communities and human health is an important for future nursing research.

REFERENCES

American Petroleum Institute. (n.d.). *Marcellus shale.* https://www.api.org/oil-and-natural-gas/energy-primers/hydraulic-fracturing/marcellus-shale

Ezani, E., Masey, N., Gillespie, J., Beattie, T. K., Shipton, Z. K., & Beverland, I. J. (2018). Measurement of diesel combustion-related air pollution downwind of an experimental unconventional natural gas operations site. *Atmospheric Environment, 189,* 30-40. doi:10.1016/j.atmosenv.2018.06.032

Environmental Protection Agency. (2021, February 19). *Local renewable energy benefits and resources.* https://www.epa.gov/statelocalenergy/local-renewable-energy-benefits-and-resources

Partnership for Policy Integrity (n.d.). *Carbon emissions from burning biomass for energy.* https://www.pfpi.net/wp-content/uploads/2011/04/PFPI-biomass-carbon-accounting-overview_April.pdf

Penn, I. (2020, July 6). *The next energy battle: Renewables vs. natural gas.* The New York Times.

U.S. Department of Energy (n.d.). *Advantages and challenges of wind energy.* https://www.energy.gov/eere/wind/advantages-and-challenges-wind-energy

U.S. Department of Energy (n.d.). *Geothermal FAQs.* Retrieved https://www.energy.gov/eere/geothermal/geothermal-faqs#environmental_impacts_of_geothermal_energy

U.S. Department of Energy (n.d.). How does solar work? https://www.energy.gov/eere/solar/how-does-solar-work

U.S. Energy Information Administration - eia - independent statistics and analysis. (2020, May 7). https://www.eia.gov/energyexplained/us-energy-facts/

U.S. Energy Information Administration. (2020, December 9). *EIA independent statistics and analysis.* https://www.eia.gov/energyexplained/biomass/biomass-and-the-environment.php

THE HEALTH IMPACTS OF UNCONVENTIONAL NATURAL GAS DEVELOPMENT

Kelly A. Kuhns, PhD, RN, CNE
Professor and Chair
Millersville University
Department of Nursing

Since the 1990s, unconventional natural gas development (UNGD) activities have increased across the United States. In 2000, there were approximately 26,000 hydraulic fracturing wells in the US and by 2015 there were more than 300,000 (Xu, Zhang, Carrillo, Zhong, Kan, & Zhang, 2019). As of 2019, nearly 18 million Americans live within one mile of an active oil or gas well (Concerned Health Professionals of New York & Physicians for Social Responsibility, 2019). UNGD includes the entire process from choosing the site for the drilling (fracking) to the delivery of the gas to the consumer. Drilling and associated industrial activities are often in close to residential areas including schools, playgrounds, and farms. People living in regions where UNGD is occurring have reported experiencing health effects that they attribute to UNGD activities. The purpose of this chapter is to provide an overview of the process involved in UNGD and the emerging issues related to health and the environment that nurses need to consider when assessing their clients for possible environmental exposures.

OVERVIEW OF THE PROCESS OF UNGD

The process of UNGD includes hydraulic fracturing or fracking. UNGD involves a series of steps and development including 1) building of the well pad and local infrastructure; 2) drilling and construction of the pipelines and other facilities; 3) the actual hydraulic fracturing; 4) the flow back of gas, fluids, and other contaminants; and 5) connection to a system of distribution, such as a pipeline. At each step of this process, there are significant environmental risks and impacts (Adgate, Goldstein, & McKenzie, 2014).

The fracking process begins with dynamite detonations to identify the geological formations under the surface prior to the drilling. The initial drilling is done vertically down to a distance of approximately 8000 feet. After the vertical shaft is completed, horizontal shafts are drilled. Approximately 2-5 million gallons of water mixed with chemicals and propping materials, such as sand, are injected under high pressure down the well and out into the horizontal shafts. The high pressure is needed to create openings, or fractures, in the gas-bearing rock. The propping material enables the fractures in the rock to remain open and provide a way for the trapped gas to

flow out of the horizontal shafts into the well. The released gas that flows into the well also contains wastewater. The wastewater includes the chemical mixture and salts injected into the well, as well as the heavy metals, hydrocarbons, radioactive materials, and other substances from deep under the surface of the earth. At the well, the gas and the wastewater are separated, and the wastewater is stored in open pits or in tanks near the well (Adgate, Goldstein, & McKenzie, 2014). Sometimes the open pits, or impoundments, are lined with black plastic; however, this does not fully prevent leaching of water and chemicals into the surrounding soil. Misters are commonly used in these impoundments to spray the wastewater into the air to aid in evaporation. Any wastewater that remains is moved via tanker trucks to be disposed of in deep injection well sites, often in another state or miles from where the drilling took place. There is a growing body of evidence linking an increase in earthquakes related to fracking, particularly with the disposal of wastewater in deep injection well sites. An estimated 60% of the water injected into the well head during the drilling process will come back with the gas. This growing volume of wastewater may also be recycled to be used in multiple wells (Adgate, Goldstein, & McKenzie, 2014).

Drilling is a 24-hour/7 day per week operation. There is constant activity related to the drilling site including transportation of materials, machinery, water, sand, and chemicals by diesel trucks (Xu & Xu, 2020). Often the drilling sites are in rural regions. It is not unusual for these diesel trucks to have to travel over single lane, dirt roads to and from the drilling site. Activities at the drilling site include gas production and onsite condensing stations. After well development is completed, flaring is often used as a controlled burning of natural gas at the well site to test and stabilize the well. Flaring can last for several days or weeks. This process of burning natural gas is also used during emergencies at processing plants and compressor stations or to take care of small amounts of waste gas. Flaring involves bright columns of flames shooting into the sky associated with continuous noise, often 24 hours per day. Additional components of UNGD include compressor stations which are used to maintain pressure and velocity of the natural gas to keep the gas flowing in the pipelines to distant ports and refineries. Pipelines can run for hundreds of miles through residential and rural areas to the final destination. Herbicides are often used to control the vegetation along the pipelines. The capacity of pipelines to transport the products from the site of extraction to market is augmented by railroad tank cars. These tank cars carrying flammable fluids pose a risk in the event of puncture or accident (Gorski & Schwartz, 2019).

In addition to the process for natural gas drilling, collection, and distribution, ethane cracker plants are being built to transform the ethane, a component of natural gas, into plastic products. Using extreme heat methods, these plants break the molecular bonds in ethane to produce ethylene, which can be processed into resin to create plastics. These plants emit tons of toxic air pollution each year. Cracker plants release 484 tons of carcinogenic VOCs (volatile organic compounds) such as benzene and toluene, and 159 tons of fine particles (PM 2.5) into the air annually (Baumgardner, 2017). Not only do these plants create additional environmental impacts through their processes and emissions, they also create additional (potentially inflated) need for more natural gas. Further, they also have the added impact of contributing to the continued dependence on plastic products (Baumgardner, 2017).

OVERVIEW OF CHEMICALS AND POLLUTANTS ASSOCIATED WITH UNGD

The exact chemical composition of fracking fluid is proprietary information and because of this, specific chemicals cannot be identified at any single drilling site. Using EPA data, Elliot, Trinh, Ma, Leaderer, Ward, and Deziel (2017) identified 1177 distinct chemical compounds used in the fracking process. They further noted that typically 15 – 100 million liters of fluid may be used for each individual well, with more than 114,00 liters of the fluid being chemical additives. The chemical additives include biocides, surfactants, and anti-corrosive agents. Of the 1177 contaminants identified, 91% (1066) had not been previously examined for possible carcinogenicity. Among those compounds that had been evaluated (111), 14 were known human carcinogens, six were probable human carcinogens, and 29 were possible human carcinogens. At least 20 of the compounds used in the fracking process have been linked to the development of leukemia. In addition, at least 74 identified fracking compounds are known to have negative reproductive effects (Inayat Hussain, Fukumura, Aziz, Jin, Jin, Gracia-Milian, Vasiliou, and Deziel 2018). See Figure 1 for the water and chemical cycle in fracking development. .

Looking beyond cancer and reproductive toxins, chemical compounds used in fracking fluid have been identified to result in adverse health effects involving the integument, respiratory, cardiovascular, gastrointestinal, nervous, and endocrine systems. Different times and lengths of exposures to these chemicals can result in different symptoms and diseases. Epidemiological studies have shown that some cancers take years to develop after

exposures to carcinogens used in other industries. It is well-documented that endocrine disruptors may take a generation or generations to manifest their effect on human and animal reproduction (Bergem et al., 2013).

Due to the vast number of chemicals used in fracking, a full discussion of each is beyond the scope of this chapter, rather, just a few of the hundreds of chemicals will be highlighted. Additional information about these pollutants can be found in the EPA Health Effects Notebook (EPA, 2016). *Benzene* (EPA, 2016) is a known carcinogen and reproductive toxin with chronic exposure. Further, acute exposure may result in dizziness, headaches, topical irritation and even unconsciousness. *Toulene* (EPA, 2016) is considered a "potential occupational carcinogen" and is associated with euphoria, hallucinations, dizziness, slurred speech, respiratory symptoms, depression, and coma and death with large acute exposures. Chronic exposures to toluene may result in liver, kidney and neurological damage, contact dermatitis, and is considered a possible teratogen. *Xylene isomers* (EPA, 2016) have been known to cause irritation of the eyes, nose, throat and gastrointestinal and neurological symptoms with acute exposure. Long-term exposure has been known to result in headaches, tremors, fatigue, dizziness, lack of coordination, as well as respiratory, kidney and cardiovascular disease. In addition, developmental effects and maternal toxicity have been documented in relation to these isomers. *Cadmium* (EPA, 2016) is often released with the flaring of drill sites. Evidence has shown a single high-level exposure to cadmium can result in long-lasting respiratory injury.

Fine particulate matter, a result of silica dust and carbon monoxide, has also been identified in and around drilling sites (OSHA-NIOSH, 2012). Crystalline silica is a known lung carcinogen. Silicosis develops after chronic exposure. Inhalation of silica dust is associated with chronic obstructive pulmonary disease, chronic renal disease, and autoimmune diseases. Diesel exhaust is associated with human health hazards (Hesterberg, Long, Bunn, Lapin, McClellan, & Valberg, 2012). Long term inhalation is "likely" to result in a lung cancer risk to humans as well as cause lung disease. Acute, short term exposures can result in irritation and inflammation as well as cause an exacerbation of pre-existing conditions such as allergies, bronchitis, and asthma. Diesel exhaust also contributes to the dissemination of other toxins such as fine particulates and nitrogen oxides.

ENVIRONMENTAL HEALTH ISSUES ASSOCIATED WITH UNGD

The environmental health issues surrounding the process of UNGD are complex. Impacts have been identified on public health, animal health, air and water quality, and crime incidence (Mayer, 2017). There are three major sources of exposure to chemicals and other potential health hazards associated with UNGD. Individuals can be exposed through contact with contaminated air, water, or soil. Negative health impacts have been noted among those living within several thousand feet of drilling stations. However, most state regulations, which vary widely, allow drilling to occur as close to 300 – 500 feet from residential areas (Mayer, 2017).

Sources of Exposure

Potential sources of air contamination include fine particles of silica dust from the sand used in the fracking fluid, diesel exhaust, emission from the well head, flaring off of the methane, evaporation of wastewater from impoundments, venting of condensation tanks during filling, compression stations emissions, and herbicide spraying to control vegetation along pipelines. More than 200 airborne chemical contaminants have been found near fracking sites, with 61 of them identified as hazardous air pollutants (including carcinogens) and another 26 identified as endocrine-disrupting compounds. Further, the volatile organic compounds (VOCs) used and produced in fracking, along with nitrogen oxides are leading to increases in ground level ozone. Individuals living near industrial sites may experience air contaminated by increased traffic from diesel trucks and the fine particulates of silica dust from the sand used in the fracking fluids (Mayer, 2017; Saberi, Propert, Powers, Emmett, & Green-Mckenzie, 2014). A potential source of water and ground soil contamination includes leakage that seeps from impoundments into the ground soil. Contaminated soil can affect food supply in the form of crops and meat production through undetected animal exposure. Because animals reproduce more frequently than humans, animal health can be an early indication of potential impacts of UNGD on human health (Bamberger & Oswald, 2012).

Health Effects

In recent years, a great deal of evidence has emerged documenting the connection between UNGD and specific health impacts. The most commonly reported symptoms include sleep disruption, headache, throat irritation, stress or anxiety, cough, shortness of breath, sinus problems, fatigue, nausea, and wheezing, (Weinberger, Greiner, Walleigh, & Brown, 2017). Other reported impacts include burning of the eyes, decreased ability to smell, bleeding from the nose, "a sweet metallic taste" in the mouth, and a gradual decrease in the ability to taste. Commonly reported dermatological signs and symptoms include a burning sensation, lesions, rashes, and chemical burns. Pulmonary complaints include an increase in the symptoms of chronic conditions such as asthma and chronic obstructive pulmonary disease. Increased drilling in areas has been linked to significant increases in the number of childhood asthma-related hospitalizations, with this effect lasting for up to eight years after drilling started in a community (Willis et al., 2018). Overall increases in number and severity of asthma exacerbations in all age groups has also been identified (Rasmussen et al., 2016). Further, higher rates of pneumonia in the elderly have been associated with UNGD (Peng et al., 2016). Cardiovascular impacts, including increased blood pressure and increased risk of heart disease have also been documented (McKenzie et al., 2019). Neurologically, individuals have reported headache, migraines, dizziness, and confusion (Tustin et al., 2017).

Generalized psychological impacts have also been noted by numerous researchers (Fisher et al., 2018; Elliot et al., 2018; McDermott-Levy & Garcia, 2016). Residents in areas of UNGD reported increased general stress and uncertainty, social stress, fear related to water and air contamination, fatigue, concerns about their physical health, and frustrations with increased traffic congestion. Further, residents have reported concerns related to the future of their community, lack of "peace" in the community due to constant noise and disruption, a generalized sense of powerlessness, and mistrust of

Figure I

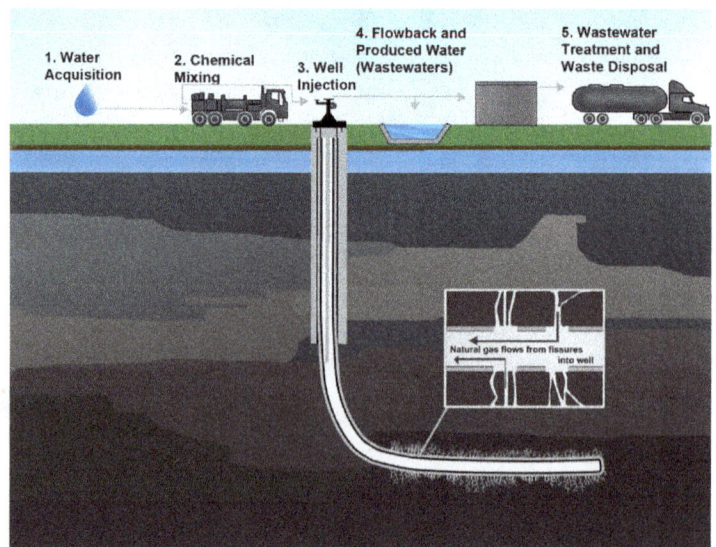

Image from U.S. Environmental Protection Agency (reproduced as part of the public domain).

elected/government officials. (Please see the chapter on noise in this unit.)

Increases in maternal antenatal anxiety and depression, as well as increases in adverse birth outcomes have also been correlated with areas of UNGD (Casey et al., 2019). Further, pre-term births, miscarriages, low birth weight, birth defects, diminished sperm quality and fertility, and endocrine disruption have all been associated with UNGD (Balise et al., 2016).

ENVIRONMENTAL HEALTH CONCERNS FOR SPECIAL POPULATIONS

Young children, pregnant people, and older adults are at greater risk for exposures to environmental toxins. More than 1.4 million children and 1.1 million elderly US residents live within one mile of an active drilling site. Due to their smaller stature, faster metabolism rate, and faster breathing rate, children are more vulnerable to environmental toxins. Associations between children living near high traffic areas and childhood asthma have been reported (Kim et al., 2012). Childbearing age people who can become pregnant and pregnant people are also vulnerable to these toxins. Low birth weight, small for gestational age, and low APGAR scores have been reported in births of women living near UNGD activities. Also, congenital heart defects and a trend toward neural tube defects have been found in mothers living near UNGD activity (McKenzie et al., 2014).

Hospitalization rates for female genitourinary problems such as kidney infections, calculus of ureter, and urinary tract infections have been noted to significantly increase in areas of UNGD (Denham et al., 2019). Older adults who tend to have chronic illnesses are also at a higher risk for experiencing negative health effects related to UNGD. Exposure to the ground level ozone, increased diesel fumes and other air contaminants have the potential to further aggravate chronic lung problems. Long term exposure has been reported to increase the risk of cancer of the lung. Peng, Meyerhoefer, and Chou (2017) identified that elderly living in areas of UNGD experienced significantly higher rates of hospitalization due to pneumonia.

Finally, in general, minorities may be more adversely affected by UNGD. Zwickl (2019) identified that African Americans were disproportionately more likely to live near drilling sites, placing this group at a greater risk for the negative health impacts. Zwikcl noted that the same seems to be true for Hispanic populations, though the evidence was less robust. Consequently, UNGD is an environmental justice issue.

COMMUNITY HEALTH ISSUES RELATED TO UNGD

Weber, Geigle, and Barkdull (2014) reported changes in local communities brought about the "boom and bust" cycles of the drilling activities. As an example, North Dakota has experienced one of the largest economic booms in the country due to the UNGD. Many community residents recognize the increase in jobs during "gas booms" but are also quick to note that many of the jobs are filled by individuals not from the local area. Further, as reported by McDermott-Levy and Garcia (2016), community members worry about the future of their communities, as well as experience mistrust of elected officials.

UNGD in the community will likely also impact the local built environment. Changes in traffic patterns and volume often lead to increases in motor vehicle accidents (Gorski & Schwartz, 2019). Xu and Xu (2020) identified an 8% increase in fatal crashes, with the majority involving a heavy truck from the fracking industry and a passenger car. Along with increases in accidents, including both motor vehicle and job site incidents, a corresponding increase in emergency response calls and local healthcare infrastructure needs has been noted (Ward, et al., 2014).

Crime rates in counties with both high (at least 75 wells) and low (less than 75 wells) fracking activity have been shown to significantly increase. In particular, violent crimes, such as rape and aggravated assault have been shown to significantly increase, when compared to counties without UNGD. In Pennsylvania, cases of sexually transmitted infections were found to be higher in rural counties where UNGD occurred compared to rural counties where no UNGD was occurring (Ward et al., 2014). More recently, Komarek and Tesh (2017) identified that increased fracking activity in a region was associated with increased rates of gonorrhea.

IMPLICATIONS FOR NURSES

The 2010 edition of the American Nurses Association (ANA) publication, Nursing: Scope and Standards of Practice, included a new Standard 16: Environmental Health. This Standard mandated that environmental health knowledge and skills are a requirement for all nurses at the entry level of practice and this has been supported in the third edition in 2015. Because the process of UNGD is a relatively new environmental health concern, nursing education at both the entry level and advanced practice level may not include information about the need to assess possible environmental exposure as a cause of presenting illnesses.

Clinical Practice

For all levels of nursing, it is important to assess if the client is living near or working near or with oil and gas drilling activities; if so, a more in-depth assessment needs to be completed. This screening may include an individual exposure health assessment, a home exposure assessment, and a residential environmental screening. In rural areas, special consideration must be given if the water source is well water and must include questions about animal exposure such as livestock and health of pets.

Research

Research in the area of the health impact of UNGD has been steadily increasing, with numerous published systematic reviews and analyses available. More than half of the peer-reviewed literature on the health impacts of UNGD have been published in the last decade (Hays & Shonkoff, 2016). As this body of evidence continues to develop, nurses must remain abreast of the research trends, as well as communicate these findings to peers, colleagues, and the general public. Research must continue to examine the health, economic, social, and long-term greenhouse effects of UNGD. Without such studies, humans, animals, and the earth will potentially be at great risk now, in the future, and for generations to come. Mayer (2017) identified seven general areas of research that must be addressed as we move forward; in particular looking at long-term quality of life across communities affected by UNGD. Nurses must develop research questions and investigate the health impacts of UNGD and strategies to protect the health of populations.

Advocacy

Nurses and other health care providers have an ethical obligation to "first do no harm" and to promote disease prevention and health promotion interventions. When there is an absence of evidence-based studies, the Precautionary Principle serves as a guide to practice. The Precautionary Principle states "When an activity raises threats of harm to human health or the environment, precautionary measures should be taken even if some cause and effect relationships are not fully established scientifically" (Wingspread, 1998). The American Nurses Association adopted the Precautionary Principle in 2003 and the importance of nursing's role in environmental health issues was further clarified in the ANA Principles for Environmental Health for Nursing Practice guidelines (ANA, 2007). Nurses play a vital role in the advocacy of health for individuals, families, and communities. In this role, the nurse has a great deal to contribute by staying informed of environmental health issues, meeting with elected officials, taking part in community meetings, and sharing information about health and safety issues in the community.

UNGD AS A GLOBAL HEALTH PHENOMENON

Concern about environmental health and UNGD is a global issue. Numerous countries including France, Bulgaria, Austria, Luxembourg, the Flanders region of Belgium, Scotland, Wales, Northern Ireland, Germany, several states in Australia, several Canadian territories, along with many others, have all banned fracking via legislative initiatives. In the United States, Vermont, New York, numerous counties in California, Maryland, Washington, and Oregon have banned fracking; numerous other states and localities have pending legislation to ban fracking ((Townsend, 2020)

SUMMARY

The environmental health concerns involved in UNGD are complex. A growing body of literature continues to provide more evidence of the link between UNGD and significant health impacts. Environmental health concerns related to UNGD are a global health concern and not limited to drilling in the United States. Contamination concerns are not from one source, but from multiple routes (non-point source) including possible contamination from air, water, and ground sources. The profession of nursing is charged with having environmental health knowledge and skills. Nurses are held to the standard of including environmental health knowledge and skills in their practice which includes assessment for environmental health concerns.

ONLINE RESOURCES

Since early 2012, the Southwest Pennsylvania Environmental Health Project (SWPA-EHP) has been in operation in Southwestern Pennsylvania, an area which has experienced a proliferation of natural gas drilling. The purpose of the Environmental Health Project is to provide education and referrals to area residents experiencing adverse health and resources to health care providers in the areas.

State Impact PA has developed a broad range of resources regarding the many impacts of fracking.

The National Library of Medicine offers environmental health and toxicology data that can be used to examine the toxicology of specific chemicals used in fracking (https://medlineplus.gov/poisoningtoxicologyenvironmentalhealth.html). In addition, EJScreen by the Environmental Protection Agency, offers a mapping tools to examine indicators such as air quality, water quality, and proximity to hazardous waste sites by location. It can be found at: https://www.epa.gov/ejscreen/overview-environmental-indicators-ejscreen.

REFERENCES

Adgate, J. L., Goldstein, B. D., McKenzie, L. M. (2014). Potential public health hazards, exposures and h e a l t h effects form unconventional natural gas development. *Environmental Science & Technology, 48*, 8307-8320. Dx.doi.org/10.1021/es404621d

American Nurses Association (ANA) (2007). *ANA's principles for environmental health for nursing practice with implementation strategies.* American Nurses Association.

American Nurses Association. (2015). *Nursing: scope and standards of practice* (3rd ed.). American Nurses Association.

Balise, V. D., Meng, C., Cornelius-Green, J. N., Kassotis, C. D., Kennedy, R., & Nagel, S. C. (2016). Systematic review of the association between oil and natural gas extraction processes and human reproduction. *Fertility and Sterility, 106*(4), 795 – 819. https://doi.org/10.1016/j.fertnstert.2016.07.1099

Bamberger, M. & Oswald, R. E. (2012). Impacts of gas drilling on human and animal health. *New Solutions, 22*(1), 51-77. doi: 10.2190/NS.22.1.e.

Baumgardner, T. (2017, April 6). *Your health vs. cracker plant jobs.* Pittsburgh Post-Gazette. https://www.post-gazette.com/opinion/Op-Ed/2017/04/06/Your-health-vs-cracker-plant-jobs/stories/201704300020?pgpageversion=pgevoke

Bergam, A., Heindel, , J. J., Kasten, T., Kidd, K. A., Jobling, S., Neira, M., Zoeller, R. T., Becher, G., Bjerregaard, P., Bornma, R., Brandt, I., Kortenkamp, A., Muir, D., Disse, M. B., Ochieng, R., Skakkebaek, N. E., Bylehn, A. S., Iguchi.T., Toppari, J., & Woodruff, T. J. (2013). The impact of endocrine disruption: A consensus statement on the state of the science. *Environmental Health Perspectives, 121*(4), A104-A106. https://doi.org/10.1289/ehp.1205448

Casey, J. A., Goin, D. E., Rudolph, K. E., Schwartz, B. S., Mercer, D., Elser, H., Eisen, E. A., & Morello-Frosch, R. (2019). Unconventional natural gas development and adverse birth outcomes in Pennsylvania: The potential mediating role of antenatal anxiety and depression. *Environmental Research, 177.* https://doi.org/10.1016/j.envres.2019.108598

Concerned Health Professionals of New York, & Physicians for Social Responsibility. (2019, June). *Compendium of scientific, medical, and media findings demonstrating risks and harms of fracking (unconventional gas and oil extraction) (6th ed.).* http://concernedhealthny.org/compendium/

Denham. A., Willis, M., Zavez, A., & Hill, E. (2019). Unconventional natural gas development and hospitalizations: evidence from Pennsylvania, United States, 2003 – 2014. *Public Health, 168*, 17-25. https://doi.org/10.1016/j.puhe.2018.11.020

Elliott, E. G., Ma, X., Leaderer, B. P., McKay, L. A., Pedersen, C. J., Wang, C., Gerber, C. J., Wright, T. J., Summer, A. J., Brennan, M., Silva, G. S., Warren, J. L., Plata, D. L., & Deziel, N. C. (2018) A community-based evaluation of proximity to unconventional oil and gas well, drinking water contaminants, and health symptoms in Ohio. *Environmental Research, 167*, 550 – 557. https://doi.org/10.1016/j.envres.2018.08.022

Elliott, E.G., Trinh, P, Ma, X., Leaderer, B. P., Ward, M. H., Deziel, N. C. (2017). Unconventional oil and gas development and risk of childhood leukemia: Assessing the evidence. *Science of the Total Environment, 576*, 138 – 147. https://doi.org/10.1016/j.scitotenv.2016.10.072

EPA (2016). *EPA health effects notebook.* https://www.epa.gov/haps/health-effects-notebook-hazardous-air-pollutants

Fisher, M. P., Mayer, A., Vollet, K., Hill, E. L., & Haynes, E. N. (2018). Psychosocial implications of unconventional natural gas development: Quality of life in Ohio's Guernsey and Noble counties. *Journal of Environmental Psychology, 55*, 90–98. https://doi.org/10.1016/j.jenvp.2017.12.008

Gorski, I. & Schwartz, B. S. (2019). *Environmental health concerns from unconventional natural gas development.* Global Public Health: Oxford Research Encyclopedia. DOI: 10.1093/acrefore/9780190632366.013.44

Hays J., & Shonkoff, B .C. S. (2016). Toward an understanding of the environmental and public health impacts of unconventional natural gas development: A categorical assessment of the peer-reviewed scientific literature, 2009 – 2015. *PLOS One, 11*(4), e0154164. Doi.10.1371/journal.pone.0154164

Hesterberg, T. W., Long, C. M., Bunn, W. B., Lapin, C. A., McClellan, R. O., & Valberg, P. A. (2012). Health effects research and regulation of diesel exhaust: An historical overview focused on lung cancer risk. Inhalation *Toxicology, 24, sup1*, 1-45. DOI: 10.3109/08958378.2012.691913

Inayat-Hussain, S. H., Fukumura, M., Aziz, A. M., Jin, C.M., Jin, L.W., Garcia-Milian, R., Vasiliou, V., & Deziel, N.C. (2018). Prioritization of reproductive toxicants in unconventional oil and gas operations using a multi-country regulatory data-drive hazards assessment. *Environment International, 117*, 348-358. https://doi.org/10.1016/j.envint.2018.05.010

Kim, K., Kabir, E., & Kabir, S. (2015) A review on the human health impact of airborne particulate matter. *Environment International, 74*, 136-143. https://doi.org/10.1016/j.envint.2014.10.005

Komarek, T. & Cseh, A. (2017). Fracking and public health: Evidence from gonorrhea incidence in the Marcellus Shale region. *Journal of Public Health Policy, 38*(4), 464-481. doi.org/10.1057/s41271-017-0089-5

Mayer, A. (2017). Quality of life and unconventional oil and gas development: Towards a comprehensive impact model for host communities. *The Extractive Industries and Society, 4*, 923-930. https://doi.org/10.1016/j.exis.2017.10.009

McDermott-Levy, R. & Garcia, V. (2016). Health concerns of Northeastern Pennsylvania residents living in an unconventional oil and gas development county. *Public Health Nursing, 33*(6), 502 – 510. Doi:10.1111/phn.12265

McKenzie, L. M., Crooks, J., Peel, J. L., Blair, B. D., Brindley, S., Allshouse, W. B., Malin, S., & Adgate, J.L. (2019). Relationships between indicators of cardiovascular disease and intensity of oil and natural gas activity in Northeastern Colorado. *Environmental Research, 170*, 56-64. https://doi.org/10.1016/j.envres.2018.12.004

OSHA-NIOSH (2012). *Worker Exposure to silica during hydraulic fracturing*. Hazard Alert. https://www.osha.gov/dts/hazardalerts/hydraulic_frac_hazard_alert.html

Peng, L., Meyerhoefer, C., & Chou, S. (2018). The health implication of unconventional natural gas development in Pennsylvania. *Health Economics, 27*, 956-983 doi.org/10.1002/hec.3649

Rasmussen, S. G., Ogburn, E. L., McCormack, M., Casey, J.A., Bandeen-Roche, K., Mercer, D. G., & Schwartz, B. S. (2016). Association between unconventional natural gas development in the Marcellus Shale and asthma exacerbations. *JAMA Internal Medicine, 176*(9), 1334- 1143. doi: 10.1001/jamainternmed.2016.2436.

Saberi, P., Propert, K. J., Powers, M., Emmett, E., Green-McKenzie, J. (2014). Field survey of health perception and complaints of Pennsylvania residents in the Marcellus Shale region. *International Journal of Research and Public Health, 11*(6), 6517-6527. https://doi.org/10.3390/ijerph110606517

Townsend, D. (2020). *The legal status of fracking worldwide: An environmental law and human rights perspective*. The Global Network for Human Rights and the Environment. https://gnhre.org/2020/01/06/the-legal-status-of-fracking-worldwide-an-environmental-law-and-human-rights-perspective/

Tustin., A. W., Hirsch, A. G., Rasmussen, S. G., Casey, J. A., Bandeen-Roche, K., & Schwartz, B.S. (2017). Associations between unconventional natural gas development and nasal and sinus, migraine headache, and fatigue symptoms in Pennsylvania. *Environmental Health Perspectives, 125*(2), 189 – 197. https://doi.org/10.1289/EHP281

Ward, S., Polson, D., & Price, M. (2014). *Measuring the cost and benefits of natural gas development in Tioga county, Pennsylvania: A case study*. Keystone Research Center and PA Budget and Policy Center. https://pennbpc.org/sites/pennbpc.org/files/tiogaCASESTUDY.pdf

Weber, B. A., Geigle, J., & Barkdull, C. (2014). Rural North Dakota's oil boom and its impact on social services. *Social Work, 59*(1), 62-72. https://doi.org/10.1093/sw/swt068

Weinberger, B., Greiner, L. H., Walleigh, L., & Brown, D. (2017). Health symptoms in residents living near shale gas activity: A retrospective record review from the Environmental Health Project. *Preventative Medicine Reports, 8*, 112–115. https://doi.org/10.1016/j.pmedr.2017.09.002

Willis, M.D., Jusko, T.A., Halterman, J. S., & Hill, E. L. (2018). Unconventional natural gas development and pediatric asthma hospitalizations in Pennsylvania. *Environmental Research, 166*, 402–408. https://doi.org/10.1016/j.envres.2018.06.022

Wingspread (1998). *Precautionary principle.* http://www.gdrc.org/u-gov/precaution-3.html

Xu, M. & Xu, Y. (2020). Fraccident: The impact of fracking on road traffic deaths. *Journal of Environmental Economics and Management, 101*, https://doi.org/10.1016/j.jeem.2020.102303

Xu, X., Zhang, X., Carrillo, G., Zhong, Y., Kan, H., Zhang, B. (2019) A systematic assessment of carcinogenicity of chemicals in hydraulic-fracturing fluids and flowback water. *Environmental Pollution, 251*, 128 – 136. https://doi.org/10.1016/j.envpol.2019.04.016

Zwickl, K. (2019). The demographics of fracking: A spatial analysis of four U.S. states. *Ecological Economics, 161*, 202-215. https://doi.org/10.1016/j.ecolecon.2019.02.001

FRACKING CASE STUDY: THE GORDIS FAMILY OF NORTHEASTERN PENNSYLVANIA*

Ruth McDermott-Levy, PhD, MPH, RN, FAAN
Professor
Co-Director, Mid-Atlantic Center for Children's Health and the Environment
Villanova University
M. Louise Fitzpatrick College of Nursing

The Gordis family heard them coming. Suddenly, their quiet country road was no longer quiet. Trucks carrying drilling equipment, millions of gallons of water, fracking chemicals, and the drilling crews passing their home seven days a week, all day, and all night. The first thing, Marica Gordis noted was noise and then the odor of diesel from the trucks. She and her 14-year-old son, Dylan, were having trouble sleeping from the noise of trucks driving by all night long. Her husband, Bob, and her 11-year-old daughter, Lucy, did not have any problems sleeping.

Marcia Gordis had spent the previous 5 years working with a coalition of other community members trying to get zoning regulations passed that restricted unconventional natural gas (UNG) drilling in her quiet Northeastern Pennsylvania community. But the gas companies' lawyers were able to thwart the efforts of the community members. Marcia worked very hard with the coalition that her community formed. All the people in the coalition had "visits" from mysterious white cars parked in their driveways for an hour or so. The cars would finally drive off when the homeowner called the police, and the patrol car would come by. People in the community suspected that the white car drivers were from the gas drilling companies that were trying to intimidate people who were resistant to gas development in the region.

Now, her neighbor signed a lease to allow drilling on his property and the Gordis family had to live through this as their rural community began to look like an industrial zone. After a week of sleepless nights Marcia and Dylan were becoming irritable. Dylan was getting in trouble at school and Marcia had been receiving calls from Dylan's teachers.

Two weeks after the trucks arrived, the drilling started. Marcia assumed this happened because when she was outside tending to her vegetable garden, she could smell a sweet strong odor in the air. Her eyes and throat burned a bit, so she went in the house. Later that night, Marcia could hear Lucy coughing. Marcia went to check on Lucy and found her wheezing and beginning an asthma attack. Marcia reached for Lucy's inhalers and could see the lights of the drilling crew and the flames from the "flaring" that

occurs to burn off the excess methane. Lucy was breathing better after her rescue medications, so everyone returned to bed.

The next morning, once the children were off to school, Marcia began answering her emails for the rental properties that she managed. Marcia noted that she had been very busy with rental properties since fracking had begun in her area and the cost to rent a house had more than doubled. Once her rental emails were answered, she started searching the internet for more information about living near a fracking well. She found the Southwest Pennsylvania Environmental Health Project (EHP) (https://www.environmentalhealthproject.org/) that is located across the state. She learned that constant noise and light can affect her health (see the chapter on Noise in the Environmental Health Sciences Unit). According to the EHP site, exposure to noise, light, and constant vibrations of heavy machinery can cause:

- Headaches

- Hearing problems

- Increases in blood pressure

- Problems sleeping

- Stress and anxiety

Marcia, thought, "Well, at least I have an explanation for Dylan's behavior at school and the way I have been feeling." She went on to read about the impacts of fracking on the air quality and found that there was a relationship between the drilling of the wells and the episode of burning eyes and scratchy throat. As she read more, she learned that her well water (see Water Quality in the Environmental Sciences Unit) could be threatened by the UNG wells on her neighbor's property and there was a risk of soil contamination on her property. Marcia discussed these things with Bob when he returned from work later that evening. They both agreed to have their well water tested for contamination from fracking.

The following week, Lucy had a check-up with the nurse practitioner (NP). Maria told the NP about the Lucy's asthma episode and the new fracking wells near her home. The NP was aware of the risks to air and water quality from fracking and the stress it can cause for community members. The NP reviewed Lucy's medications, added another rescue medication, and taught Lucy and Marcia ways to reduce risk of air pollution, such as closing windows using air purifiers and taking steps to reduce indoor air pollutants (see Air Quality chapter the Environmental Sciences Unit).

At the end of the visit with the NP, Marcia stated, "Thank you, what you told us is helpful. But we need to stop this activity to protect everyone, including the gas workers." The NP agreed and shared that policy change would make a big difference. The NP also shared that nurses and other health providers are advocating for policies to protect communities from the risks of fracking. Among those organizations are the Alliance of Nurses for Healthy Environments, Concerned Health Professionals of Pennsylvania, and Concerned Health Professionals of New York. Marcia shared that she would be letting her coalition know about these groups and reaching out to see how the community and health care providers groups might work together to protect the health of everyone in the community.

*The case is a composite of media reports (newspaper, radio), peer-reviewed literature, and the author's research in unconventional gas development communities. The names are made up by the author of the case. The Gordis family is fictional.

FURTHER READING

McDermott-Levy, R. & Garcia, V. (2016). Health concerns of Northeastern Pennsylvania residents living in an unconventional oil and gas development county. *Public Health Nursing, 33*(6), 502-510. doi: 10.1111/phn.12265

Peng, L., Meyerhoefer, C. & Chou, S-Y. (2018). The health implications of unconventional natural gas development in Pennsylvania. *Health Economics, 26*(6), 956-983. https://doi.org/10.1002/hec.3649

Powers, M., Saberi, P., Pepino, R. et al. (2015). Popular epidemiology and "Fracking": Citizens' concerns regarding the economic, environmental, health and social impacts of unconventional natural gas drilling operations. *Journal of Community Health 40,* 534–541. https://doi.org/10.1007/s10900-014-9968-x

ADDITIONAL RESOURCES

Concerned Health Professionals of New York: https://concernedhealthny.org/

Physicians for Social Responsibility – Pennsylvania: Fracking and Health https://www.psrpa.org/environmental-health

Southwest Pennsylvania Environmental Health Project https://www.environmentalhealthproject.org/

ENDOCRINE DISRUPTORS

Sahar Nouredini, PhD, RN, CNS
California State University East Bay
Nursing

Juleen Lam, PhD, MHS, MS
California State University East Bay
Department of Health Sciences

ENDOCRINE DISRUPTORS

The endocrine system is a series of glands that produce hormones that regulate various systems in our body. These hormones control a variety of bodily functions including metabolism, growth, mood, sleep, reproduction and sexual function. Endocrine disrupting chemicals (EDCs) are chemicals that interfere with hormone function through a variety of methods, including: mimicking naturally occurring hormones, binding to a hormone receptor thus blocking a naturally occurring hormone from binding to the receptor or by interfering with the production of natural hormones and receptors. Because the endocrine system is responsible for regulating so many of our body systems, when it is impaired, it can increasing risk for a variety of diseases. There is increasing evidence that exposure to EDC's increase risk for obesity and diabetes, female and male reproduction, hormone-sensitive cancers in females, prostate cancer, thyroid, and neurodevelopmental and neuroendocrine system disorders (Gore et al., 2015)

EDCs are ubiquitous and exposure often begins in the womb. One study of pregnant people in the United States found that 99-100% of the women were exposed to EDCs (Woodruff, Zota, Schwartz, 2011). As many as 1,000 chemicals of the 85,000 currently on the market are classified as EDCs. However, this number might be much higher because many chemicals currently in use have not been sufficiently tested. Common sources of EDCs include phthalates, polybrominated diphenyl ethers (PBDEs) such as brominated flame retardants (perflourochemicals) found in clothing, bedding and electronics, alkylphenols, and pesticides. Phthalates (used to make products fragrant and pliable) are common in food packaging, children's products and personal care products. The pesticide chlorpyrifos that has been cited for human safety concerns is a common insecticide used in commercial agriculture. Other pesticides that are known EDCs include DDT, 2,4-D glycophosphate and atrazine. Banned EDCs such as PCBs are still present in electronics, insulation and paints and the health effects of the pesticide DDT are still present in the environment (Gore et al, 2014). Recent research suggests that

nanomaterials also might cause endocrine damage (Priyam, Singh & Gehlout, 2018). The Endocrine Society's Introduction to Endocrine Disrupting Chemicals is a useful guide to better understand EDCs. See Figure 1

Figure 1

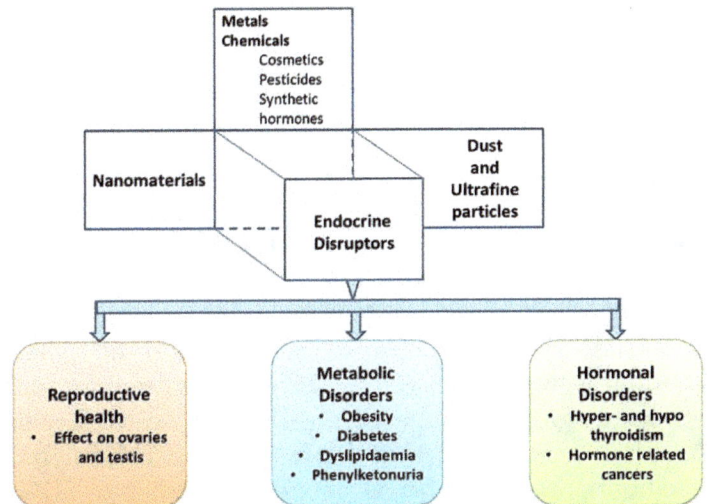

Source: Priyam A, Singh PP and Gehlout S (2018) Role of Endocrine-Disrupting Engineered Nanomaterials in the Pathogenesis of Type 2 Diabetes Mellitus. Front. Endocrinol. 9:704. doi: 10.3389/fendo.2018.00704

below.

BPA is one of the more well-known EDCs that has been linked to a variety of health issues including infertility, various reproductive system disorders, neurodevelopmental and cardiovascular diseases (Gore et al., 2014). It is commonly found in canned food lining and rigid plastic food containers, and, while its use has been phased out or banned in some products, the CDC estimates that 96% of the American population would test positive for BPA exposure (Gore et al., 2014). This can be because of continued exposure through non-food sources and environmental contamination from discarded plastics. Furthermore, exposure to BPA is not evenly distributed across the population as African Americans and people with lower income levels have been shown to have higher BPA body burden compared to their counterparts (Ruiz, Becerra, Jagai, Ard & Sargis, 2018).

ROLE OF THE NURSE IN REDUCING EDC EXPOSURE

Nurses can play a key role in helping to prevent exposure to EDCs. At the individual level, nurses working in clinical settings would benefit from being informed about EDCs in order to incorporate that knowledge when providing assessment, and education focusing on sources of EDCs in the home environment and the use of safer alternatives. For example, the hormone, insulin, regulates our blood sugar. When insulin production and delivery is impeded by EDCs, it can increase risk for insulin resistance or diabetes. Being able to identify and thus eliminate sources of exposure to EDC's has the potential to reduce the burden of endocrine diseases, such as diabetes (Ruiz, et al., 2018).

While working at the individual level is essential, it is not enough. Other actions that nurses can engage in at the community and policy level include collaborating with other disciplines in finding safer alternatives and pushing for policy change. For example, within the healthcare setting, EDCs are found in medical devices, gloves, cleaning products, textiles, flooring and IV tubing and bags (Healthcare without Harm, 2018). Hospitals in European countries have been able to phase out some EDCs (Healthcare without Harm, 2018), thus nurses can advocate for green purchasing options within their healthcare settings. Healthcare without Harm has additional resources that elaborate on sources of EDCs and ways to reduce EDC exposure in the healthcare environment. Getting involved in policy and advocacy can be achieved by working with organizations that specifically focus on endocrine disruptor research and policy. The endocrine disruption exchange and International POPs (Persistent Organic Pollutant) Elimination Network are good resources to reach out to. For additional resources about EDC sources, alternatives and policy, please see Table 1.

Table 1: Additional resources to learn more about endocrine disruptors

Website	Resource Description
https://www.nrdc.org/stories/9-ways-avoid-hormone-disrupting-chemicals	9 ways to avoid hormone disrupting chemicals Source: NRDC
https://www.ewg.org/research/dirty-dozen-list-endocrine-disruptors	Dirty dozen list of endocrine disruptors- List of 12 most offensive EDCs and sources Source: Environmental Working Group
https://www.youtube.com/watch?v=ibfAF66JzFE	Endocrine disrupting chemicals- Brief video overview about EDC Source: Hormone Health Network
https://endocrinedisruption.org	The endocrine disruption exchange- TEDX provides list of potential EDCs, links to webinars and systematic reviews.
https://www.endocrine.org/-/media/endosociety/files/advocacy-and-outreach/important-documents/introduction-to-endocrine-disrupting-chemicals.pdf?la=en	Introduction To Endocrine Disrupting Chemicals (EDCs) A Guide For Public Interest Organizations And Policy-Makers An introductory guide to EDCs specifically targeted towards policy makers and public interest organizations. Source: IPEN and Endocrine Society
https://noharm-europe.org/issues/europe/edcs-infographic	Non-toxic healthcare-reducing risk with safer alternatives List of EDCs in healthcare environment and available alternatives to EDCs in infographic form. Source: Healthcare without Harm
https://www.epa.gov/saferchoice	EPA safer choice program Helps to find products that perform and are safer for human health and the environment. Source: EPA
https://endocrinedisruption.org/interactive-tools/endocrine-disruption-audio-and-video	Links to presentations and videos on endocrine disruptors Source: TEDX

https://www.niehs.nih.gov/health/materials/endocrine_disruptors_508.pdf	Endocrine Disruptors and Your Health Source: NIEHS

impact of chemicals in animals cannot be determined for the fetus, infant, child or along the life span. (Gore et al, 2014). This can make regulation of EDCs very challenging. Other challenges to assessing risk and developing policy are listed in Table 2.

REGULATION OF CHEMICALS

The Environmental Protection Agency (EPA) is charged with regulating chemicals to protect the environment and to protect human health. Such regulation is led by specific offices within the federal agency. For example, the Office of Chemical Safety and Pollution Prevention protects risks from pesticides and toxic chemicals through federal laws such as the Federal Insecticide, Fungicide, and Rodenticide Act (FIFRA), the Federal Food, Drug and Cosmetic Act (FFDCA) and Toxic Substances Control Act (TSCA) (EPA, 2021).

EDC PROPERTIES AND THE CHALLENGES OF REGULATION

Some EDCs are persistent and bioaccumulate, particularly in fatty tissue. Babies and fetuses are exposed to EDCs via transmission through the placenta and breast milk. Furthermore, EDC exposure can change genes, potentially impacting the health of future generations. Harmful effects of EDCs can occur at very low and very high levels, with the dose response following a U-shaped curve (Calabrese & Baldwin, 2003). This can make regulation of EDCs very challenging. Traditional approaches to chemical testing are problematic when applied to the testing for EDCs. Most chemical testing measures the effect of one chemical at time but most people alive today have had many exposures to a variety of chemicals produced since the 1940s and interactive effects must be considered in the human body. Testing is based upon the assumption that there is a safe level for a chemical in the human body however science has not shown that any level is actually safe in humans. Finally, most tests are conducted in adult animals and the

TSCA OVERVIEW

Most people interact with hundreds of different products and materials (such as toys, clothing, cosmetics, lotions, electronics, furniture cleaning products, cars, building materials, food, food storage containers, etc.) every day in their homes, schools, and workplaces without giving a second thought to the potentially harmful chemicals contained within them. However, with more than 85,000

Table 2: Traditional concepts in chemical testing and why they are inadequate to determine endocrine disrupting activity

Traditional Approach to Chemical Testing: 'The Dose is the Poison'	Why this approach is insufficient for Endocrine-Disrupting Chemicals
Tests individual chemicals one at a time	Every person in the world now carries a body burden of chemicals that did not exist before 1940. Many more are being produced and released into the environment each year. Testing chemicals one at a time can't keep pace with exposure and doesn't take into account how combinations of chemicals within the body are impacting human development or health.
Assumes individual chemicals have a "safe or acceptable" level of exposure below which there are no adverse effects	The endocrine system regulates virtually every aspect of human health from development in the womb, to growth, to reproduction, and overall health. Recent science shows that even very small amounts of these chemicals or mixtures of these chemicals disrupt the endocrine system, reducing intelligence, disrupting reproductive systems, and causing other health problems. There may, in fact, be no safe level, especially when individuals have hundreds of these chemicals in their bodies.
Tests are focused on adult animals	Hormones regulate body systems beginning in the womb and throughout life. Tests conducted only on adult animals can't capture the impact of chemicals on the endocrine system throughout the body's life cycle.
Presumes doses below the amounts which cause test animals to die or develop a target disease (usually cancer) are 'safe'	Endocrine-disrupting chemicals have many impacts beyond death or disease.

Source: Endocrine Society and IPEN report an Introduction to Endocrine Disrupting Chemicals (EDCs) A Guide for Public Interest Organizations and Policy Makers

chemicals currently registered for commercial use in the United States, and 2,000 more being introduced each year, exposures to these chemicals is virtually certain (CA DTSC, 2007).

Research reveals numerous chemicals used in these products can be measured in the bodies of adults, pregnant people, children and newborns, including polybrominated diphenyl ethers (PBDEs, used as chemical flame retardants in furniture and building materials), Bisphenol A (BPA, used in plastics and resins), perchlorate (used in explosives and fireworks, and per- and poly-fluoroalkyl substances (PFAS, used to make carpet and clothing stain-resistant and non-stick cookware). These chemicals have been linked with a variety of adverse human health effects including neurodevelopmental disorders such as ADHD and autism, reproductive issues such as birth defects and low birth weight, endocrine disruption such as hypothyroidism, and cancer.

The major legislation regulating chemicals in the United States is the Toxic Substances Control Act (TSCA), enacted in 1976 (15 U.S.C. Secs 2601 et seq.). This law was intended to protect the public from toxic exposures by regulating the use of harmful chemicals in everyday products, but instead it proved over the next four decades to be weak and highly ineffective. Of the tens of thousands of chemicals on the market, 62,000 chemicals already on the market when the law was passed were grandfathered in and deemed "safe" unless the Environmental Protection Agency (EPA) later determined. Since then, only a couple hundred chemicals have since been evaluated for safety by the EPA, and only five chemicals or classes of chemicals have actually been banned (GAO, 2005). Complex and cumbersome administrative burdens, data limitations, requirements to consider financial implications to industry, and recurring corporate lawsuits created such roadblocks that it became virtually impossible for EPA to ban or regulate any chemicals, even when strong scientific evidence of danger was present. An example of the clear inadequacies of TSCA was the failure of EPA in 1989 to ban asbestos, a known human carcinogen, after being overruled by the courts after industry groups sued (Stadler, 1993).

After years of criticism, debate, and different versions of proposed amendments, on June 22, 2016 President Obama signed the Frank R. Lautenberg Chemical Safety for the 21st Century Act ("Lautenberg Act"), the first major overhaul of TSCA since its original passage. The Lautenberg Act offered several tools that increased the ability of EPA to act on harmful chemicals. The EPA announced on January 14, 2021 that the final evaluation of the first 10 chemicals that were mandated for risk

Website	Description
https://www.edf.org/sites/default/files/denison-primer-on-lautenberg-act.pdf	Environmental Defense Fund Primer on TSCA
https://ucsf.app.box.com/v/lb2018	UCSF press kit on TSCA
https://www.epa.gov/laws-regulations/summary-toxic-substances-control-act	EPA summary of TSCA and link to full text of TSCA

evaluation after passage of the Lautenberg Act was completed. (EPA, 2021). However, the Environmental Defense Fund argues that steps to examine the risk of chemicals and take action were blocked or ignored during the years of the Trump administration allowing for major toxic emissions and hazards to health to occur (Environmental Defense Fund, 2019).

CASE STUDY: TSCA CHEMICAL HBCD AND ENDOCRINE DISRUPTION

One of the first ten TSCA chemicals EPA is evaluating under the Lautenberg Amendment is hexabromocyclododecane (HBCD), a chemical commonly used as a flame retardant. HBCD can be found in a number of different products, including:

- Expanded (EPS) and extruded (XPS) polystyrene foam

- Foam boards and insulation

- Textiles

- High impact polystyrene (HIPS), used in toys, plastic cups, shipping and packing material, refrigerator linings, televisions, wire and cable applications

Globally, HBCD use has decreased subsequent to a ban implemented in 2013 (Stockholm Convention, 2012) by several industrial countries. However, it is still heavily produced and used in the US, who signed but has not yet ratified the agreement. In the U.S., HBCD produced and imported an estimated 1-10 million pounds in 2015 alone (EPA, 2017). HBCD is added to consumer products rather than bonded to them, and therefore will slowly be released into the environment through all phases of the production and life cycle of these products. Due to its high production volumes and persistency in air, water, and soil there is high potential for human exposure and resulting adverse health effects (EPA, 2015).

People who may be exposed include workers in HBCD manufacturing and processing industries and people using commercial and consumer products containing HBCD. Pregnant people/ developing fetus/children may be more susceptible to adverse health effects (EPA, 2015). HBCD has been detected in indoor air and dust (Abdallah et al., 2008), outdoor air (Jo et al., 2017), soil (Meng et al., 2011, Desborough et al., 2016), human serum and breastmilk (Carnigan et al., 2012, Rawn et al., 2014), and lake sediments (Harrad et al., 2009a, Yang et al., 2012). It can also bioconcentrate and biomagnify in fish and wildlife (Covaci et al. 2009, Harrad et al. 2009b, Johnson-Restrepo et al. 2008).

Animal studies indicate that HBCD is toxic, especially in the liver, immune system, on serum thyroid hormone (TH concentrations), interference with thyroid hormone signalling, and TH-dependent developmental processes (Canton et al., 2008, Germer et al., 2006, van der Ven et al., 2006). HBCD exposures lower thyroxine (T4) hormone levels with increased levels of thyroid stimulating hormones in rat and, in female rats, reduce the number of ovarian primordial follicles (Ema et al., 2008). Prenatal and neonatal exposure to HBCDs in rodents has been shown to decrease TSH levels and alter spontaneous behavior even at low exposures (Saegusa et al., 2009, Ema et al., 2008, Eriksson et al., 2006). The few human studies investigating HBCD health effects that exist demonstrate adverse effects from HBCD prenatal exposure on sexual and psychomotor development (Meijer et al., 2008).

Hypothyroidism can negatively affect neurological development, energy metabolism, early development and can lead to heart failure (Miller et al., 2016). In particular, normal thyroid functions are a necessity for healthy neonatal development, particularly the brain, and so prenatal exposures to HBCD could result in serious health outcomes such as neurotoxicity or infertility (Roze et al., 2009, Hond et al., 2015).

In September 2020 the EPA published their final risk evaluation of HBCD for the TSCA review. From what you have read in this case study and your examination of the EPA risk evaluation what concerns do you have for human health? Will you sign up for email alerts to keep following this chemical of concern?

Case study developed by Dr. Juleen Lam (2019)

REFERENCES

15 U.S.Code Subchapter I – Control of Toxic Substances Secs 2601 et seq. 1976. Toxic Substances Control Act.

Abdallah M.A., Sharkey M., Berresheim H., & Harrad S. (2018). Hexabromocyclododecane in polystyrene packaging: A downside of recycling? Chemosphere, 199, 612-616.

Calabrese, E.A. & Baldwin, L.A. (2003). Toxicology rethinks its central belief. Nature, 421(6924), 691-2.

California Department of Toxic Substances Control (CA DTSC). (2007). Emerging Chemicals of Concern. https://www.dtsc.ca.gov/AssessingRisk/EmergingContaminants.cfm.

Cantón R. F., Peijnenburg A. A., Hoogenboom R. L., Piersma A. H., van der Ven L. T., van den Berg M., & Heneweer M. (2008). Subacute Effects of Hexabromocyclododecane (HBCD) on Hepatic Gene Expression Profiles in Rats. Toxicology and Applied Pharmacology, 231(2), 267-72.

Carignan C. C., Abdallah M. A., Wu N., Heiger-Bernays W., McClean M. D., Harrad S., & Webster T. F. (2012). Predictors of tetrabromobisphenol-A (TBBP-A) and hexabromocyclododecanes (HBCD) in milk from Boston mothers. Environmental Science & Technology, 46(21), 12146-53.

Costa L.G., & Giordano G. (2007). Developmental neurotoxicity of polybrominated diphenyl ether (PBDE) flame retardants. Neurotoxicology, 28(6), 1047-67.

Covaci A., Voorspoels S., Abdallah M.A., Geens T., Harrad S., & Law, R.J. (2009). Analytical and Environmental Aspects of the Flame Retardant Tetrabromobisphenol-A and its Derivatives. Journal of Chromatography A. 1216(3):346-63.

Desborough J., Evans T., Müller J., & Harrad S. (2016). Polychlorinated biphenyls (PCBs), hexabromocyclododecanes (HBCDDs) and degradation products in topsoil from Australia and the United Kingdom. Emerging Contaminants, 2(1), 37-41.

Den Hond E., Tournaye H., De Sutter P., Ombelet W., Baeyens W., Covaci A., Cox B., Nawrot T.S., Van Larebeke N., & D'Hooghe T. (2015). Human exposure to endocrine disrupting chemicals and fertility: A case-control study in male subfertility patients. Environment International, 84, 154-60.

Ema M., Fujii S., Hirata-Koizumi M., & Matsumoto M. (2008). Two-generation reproductive toxicity study of the flame retardant hexabromocyclododecane in rats. Reproductive Toxicology, 25(3), 335-51.

Environmental Defense Fund (2019). Toxic consequences of Trump's chemical safety attacks. https://www.edf.org/health/toxic-consequences-trumps-chemical-safety-attacks.

Environmental Protection Agency (EPA). *EPA completes first ten risk evaluations.* https://www.epa.gov/newsreleases/epa-completes-first-10-risk-evaluations-reaching-major-chemical-safety-milestone.

Environmental Protection Agency (EPA) (2021). *About the Office of Chemical Safety and Pollution Protection.* https://www.epa.gov/aboutepa/about-office-chemical-safety-and-pollution-prevention-ocspp.

Eriksson P., Fischer C., Wallin M., Jakobsson E., & Fredriksson A. (2006). Impaired behaviour, learning and memory in adult mice neonatally exposed to hexabromocyclododecane (HBCDD). *Environmental Toxicology and Pharmacology, 21*(3), 317-22.

Germer S., Piersma A.H., Van der Ven L., Kamyschnikow A., Fery Y., Schmitz H.J., & Schrenk D. (2006). Subacute effects of the brominated flame retardants hexabromocyclododecane and tetrabromobisphenol A on hepatic cytochrome P450 levels in rats. *Toxicology. 218*(2-3):229-36.

Gore, A. C., Crews, D., Doan, L. L., La Merrill, M., Patisaul, H., & Zota, A. (2014). *An introduction to endocrine disrupting chemicals (EDCs): A guide for public interest organizations and policy makers.* https://www.endocrine.org/-/media/endosociety/files/advocacy-and-outreach/important-documents/introduction-to-endocrine-disrupting-chemicals.pdf?la=en.

Gore, A. C., Chappell, V. A., Fenton, S. E., Flaws, J. A., Nadal, A., Prins, G. S., ... Zoeller, R. T. (2015). EDC-2: The ndocrine Society's Second Scientific Statement on Endocrine-Disrupting Chemicals. *Endocrine Reviews, 36*(6), E1–E150. doi:10.1210/er.2015-1010.

Harrad S., Abdallah M. A., & Covaci A. (2009a). Causes of variability in concentrations and diastereomer patterns of hexabromocyclododecanes in indoor dust. *Environment International, 35*(3), 573-9.

Harrad S., Abdallah, M. A., Rose N. L., Turner S. D., & Davidson T.A. (2009b). Current-Use brominated flame retardants in water, sediment, and fish from English Lakes. *Environmental Science & Technology. 43*(24):9077-83.

Healthcare Without Harm. (2018). *EDCs infographic.* https://noharm-europe.org/issues/europe/edcs-infographic.

Jo H., Son M. H., Seo S. H., & Chang, Y .S. (2017). Matrix-specific distribution and diastereomeric profiles of hexabromocyclododecane (hbcd) in a multimedia environment: Air, soil, sludge, sediment, and fish. *Environmental Pollution, 226,* 515-522.

Johnson-Restrepo B., Adams D. H., & Kannan K. 2008. Tetrabromobisphenol A (TBBPA) and hexabromocyclododecanes (HBCDs) in tissues of humans, dolphins, and sharks from the United States. *Chemosphere, 70*(11)1935-44.

Meijer L., Weiss J., Van Velzen M., Brouwer A., Bergman Å.K., & Sauer P.J. (2008). Serum Concentrations of neutral and phenolic organohalogens in pregnant women and some of their infants in the Netherlands. *Environmental Science & Technology, 42*(9), 3428-33.

Meng X. Z., Duan Y. P., Yang C, Pan Z.Y., Wen Z. H., & Chen L. (2011). Occurrence, sources, and inventory of hexabromocyclododecanes (HBCDs) in soils from Chongming Island, the Yangtze River Delta (YRD). *Chemosphere, 82*(5):725-31.

Miller I., Serchi T., Cambier S., Diepenbroek C., Renaut J., Van der Berg J. H., Kwadijk C., Gutleb A. C., Rijntjes E., & Murk A. J. (2016). Hexabromocyclododecane (HBCD) induced changes in the liver proteome of eu-and hypothyroid female rats. *Toxicology Letters, 245,* 40-51.

Priyam, A., Singh, P. P., & Gehlout, S. (2018). Role of endocrine-disrupting engineered nanomaterials in the pathogenesis of type 2 diabetes mellitus. *Endocrinology, 9,* 704. doi: 10.3389/fendo.2018.00704.

Rawn D. F., Gaertner D. W., Weber D., Curran I. H., Cooke G. M., & Goodyer C. G. (2014). Hexabromocyclododecane concentrations in Canadian human fetal liver and placental tissues. *Science of The Total Environment, 468,* 622-9.

Roze E., Meijer L., Bakker A., Van Braeckel K. N., Sauer P. J., & Bos, A. F. (2009). Prenatal exposure to organohalogens, including brominated flame retardants, influences motor, cognitive, and behavioral performance at school age. *Environmental Health Perspectives, 117*(12):1953.

Ruiz, D., Becerra, M., Jagai, J. S., Ard, K., & Sargis, R. M. (2018). Disparities in environmental exposures to endocrine-disrupting chemicals and diabetes risk in vulnerable populations. *Diabetes Care, 41*(1), 193–205. doi:10.2337/dc16-2765.

Saegusa Y., Fujimoto H., Woo G.H., Inoue K., Takahashi M., Mitsumori K., Hirose M., Nishikawa A., Shibutani M. (2009). Developmental toxicity of brominated flame retardants, tetrabromobisphenol a and 1, 2, 5, 6, 9, 10-hexabromocyclododecane, in rat offspring after maternal exposure from mid-gestation through lactation. *Reproductive Toxicology, 28*(4), 456-67.

Stadler L. (1993. Corrosion Proof Fittings v. EPA: Asbestos in the Fifth Circuit--A battle of unreasonableness. *Tulane Environmental Law Journal, 6*(2):423-428.

Stockholm Convention on Persistent Organic Pollutants, United Nations Environment Programme. 2013. *Amendment to Annex A, Decision SC-5/3.*http://www.pops.int/Portals/0/download.aspx?d=UNEP-POPS-COP.5-SC-5-3.English.pdf.

U.S. Environmental Protection Agency (EPA), Office of Chemical Safety and Pollution Prevention (OCSP). (2015). *TSCA work plan chemical problem formulation and initial assessment: cyclic aliphatic bromide cluster (HBCD).*https://www.epa.gov/sites/production/files/2015-09/documents/hbcd_problem_formulation.pdf.

U.S. Environmental Protection Agency (EPA), Office of Chemical Safety and Pollution Prevention (OCSP). (2017). *Preliminary information on manufacturing, processing, distribution, use, and disposal: cyclic aliphatic bromide cluster (HBCD).* https://www.epa.gov/sites/production/files/2017-02/documents/hbcd.pdf.

U.S. Environmental Protection Agency (EPA). (2018). *2018 annual plan for chemical risk evaluations under TSCA.* https://www.epa.gov/sites/production/files/2018-01/documents/2018_annual_risk_evaluation_plan_final.pdf.

U.S. Government Accountability Office (GAO). (2005). *Chemical regulation: Options exist to improve EPA's ability to assess health risks and manage its chemical review program, June 2005, GAO-05-458.* https://www.gao.gov/new.items/d05458.pdf.

Van der Ven L. T., Verhoef A., Van De Kuil T., Slob W., Leonards P. E., Visser T. J., Hamers T., Herlin M., Håkansson H., Olausson H., & Piersma A .H. (2006). A 28-day oral dose toxicity study enhanced to detect endocrine effects of hexabromocyclododecane in Wistar rats. *Toxicological Sciences, 94*(2), 281-92.

Woodruff, T. J., Zota, A. R., & Schwartz, J. M. (2011). Environmental chemicals in pregnant women in the United States: NHANES 2003-2004. *Environmental Health Perspectives, 119*(6), 878–885. doi:10.1289/ehp.1002727.

Yang, R., Wei, H., Guo, J., & Li, A. (2012). Emerging brominated flame retardants in the sediment of the Great Lakes. *Environmental Science & Technology, 46*(6), 3119-26.

A NEW FORM OF ENVIRONMENTAL POLLUTION: WIRELESS AND NON-IONIZING ELECTROMAGNETIC FIELDS

Catherine Dodd PhD, RN, FAAN
Environmental Health Consultant
Former Chief of Staff for Speaker Nancy Pelosi
Former Deputy Chief of Staff for Health and Human Services to San Francisco Mayor (now CA Governor Newsom)
Former Director Region IX USDHHS under President Clinton.

Theodora Scarato, MSW
Executive Director
Environmental Health Trust

The wireless revolution and the expansion of the internet of things is rapidly increasing our exposure to non-ionizing electromagnetic fields (EMFs) now considered a new form of environmental pollution (Russell, 2018, Bandara & Carpenter, 2018). Health and medical professionals recommend that we reduce these EMF exposures because of a growing body of research that documents adverse biological effects from low level exposures (Miller, 2019).

This chapter will introduce what EMFs are, how people are exposed, science documenting health effects of exposure, U.S. and international policy on protection from EMFs and nursing implications for clinical practice and advocacy in concert with ANA's principles.

WHAT ARE EMFS?

EMFs are invisible energy waves consisting of electric and magnetic fields. For thousands of years, humans have been exposed to natural EMFs - such as the magnetic field of the earth and light from the sun. However, exposure to human-made EMFs are a relatively recent phenomenon and the more complex data carrying signals of cellular networks have been found to have significant biologic effects. (Panagopoulos, 2015).

Humans are electrical beings. Our cells communicate with tiny electrical impulses which affect our heart, our brain, our nervous system, and our endocrine system. In health care, these electrical impulses are recorded as electric waves on electrocardiograms and electroencephalograms.

IONIZING RADIATION VERSUS NON-IONIZING RADIATION

Electromagnetic fields include two types of radiation: ionizing and non-ionizing. Ionizing radiation has intense high energy, high frequency waves which can remove electrons from atoms or "ionize them" causing cellular damage and directly breaking DNA. Ionizing radiation is known to cause cancer.

Ionizing radiation is used in healthcare both diagnostically (e.g. x-rays and CT scans), and therapeutically to reduce tumors (radiation treatment). Protective precautions such as lead shields and minimizing exposure are required. Health care institutions have procedures for nurses and other staff who with patients receiving ionizing radiation therapy to minimize the health care providers' exposures (Kaiser, 2001).

In contrast, non-ionizing radiation (e.g. Wi-Fi, wireless networks, cell tower radiation) has much lower energy and lower frequency waves. Decades ago, cell phones and wireless networks were brought to market without long term safety studies because the frequencies were non-ionizing and assumed to be safe. While non-ionizing radiation is not thought to cause DNA damage in the same way that ionizing radiation does, recent studies indicate that DNA damage and other adverse health

---

The American Nurses Association Principles of Environmental Health for Nursing Practice were based on a Foundation of Principles including (among them):Human health is linked to the quality of the environment.

- A healthy environment is a universal need and fundamental human right.

- Current generations should meet their needs without compromising the ability of future generations to meet their own needs.

- Pollution prevention should occur at its source. The concern of nurses is the promotion, maintenance, and restoration of people's health.

- Nurses have an obligation to address health disparities and environmental injustice. The nurse collaborates with other professionals, policy makers, advocacy groups, and the public in promoting local, state, national, and international efforts to meet health needs.

(ANA's Principles of Environmental Health for Nursing Practice with Implementation Strategies, 2007)

Reproduced with permission of the American Nurses Association

effects can result from non-ionizing radiation, via a more complex indirect process (Lai, 2021, Panagopoulos et al., 2021).

There are two main categories of non-ionizing EMF's of scientific research conducted to identify possible biological and environmental effects for over four decades.

- Magnetic Field Extremely Low Frequency (ELF-EMFs)- which are generated anywhere electricity flows such as powerlines, electrical wiring and charging cords.

- Radiofrequency (RF- EMFs) - also known as Radiofrequency Radiation (RFR) -which are the data/information carrying waves of cell phones and wireless networks (Moon, 2020).

In this chapter, unless otherwise noted, the acronym "EMF refers to both ELF and RFF.

WHY ARE EMF EXPOSURES IMPORTANT?

A large and increasing body of research in both human and animal studies have found that even legally allowed low level exposures are linked to a myriad of harmful biological effects including cancer, DNA damage and impacts to reproduction, nervous system and brain development (Bandara & Carpenter, 2018). The effects of new technology on human health are challenging to study because there is no unexposed control group in humans (Russell, 2018.)

SOURCES OF EMF EXPOSURES

Home and School Exposures

People are directly and indirectly exposed to EMFs from cell phones, computers, smart electronics and the myriad of Wi-Fi networks in their homes, workplaces and schools (see table 1). The use of wireless electronics by every age group continues to increase each year (Common Sense Media, 2019). Many school districts have robust Wi-Fi networks and students now use computers in school and at home for hours a day.

The use of electronics close to the body -e.g. laptops on laps, cell phones carried in a pocket or bra- create two kinds of intense EMF exposures to the body part closest

to the device- RF from the wireless and ELF from the electricity. In addition, ELF exposures are elevated near charging cell phones, appliances, and electronics (Behrens et al., 2004).

Occupational Exposures

Cell phones, and wireless networks are common in today's workplace -e.g. in hospitals, schools, retail, transportation and numerous industries. There is a critical need to gather health data on these exposures (Stam, 2021). For example, many delivery drivers use cell phones and tablets to track packages and hospital workers often have a cell phone in their pocket, a walkie talkie clipped to their chest, and they use numerous wireless devices over the course of one day.

Cell tower/antenna maintenance workers, physical therapists using diathermy, and operators of dielectric welders have elevated EMF exposures. The latter two directly use high frequency EMFs to generate heat produced by EMFs (Aniołczyk et al., 2015). Overexposure has been documented to induced central nervous system demyelinating disease mimicking Multiple Sclerosis (Raefsky et al., 2020). Although U.S. National Institute for Occupational Safety and Health (NIOSH) scientists developed recommendations to reduce EMF, they were never implemented (Bowman, 2016).

Figure 1

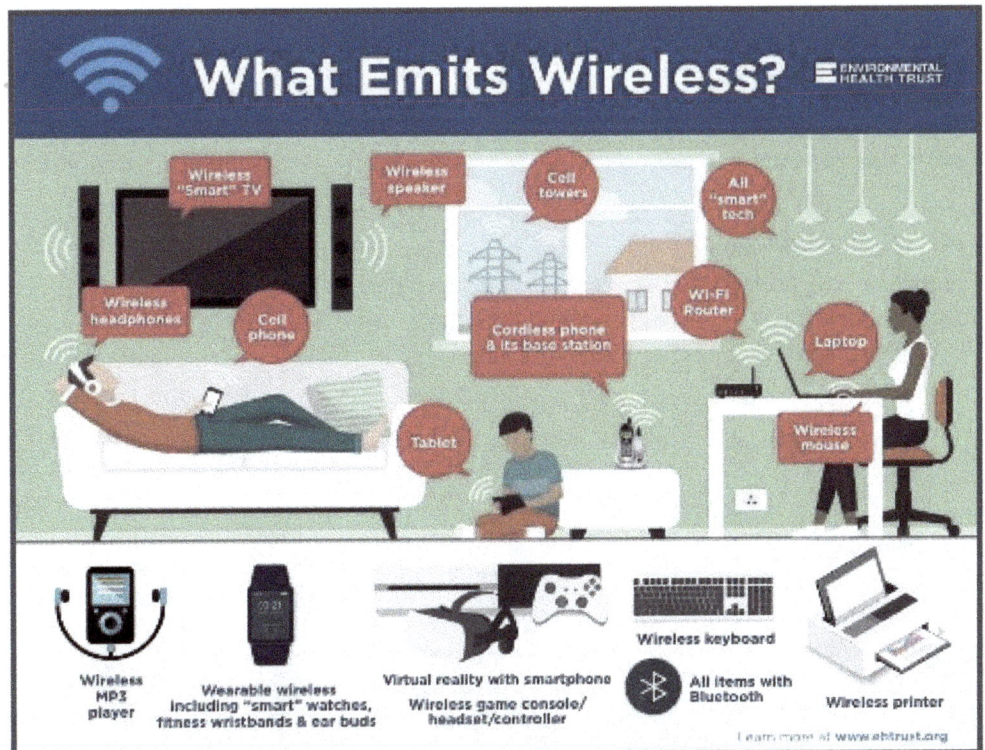

Used with permission from Environmental Health Trust

Table 1: Types and sources of EMF exposures

First-Hand Exposure (Devices Used Close to the Body)	Second-Hand Exposure (Devices and Networks Inside Homes, Schools and Buildings)	Environmental Exposure
ELF- EMF and Magnetic fields (*Also emit RF if wireless)		
• Cell phones, tablets and laptops * • Electric blankets • Charging phones and electronics * • Alarm clocks and radios plugged in directly near the body such as near beds	• Wiring errors in electrical systems • Electric cars **Occupational sources** • Microwave ovens • Welding equipment • Appliances • Electrical equipment • Motors	• High-voltage power lines • Power cables • Electrical transformers • Substations • Railways and electric trains
RF-EMF		
• Cell phones • Cordless phones • Wi-Fi tablets, laptops & computers • Walkie talkies • Wearable technology • Smart watches • Wireless keyboard and mouse • Bluetooth • Wireless Toys	• Wi-Fi networks • Wi-Fi routers • Cordless phone base station • Wireless devices such as: • Baby monitors • Gaming consoles • Speakers • Security systems/hubs- doorbells with cameras • Virtual Assistants • Wireless printers	• Cell towers • Small cell towers aka: Personal Wireless Facilities • Antennas mounted on buildings • Smart Meter networks

Environmental Exposures

Environmental exposures to non-ionizing EMFs have dramatically increased over the last few decades (Bandara& Carpenter, 2018). People who live near high voltage powerlines and substations may have elevated ELF-EMF throughout their home (Gagsek et al., 2013, Amoon et al., 2020).

Cell tower networks are a significant source of a person's daily RF-EMF exposure, especially in urban areas (Sagar et al., 2018). Cell tower RF-EMF penetrates into homes, especially through windows facing the beam of a nearby wireless antenna (Hardell et al., 2018). The newest generations of wireless - 4G and 5G- will increase RF-EMF as these networks consist of thousands of new "small" cell towers built closer to homes (El Hajj and Naous, 2020, Mzloum et al., 2019). It is estimated that 800,000 new cell towers will be needed in the U.S. (Shepardson, 2018). Researchers caution that increasing cell antennas closer to the ground, close to homes and schools will increase ambient RF exposures to people (Frank 2021, Koppel et al 2022, Pearce 2020).

WHO ARE MOST VULNERABLE TO HEALTH EFFECTS OF EMFS?

Children

When cell phones first came on the market, no one could imagine the need for a child to use one. Now they are a favorite toy and used as babysitters. Children are uniquely vulnerable to EMFs just as they are to other environmental toxins. As wireless technology is now ubiquitous, children will receive a greater cumulative exposure than today's adults, with exposure starting before they are born (Miller et al., 2019). Both their ongoing physical development and physiology put them at greater risk.

• Children absorb proportionally higher doses of cell phone RF-EMF in the eyes and critical brain regions than adults due to their smaller heads, thinner undeveloped skulls and the higher water content in both their bodies and brain (Fernandez et al., 2018).

- Children's developing brains are more susceptible to neurotoxic exposures (Redmayne and Johansson, 2014 and 2015).

- Children have more active stem cells and stem cells have been found to be more sensitive to RF-EMF exposure (Markova et al., 2010).

- Safety limits for RF-EMF from cell phones and cell towers are outdated as they were set over two decades ago in 1996 and are based on the body of a large adult, not a child (Gandhi et al., 2012).

Researchers at Penn State Medical Center found reducing EMFs improved health outcomes in preterm infants (Passi et al., 2017). NICU equipment is linked to various impacts to the autonomic nervous system including melatonin

Figure 2

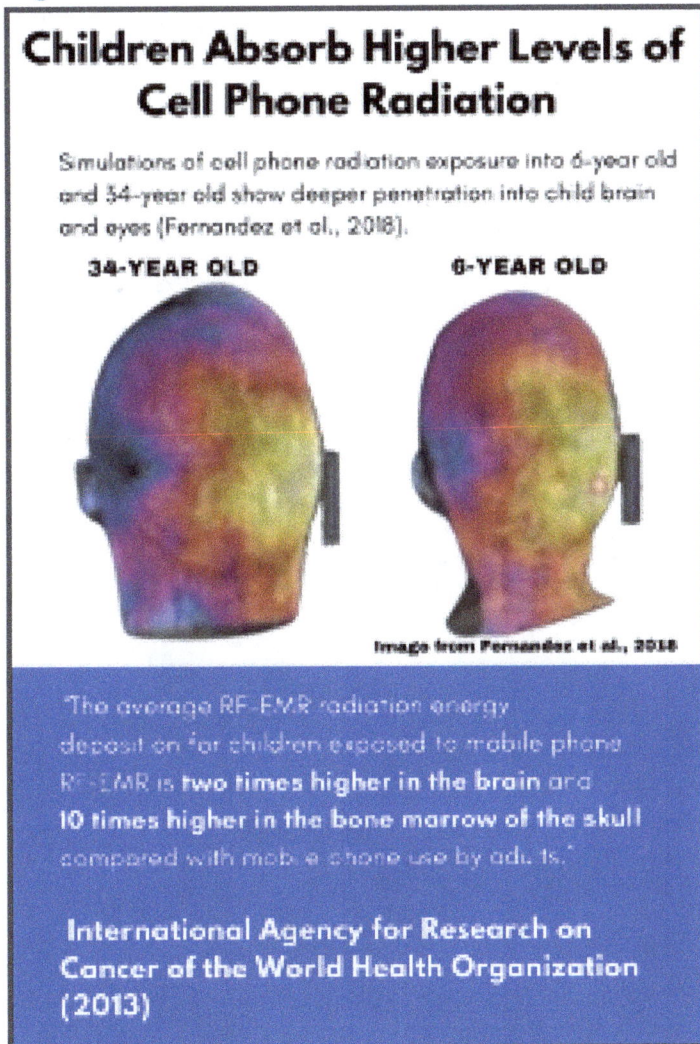

Children Absorb Higher Levels of Cell Phone Radiation

Simulations of cell phone radiation exposure into 6-year old and 34-year old show deeper penetration into child brain and eyes (Fernandez et al., 2018).

34-YEAR OLD   6-YEAR OLD

Image from Fernandez et al., 2018

"The average RF-EMR radiation energy deposition for children exposed to mobile phone RF-EMR is **two times higher in the brain** and **10 times higher in the bone marrow of the skull** compared with mobile phone use by adults."

International Agency for Research on Cancer of the World Health Organization (2013)

Used with permission from Environmental Health Trust and Professor Claudio Fernandez.

production and heart rate and a 2017 review concluded that incubators should be redesigned to reduce exposure to the babies and caregivers (Bellieni et al., 2017).

Pregnancy

As with other environmental toxins, the developing fetus is particularly sensitive to exposure during critical developmental windows. Although more research needs to be done to fully understand the risk during windows of vulnerability, research on pregnant people has linked prenatal cell phone radiation exposure to oxidative stress and DNA damage in cord blood (Bektas et al., 2021); increased risk for miscarriage (Mahmoudabadi et al., 2015), lower birth weight (Lu et al., 2017), fetal growth impacts (Boileau et al., 2020), and preterm birth (Tsarna et al., 2019); as well as emotional/behavioral problems (Divan et al., 2012, Sudan et al., 2016) and hyperactivity (Birks et al., 2017) in their children. Animal studies have linked prenatal wireless exposure to DNA damage (Smith-Roe et al., 2020), brain damage (Tan et al., 2017), memory problems (Shahin et al., 2018) and hyperactivity (Aldad et al., 2012).

A Kaiser Foundation Research Institute team took measurements of the magnetic field ELF-EMF exposure of pregnant people and followed their pregnancies and subsequent birth and health of their children over time. They published a series of studies documenting links between higher prenatal magnetic field exposure (ELF-EMF) and miscarriage (Li et al., 2017) as well as ADHD (Li et al., 2020), obesity (Li et al., 2012), and asthma (Li et al., 2011) in children exposed prenatally.

Watch BabySafe Project press conference where Hugh Taylor MD, Chief of OBGYN at Yale Medicine and Devra Davis PhD, MPH presented on the scientific basis for the recommendations to reduce exposure.

PHYSIOLOGICAL IMPACTS OF ELECTROMAGNETIC FIELDS

Oxidative Stress and Preexisting Conditions

Reviews of animal and cell studies consistently find even very low EMF exposure associated with increased oxidative stress. Oxidative stress plays a role in the development of many diseases, such as cancer, diabetes, immune and neurodegenerative syndromes. The young, old and/or medically compromised individuals, whose immune system and defense mechanisms are already compromised, are more likely to experience health effects from the increased oxidative stress (Yakymenko et al., 2015, Schuermann & Mevissen, 2021).

Cancer

Researchers have long studied EMFs for their relationship to causation. In 2002, magnetic field ELF-EMF was classified by the World Health Organization International Agency for Research on Cancer (WHO/IARC) as a Group 2B possible carcinogen due to research findings that showed a relationship between residential exposure and increased childhood leukemia risk (WHO/IARC 2002). This association continues to be reported in more recent studies (Carpenter 2019, Seomun et al., 2021).

In 2011, the WHO/IARC concluded that wireless radiofrequency radiation (RF-EMF) was a Group 2B possible carcinogen largely based on studies of long term cell phone users with increased tumors-glioblastomas and acoustic neuromas (WHO/ IARC 2011). Several international experts conclude RF-EMF is a proven Group I human carcinogen (Miller et al., 2018, Peleg et al., 2018 Carlberg and Hardell 2017, Belpomme et al., 2018).

Examples of new scientific research that finds a carcinogenic effect for RF-EMF include:

• Two major animal studies investigating long-term exposure found the same tumors as found in human studies (U.S. National Toxicology Program, 2018, Falcioni et al., 2018).

• A 2020 meta-analysis linked cumulative cell phone use over 1000 hours increased tumor risk (Choi et al., 2020).

• Studies have found women who carry cellphones in the bra have elevated breast cancer risk (West et al., 2013, Shih et al., 2020).

• A Yale study funded by the American Cancer Society found elevated thyroid cancer risk in heavy cell phone users with specific genetic susceptibilities (Luo et al., 2020).

Reproduction

Systematic reviews associate RF-EMF with impacts to sperm (Kim et al., 2021, Yu et al., 2021) and decreased testosterone (Maluin et al., 2021) leading many researchers to conclude "it is recommended to keep the cell phone away from the pelvis as much as possible" (Hassanzadeh-Taheri et al., 2021).

Nervous System Impacts

The nervous system is sensitive to EMFs (Bertagna et al., 2021). Cell phone radiation has been found to alter brain activity (Volkow et al., 2011, Bin et al., 2014), impact neurotransmitters and alter neuron development (Kaplan et al., 2015, Li et al., 2021, Chen et al., 2021). Teenagers were found to experience memory damage to the area of the brain most exposed to cell phone radiation after just one year (Foerster et al., 2018).

Experimental animal research has found a variety of RF-EMF impacts especially in the brain regions critical to memory and learning (Sonmez, et al., 2010, Dasdag et al., 2015, Shahin et al., 2018, Obajuluwa et al., 2017, Tan et al., 2021, Hasan et al., 2021).

Electromagnetic Hypersensitivity

In 2021, scientists published a consensus statement calling for the acknowledgement of electrohypersensitivity as a distinct neuropathological disorder (Belpomme et al., 2021) and exposure to non-ionizing radiation has a series of ICD 10 codes.

Electromagnetic hypersensitivity (EHS) is characterized by the development of numerous symptoms linked to EMF exposure including: headaches, sleeping problems, concentration problems, nosebleeds, unexplained skin rashes, digestive problems, neurological problems, heart palpitations and disabling fatigue (Belyaev et al., 2016).

Synergistic Effects

EMFs can add to our total body burden of carcinogens. Research has found that EMF exposure can act synergistically with other environmental pollutants potentiating harmful effects (Kostoff and Lau, 2017). For example, prenatal and postnatal mobile phone exposure has been linked to greater neurobehavioral effects in children with elevated lead levels (Choi et al., 2017, Byun et al., 2017).

It is challenging to isolate an association epidemiologically because there is no unexposed control group (Russell, 2018.) Scientists must therefore rely on animal experiments which are carefully controlled to understand if the effects are caused by the exposure.

Animal studies have found combining ELF-EMF exposure with known carcinogens can increase tumors (Soffritti et al., 2016, Soffritti et al., 2016). EMFs can increase permeability of the blood brain barrier, thus, allowing more toxic agents to reach the brain (Sirav and Seyhan, 2016, Tang et al., 2015).

EMFs and the Environment

There are reports that the proliferation of cell antennas will have numerous environmental effects. Analysis are accumulating that electricity and energy consumption of 5G and new wireless networks will contribute to greenhouse gasses and exacerbate climate change (The Shift Project, 2019, Williams et al, 2022).

Further, trees are critical to a healthy environment. They filter toxic chemicals from the air, reduce ground-level ozone and absorb carbon dioxide emissions that are driving climate change (Terzaghi et al., 2020, Bastin et al., 2019). There are studies finding that cell antenna RF- EMF can injure trees (Waldmann-Selsam, C., et al., 2016, Breunig, 2017, Haggerty, 2010) and impact plant growth (Halgamuge, 2017, Pall, 2016).

A 2021 research review on effects to wildlife published in Reviews on Environmental Health references more than 1,200 scientific references which found impacts to wildlife, including pollinators, from even very low intensities of non-ionizing EMFs including impacts to orientation and migration, reproduction, mating, nest, den building and survivorship (Levitt et al., 2021a, b, c). The authors assert that the current body of science should trigger urgent protective regulatory action to protect wildlife.

A COMPLEX SCIENCE WITH LIMITED PROTECTIVE FEDERAL REGULATION AND HEAVY INDUSTRY INFLUENCE

U.S. and international scientists are calling for an update to the 1996 federal regulations and the need for independent research reviews in order to ensure the public is protected (Hardell & Carlberg, 2020). Similar to other environmental pollutants, literature reviews show conflicting results and industry funding has long been found to influence the results both in ELF and RF research (Hardell et al., 2006, Carpenter 2019, Huss et al., 2017). The official reports of many authorities have been criticized as having major conflicts of interest (Hardell 2017, Buchner & Rivasi, 2020).

The book, "Captured Agency" (Alster, 2015) identified a "revolving door" between industry, Congress and the Federal Communications Commission. The investigation compared the tactics of the wireless industry to Big Tobacco citing the heavy industry lobbying, the funding of science that shows no effect and the massive public relations campaigns designed to attack the credibility of the science and of scientists who do find harmful effects.

U.S. Policy

The Federal Communications Commission (FCC) established human exposure limits for cell phones and cellular network RF-EMF in 1996 and they have not been updated despite the dramatic changes in wireless communications in the last 25 years. The FCC is not a health agency and does not have medical or public health experts on staff. In 2021, a federal court ruled that the

FCC needed to reexamine their decision to retain the 1996 limits (No. 20-1025, 2021). To date, governmental health and environmental agencies such as the Environmental Protection Agency (EPA), the Food and Drug Administration (FDA), the Department of Health and Human Services and National Cancer Institutes have not reviewed the totality of the latest science on health effects of EMFs.

In 2018, the U.S. National Toxicology Program (NTP) found "clear evidence of cancer" and DNA damage in a large-scale animal study designed to evaluate the effects of long term exposure to radio frequency radiation from cell phones (U.S. National Toxicology Program, 2018). Although the FDA requested the studies, they rejected the study conclusions. Research analyzing the NTP findings conclude U.S safety limits need to be strengthened by 200 to 400 times to protect children according to current risk assessment guidelines (Uche & Naidenko ., 2021).

The American Academy of Pediatrics has long recommended that FCC limits be updated to protect children and pregnant people (AAP, 2012 & 2013). In addition, cell phones and electronics are not tested the way people use devices today- in body contact positions. Although it is now commonplace to see children watching videos with a cell phones pressed against their chest, research has found that when phones are tested for exposure levels in body contact positions, they can exceed government limits up to 11 times the FCC limit (Gandhi, 2019). Pregnant people rest cell phones laptops on their abdomens, and research finds these positions create RF-EMF exposures into the fetal brain (Cabot et al., 2014) and can induce ELF-EMF in the fetus Bellieni et al., 2012).

Magnetic and ELF Safety Limits

The United States has no federal safety limit for magnetic fields or ELF-EMF. In contrast, over a dozen countries have some level of protective policy in place and they limit building homes in areas with magnetic field levels higher than the levels associated with childhood leukemia (Stam, 2018).

State and Local Policies

In the US, many states and localities have enacted laws related to Cell/Tower/Antenna placement. Physicians for Safe Technology and the Environmental Health Trust track state legislation and local ordinances. In 2020, the New Hampshire State Commission on 5G issued 15 recommendations which included several recommendations including large setbacks to distance cell

Figure 3

U.S. Policy and Recommendations on Cell Phones, Cell Towers and Wi-Fi

School Districts

"Best Practices" posted in classrooms – to turn Wi-Fi off when not in use.
- Onteora NY
- Ashland, MA

Information on how to reduce wireless.
- Worcester MA
- Montgomery County MD

Ban on Cell Towers
- Palo Alto Unified CA
- Los Angeles CA
- West Linn-Wilsonville OR
- Montgomery County MD
- Prince George's MD
- Portland OR

Teacher Unions

New York State United Teachers
- Resolution "Hazards of Wireless Radiation Emission"and "Best Practices" recommend wired ethernet connections.
- Webinar "Risks of wireless technologies and protecting children and staff in schools."

United Educators of San Francisco CA
- Resolution on Safer Technology calls for the California cell phone advisory on how to reduce cell phone exposure be disseminated to students and staff.
- Webinars on reducing RF exposure

State Public Health Departments

California Cell Phone Advisory (2017)
- Explains how to reduce cell phone exposure- especially for children.

Connecticut Cell Phone Advisory (2015)
- States that it "is wise" to reduce cellphone radiation to brain.

North Carolina Department of Occupational & Environmental Epidemiology
- Lists the American Academy of Pediatrics recommendations to reduce cell phone radiation

Cell Tower Setbacks

Numerous cities restrict cell antennas near homes with setbacks and strict ordinances including: Los Altos, Petaluma, Mill Valley, Malibu, Santa Barbara, Nevada City, Suisin, Calabasas, San Clemente, Westlake, Sonoma, Sebastopol, San Rafael, Ross Valley, Encinitas, Fairfax, Palo Alto, Walnut City and San Diego County CA, Ithaca and Scarsdale NY, Randolph, Great Barrington and Stockbridge MA

As an example, the **Los Altos City ordinance prohibits installation of small cells on public utility easements in residential** and has a 500 ft school setback. San Diego County does not allow small cells within 1,000 feet of schools, child care centers, hospitals, or churches.

Cell Phone Right To Know Laws

San Francisco CA (2010) & Berkeley CA (2015)
- Informed consumers that phones emit radiation and should not be in body contact.
- Passed but not implemented after wireless industry lawsuits.

Maryland State Council

Council on Children's Environmental Health Report (2017)
- Install wired networks instead of Wi-Fi when building schools.
- Reduce wireless exposure in schools.

New Jersey Education Association

Recommendations (2016)
- Hard wire devices, printers, projectors and boards.
- Use hard-wired phones instead of cell or cordless phones.
- Put devices in airplane mode.

New Hampshire State

2020: Final Report of Commission on Health & Environmental Effects of 5G
15 recommendations include:
- An independent federal study of health effects
- Educational campaign to reduce public exposure.
- Replace Wi-Fi with wired in schools and libraries.
- Setbacks for antennas from schools and homes
- Measure cell network radiation levels.
- Establish wireless radiation limits to protect trees, plants, wildlife and insects.
- Require software changes to reduce emissions.
- Establish wireless radiation-free zones.
- An environmental impact assessment on 5G.

Resolutions Halt 5G and/or Study Health Effects
- Hawai'i County HI
- Easton CT
- Farragut TN
- Hallandale FL
- Keene NH
- Carmel City IN

Proclamations Cell Phone Radiation
- Portland ME
- Pembroke Pines FL
- Jackson Hole WY

EMF Hypersensitivity
- Alabama
- Colorado
- Connecticut
- Broward County FL

ENVIRONMENTAL HEALTH TRUST

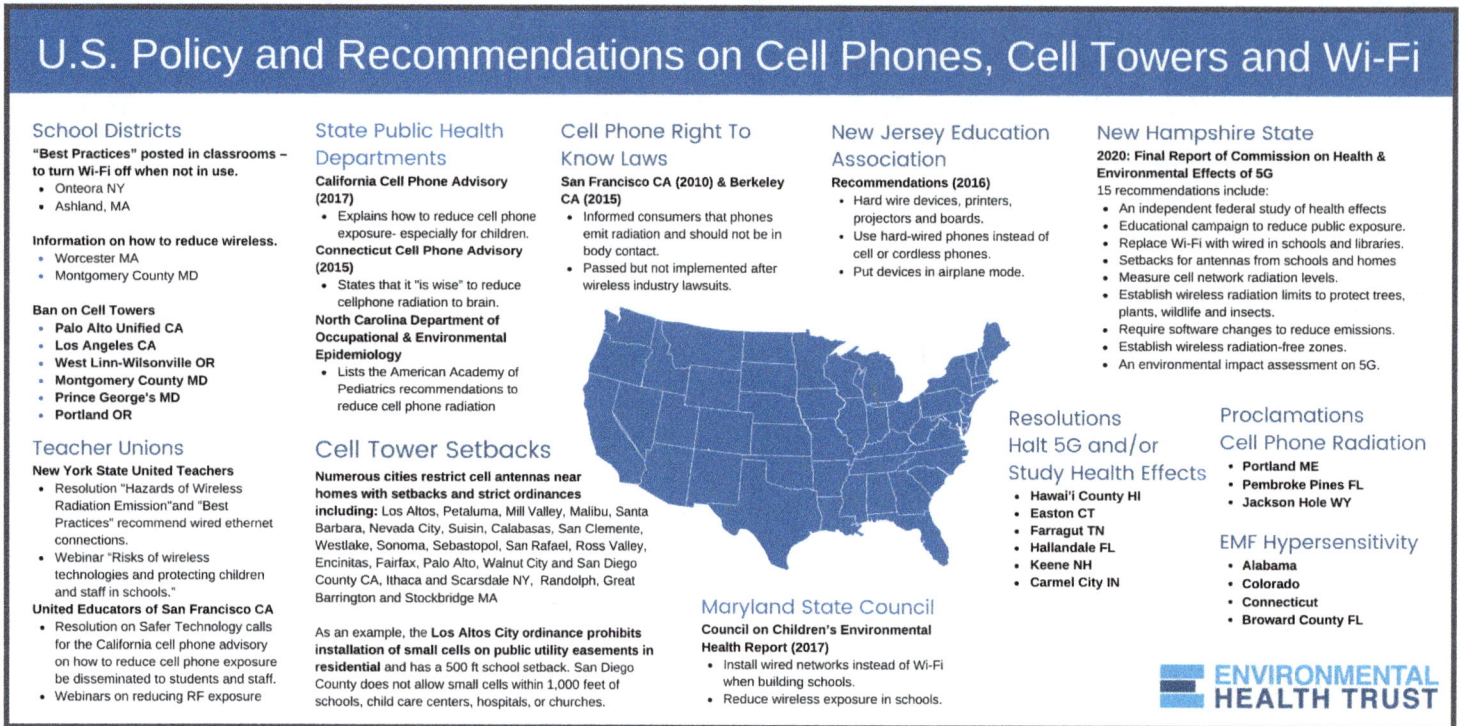

Used with permission from Environmental Health Trust

antennas from homes and schools, replacing Wi-Fi with wired in schools and a public health campaign to educate families. In 2023, Massachusetts state legislature proposed a bill (H.2158) that would recognize electromagnetic sensitivity (EMS) as a disease that is a public health issue and establish a state-wide EMS disease registry.

International Policies and Actions

Internationally governments have policies and regulations in place to inform the public and reduce exposures. Numerous scientists, medical and public health professionals have issued appeals and recommendations on the need to reduce exposure to electromagnetic radiation and pause the proliferation of new untested networks (EMF Scientists Appeal, 2015, Di Ciaula, 2018, Mallery-Blythe, 2020, Nyberg & Hardell, 2017)

- Switzerland, Italy, China, Russia, India, Israel and several European countries have far more stringent cell tower radiation emission limits compared to the US FCC and many define homes, schools and kindergartens as "sensitive areas" (Stam, 2017).

- Over a dozen countries have clear recommendations that people reduce exposure to cell phone radiation, especially for children (Redmayne, 2016, EHT, 2021).

- France has several policies including: limiting Wi-Fi in classrooms, banning the sale of cell phones designed for young children, banning advertisements aimed at children under 14 years old. Consumers are informed with instructions to use speakerphone, limit children's use and "keep away from the belly of pregnant people and lower abdomen of adolescents."

- Cyprus and French Polynesia have multimedia public education campaigns (EHT, 2021).

- A major hospital in Cyprus removed Wi-Fi from the pediatric Intensive Care Unit and Neonatal units (Cyprus Committee on Environment and Children's Health, 2019).

IMPLICATIONS FOR NURSING PRACTICE

In 1992, the International Council of Nurses made environmental health, preventing illness by eliminating environmental toxins a priority (as cited in ANA's Principles of Environmental Health for Nursing Practice with Implementation Strategies 2007). Nurses can protect human health and the environment through prevention, clinical practice, and advocacy.

Prevention

Nurses are trusted advisors. Nurses must first protect themselves and their families, their patients, and their communities by learning how to decrease exposures to EMFs. Small lifestyle changes can significantly reduce cellular damage of our total lifetime exposure. We can then educate our patients- especially parents and vulnerable populations. Nurses can work in coalition with other groups to educate why and how to reduce EMF exposures in the workplace, schools, and communities. People need to know how to eliminate unnecessary sources of EMFs and choose safe alternatives. Tips and checklists follow.

Clinical Practice

Nurses can integrate their understanding of EMFs into their clinical practice and include interview questions about technology use and EMF exposure in their assessments. When patients present with EHS symptoms, such as headache, insomnia, irritability, they should be further assessed for EMF sensitivity.

Helpful resources include:

- Physicians for Safe Technology EHS information includes Clinical Interview Questions

- Austrian Medical Association EMF Guidelines Has algorithms and a sample patient questionnaire.

- The Environmental Health Clinic, Women's College Hospital at the University of Toronto Practice Guidelines for Diagnosis and Treatment (Bray, 2020)

- EMF Medical Conference 2021 offers CME Online

- Electrosensitivity Society Providers in US and Canada

ADVOCACY

Protecting Health Requires Nurses To Be Advocates for Systematic Policy Change

Just as with other environmental issues, nurses have a responsibility to act to protect individuals and communities by supporting meaningful policy change.

Nurses bring credibility on health issues to advocacy and our voices are important in developing protective policy. Working in coalition with other organizations always strengthens the message (e.g parent groups, environmental organizations, faith-based organizations, etc.).

- Nursing organizations can adopt resolutions or policy positions on wireless and EMF exposures. See the resolution of the California Medical Association.

- Nurses can join "safe tech" organizations and coalitions to support policies that reduce EMF exposures in our workplaces, schools, and communities. These include the citing of small cell antennas in neighborhood and sensitive areas and advocate for wired internet

connection to and into the building: FASTER, SAFER, RELIABLE, and if it is a municipal/community partnership, it will eliminate the digital divide. Learn more at: SafeG.net

- Nurses and nursing organizations fighting climate change can lobby elected officials to take into account the carbon footprint of wireless technology. Download Environmental Health Trust's Fact sheet on 5G and Climate Change which describes research showing escalating energy consumption from 5G networks.

- As environmental health advocates, nurses can educate and work with schools, parents, teachers, and unions to reduce EMF exposures in schools, replace Wi-Fi with wired internet connections and ensure cell towers are not built near schools or daycare centers.

RESOURCES

Resources for Safe Schools

Environmental Health Trust
Physicians for Safe Technology

Santa Clara Medical Association

Wi-fi In Schools: Are We playing It Safe With Our Kids?
Shallow Minds: How the Internet and Wi Fi in Schools Can Affect Learning

How To Reduce EMFs in Schools

New Jersey Education Association Article, PDF of Recommendations
Maryland State Children's Environmental Health and Protection Advisory Council
Collaborative for High Performance Schools Low EMF Criteria
Grassroots Environmental Education
Environmental Health Trust Checklist for Schools

Websites

Environmental Health Trust
Environmental Working Group
Physicians for Safe Technology
Americans for Responsible Technology
Dr. Joel Moskowitz, UC Berkeley School of Public Health, Director, Center for Family and Community Health

Educational Webinars

Dr. Joel Moskowitz "Health Effects of Cell Phones and Wireless: Implications for 5G" Center for Occupational and Environmental Health Webinar
Dr. Devra Davis "Children, Wireless Radiation and Health" Cyprus Pediatric Symposium

Table 2: Ways to reduce exposure to cell phone radiation

American Academy of Pediatrics Reducing Cell Phone Radiation Recommendations

- Prefer texting to voice calls
- Use cell phones in speaker mode or hands-free.
- Hold cell phone at a distance from head.
- Make only short or essential calls on cell phones.
- Avoid carrying your phone against the body like in a pocket, sock, or bra.
- Do not talk on the phone or text while driving.
- If you plan to watch a movie on your device, download it first, then switch to airplane mode while you watch in order to avoid unnecessary radiation exposure.
- Minimize use in areas of low signal (i.e. how many bars you have). The weaker your cell signal, the harder your phone has to work and the more radiation it gives off.
- Avoid making calls in cars, elevators, trains, and buses. The cell phone works harder to get a signal through metal, so the power level increases.
- Remember that cell phones are not toys or teething items.

(American Academy of Pediatrics, 2016)

Resources on How To Reduce Cell Phone Radiation

- EHT Steps to Reduce Cell Phone Radiation
- Cell Phone Tip Card from Grassroots Environmental Education
- Downloadable Posters on Reducing Cell Phone Radiation

Reducing EMFs During Pregnancy

During pregnancy, new parents are highly motivated to learn everything they can to have a healthy baby. This is a great opportunity for nurses to give parents information.

The Baby Safe Project website includes five simple ways to reduce exposure, downloadable brochures in French and Spanish.

Reducing EMFs at Home

- Replace cordless phones with corded telephones
- Minimize wireless use. Start by turning Wi-Fi off at night. Then install wired ethernet connections instead of Wi-Fi.

Reducing EMFs at Home (Cont.)

- Use wired mouse, keyboard, speaker, and printer.
- Use wired alarm systems and doorbells not wireless
- Keep devices on a table off the lap/body.
- Do not use wireless speakers or virtual assistants.
- Keep mobile devices and chargers out of bedrooms.
- Eliminate baby monitors and wireless cameras.
- Refuse Smart meters and request analog, non-wireless utility (water, electricity, gas) meter options.
- Safe Technology at Home
- Checklist for Reducing EMF at Home
- How to Connect Your Laptop with Ethernet Instead of Wi-Fi

Tips for Reducing Magnetic Field EMF

- Use tablets, laptops and electronics on a table, not the lap.
- Do not use a cell phone or device while it is charging.
- Charge phones and devices away from beds and away from your body.
- Remove screens and electronics from the bedroom - especially around your bed and the crib.
- Avoid sleeping with electric blankets and heating pads.
- Ensure you are not sleeping against a wall with the utility meter on the other side.
- Get magnetic field measurements, especially if you live close to high voltage power lines.
- Building science and radiofrequency radiation: What makes smart and healthy buildings: Reduce EMF
- Collaborative for High Performance Schools Reduce RF and Low EMF Criteria
- How to Reduce EMF in Schools
- Safe Tech for Kids: What to do about children's increased use of technology during Covid-19

Expert Webinar "What Environmental Health Leaders Need to Know"

Downloads/Printables

EHT Posters and Factsheets

American Academy of Pediatrics Letters

Santa Clara Medical Organization

Books

Dunkley, V. (2015). Reset your child's brain: A four-week plan to end meltdowns, raise grades, and boost social skills by reversing the effects of electronic screen-time. New World Library.

Cohen, A.,& vom Saal, F.S. (2020). *Non-toxic: Guide to living healthy in a chemical world.* Oxford University Press.

Davis et al, (2018). Chapter 10: Microwave/Radiofrequency Radiation and Human Health: Clinical Management in the Digital Age, in Integrative Environmental Medicine Oxford University Press

REFERENCES

Aldad, T. S., Gan, G., Gao, X.-B., & Taylor, H. S. (2012). Fetal radiofrequency radiation exposure from 800-1900 mhz-rated cellular telephones affects neurodevelopment and behavior in mice. *Scientific Reports*, 2(1), 312. https://doi.org/10.1038/srep00312

Alster, N. (2015). *Captured agency: How the Federal Communications Commission is dominated by the industries it presumably regulates.* Harvard University. https://ethics.harvard.edu/files/center-for-ethics/files/capturedagency_alster.pdf

American Academy of Pediatrics. (2016). *Cell phone radiation & children's health: What parents need to know.* HealthyChildren.Org. https://www.healthychildren.org/English/safety-prevention/all-around/Pages/Cell-Phone-Radiation-Childrens-Health.aspx

Amoon, A. T., Swanson, J., Vergara, X., & Kheifets, L. (2020). Relationship between distance to overhead power lines and calculated fields in two studies. *Journal of Radiological Protection: Official Journal of the Society for Radiological Protection*, 40(2), 431–443. https://doi.org/10.1088/1361-6498/ab7730

ANA. (2007). *ANA's principles of environmental health for nursing practice with implementation strategies.* ANA. http://ojin.nursingworld.org/MainMenuCategories/WorkplaceSafety/Healthy-Nurse/ANAsPrinciplesofEnvironmentalHealthforNursingPractice.pdf

Arfin, S., Jha, N. K., Jha, S. K., Kesari, K. K., Ruokolainen, J., Roychoudhury, S., Rathi, B., & Kumar, D. (2021). Oxidative stress in cancer cell metabolism. *Antioxidants*, 10(5), 642. https://doi.org/10.3390/antiox10050642

Austrian Medical Association's EMF & Working Group. (2012). *Guideline of the Austrian Medical Association for the diagnosis and treatment of EMF related health problems and illnesses (EMF syndrome).* Austrian Medical Association. https://ehtrust.org/wp-content/uploads/The-Austrian-Medical-Association-Guidelines-for-Diagnosis-and-Treatment-of-EMF-related-Health-Problems.pdf

Bandara, P., & Carpenter, D. O. (2018a). Planetary electromagnetic pollution: It is time to assess its impact. *The Lancet Planetary Health*, 2(12), e512–e514.

Bandara, P., & Carpenter, D. O. (2018b). Planetary electromagnetic pollution: It is time to assess its impact. *The Lancet Planetary Health*, 2(12), e512–e514. https://doi.org/10.1016/S2542-5196(18)30221-3

Bastin, J.-F., Finegold, Y., Garcia, C., Mollicone, D., Rezende, M., Routh, D., Zohner, C. M., & Crowther, T. W. (2019). The global tree restoration potential. *Science*, 365(6448), 76–79. https://doi.org/10.1126/science.aax0848

Behrens, T., Terschüren, C., Kaune, W. T., & Hoffmann, W. (2004). Quantification of lifetime accumulated ELF-EMF exposure from household appliances in the context of a retrospective epidemiological case–control study. *Journal of Exposure Science & Environmental Epidemiology*, 14(2), 144–153. https://doi.org/10.1038/sj.jea.7500305

Bektas, H., Bektas, M. S., & Dasdag, S. (2018). Effects of mobile phone exposure on biochemical parameters of cord blood: A preliminary study. *Electromagnetic Biology and Medicine*, 37(4), 184–191. https://doi.org/10.1080/15368378.2018.1499033

Bellieni, C. V., Acampa, M., Maffei, M., Maffei, S., Perrone, S., Pinto, I., Stacchini, N., & Buonocore, G. (2008). Electromagnetic fields produced by incubators influence heart rate variability in newborns. *Archives of Disease in Childhood - Fetal and Neonatal Edition*, 93(4), F298–F301. https://doi.org/10.1136/adc.2007.132738

Bellieni, C.V., Nardi, V., Buonocore, G., Di Fabio, S., Pinto, I., & Verrotti, A. (2019). Electromagnetic fields in neonatal incubators: The reasons for an alert. *The Journal of Maternal-Fetal & Neonatal Medicine*, 32(4), 695–699. https://doi.org/10.1080/14767058.2017.1390559

Bellieni, C. V., Pinto, I., Bogi, A., Zoppetti, N., Andreuccetti, D., & Buonocore, G. (2012). Exposure to electromagnetic fields from laptop use of "laptop" computers. *Archives of Environmental & Occupational Health*, 67(1), 31–36. https://doi.org/10.1080/19338244.2011.564232

Bellieni, C.V., Tei, M., Iacoponi, F., Tataranno, M. L., Negro, S., Proietti, F., Longini, M., Perrone, S., & Buonocore, G. (2012). Is newborn melatonin production influenced by magnetic fields produced by incubators? *Early Human Development*, 88(8), 707–710. https://doi.org/10.1016/j.earlhumdev.2012.02.015

Belpomme, D., Carlo, G. L., Irigaray, P., Carpenter, D. O., Hardell, L., Kundi, M., Belyaev, I., Havas, M., Adlkofer, F., Heuser, G., Miller, A. B., Caccamo, D., De Luca, C., von Klitzing, L., Pall, M. L., Bandara, P., Stein, Y., Sage, C., Soffritti,

M., ... Vorst, A. V. (2021). The critical importance of molecular biomarkers and imaging in the study of electrohypersensitivity. A scientific consensus international report. *International Journal of Molecular Sciences*, 22(14), 7321. https://doi.org/10.3390/ijms22147321

Belpomme, D., Hardell, L., Belyaev, I., Burgio, E., & Carpenter, D. O. (2018). Thermal and non-thermal health effects of low intensity non-ionizing radiation: An international perspective. *Environmental Pollution*, 242, 643–658. https://doi.org/10.1016/j.envpol.2018.07.019

Belyaev, I., Dean, A., Eger, H., Hubmann, G., Jandrisovits, R., Kern, M., Kundi, M., Moshammer, H., Lercher, P., Müller, K., Oberfeld, G., Ohnsorge, P., Pelzmann, P., Scheingraber, C., & Thill, R. (2016). EUROPAEM EMF Guideline 2016 for the prevention, diagnosis and treatment of EMF-related health problems and illnesses. *Reviews on Environmental Health*, 31(3), 363–397. https://doi.org/10.1515/reveh-2016-0011

Bertagna, F., Lewis, R., Silva, S. R. P., McFadden, J., & Jeevaratnam, K. (2021). Effects of electromagnetic fields on neuronal ion channels: A systematic review. *Annals of the New York Academy of Sciences*, 1499(1), 82–103. https://doi.org/10.1111/nyas.14597

Bin, L., Chen, Z., Wu, T., Shao, Q., Yan, D., Ma, L., Lu, K., & Xie, Y. (2014). The alteration of spontaneous low frequency oscillations caused by acute electromagnetic fields exposure. *Clinical Neurophysiology*, 125(2), 277–286. https://doi.org/10.1016/j.clinph.2013.07.018

Birks, L., Guxens, M., Papadopoulou, E., Alexander, J., Ballester, F., Estarlich, M., Gallastegi, M., Ha, M., Haugen, M., Huss, A., Kheifets, L., Lim, H., Olsen, J., Santa-Marina, L., Sudan, M., Vermeulen, R., Vrijkotte, T., Cardis, E., & Vrijheid, M. (2017). Maternal cell phone use during pregnancy and child behavioral problems in five birth cohorts. *Environment International*, 104, 122–131. https://doi.org/10.1016/j.envint.2017.03.024

Boileau, N., Margueritte, F., Gauthier, T., Boukeffa, N., Preux, P.-M., Labrunie, A., & Aubard, Y. (2020). Mobile phone use during pregnancy: Which association with fetal growth? *Journal of Gynecology Obstetrics and Human Reproduction*, 49(8), 101852. https://doi.org/10.1016/j.jogoh.2020.101852

Bray, R. I. (2020). *PRELIMINARY Clinical Practice Guidelines in the Diagnosis and Management of Electromagnetic Field Hypersensitivity (EHS)*. Women's College Hospital. https://www.womenscollegehospital.ca/assets/pdf/environmental/Preliminary%20Clinical%20Guidelines%20%20for%20EHS.pdf

Breunig, H. (2017). *Tree damage caused by mobile phone base stations An observation guide*. Kompetenzinitiative.com.

https://kompetenzinitiative.com/wp-content/uploads/2019/08/2017_Observation_Guide_ENG_FINAL_RED.pdf

Buchner, K., & Rivasi, M. (2020). The International Commission on Non-Ionizing Radiation Protection: Conflicts of interest, corporate capture and the push for 5G. https://prodstoragehoeringspo.blob.core.windows.net/7ab5abc7-2a10-4e10-a443-a92218e6df72/Underbilag%2013%20ICNIRP-report-FINAL-19-JUNE-2020.pdf

Byun, Y.-H., Ha, M., Kwon, H.-J., Hong, Y.-C., Leem, J.-H., Sakong, J., Kim, S. Y., Lee, C. G., Kang, D., Choi, H.-D., & Kim, N. (2013). Mobile phone use, blood lead levels, and attention deficit hyperactivity symptoms in children: A longitudinal study. *PLOS ONE*, 8(3), e59742. https://doi.org/10.1371/journal.pone.0059742

Cabot, E., Christ, A., Bühlmann, B., Zefferer, M., Chavannes, N., Bakker, J. F., van Rhoon, G. C., & Kuster, N. (2014). Quantification of RF-exposure of the fetus using anatomical CAD-models in three different gestational stages. *Health Physics*, 107(5), 369–381. https://doi.org/10.1097/HP.0000000000000129

Capstick, M. H., Kuehn, S., Berdinas-Torres, V., Gong, Y., Wilson, P. F., Ladbury, J. M., Koepke, G., McCormick, D. L., Gauger, J., Melnick, R. L., & Kuster, N. (2017). A radio frequency radiation exposure system for rodents based on reverberation chambers. *IEEE Transactions on Electromagnetic Compatibility*, 59(4), 1041–1052. https://doi.org/10.1109/TEMC.2017.2649885

Carlberg, M., & Hardell, L. (2017). Evaluation of mobile phone and cordless phone use and glioma risk using the Bradford Hill Viewpoints from 1965 on association or causation. *BioMed Research International*, 2017, e9218486. https://doi.org/10.1155/2017/9218486

Carpenter, D. O. (2019a). Extremely low frequency electromagnetic fields and cancer: How source of funding affects results. *Environmental Research*, 178, 108688. https://doi.org/10.1016/j.envres.2019.108688

Carpenter, D. O. (2019b). Extremely low frequency electromagnetic fields and cancer: How source of funding affects results. *Environmental Research*, 178, 108688. https://doi.org/10.1016/j.envres.2019.108688

Choi, K.-H., Ha, M., Ha, E.-H., Park, H., Kim, Y., Hong, Y.-C., Lee, A.-K., Hwa Kwon, J., Choi, H.-D., Kim, N., Kim, S., & Park, C. (2017). Neurodevelopment for the first three years following prenatal mobile phone use, radio frequency radiation and lead exposure. *Environmental*

Research, 156, 810–817. https://doi.org/10.1016/j.envres.2017.04.029

Choi, Y.-J., Moskowitz, J. M., Myung, S.-K., Lee, Y.-R., & Hong, Y.-C. (2020). Cellular phone use and risk of tumors: systematic review and meta-analysis. International Journal of Environmental Research and Public Health, 17(21), 8079. https://doi.org/10.3390/ijerph17218079

Clegg, F. M., Sears, M., Friesen, M., Scarato, T., Metzinger, R., Russell, C., Stadtner, A., & Miller, A. B. (2020). Building science and radiofrequency radiation: What makes smart and healthy buildings. Building and Environment, 176, 106324. https://doi.org/10.1016/j.buildenv.2019.106324

Cyprus Committee on Environment and Children's Health. (2019). PRESS RELEASE "Living with Technology, Children's Health Remains their Inexplicable Right and our Own Obligation". Cyprus Committee on Environment and Children's Health. https://ehtrust.org/wp-content/uploads/PRESS-RELEASE-Cyprus-2019-Campaign-3.pdf

Dasdag, S., Akdag, M. Z., Erdal, M. E., Erdal, N., Ay, O. I., Ay, M. E., Yilmaz, S. G., Tasdelen, B., & Yegin, K. (2015). Effects of 2.4 GHz radiofrequency radiation emitted from Wi-Fi equipment on microRNA expression in brain tissue. International Journal of Radiation Biology, 91(7), 555–561. https://doi.org/10.3109/09553002.2015.1028599

Di Ciaula, A. (2018). 5G networks in European Countries: Appeal for a standstill in the respect of the precautionary principle. International Society of Doctors for Environment. https://www.isde.org/5G_appeal.pdf

Directorate-General for Parliamentary Research Services (European Parliament), & Belpoggi, F. (2021). Health impact of 5G: Current state of knowledge of 5G related carcinogenic and reproductive/developmental hazards as they emerge from epidemiological studies and in vivo experimental studies. Publications Office of the European Union. https://data.europa.eu/doi/10.2861/657478

Divan, H. A., Kheifets, L., Obel, C., & Olsen, J. (2012). Cell phone use and behavioural problems in young children. J Epidemiol Community Health, 66(6), 524–529. https://doi.org/10.1136/jech.2010.115402

El-Hajj, A. M., & Naous, T. (2020). Radiation analysis in a gradual 5g network deployment strategy. 2020 IEEE 3rd 5G World Forum (5GWF), 448–453. https://doi.org/10.1109/5GWF49715.2020.9221314

ENVIRONMENTAL HEALTH TRUST, ET AL., PETITIONERS v. FEDERAL COMMUNICATIONS COMMISSION AND UNITED STATES OF AMERICA, RESPONDENTS, No. 20-1025, Consolidated with 20-1138 (United States Court of Appeals FOR THE DISTRICT OF COLUMBIA CIRCUIT August 13, 2021). https://www.cadc.uscourts.gov/internet/opinions.nsf/FB976465BF00F8BD85258730004EFDF7/$file/20-1025-1910111.pdf

Falcioni, L., Bua, L., Tibaldi, E., Lauriola, M., De Angelis, L., Gnudi, F., Mandrioli, D., Manservigi, M., Manservisi, F., Manzoli, I., Menghetti, I., Montella, R., Panzacchi, S., Sgargi, D., Strollo, V., Vornoli, A., & Belpoggi, F. (2018). Report of final results regarding brain and heart tumors in Sprague-Dawley rats exposed from prenatal life until natural death to mobile phone radiofrequency field representative of a 1.8 GHz GSM base station environmental emission. Environmental Research, 165, 496–503. https://doi.org/10.1016/j.envres.2018.01.037

Fernández, C., de Salles, A. A., Sears, M. E., Morris, R. D., & Davis, D. L. (2018). Absorption of wireless radiation in the child versus adult brain and eye from cell phone conversation or virtual reality. Environmental Research, 167, 694–699. https://doi.org/10.1016/j.envres.2018.05.013

Frank JW. (2021) Electromagnetic fields, 5G and health: what about the precautionary principle?. Epidemiology of Community Health, 75, 562-566. 10.1136/jech-2019-213595

Foerster, M., Thielens, A., Joseph, W., Eeftens, M., & R, öösli M. (n.d.). A prospective cohort study of adolescents' memory performance and individual brain dose of microwave radiation from wireless communication. Environmental Health Perspectives, 126(7), 077007. https://doi.org/10.1289/EHP2427

Fragopoulou, A. F., Polyzos, A., Papadopoulou, M.-D., Sansone, A., Manta, A. K., Balafas, E., Kostomitsopoulos, N., Skouroliakou, A., Chatgilialoglu, C., Georgakilas, A., Stravopodis, D. J., Ferreri, C., Thanos, D., & Margaritis, L. H. (2018). Hippocampal lipidome and transcriptome profile alterations triggered by acute exposure of mice to GSM 1800 MHz mobile phone radiation: An exploratory study. Brain and Behavior, 8(6), e01001. https://doi.org/10.1002/brb3.1001

Gajšek, P., Ravazzani, P., Grellier, J., Samaras, T., Bakos, J., & Thuróczy, G. (2016). Review of studies concerning electromagnetic field (EMF) exposure assessment in Europe: Low frequency fields (50 Hz-100 kHz). International Journal of Environmental Research and Public Health, 13(9), E875. https://doi.org/10.3390/ijerph13090875

Gandhi, O. P. (2019). Microwave emissions from cell phones exceed safety limits in Europe and the US when touching the body. IEEE Access, 7, 47050–47052. https://doi.org/10.1109/ACCESS.2019.2906017

Gandhi, O. P., Morgan, L. L., de Salles, A. A., Han, Y.-Y., Herberman, R. B., & Davis, D. L. (2012b). Exposure limits: The underestimation of absorbed cell phone radiation, especially in children. *Electromagnetic Biology and Medicine*, 31(1), 34–51. https://doi.org/10.3109/15368378.2011.622827

Gong, Y., Capstick, M. H., Kuehn, S., Wilson, P. F., Ladbury, J. M., Koepke, G., McCormick, D. L., Melnick, R. L., & Kuster, N. (2017). Life-time dosimetric assessment for mice and rats exposed in reverberation chambers for the two-year NTP cancer bioassay study on cell phone radiation. *IEEE Transactions on Electromagnetic Compatibility*, 59(6), 1798–1808. https://doi.org/10.1109/TEMC.2017.2665039

Haggerty, K. (2010). Adverse influence of radio frequency background on trembling aspen seedlings: Preliminary observations. *International Journal of Forestry Research*, 2010, e836278. https://doi.org/10.1155/2010/836278

Halgamuge, M. N. (2017). Review: Weak radiofrequency radiation exposure from mobile phone radiation on plants. *Electromagnetic Biology and Medicine*, 36(2), 213–235. https://doi.org/10.1080/15368378.2016.1220389

Hardell, L. (2017). World Health Organization, radiofrequency radiation and health—A hard nut to crack (Review). *International Journal of Oncology*, 51(2), 405–413. https://doi.org/10.3892/ijo.2017.4046

Hardell, L., & Carlberg, M. (2020). [Comment] Health risks from radiofrequency radiation, including 5G, should be assessed by experts with no conflicts of interest. *Oncology Letters*, 20(4), 1–1. https://doi.org/10.3892/ol.2020.11876

Hardell, L., & Carlberg, M. (2013). Use of mobile and cordless phones and survival of patients with Glioma. *Neuroepidemiology*, 40(2), 101–108. https://doi.org/10.1159/000341905

Hardell, L., Walker, M. J., Walhjalt, B., Friedman, L. S., & Richter, E. D. (2007). Secret ties to industry and conflicting interests in cancer research. *American Journal of Industrial Medicine*, 50(3), 227–233. https://doi.org/10.1002/ajim.20357

Hardell L, Carlberg M, Hedendahl LK. (2018). Radiofrequency radiation from nearby base stations gives high levels in an apartment in Stockholm, Sweden: A case report. *Oncology Letters*, 15(5), 7871-7883. https://doi.org/10.3892/ol.2018.8285

Hasan, I., Rubayet Jahan, M., Nabiul Islam, M., & Rafiqul Islam, M. (2022). Effect of 2400 MHz mobile phone radiation exposure on the behavior and hippocampus morphology in Swiss mouse model. *Saudi Journal of Biological Sciences*, 29(1), 102–110. https://doi.org/10.1016/j.sjbs.2021.08.063

Hassanzadeh-Taheri, M., Khalili, M. A., Hosseininejad Mohebati, A., Zardast, M., Hosseini, M., Palmerini, M. G., & Doostabadi, M. R. (2021). The detrimental effect of cell phone radiation on sperm biological characteristics in normozoospermic. *Andrologia*, e14257. https://doi.org/10.1111/and.14257

Huss, A., Egger, M., Hug, K., Huwiler-Müntener, K., & Röösli, M. (2007). Source of Funding and Results of Studies of Health Effects of Mobile Phone Use: Systematic Review of Experimental Studies. *Environmental Health Perspectives*, 115(1), 1. https://doi.org/10.1289/ehp.9149

IARC. (n.d.). *Non-ionizing radiation, Part 1: Static and extremely low-frequency (ELF) electric and magnetic fields.* https://publications.iarc.fr/Book-And-Report-Series/Iarc-Monographs-On-The-Identification-Of-Carcinogenic-Hazards-To-Humans/Non-ionizing-Radiation-Part-1-Static-And-Extremely-Low-frequency-ELF-Electric-And-Magnetic-Fields-2002

IARC Working Group on the Evaluation of Carcinogenic Risks to Humans. (2013). *Non-ionizing radiation, Part 2: Radiofrequency electromagnetic fields.* World Health Organization, International Agency for Research on Cancer. https://www.ncbi.nlm.nih.gov/books/NBK304630/

IARC. (2011). *IARC classifies radiofrequency electromagnetic fields as possibly carcinogenic to humans.* World Health Organization. https://www.iarc.who.int/wp-content/uploads/2018/07/pr208_E.pdf

Jimenez, H., Blackman, C., Lesser, G., Debinski, W., Chan, M., Sharma, S., ... & Pasche, B. (2018). Use of non-ionizing electromagnetic fields for the treatment of cancer. *Frontiers in Bioscience (Landmark Ed)*, 23(2), 284-97.. https://doi.org/10.2741/4591

Kaiser Permanente. (2001). *Radiation safety for nurses.* Kaiser Permanente Medical Care Program, Southern California Region. https://kpnursing.org/_SCAL/professionaldevelopment/orientation/LAMC/rs_nurse.pdf

Kim, S., Han, D., Ryu, J., Kim, K., & Kim, Y. H. (2021). Effects of mobile phone usage on sperm quality - No time-dependent relationship on usage: A systematic review and updated meta-analysis. *Environmental Research*, 202, 111784. https://doi.org/10.1016/j.envres.2021.111784

Koppel T, Ahonen M, Carlberg M, Hardell L. (2022). Very high radiofrequency radiation at Skeppsbron in Stockholm, Sweden from mobile phone base station antennas positioned close to pedestrians' heads. *Environmental*

Research. Epub ahead of print. https://doi.org/10.1016/j.envres.2021.112627

Kostoff, R. N., & Lau, C. G. Y. (2017). Modified Health Effects of Non-ionizing Electromagnetic Radiation Combined with Other Agents Reported in the Biomedical Literature. In C. D. Geddes (Ed.), *Microwave Effects on DNA and Proteins* (pp. 97–157). Springer International Publishing. https://doi.org/10.1007/978-3-319-50289-2_4

Lai, H. (2021). Genetic effects of non-ionizing electromagnetic fields. *Electromagnetic Biology and Medicine*, 40(2), 264–273. https://doi.org/10.1080/15368378.2021.1881866

Lerchl, A., Klose, M., Grote, K., Wilhelm, A. F. X., Spathmann, O., Fiedler, T., Streckert, J., Hansen, V., & Clemens, M. (2015). Tumor promotion by exposure to radiofrequency electromagnetic fields below exposure limits for humans. *Biochemical and Biophysical Research Communications*, 459(4), 585–590. https://doi.org/10.1016/j.bbrc.2015.02.151

Levitt, B. B., Lai, H. C., & Manville, A. M. (2021a). Effects of non-ionizing electromagnetic fields on flora and fauna, part 1. Rising ambient EMF levels in the environment. *Reviews on Environmental Health*. https://doi.org/10.1515/reveh-2021-0026

Levitt, B. B., Lai, H. C., & Manville, A. M. (2021b). Effects of non-ionizing electromagnetic fields on flora and fauna, Part 2 impacts: How species interact with natural and man-made EMF. *Reviews on Environmental Health*. https://doi.org/10.1515/reveh-2021-0050

Levitt, B. B., Lai, H. C., & Manville, A. M. (2021c). Effects of non-ionizing electromagnetic fields on flora and fauna, Part 3. Exposure standards, public policy, laws, and future directions. *Reviews on Environmental Health*. https://doi.org/10.1515/reveh-2021-0083

Li, D.-K., Chen, H., Ferber, J. R., Hirst, A. K., & Odouli, R. (2020). Association between maternal exposure to magnetic field nonionizing radiation during pregnancy and risk of attention-deficit/hyperactivity disorder in offspring in a longitudinal birth cohort. *JAMA Network Open, 3*(3), e201417. https://doi.org/10.1001/jamanetworkopen.2020.1417

Li, D.-K., Chen, H., Ferber, J. R., Odouli, R., & Quesenberry, C. (2017). Exposure to magnetic field non-ionizing radiation and the risk of miscarriage: A prospective cohort study. *Scientific Reports*, 7(1), 17541. https://doi.org/10.1038/s41598-017-16623-8

Li, D.-K., Chen, H., & Odouli, R. (2011). Maternal exposure to magnetic fields during pregnancy in relation to the risk of asthma in offspring. *Archives of Pediatrics & Adolescent Medicine*, 165(10), 945–950. https://doi.org/10.1001/archpediatrics.2011.135

Li, D.-K., Ferber, J. R., Odouli, R., & Quesenberry, C. P. (2012). A prospective study of in-utero exposure to magnetic fields and the risk of childhood obesity. *Scientific Reports*, 2(1), 540. https://doi.org/10.1038/srep00540

Lu, X., Oda, M., Ohba, T., Mitsubuchi, H., Masuda, S., & Katoh, T. (2017). Association of excessive mobile phone use during pregnancy with birth weight: An adjunct study in Kumamoto of Japan Environment and Children's Study. *Environmental Health and Preventive Medicine*, 22(1), 52. https://doi.org/10.1186/s12199-017-0656-1

Luo, J., Li, H., Deziel, N. C., Huang, H., Zhao, N., Ma, S., Ni, X., Udelsman, R., & Zhang, Y. (2020). Genetic susceptibility may modify the association between cell phone use and thyroid cancer: A population-based case-control study in Connecticut. *Environmental Research*, 182, 109013. https://doi.org/10.1016/j.envres.2019.109013

Mahmoudabadi, F. S., Ziaei, S., Firoozabadi, M., & Kazemnejad, A. (2015). Use of mobile phone during pregnancy and the risk of spontaneous abortion. *Journal of Environmental Health Science and Engineering*, 13(1), 34. https://doi.org/10.1186/s40201-015-0193-z

Mallery-Blythe, E. (2020). *2020 Consensus Statement of UK and International Medical and Scientific Experts and Practitioners on Health Effects of Non-Ionising Radiation (NIR).* Physicians' Health Initiative for Radiation and Environment (PHIRE), British Society for Ecological Medicine (BSEM). https://phiremedical.org/wp-content/uploads/2020/11/2020-Non-Ionising-Radiation-Consensus-Statement.pdf

Maluin, S. M., Osman, K., Jaffar, F. H. F., & Ibrahim, S. F. (2021). Effect of radiation emitted by wireless devices on male reproductive hormones: A systematic review. *Frontiers in Physiology*, 12, 1568. https://doi.org/10.3389/fphys.2021.732420

Markovà, E., Malmgren, L. O. G., & Belyaev, I. Y. (2010). Microwaves from mobile phones inhibit 53BP1 focus formation in human stem cells more strongly than in differentiated cells: possible mechanistic link to cancer risk. . *Environmental Health Perspectives*, 118(3), 394. https://doi.org/10.1289/ehp.0900781

Mazloum, T., Aerts, S., Joseph, W., & Wiart, J. (2019). RF-EMF exposure induced by mobile phones operating in LTE small cells in two different urban cities. *Annals of Telecommunications*, 74(1), 35–42. https://doi.org/10.1007/s12243-018-0680-1

McInerny, T. K. (2012a, July 12). *American Academy of Pediatrics to The Honorable Julius Genachowski* [Letter]. https://ehtrust.org/wp-content/uploads/American-Academy-of-Pediatrics-Letters-to-FCC-and-Congress-.pdf

McInerny, T. K. (2012b, December 12). *American Academy of Pediatrics to The Honorable Dennis Kucinich; support of H.R. 6358, the Cell Phone Right to Know Act* [Letter]. https://ehtrust.org/wp-content/uploads/American-Academy-of-Pediatrics-Letters-to-FCC-and-Congress-.pdf

McInerny, T. K. (2013, August 20). *American Academy of Pediatrics to The Honorable Mignon L. Clyburn and The Honorable Dr. Margaret A. Hamburg; comment on the Proposed Rule "Reassessment of Exposure to Radiofrequency Electromagnetic Fields Limits and Policies" published in the Federal Register on June 4, 2013.* https://ehtrust.org/wp-content/uploads/American-Academy-of-Pediatrics-Letters-to-FCC-and-Congress-.pdf

Melnick, R. L. (2019). Commentary on the utility of the National Toxicology Program study on cell phone radiofrequency radiation data for assessing human health risks despite unfounded criticisms aimed at minimizing the findings of adverse health effects. *Environmental Research, 168,* 1–6. https://doi.org/10.1016/j.envres.2018.09.010

Miller, A. B., Morgan, L. L., Udasin, I., & Davis, D. L. (2018). Cancer epidemiology update, following the 2011 IARC evaluation of radiofrequency electromagnetic fields (Monograph 102). *Environmental Research, 167,* 673–683. https://doi.org/10.1016/j.envres.2018.06.043

Miller, A. B., Sears, M. E., Morgan, L. L., Davis, D. L., Hardell, L., Oremus, M., & Soskolne, C. L. (2019). Risks to health and well-being from radio-frequency radiation emitted by cell phones and other wireless devices. *Frontiers in Public Health, 7,* 223. https://doi.org/10.3389/fpubh.2019.00223

Moon, J.-H. (2020). Health effects of electromagnetic fields on children. *Clinical and Experimental Pediatrics, 63*(11), 422. https://doi.org/10.3345/cep.2019.01494

Nittby, H., Brun, A., Eberhardt, J., Malmgren, L., Persson, B. R. R., & Salford, L. G. (2009). Increased blood–brain barrier permeability in mammalian brain 7 days after exposure to the radiation from a GSM-900 mobile phone. *Pathophysiology, 16*(2), 103–112. https://doi.org/10.1016/j.pathophys.2009.01.001

Nyberg, R., & Hardell, L. (2017). *5G Appeal.* http://www.5gappeal.eu/scientists-and-doctors-warn-of-potential-serious-health-effects-of-5g/

Ordinance of the Federal Minister for Labor, Social Affairs and Consumer Protection, with which the ordinance on the protection of workers from exposure to electromagnetic fields (Ordinance on Electromagnetic Fields—VEMF) is enacted and with which the Ordinance on Health Monitoring at Work 2014 and the regulation on employment bans and restrictions for young people will be amended, no. Federal Law Gazette II No. 179/2016 (2016), Federal Law Gazette authentic from 2004. https://www.ris.bka.gv.at/eli/bgbl/II/2016/179/20160707

Pall, M. L. (2016). Electromagnetic fields act similarly in plants as in animals: Probable activation of calcium channels via their voltage sensor. *Current Chemical Biology, 10*(1), 74–82. DOI: 10.2174/2212796810666160419160433

Panagopoulos, D. J., Johansson, O., & Carlo, G. L. (2015). Polarization: a key difference between man-made and natural electromagnetic fields, in regard to biological activity. *Scientific Reports, 5*(1), 14914. https://doi.org/10.1038/srep14914

Panagopoulos, D. J., Karabarbounis, A., Yakymenko, I., & Chrousos, G. P. (2021). Human-made electromagnetic fields: Ion forced-oscillation and voltage-gated ion channel dysfunction, oxidative stress and DNA damage (Review). *International Journal of Oncology, 59*(5), 1–16. https://doi.org/10.3892/ijo.2021.5272

Passi, R., Doheny, K. K., Gordin, Y., Hinssen, H., & Palmer, C. (2017). Electrical Grounding Improves Vagal Tone in Preterm Infants. *Neonatology, 112*(2), 187–192. https://doi.org/10.1159/000475744

Pearce JM. (2020). Limiting liability with positioning to minimize negative health effects of cellular phone towers. *Environmental Research, 181.* 10.1016/j.envres.2019.108845

Peleg, M., Nativ, O., & Richter, E. D. (2018). Radio frequency radiation-related cancer: Assessing causation in the occupational/military setting. *Environmental Research, 163,* 123–133. https://doi.org/10.1016/j.envres.2018.01.003

Physicians for Safe Technology. (n.d.). *Patient questionnaire electrosensitivity.* Environmental Health Trust. https://ehtrust.org/wp-content/uploads/patient-questionnaire-electrohypersensitivity-print-pdf-2.pdf

Raefsky, S. M., Chaudhari, A., & Sy, M. Y. (2020). Delayed-onset multiphasic demyelinating lesions after high dose radiofrequency electromagnetic field exposure: A multiple sclerosis (MS) mimic. *Multiple Sclerosis and Related Disorders, 45.* https://doi.org/10.1016/j.msard.2020.102318

Redazione, L. (2015). International Appeal: Scientists call for protection from non-ionizing electromagnetic field exposure. *European Journal of Oncology and Environmental Health, 20*(3/4), 180–182.

Redmayne, M. (2016). International policy and advisory response regarding children's exposure to radio frequency electromagnetic fields (RF-EMF). *Electromagnetic Biology and Medicine*, 35(2), 176–185. https://doi.org/10.3109/15368378.2015.1038832

Redmayne, M., & Johansson, O. (2014). Could myelin damage from radiofrequency electromagnetic field exposure help explain the functional impairment electrohypersensitivity? A review of the evidence. *Journal of Toxicology and Environmental Health. Part B, Critical Reviews*, 17(5), 247–258. https://doi.org/10.1080/10937404.2014.923356

Redmayne, M., & Johansson, O. (2015). Radiofrequency exposure in young and old: Different sensitivities in light of age-relevant natural differences. *Reviews on Environmental Health*, 30(4), 323–335. https://doi.org/10.1515/reveh-2015-0030

Rideout, V., & Robb, M. B. (2019). *The Common Sense census: Media use by tweens and teens,*. Common Sense Media. https://www.commonsensemedia.org/sites/default/files/uploads/research/2019-census-8-to-18-full-report-updated.pdf

Russell, C. L. (2018). 5 G wireless telecommunications expansion: Public health and environmental implications. *Environmental Research*, 165, 484–495. https://doi.org/10.1016/j.envres.2018.01.016

Sagar, S., Adem, S. M., Struchen, B., Loughran, S. P., Brunjes, M. E., Arangua, L., Dalvie, M. A., Croft, R. J., Jerrett, M., Moskowitz, J. M., Kuo, T., & Röösli, M. (2018). Comparison of radiofrequency electromagnetic field exposure levels in different everyday microenvironments in an international context. *Environment International*, 114, 297–306. https://doi.org/10.1016/j.envint.2018.02.036

Schuermann, D., & Mevissen, M. (2021). Manmade electromagnetic fields and oxidative stress—biological effects and consequences for health. *International Journal of Molecular Sciences*, 22(7), 3772. https://doi.org/10.3390/ijms22073772

Seomun, G., Lee, J., & Park, J. (2021). Exposure to extremely low-frequency magnetic fields and childhood cancer: A systematic review and meta-analysis. *PLOS ONE*, 16(5), e0251628. https://doi.org/10.1371/journal.pone.0251628

Shahin, S., Banerjee, S., Swarup, V., Singh, S. P., & Chaturvedi, C. M. (2018a). From the cover: 2.45-GHz microwave radiation impairs hippocampal learning and spatial memory: Involvement of local stress mechanism-induced suppression of iGluR/ERK/CREB signaling. *Toxicological Sciences*, 161(2), 349–374. https://doi.org/10.1093/toxsci/kfx221

Shepardson, D. (2018, September 28). *Trump Administration looks to speed 5G networks, ease hurdles.* Reuters. https://www.reuters.com/article/ctech-us-usa-tech-5g-idCAKCN1M82UN-OCATC

Shih, Y.-W., Hung, C.-S., Huang, C.-C., Chou, K.-R., Niu, S.-F., Chan, S., & Tsai, H.-T. (2020). The association between smartphone use and breast cancer risk among Taiwanese women: a case-control study. *Cancer Management and Research*, 12, 10799. https://doi.org/10.2147/CMAR.S267415

Singh, K. V., Gautam, R., Meena, R., Nirala, J. P., Jha, S. K., & Rajamani, P. (2020). Effect of mobile phone radiation on oxidative stress, inflammatory response, and contextual fear memory in Wistar rat. *Environmental Science and Pollution Research*, 27(16), 19340–19351. https://doi.org/10.1007/s11356-020-07916-z

Sırav, B., & Seyhan, N. (2016). Effects of GSM modulated radio-frequency electromagnetic radiation on permeability of blood–brain barrier in male & female rats. *Journal of Chemical Neuroanatomy*, 75, 123–127. https://doi.org/10.1016/j.jchemneu.2015.12.010

Smith, M. T., Guyton, K. Z., Gibbons, C. F., Fritz, J. M., Portier, C. J., Rusyn, I., DeMarini, D. M., Caldwell, J. C., Kavlock, R. J., Lambert, P. F., Hecht, S. S., Bucher, J. R., Stewart, B. W., Baan, R. A., Cogliano, V. J., & Straif, K. (2016). Key characteristics of carcinogens as a basis for organizing data on mechanisms of carcinogenesis. *Environmental Health Perspectives*, 124(6), 713–721. https://doi.org/10.1289/ehp.1509912

Smith-Roe, S. L., Wyde, M. E., Stout, M. D., Winters, J. W., Hobbs, C. A., Shepard, K. G., Green, A. S., Kissling, G. E., Shockley, K. R., Tice, R. R., Bucher, J. R., & Witt, K. L. (2020). Evaluation of the genotoxicity of cell phone radiofrequency radiation in male and female rats and mice following subchronic exposure. *Environmental and Molecular Mutagenesis*, 61(2), 276–290. https://doi.org/10.1002/em.22343

Soffritti, M., Tibaldi, E., Padovani, M., Hoel, D. G., Giuliani, L., Bua, L., Lauriola, M., Falcioni, L., Manservigi, M., Manservisi, F., & Belpoggi, F. (2016). Synergism between sinusoidal-50 Hz magnetic field and formaldehyde in triggering carcinogenic effects in male Sprague–Dawley rats. *American Journal of Industrial Medicine*, 59(7), 509–521. https://doi.org/10.1002/ajim.22598

Soffritti, M., Tibaldi, E., Padovani, M., Hoel, D. G., Giuliani, L., Bua, L., Lauriola, M., Falcioni, L., Manservigi, M., Manservisi,

F., Panzacchi, S., & Belpoggi, F. (2016). Life-span exposure to sinusoidal-50 Hz magnetic field and acute low-dose γ radiation induce carcinogenic effects in Sprague-Dawley rats. *International Journal of Radiation Biology*, 92(4), 202–214. https://doi.org/10.3109/09553002.2016.1144942

Sonmez, O. F., Odaci, E., Bas, O., & Kaplan, S. (2010). Purkinje cell number decreases in the adult female rat cerebellum following exposure to 900 MHz electromagnetic field. *Brain Research*, 1356, 95–101. https://doi.org/10.1016/j.brainres.2010.07.103

Stam, R. (2022). Occupational exposure to radiofrequency electromagnetic fields. *Industrial Health*, adv pub. https://doi.org/10.2486/indhealth.2021-0129

Stam, R. (2017). *Comparison of international policies on electromagnetic fields*. National Institute for Public Health and the Environment, RIVM. https://www.rivm.nl/sites/default/files/2018-11/Comparison%20of%20international%20policies%20on%20electromagnetic%20fields%202018.pdf

Sudan, M., Olsen, J., Arah, O. A., Obel, C., & Kheifets, L. (2016). Prospective cohort analysis of cellphone use and emotional and behavioural difficulties in children. *Journal of Epidemiology and Community Health*, 70(12), 1207–1213. https://doi.org/10.1136/jech-2016-207419

Tan, S., Wang, H., Xu, X., Zhao, L., Zhang, J., Dong, J., Yao, B., Wang, H., Hao, Y., Zhou, H., Gao, Y., & Peng, R. (2021). Acute effects of 2.856 GHz and 1.5 GHz microwaves on spatial memory abilities and CREB-related pathways. *Scientific Reports*, 11(1), 12348. https://doi.org/10.1038/s41598-021-91622-4

Tan, S., Wang, H., Xu, X., Zhao, L., Zhang, J., Dong, J., Yao, B., Wang, H., Zhou, H., Gao, Y., & Peng, R. (2017). Study on dose-dependent, frequency-dependent, and accumulative effects of 1.5 GHz and 2.856 GHz microwave on cognitive functions in Wistar rats. *Scientific Reports*, 7(1), 10781. https://doi.org/10.1038/s41598-017-11420-9

Tang, J., Zhang, Y., Yang, L., Chen, Q., Tan, L., Zuo, S., Feng, H., Chen, Z., & Zhu, G. (2015). Exposure to 900MHz electromagnetic fields activates the mkp-1/ERK pathway and causes blood-brain barrier damage and cognitive impairment in rats. *Brain Research*, 1601, 92–101. https://doi.org/10.1016/j.brainres.2015.01.019

Terzaghi, E., De Nicola, F., Cerabolini, B. E. L., Posada-Baquero, R., Ortega-Calvo, J.-J., & Di Guardo, A. (2020). Role of photo- and biodegradation of two PAHs on leaves: Modelling the impact on air quality ecosystem services provided by urban trees. *Science of The Total Environment*, 739, 139893. https://doi.org/10.1016/j.scitotenv.2020.139893

The Shift Project. (2019, March 5). *"Lean ICT: Towards Digital Sobriety": Our new report*. The Shift Project. https://theshiftproject.org/en/article/lean-ict-our-new-report/

Tsarna, E., Reedijk, M., Birks, L. E., Guxens, M., Ballester, F., Ha, M., Jiménez-Zabala, A., Kheifets, L., Lertxundi, A., Lim, H.-R., Olsen, J., González Safont, L., Sudan, M., Cardis, E., Vrijheid, M., Vrijkotte, T., Huss, A., & Vermeulen, R. (2019). Associations of maternal cell-phone use during pregnancy with pregnancy duration and fetal growth in 4 birth cohorts. *American Journal of Epidemiology*, 188(7), 1270–1280. https://doi.org/10.1093/aje/kwz092

Uche, U. I., & Naidenko, O. V. (2021). Development of health-based exposure limits for radiofrequency radiation from wireless devices using a benchmark dose approach. *Environmental Health*, 20(1), 84. https://doi.org/10.1186/s12940-021-00768-1

Volkow, N. D., Tomasi, D., Wang, G.-J., Vaska, P., Fowler, J. S., Telang, F., Alexoff, D., Logan, J., & Wong, C. (2011). Effects of cell phone radiofrequency signal exposure on brain glucose metabolism. *JAMA : The Journal of the American Medical Association*, 305(8), 808. https://doi.org/10.1001/jama.2011.186

Waldmann-Selsam, C., Balmori-de la Puente, A., Breunig, H., & Balmori, A. (2016). Radiofrequency radiation injures trees around mobile phone base stations. *Science of The Total Environment*, 572, 554–569. https://doi.org/10.1016/j.scitotenv.2016.08.045

West, J. G., Kapoor, N. S., Liao, S.-Y., Chen, J. W., Bailey, L., & Nagourney, R. A. (2013). Multifocal breast cancer in young women with prolonged contact between their breasts and their cellular phones. *Case Reports in Medicine*, 2013, e354682. https://doi.org/10.1155/2013/354682

Williams, D. A., Xu, H., & Cancelas, J. A. (2006). Children are not little adults: Just ask their hematopoietic stem cells. *Journal of Clinical Investigation*, 116(10), 2593. https://doi.org/10.1172/JCI30083

Wyde, M., Cesta, M., Blystone, C., Elmore, S., Foster, P., Hooth, M., Kissling, G., Malarkey, D., Sills, R., Stout, M., Walker, N., Witt, K., Wolfe, M., & Bucher, J. (2016). *Report of Partial Findings from the National Toxicology Program Carcinogenesis Studies of Cell Phone Radiofrequency Radiation in Hsd: Sprague Dawley ® Sd Rats (Whole Body Exposure)* [Preprint]. Cancer Biology. https://doi.org/10.1101/055699

Wyde, M. E., Horn, T. L., Capstick, M. H., Ladbury, J. M., Koepke, G., Wilson, P. F., Kissling, G. E., Stout, M. D., Kuster, N., Melnick, R. L., Gauger, J., Bucher, J. R., & McCormick, D.

L. (2018). Effect of cell phone radiofrequency radiation on body temperature in rodents: Pilot studies of the National Toxicology Program's reverberation chamber exposure system. *Bioelectromagnetics, 39*(3), 190–199. https://doi.org/10.1002/bem.22116

Yakymenko, I., Tsybulin, O., Sidorik, E., Henshel, D., Kyrylenko, O., & Kyrylenko, S. (2016). Oxidative mechanisms of biological activity of low-intensity radiofrequency radiation. *Electromagnetic Biology and Medicine, 35*(2), 186–202. https://doi.org/10.3109/15368378.2015.1043557

Yu, G., Bai, Z., Song, C., Cheng, Q., Wang, G., Tang, Z., & Yang, S. (2021). Current progress on the effect of mobile phone radiation on sperm quality: An updated systematic review and meta-analysis of human and animal studies. *Environmental Pollution, 282*, 116952. https://doi.org/10.1016/j.envpol.2021.116952

Unit IV:
Practice Settings

INTRODUCTION

Nursing is known as the caring profession. It is imperative that nurses not only care for the patients and communities that they serve, but also for our environment. The American Nurses Association (ANA) called on all registered nurses to have a working understanding of environmental exposures, the impact on human health and to apply this information into our practice (2007). Nurses are present in nearly every community and work in a variety of settings. As the most trusted profession, nurses have a tremendous opportunity to impact the health of population and the planet by advocating for a healthier environment and healthier people. After all, to have healthy people we need a healthy planet.

This section of *Environmental Health in Nursing* provides many opportunities to learn about the variety of ways nurses can be involved in promoting a healthier environment. For example, a review of the food sources in hospitals to provide healthier options or hosting farmer's markets on a healthcare facility's campus can provide fresh produce not only for the staff, but also the community. Nurses positioned on purchasing committees can review personal care products such as soaps, lotions and shampoo and find safer options with fewer chemicals of concern. These and many other strategies are consistent with the ANA's Nursing: Scope and Standards of Practice, 4th edition (2021), specifically Standard 18 which notes the nurses' role in environmental health and practice.

Each one of the nurses included in this section is an inspiration in their contribution to a healthier environment. Be inspired to work within your full scope of practice and include environmental health not only into your care, but into your daily life to protect yourself, your family, colleagues, patients, and communities.

REFERENCES

American Nurses Association (ANA). (2007). *Principles of environmental health for nursing practice with implementation strategies*. American Nurses Association.

American Nurses Association (ANA). (2015). *Nursing: Scope and standards of practice* (3rd ed.). American Nurses Association.

American Nurses Association (ANA). (2021). *Nursing: Scope and standards of Practice* (4th ed.). American Nurses Association.

NURSE EXPOSURE IN WORK

Barbara Sattler, RN, DrPH, FAAN
Emeritus Professor
University of San Francisco

Over 60% of nurses in the U.S. work in a hospital setting. While our mission in hospitals is to provide healing environments, the methods of healing often result in chemical, biological, and radiological exposures to the patients and hospital employees. This section will review some of the potential exposures that nurses experience and ways in which nurses are engaging in environmental health changes that are not just decreasing exposures but actually promoting health.

In the past few years, there have been studies that have helped us to understand the importance of addressing our own workplace environments.

The Nurses' Exposure Study showed us that there are a number of increased risks for disease (asthma, infertility, cancer, and others) that may be associated with chemical and radiological exposures in hospitals.

The Nurse and Physician Body Burden Studies found measurable amounts of toxic chemicals that are commonly found in hospitals in the blood and urine of doctors and nurses.

In a 2011 study, using the National Health Study II, Lawson et al, found an increased risk of miscarriage in nurses who were exposed to chemotherapeutic agents, sterilants, or x-Rays. Read the abstract here.

These studies help us to understand that the chemicals and processes that we use in health care create clear and present risks to our health.

WORKING THE GREEN SHIFT

Occupational and environmental health has not received much attention in nursing curriculum and therefore nurses have lacked the skills to both assess occupational/environmental risks and to reduce or eliminate them. In the last decade or more, some nurses from around the country have begun to look at their hospitals through a new occupational and environmental lens. They have seen unnecessary exposures to toxic cleaning products, batteries that are being tossed in the trash, and product-selection based on lowest cost with little attention paid to potentially harmful exposures to patients and staff. These nurses noted that hospital waste was not segregated, not recycled (nor composted) – practices that they did at home. And they started to question these old workplace practices and bring new and sustainable practices to their hospitals – occupationally and environmentally healthy practices.

This section of the text will guide the reader through a range of issues associated with environmental health and sustainability in health care. It will also help the reader to understand how positive changes are being made – how Green Teams are being created, new collaborators are being found throughout the facility, including housekeeping and dietary services, and how changes in purchasing decisions can have a huge impact on health.

(Note: it will not cover needle stick injuries, lifting policies, workplace violence, nor bloodborne pathogen exposures – all of which are critical occupational health issues in nursing. For more information on these issues, we refer you to the American Nurses Association's Center for Occupational and Environmental Health site).

REFERENCES

Environmental Working Group. (2007). *Nurses' health: Nurses' exposure.* http://www.ewg.org/research/nurses-health/nurses-exposure

Wilding BC., Curtis K., & Welker-Hood K. (2009). *Hazardous chemicals in health care: A snapshot of chemicals in doctors and nurses.* http://www.psr.org/resources/hazardous-chemicals-in-health.html

HAZARDOUS EXPOSURES IN HEALTHCARE
Barbara Sattler, RN, DrPH, FAAN
Emeritus Professor
University of San Francisco

While hospitals and other healthcare facilities are meant to be places of healing, many of the chemicals and products used in healthcare can have negative impacts on the health of patients, visitors, nurses, and staff.

MERCURY

Most hospitals have replaced their mercury thermometers with digital, mercury-free ones. This process occurred because nurses and others discovered the dangers posed by mercury. A conscious effort was made to substitute the mercury containing devices and provide a healthier choice for one that posed a hazard. Mercury-containing products are particularly problematic if they are incinerated. When the mercury that is released into the air from incinerator emissions lands on bodies of water, a set of processes occur that result in mercury-contaminated fish. Below is an illustration of the "fate and transport" of mercury (Figure 1).

Mercury is a powerful neurotoxicant, linked to health effects in humans and animals. Long-term exposure to mercury can cause effects which develop gradually making

identification of exposure difficult. Mercury exposure may cause shaking of the hands, eyelids, lips, tongue, or jaw. It may cause headaches, trouble sleeping, personality change, memory loss, irritability, indecisiveness and loss of intelligence. It can also cause skin rash, sores in the mouth, or sore and swollen gums. Many of these symptoms go away when the exposure to mercury stops. Mercury is excreted in urine.

KEY RESOURCES

* EWG's Fish List page on website of Environmental Working Group lists mercury levels in fish and other seafood

* Global Movement for Mercury-Free Health Care Report (pdf)

* Making Medicine Mercury Free (pdf)

* The Mercury Problem: Fast Facts (pdf)

* Mercury-Free Health Care website, a WHO-HCWH Global Initiative

* Mercury Policy Project website

* Mercury Thermometers and Your Family's Health (pdf)

* Toward the Tipping Point (pdf) WHO-HCWH Global Initiative to Substitute Mercury-Based Medical Devices in Health Care and Two-Year Progress Report

PLASTICS

We use a lot of plastics in health care – IV tubing and bags, respiratory therapy tubing, dialysis tubes, etc. There are two major problems with plastics. First, is the problem with polyvinyl chloride which is the component chemical in polyvinyl chloride (PVC) plastics. This particular plastic is toxic during its manufacture when both workers and the environment can be exposed to dioxins, a family of highly toxic chemicals and one of the most carcinogenic chemicals known whose unintentional exposures are the consequence of PVC manufacture. Dioxin contamination also results when PVC products are incinerated, either in medical waste incinerators or municipal incinerators. It's important for nurses to know how and where the waste from their hospital is disposed. When PVC waste products are sent to landfills, there is no real concern regarding exposures, but consider the amount of plastic waste used in hospitals daily entering landfills. However, if PVC waste is sent to an incinerator, very unhealthy air contaminants can result.

Hard plastics are made more malleable (for use in IV bags, tubes and so on) by the addition of phthalates. Phthalates are a group of chemicals that come with a range of health

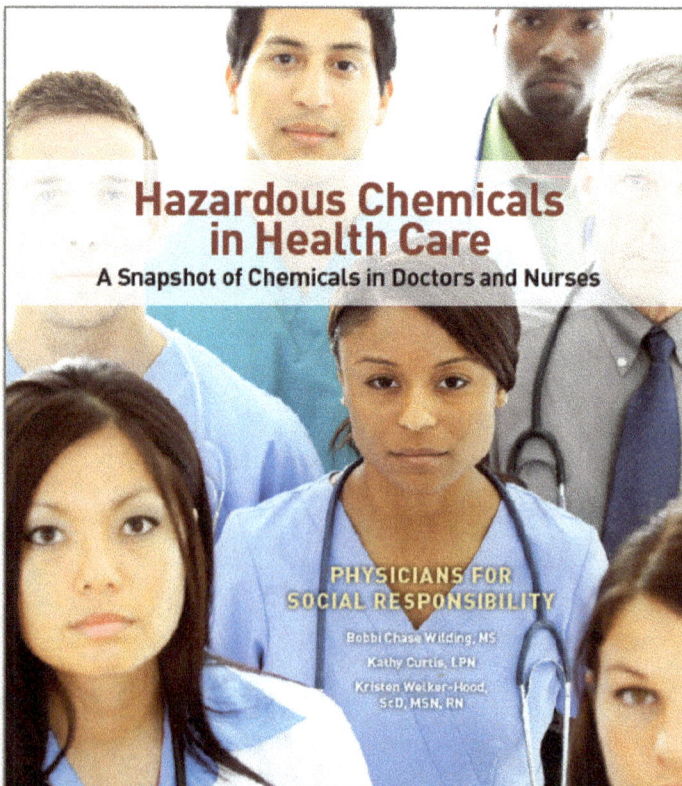

Hazardous Chemicals in Health Care
A Snapshot of Chemicals in Doctors and Nurses

PHYSICIANS FOR SOCIAL RESPONSIBILITY

Bobbi Chase Wilding, MS
Kathy Curtis, LPN
Kristen Welker-Hood, ScD, MSN, RN

effects, including endocrine disruption. The particular phthalate that is commonly found in hospital equipment is Diethylhexyl Phthalate (DEHP). Studies indicate that there is a risk of testicular problems in baby boys who are exposed to DEHP and it is further recommended that DEHP-free tubing be used in neonatal intensive care units.

Some hospitals have made the shift to DEHP-free NICUs and others are even DEHP-free throughout the hospital. DEHP-free products are now readily available and price competitive.

Health Care Without Harm has created a set of resources on Plastics and DEHP.

KEY RESOURCES

- Alternatives to PVC and DEHP

- Aggregate Exposures to Phthalates in Humans: HCWH 2002 Report (pdf)

- DEHP Exposures During the Medical Care of Infants (pdf)

- Find out more about PVC-Free Building Materials (pdf)

- Neonatal Exposure to DEHP and Opportunities for Prevention (pdf)

- Weight of the Evidence on DEHP (pdf)

- Why Health Care is Moving Away from PVC (pdf)

GREEN CLEANING IN HOSPITALS

Hospitals have to have high standards for cleaning and disinfecting. However, they can select products that are both effective AND green, as a way of decreasing exposures to patients, staff, and visitors. Green cleaning

Figure 1

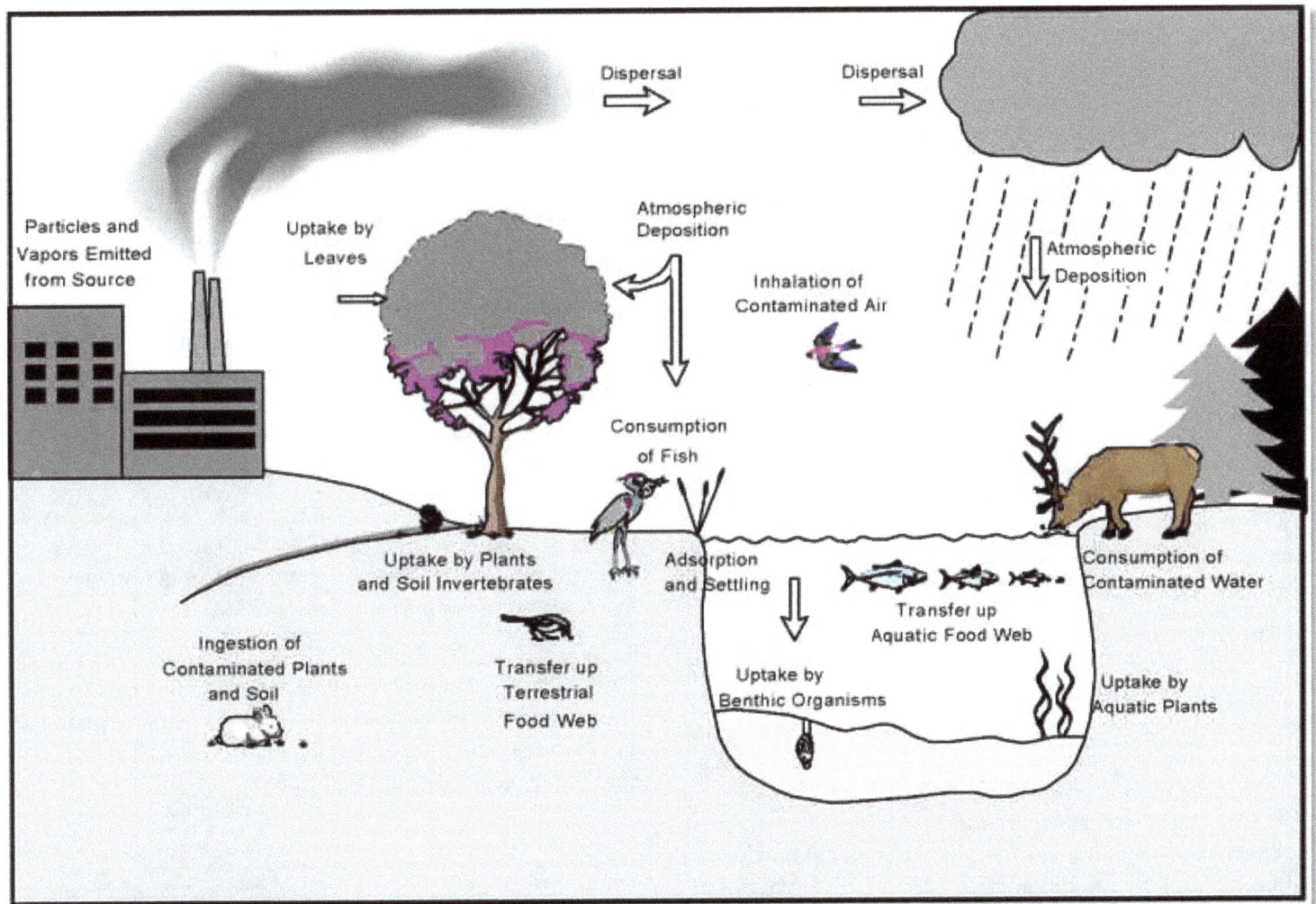

https://www.epa.gov/fera/multimedia-fate-and-transport-modeling-general
Reproduced as part of the public domain.

refers to using cleaning products that do not contain toxic chemicals (including fragrances), some of which are associated with respiratory and other health problems. Some hospitals are also addressing the paper and equipment used in cleaning processes, requiring paper products used for cleaning to contain recycled material and requiring the use of microfiber mops, which decrease water consumption.

In other hospitals, green cleaning policies have gone so far as to include specifications for cleaning versus disinfecting. It is important to understand the difference between cleaning and disinfecting. Disinfectants pose the highest risk, as they are formulated to kill bacteria. New, safer disinfectants are coming to market in the United States that are hydrogen peroxide based. Because these disinfectants break down into hydrogen and water, there is essentially no risk of adverse health effects. Some of the hydrogen peroxide-based cleaners also boast a shorter contact time that contributes to better infection prevention (Perez et al 2005).

When disinfectants or sterilants are warranted, such as cleaning a NICU warmer or incubator in-between patients, or cleaning equipment in the cath lab or operating room, it is critical for nurses and others to know how to protect themselves when using the products. Reading the safety data sheet (formerly MSDS), the chemical information sheet associated with the product, can be helpful but sometimes it is too vague. The statement "wear gloves" or "use respiratory protection when using this product" is not sufficient guidance. If that is all that is suggested on the safety data sheet, then the manufacturer needs to be called and queried about the precise type of glove and/or respirator (mask) to be used with the product.

Some manufacturers provide substantial guidance and it is then incumbent on nurses and others to make sure they are following the manufacturer's recommendations. For example, on a safety data sheet for gluteraldehyde regarding skin protection, the manufacture states:

"To protect hands and forearm wear gloves of appropriate type and length. MICRO TOUCH latex gloves are acceptable, if changed frequently (i.e. every 5 – 10 minutes) and/or double gloved. Before using other latex gloves contact the manufacturer for permeation information to determine if their gloves are suitable for use with gluteraldehyde solutions. Nitrile rubber, butyl rubber, and similar synthetic rubber gloves (i.e., ALLERGARD Synthetic Surgical Gloves, are acceptable glove materials. Do not use neoprene rubber, or polyvinyl chloride (vinyl) gloves, as gluteraldehyde may (be) rapidly absorb by these materials."

If sterilants and disinfectants are potentially hazardous to adults then we can assume that the very susceptible neonate, with its immature, developing organs will be considerably more susceptible to these hazards. For neonates that are not on independent respiratory support it is important to consider their potential exposures to cleaning chemicals, antimicrobial soaps, and disinfectants. Many hospitals use flooring materials that require extensive maintenance by stripping, waxing, etc and many of these products have been linked to respiratory problems (Rosenman et al 2003, Medina-Ramon et al 2005). In addition to looking for safer cleaning chemicals, it is important to also consider changing the surfaces to make them easier to clean. For example, the University of Maryland Medical Center is transitioning to rubber flooring, which does not require the use of wax, and hence, floor strippers. The companies producing these no-wax products are boasting less slips, trips and falls because the rubber floor is less slippery.

Many health care facilities are adopting "fragrance free" policies and these policies can extend to cleaning products. Educating housekeeping staff and others in the hospital about the true smell of clean – which is NO smell – will help them to rethink the need for pine or lemon-smelling products. Real pine and/or lemons are rarely part of the fragrances' ingredients. The word "fragrance" on a product's label can mean up to 100 additional chemicals used to create this "fresh" or "clean" scent.

REFERENCES

Medina-Ramón, M., Zock, J. P., Kogevinas, M., Sunyer, J., Torralba, Y., Borrell, A., Burgos, F., & Anto, J. M. (2005). Asthma, chronic bronchitis, and exposure to irritant agents in occupational domestic cleaning: A nested case-control study. *Occupational and Environmental Medicine, 62,* 598-606. doi:10.1136/oem.2004.017640.

Perez J., Springthorpe V. S., & Sattar S. A. (2005). Activity of selected oxidizing microbicides against the spores of Clostridium difficile: relevance to environmental control. *American Journal of Infection Control, 33*(6), 320-5.

Rosenman, K. D., Reilly, M. J., Schill, D. P., Valiante, D., Flattery, J., Harrison, R., Reinisch, F., Pechter, E., Davis, L., Tumpowsky, C. M., & Filios. M. (2003). Cleaning products and work-related asthma. *Journal of Occupational and Environ mental Medicine, 45*(5), 556-63.

ENVIRONMENTAL HEALTH IN THE SCHOOL SETTING

Linda Mendonça, DNP, MEd, RN, NCSN, PHNA-BC, FNASN
Assistant Professor, Community/Public Health Nursing
Rhode Island College
Zvart Onanian School of Nursing,
President, National Association of School Nurses

The impact that school environments have on asthma and other chronic health conditions has been ignored for too long. The school building is an environment where children and staff spend a significant amount of their time. Physical environmental stressors in schools are significant and affect children's academic achievement (Healthy Schools Network, 2015). Ensuring that schools are free of environmental hazards is a public health necessity. Capital budgets to maintain healthy schools have decreased in the United States (Healthy Schools Network, 2015) making renovations and routine maintenance difficult for many school districts.

According to a work study completed by the National Association of School Nurses (NASN), schools in the United States employ approximately 95,776 full time nurses who practice school nursing in the school setting (National Association of School Nurses , 2017). The school nurse is typically the only health care professional in the building and works collaboratively with their education counterpart provide quality evidence-based care to the school community. The role of the 21st century school nurse is complex and multi-faceted. The NASN outlines this 21st century role in a position statement that includes leadership, community/public health, care coordination and quality improvement (NASN, 2018). Addressing the physical environment of a school is something that must be on the radar and seek the attention of the school nurse to ensure a healthy environment for all occupants.

School nurses can play an important role in reducing environmental stressors and improving school environments (National Association of School Nurses, 2018). The school nurse's role includes assessment, education and advocacy. In the assessment role the school nurse might uncover issues in the home and school environment that need to be addressed. Such stressors can include allergens, bites and need for integrated pest management, toxic cleaning products, paints and solvents, and carbon monoxide, among others. Education about reducing these stressors can be directed to school teachers and staff, parents, students, and the larger community.

School nurses also monitor healthy school environments. They can support interest in environmental issues and bring pressing student health concerns to the attention of other stakeholders who can help to address them. A good reference for sources of pollutants in schools is published by the Children's Environmental Health Network (n.d.): Environmental Health in Schools. School nurses can stay informed about best practices around issues such as indoor air quality, asthma management, pesticide use, and neuro-toxins causing learning disabilities. The school nurse has the expertise to advocate for preventive environmental measures to help keep students and staff healthy and in school. Environmental health is a very important aspect of school health that tends to get overlooked, partly because the school nurse is typically the only one in the school setting with a health background. Additionally, the school nurse may be in the physical building part time and covering other schools each week. Promoting healthy school environments can help ensure that students are healthy and ready to learn and faculty and staff are ready to teach and support each child.

Another role of a school nurse is that of advocacy. The school nurse can advocate for environmental health needs and concerns in the school setting in different ways. Some examples of this may be walking through the school on a routine basis looking for any concerns, addressing those within the nurse's scope, and then following up with school administrative personnel to ensure that those concerns are addressed routinely. This can be a multidisciplinary approach by touring the building with parents, custodians, administration, and a faculty representative. Reaching out to your local, state or federal legislators with your concerns is another way to advocate for environmental health policy in schools. For example, this can occur by making a request to a local legislator to submit legislation around green cleaning in schools. Asthma awareness month in one state was recognized by a U.S. senator from that state by holding a field hearing to bring awareness around asthma in schools and the impact the school environment has on students and staff (J. Leffers, personal communication, 2015). As a school nurse you have the knowledge and field experience to testify at such hearings.

REDUCING ASTHMA IN SCHOOLS

Data demonstrating a link between school environment and asthma has been part of the focus in the implementation of Environmental Protection Agency's (EPA) Indoor Air Quality (IAQ) Tools for Schools. An unhealthy school environment consisting of mold, vermin, dust, chemicals from cleaning supplies, poor air quality, or other such hazards can trigger asthma symptoms in students and staff (Sampson, 2012). Respiratory illnesses, such as asthma, have been linked to poor indoor air quality (Massawe & Vaust, 2013). The CDC endorses the use of the EPA's guidelines to improve the IAQ and reduce asthma triggers in schools (CDC, 2018). However, according to the Centers for Disease Control and Prevention's School Health Policies and Practices Study, the proportion of schools reporting implementation of IAQ management programs dropped from 47.7% in 2012 to 46.1% in 2014 (Schools for Health Report, 2018). Intervening in the school environment can be instrumental in decreasing the impact of asthma by reducing student suffering and absenteeism, parental stress, and cost of medical care for acute asthma attacks. The EPA has focused on creating a healthy school environment across the nation and developed the Tools for Schools framework that schools can implement to improve indoor air quality. This toolkit is based on research and best practices (EPA, 2016). A study published in 2011 demonstrated the effectiveness of Tools for Schools (TfS) when implemented as part of a collaborative approach to improving the health of schools (Foscue & Harvey, 2011). Creating a healthy school environment may be able to prevent or help mitigate symptoms of illness of students, faculty, and staff.

SCHOOL NURSE ROLES IN ENVIRONMENTAL HEALTH

The school nurse can be the advocate and take a leadership role in addressing environmental health issues by encouraging schools to utilize the EPA's Indoor Air Quality Tools for Schools action kit (TfS). TfS was developed by the EPA to provide Indoor Air Quality (IAQ) guidance for schools to make voluntary changes that will reduce exposures to indoor environmental contaminants in schools. Indoor air quality TfS recommendations are based on research and best practices and more information can be located on the tool kit website.

Green cleaning is another way to help students stay healthy and in school (Balek, 2012). Green cleaning is cleaning that uses fewer toxic products to protect the health of students and staff without harming the environment. (Web resources listed in table) It also increases the lifespan of facilities, preserves the environment and ultimately saves the school money. The biggest priority with green cleaning is implementing a green cleaning program that eliminates harmful chemicals, manages volatile organic compounds (VOCs), and reduces harmful bacteria keeping students, faculty, and staff healthier.

School nurses can also play a key role in policy development at the school district level and the local, state and federal government. The use of the Precautionary Principle as a strategy to develop policy has also been described in the literature. This principle provides the justification to support safer policies when information may be lacking, but the potential health consequences of not having the policy are significant, thus justifying precautionary action (Abramson, S.L., 2018). Additionally, the SAMPRO project was mentioned by Abramson as a potential link to policy development to address indoor air quality. SAMPRO is a school-based asthma management program, developed by the American Academy of Allergy, Asthma and Immunology with the American Academy of Pediatrics, which has many components, including improving IAQ.

The American Public Health Association (APHA) outlines policy that is focused on children and environmental health. The policy calls on development and implementation of public health systems to protect children from harmful environmental exposures in the school setting. It addresses the need for the federal government's responsibility to monitor and assist with public health strategies (American Public Health Association, 2017). Having the awareness of this national resource to assist school nurses is an asset in the advocacy tool box in this environmental work.

School nurses can empower school staff to investigate environmental issues in their buildings and advocate for students through policy development which will help to create environmentally friendly schools that are sustainable. Identifying legislative champions and key stakeholders to provide recommendations for change is one-way school nurses can strategize for healthier, safer environments. Another way is to provide testimony at professional organizations meetings such as, APHA, for policy development focused on environmental health.

Additionally, it is important for the school nurse to have a strong voice for leadership decision-making that impacts the health and safety of students and staff in the school setting. The COVID-19 pandemic has provided many opportunities for school nurses to be part of the team in K-12 school reopening plans. Along with mitigation strategies impacting the school environment and implementing protocols around contact investigation/ contact tracing and testing strategies in schools, are examples of how school nurses can share their expertise in assuring a healthy school environment. Many state school nurse consultants and state school nurse organizations were part of state level leadership making sure that there was a school nursing voice as guidance for policy and protocol development. Also, at the national level the NASN was invited to meet with many key partners at the federal level to ensure a school nurse voice.

This public health crisis that the pandemic has put before us has provided opportunities as well. One being the awareness focused on the school environment. With a virus looming indoor air quality gained much attention and concern for occupants. School administrators assessed school buildings to ensure that classrooms had four to six air exchanges per hour (ACH) necessary for safe occupancy. Inspecting HVAC systems and utilization of HEPA filter units is an example of a strategy used to get to at least four air changes per hour (CDC, 2019). With this increased awareness it is important that school buildings are maintained and sustained moving forward. Climate change promoting natural disasters have the potential to impact school environments. Preparation and advocacy are key to increase awareness around these issues.

RESOURCES FOR IMPROVING SCHOOL ENVIRONMENTS

There are a number of tools and resources to help support this work. Working together with facilities managers, custodial staff and administrators using these resources is a great place to start. A list of Web resources for school nurses can be found in the table below. Healthy Schools Campaign is an independent nonprofit that believes each child deserves a healthy school. The campaign is supported by industry leaders in the manufacturing and distribution of green cleaning products and services. Another excellent resource is the Healthy Schools Network that provides resources and opportunities for advocacy efforts. The professional organization for school nurses, NASN, provides resources on environmental health in addition to their position statement mentioned earlier.

WEB RESOURCES FOR SCHOOL NURSES ON GREEN CLEANING, INDOOR AIR QUALITY AND CHILDREN'S ENVIRONMENTAL HEALTH

Green Cleaning in Schools

- https://www.healthygreenschools.org/

- http://www.phi.org/wp-content/uploads/migration/uploads/application/files/khcqbtgu01fuyi5w1owortxqfpnrwrsode32y7sbqs0cfb0uy0.pdf

- https://healthyschoolscampaign.org/issues/environment/

- http://healthyschools.org/Cleaning-For-Healthy-Schools/

- https://greenschoolsnationalnetwork.org/implement-green-cleaning-program-schools-right-way/

Indoor Air Quality (IAQ) and Environment Health:

- https://www.cehn.org/wp-content/uploads/2015/11/Environmental_Health_in_Schools13.pdf

- https://www.epa.gov/iaq-schools/indoor-air-quality-tools-schools-action-kit

- https://www.nasn.org/nasn/nasn-resources/practice-topics/environmental-health

CONCLUSION

Environmental health brings nurses back to the basics as Florence Nightingale writes in her memoirs (1860). It is important that all nurses, regardless of their type of nursing practice, must be able to incorporate environmental health principles. The school setting is no exception and environmental issues should be part of every school nurse's practice on a daily basis. School nurses must utilize their advocacy and leadership skills along with their public health expertise to be a driving force to demand a health school environment for all occupants.

REFERENCES

Abramson, S. L. (2018). Reducing environmental allergic triggers: Policy issues. *Journal of Allergy and Clinical Immunology: In Practice, 6*(1), 32-35.

American Public Health Association, (2017). *Establishing environmental public health systems for children at risk or with environmental exposures in schools.* https://apha.org/policies-and-advocacy/public-health-policy-statements/policy-database/2018/01/18/establishing-environmental-public-health-systems-for-children

Balek, B. (2012). *Taking green cleaning to schools. ISSA Today, February 2012, 16-19.* International Sanitary Supply Association. http://www.issa.com/articles/article-details/all/taking-green-cleaning-toschools#.V_rXOYXlfQw

Centers for Disease Control Asthma Surveillance Data (2018). https://www.cdc.gov/asthma/most_recent_data.htm

Centers for Disease Control Ventilation (2019). https://www.epa.gov/coronavirus/ventilation-and-coronavirus-covid-19

Children's Environmental Health Network. (n.d.) *Environmental health in schools.* www.cehn.org/our-work/policy/policy-factsheets/environmental-health-in-schools/

Foscue, K., and Harvey, M. (2011). A statewide multiagency intervention model for empowering schools to improve indoor environmental quality. *Journal of Environmental Health, 74,* 8-15.

Healthy Schools Network Inc. (2015). *Toward healthy schools 2015.* www.healthyschools.org/HealthySchools2015.pdf

IAQ Tools for Schools fact sheet. (2016). http://www.epa.gov/iaq/schools/pdfs/publications/iaqtfs_factsheet.pdf

Kats, G. (2006). *Greening America's schools: Costs and benefits.* http://www.usgbc.org/ShowFile.aspx?DocumentID=2908

Massawe, E., and Vasut, L. (2013). Promoting healthy school environments: A step-by-step framework to improve indoor air quality in Tangipahoa Parish, Louisiana. *Journal of Environmental Health, 76*(2), 22-29.

National Association of School Nurses (NASN). (2017). *Workforce Study.* https://bit.ly/2O7oZVm

National Association of School Nurses (NASN). (2018). *Environmental health in the school setting: The role of the school nurse.* NASN. https://bit.ly/3fqgorU

National Association of School Nurses. (2018). *Role of the 21st Century School Nurse.* https://www.nasn.org/nasn/advocacy/professional-practice-documents/position-statements/affiliates

Nightingale, F. (1860), *Notes on nursing: What it is and what it is not.* D. Appleton. https://digital.library.upenn.edu/women/nightingale/nursing/nursing.html

Sampson, N. (2012). Environmental justice at school: Understanding research, policy, and practice to improve our children's health. *Journal of School Health, 82*(5), 246-252

Schools for Health Report (2018). Harvard T.H. Chan School of Public Health: https://schools.forhealth.org/Harvard.Schools_For_Health.Foundations_for_Student_Success.pdf

GREEN TEAMS
Barbara Sattler, RN, DrPH, FAAN
Professor Emeritus
University of San Francisco

There are a number of names that have been given the committees/groups that have been convened at hospitals to address environmental health and sustainability. One of the most common names is the Green Team. These multidisciplinary teams are convened by nurses, administrators, and others. Their make-up can vary, but the most successful ones have representatives from the departments noted below. They can help to raise concerns, do assessments and audits, compare alternative solutions, make recommendations, and help to implement changes and then evaluate those changes.

Watch Denise Choiniere, who was the first Sustainability Manager at the University of Maryland Medical Center, describe how nurses are working on "greening" their hospitals. A great introduction to incorporating environmental health into nursing practice.

Here's the website for the University of Maryland Medical Center's Green Team

It's just one example of many green team programs. If you search the internet with the terms "hospital green teams", you'll see lots of other examples. (Note, the University of Maryland Medical Center is conveniently located on Greene Street.)

WHO'S IN CHARGE IN HOSPITALS?

Really, everyone has a part, but there are several offices/departments/individuals/committees that can be particularly important:

* Environmental Services / Housekeeping / Maintenance – often where the decisions are made about the cleaning processes and products

* Purchasing Department or Committee – make important product selection decisions

* Architects/Planners – often take the lead when building modifications, expansions, and new hospital buildings are being planned and developed

* Infection Control – should be consulted when making decisions are being made about cleaners/sterilants/disinfection products

* Occupational Health and Safety – can help provide additional support for decisions especially regarding physical equipment

* Food Services – can be instrumental in helping to bring local, sustainably-grown foods to the hospital's menu and when planning/implementing a Farmers' Market

* Public Relations – important to keep in the loop to recognize and publicize great work

* Nursing and Professional Development – a good place to help to bring speakers into the hospital to educate on environmental health and sustainability related to health care. Nursing "grand rounds", lunch-time talks, and other venues can provide great opportunities to have compelling speakers.

* GREEN TEAMS – critical organizational structures in which sustainability and environmental health can be discussed and addressed.

Some hospitals have made institutional commitments to environmental health and sustainability, even including it in their core values statement.

OCCUPATIONAL HEALTH
Julie C. Jacobson Vann, PhD, MS, RN
The University of North Carolina at Chapel Hill
School of Nursing

INTRODUCTION TO OCCUPATIONAL HEALTH

The discipline of occupational health and safety focuses on promoting safe and healthful working conditions that protect workers, the community, and the environment. The emphasis is on the whole person, including social, mental, and physical well-being. Occupational health and safety interventions span policies, systems, and personal-level approaches. One specialty area of occupational health is industrial hygiene, defined as "the science and art devoted to the anticipation, recognition, evaluation, and control of those environmental factors or stresses arising in or from the workplace that may cause sickness, impaired health and well-being, or significant discomfort among workers or among the citizens of the community" (American Industrial Hygiene Association [AIHA], 2018).

A major emphasis of occupational health and industrial hygiene is primary prevention, which involves implementing health promotion and health protection measures to prevent diseases and injuries from occurring. For example, replacing toxic chemicals used in an industrial or process with a nontoxic alternative can protect workers, family members, and the community from developing health problems and protect the environment from contamination. Another example of primary prevention is giving the influenza vaccine, as this intervention protects people from getting influenza.

Occupational health also focuses on secondary and tertiary prevention. Secondary prevention involves detecting and treating diseases or injuries early at a time when they may be more treatable or less severe. Secondary prevention often involves screening to detect an asymptomatic condition, such as conducting blood pressure screenings and intervening early. Tertiary prevention involves actions to prevent a condition from getting worse, preventing complications, or preventing disability. Examples of tertiary prevention services or interventions are rehabilitation services, case management, and/or behavior change strategies, such as motivational interviewing and health coaching.

OCCUPATIONAL HEALTH AND THE 3 PS: PEOPLE, PROFIT, AND PLANET

The concept of the Triple Bottom Line is important to occupational health. Triple Bottom Line or the 3 Ps refers to the people, profits, and the planet (University of

Hazard Category	Examples of Hazards
Safety	Slips, trips, falls, working from heights, faulty equipment, confined spaces
Biological	Blood and other body fluids, bacteria and viruses, plants, insect bites, mold
Physical	Loud noise, temperature extremes, radiation
Ergonomic	Repetition, lifting, awkward postures, use of heavy force
Chemical and Dust	Pesticides, cleaning products, asbestos, particulate matter, vapors, fumes, solvents
Work Organization	Sources of stress, workload demands, workplace violence, control over work

Source: (OSHA, n.d.-a)

Wisconsin, 2018). Entities that adopt the 3 P model exhibit corporate social responsibility rather than focus heavily on profits. This approach may involve a range of strategies, such as reducing risks to employees, reducing emissions, protecting the planet, and encouraging or incentivizing employees to volunteer to help important causes of initiatives. In the context of occupational health and safety, employers and employees who apply the triple bottom line philosophy focus on sustainability and the effect of business operations on the community and environment. These organizations may adopt eco-innovation and implement sustainable or "green" practices that protect workers, the public, and the earth.

One occupational health and safety expert wrote that: "The health and safety function must be given the same level of importance and accountability as the production function" (Plog & Quinlan, 2012) and aligns with the concept of the 3 Ps. This concept challenges occupational health and safety professionals to work within their respective organizations to promote health and safety among workers and the greater community as part of the overall mission of the organization.

INDUSTRIAL HYGIENE: PROTECT WORKERS, FAMILIES, COMMUNITY AND THE ENVIRONMENT

As stated above, industrial hygiene focuses on anticipating, recognizing, evaluating and controlling factors in the environment that create health problems "among workers or among the citizens of the community" (Plog & Quinlan,

2012, p. 3). Industrial hygiene focuses on promoting a healthy workplace and processes that protect health, and considers the immediate, short-term, and long-term health effects of hazards. An important and perhaps overlooked part of the definition of industrial hygiene is: "among citizens of the community" (AIHA, 2018). This phrase is critical because it highlights the role of occupational health professionals, including industrial hygienists, in not only protecting the health and safety of workers, but also protecting populations beyond the organization. This requires employers to implement environmentally healthy practices to protect the community and the earth from health hazards, such as toxic spills, water contamination and other sources of pollution, and climate change.

IMPORTANCE OF OCCUPATIONAL HEALTH AND INDUSTRIAL HYGIENE

Workplace illnesses and injuries are costly to society, in dollars, pain, suffering, and deaths. The United States Department of Labor (USDL, n.d.) estimates that "employers pay almost $1 billion per week for direct workers' compensation costs alone." During 2016, there were nearly 2.9 million reported nonfatal workplace injuries and illnesses in the United States (U.S.); this included approximately 892,300 severe cases that contributed to absenteeism (Bureau of Labor Statistics [BLS], 2017). In 2016, "5,190 workers died from a work-related injury in the U.S." (BLS, 2017). On a global level, "an estimated 24% of the global burden of disease and 23% of all deaths can be attributed to environmental factors (Stanhope & Lancaster, 2016, p. 218)."

It is important to emphasize that most occupational illnesses and injuries are preventable. Therefore, occupational health and safety programs and professionals offer substantial benefits to workers, employers, and society by reducing workplace injuries and illnesses, related deaths, suffering, and costs.

Pollution created by industry and other businesses, including health services organizations, also contributes significantly to health problems, deaths, environmental destruction, and costs associated with clean-up efforts (Sacramento Metropolitan Air Quality Management District, 2018). For example, "air pollution was linked to 6.5 million deaths in 2015, water pollution was linked to 1.8 million deaths and workplace pollution was linked to nearly one million deaths (Sifferlin, 2017)." Watch a brief online video about air pollution and deaths at: http://time.com/4989641/water-air-pollution-deaths/.

OCCUPATIONAL HEALTH AND THE PRECAUTIONARY PRINCIPLE

It is important for occupational health and safety professions to apply the Precautionary Principle to promote and protect health and safety of workers and the community. This principle urges that when there is evidence to suggest potential harm from an activity, substance or other exposure, there is a social responsibility to protect workers and the public from exposure to harm, even if the cause and effect relationships are not fully determined based on available scientific evidence. The Precautionary Principle involves "taking preventive action in the face of uncertainty; shifting the burden of proof to the proponents of an activity; exploring a wide range of alternatives to possibly harmful actions; and increasing public participation in decision making (Kriebel et al., 2001, p. 871)."

HIERARCHY OF CONTROLS

In the field of industrial hygiene, efforts to protect from exposures to occupational hazards are classified in a hierarchy of controls that are arranged based on level of effectiveness (National Institute for Occupational Safety and Health [NIOSH], 2018a). Often this hierarchy of controls includes three classifications: engineering controls, administrative controls, and personal protective equipment. In some models, engineering controls may also include two higher-level tiers, elimination and substitution. For example, NIOSH (2018a) has classified the "Hierarchy of Controls" as: elimination, substitution, engineering controls, administrative controls, and personal protective equipment.

Engineering controls are considered to be the first strategy to use as they involve removing, replacing or reducing the hazards. This approach not only protects workers but also may better protect the community and environment if an engineering approach involves substituting use of a toxic material with a non-toxic material. In this description, elimination and substitution are included as part of engineering controls. Engineering controls may be considered upstream preventive approaches and are likely to be more effective than relying on personal behavior changes.

Administrative controls are generally considered to be the second strategy to use. This may involve changing the work processes to limit worker exposure to some type of hazard or health threat. A few examples of administrative control strategies are to pace the work processes to reduce exposure, and to distribute work involving exposure among workers.

Personal protective equipment (PPE) is generally considered to be the third line of defense. Personal protective equipment may include uses of gloves, eyewear, helmets, ear plugs, and other types of safety equipment that protects the worker from exposures.

Read more about the hierarchy of controls at the NIOSH website at: https://www.cdc.gov/niosh/topics/hierarchy/default.html.

SELECT HEALTH PROBLEMS ASSOCIATED WITH OCCUPATIONAL EXPOSURES

Workplace illnesses and injuries can affect any part of the body. The most common problems vary by type of employment setting and role. However, some commonly occurring occupational injuries and illnesses are: allergic and irritant dermatitis, asthma, chronic obstructive pulmonary disease (COPD), fertility and pregnancy abnormalities, hearing loss, infectious diseases, low back disorders, musculoskeletal disorders of the upper extremities, and traumatic injuries (NIOSH, 2014). Some details are presented below for occupational skin disorders, the respiratory system, ears, and eyes.

OCCUPATIONAL SKIN DISORDERS

Two major types of skin problems that may occur in occupational settings are dermatosis and dermatitis. Dermatosis is a general term for "any abnormal condition of the skin (Plog & Quinlan, 2012, p. 60). Dermatitis is more specific and is limited to inflammatory conditions of the skin, such as contact dermatitis. Inflammation generally refers to a local reaction that may include redness, swelling, warmth and pain in reaction to some type of irritant, infection, injury or toxic exposure.

Direct causes of occupational skin disease

Occupational skin diseases are caused by many factors, most preventable. The common causes of occupational skin disease are: chemical, mechanical, physical, biological, and botanical. Some chemicals may be considered irritants, some are sensitizers, and some chemicals are classified as both. Mechanical injuries can be caused by friction, pressure, sharp objects or external forces. Physical causes of skin disorders include heat, cold and radiation. Sunlight is one source of skin-damaging radiation for people who work outside. Biological hazards that can affect the skin are bacteria, viruses, fungi, and parasites. Botanical hazards are some plants and wood, such as poison oak and poison ivy.

THE RESPIRATORY SYSTEM

The respiratory system can be exposed to many different types of unhealthy conditions at the workplace and in other settings. Several examples are emphysema, chronic bronchitis, and pneumoconiosis. Emphysema is a condition involving over-inflation of the alveoli, which become

damaged and enlarged, making it difficult to breathe. Emphysema can be caused by exposures such as coal dust, cadmium fumes, and cigarette smoke. Chronic bronchitis is a persistent inflammation of the bronchi. The most common cause of bronchitis is smoking; however, it can also be caused by occupational exposures, such as dusts, vapors, gases or fumes. Pneumoconiosis is a general term for various pulmonary disorders that occur from dust inhalation, such as silicosis and asbestosis. The inhalation of asbestos, for example, can lead to scarring or fibrosis in the lungs and can make lungs less resilient, thereby reducing the exchange of gas in the lungs. Asbestos exposure has been linked to severe respiratory diseases including asbestosis and, mesothelioma (lung cancer) (U.S. Department of Health and Human Services, 2016).

Inhaled contaminants

The effect that inhaled air contaminants have on the lungs and body depend on the size, solubility, and chemical reactivity of these contaminants. The size of particles affects where they may be deposited in the airway. Inhaled contaminants that adversely affect the lungs fall into three general categories: aerosols and dusts that may produce tissue reaction and/or disease; toxic gases that may injury tissue directly; and toxic aerosols or gases that enter the lungs, are absorbed into the bloodstream, are carried to other organs, or adversely affect the oxygen-carrying capacity of the blood.

THE EARS

"Occupational hearing loss is one of the most common work-related illnesses in the United States (NIOSH,

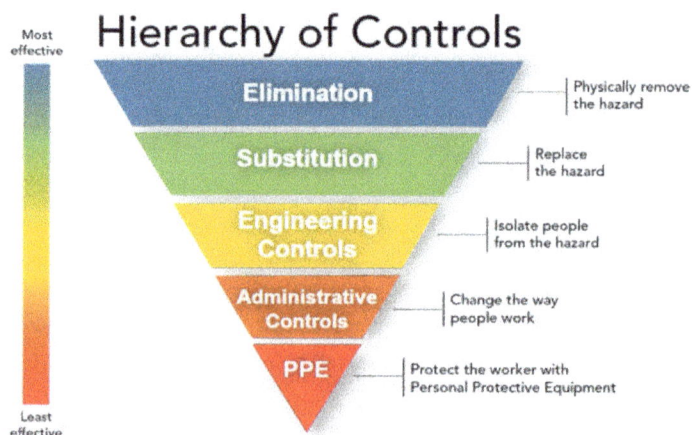

Figure 1: NIOSH, 2018a; https://www.cdc.gov/niosh/topics/hierarchy/default.html
Reproduced as part of the public domain.

2018b)." Approximately 22 million United States (U.S.) workers are exposed to hazardous noise levels at work each year; and more than 30 million workers are exposed to chemicals, some of which are ototoxic, harmful to the ear.

Noise levels of various workplace sounds.

The NIOSH has provided a list of sources of sounds in various workplaces. This "Noise Meter" provides sound levels, in decibels, for more than a dozen workplace sounds. Review this list at: https://www.cdc.gov/niosh/topics/noise/noisemeter_html/old/hp0.html

Effects of noise exposure

Noise exposure can cause temporary or permanent hearing loss and may lead to other health problems, such as high blood pressure and sleep disturbances. Noise exposure can even be harmful to a pregnancy, increasing the risk for preterm births and low birthweight infants. Ears generally can recover from brief exposures to intense sounds, however, more prolonged exposure to high decibel levels of noise can gradually damage the cochlear hair cells of the inner ear (Plog & Quinlan, 2012, p. 97), and this can result in hearing loss across the sound frequency levels. For more information about noise, see the noise chapter in Unit III: Environmental Health Sciences.

THE EYES

The eyes are at risk for physical injuries in some workplaces. Examples of these risks are being hit by blunt objects, cut by sharp objects, damaged by foreign bodies, burned by heat and/or chemicals, or damaged by radiation. The most common type of physical injury to the eye involves foreign bodies. Workers can also be exposed to chemicals that damage the eye by accidental splashing, mists, vapors, and gases. The degree of injury can range from a minor irritation, vision loss, and systemic poisoning. Chemical burns may be alkali burns, acid burns, or irritants. The most dangerous chemical burns are from alkali, such as ammonia hydroxide, fertilizers, lye, and lime. Laser lights are another hazard to the eyes, and especially the macula, as well as sunlight can damage the eyes.

Eye protective equipment may be needed in various work settings. And, for outside work, the use of sunglasses can reduce the risk of glaucoma, cataracts, and macular degeneration. For more information about eye and face protection, see: https://www.osha.gov/SLTC/eyefaceprotection/hazards.html.

CATEGORIES OF OCCUPATIONAL HAZARDS

"A hazard is a situation that poses a level of potential threat or risk, to life, health, property, or environment" (Breeding, 2011). The Occupational Safety and Health Administration (OSHA) has classified hazards as: safety, biological, physical, ergonomic, chemical and dust, and work organization (OSHA, n.d.-a). Review some examples of each type of hazard at: https://www.osha.gov/dte/grant_materials/fy10/sh-20839-10/circle_chart.pdf. A similar classification of occupational hazards is: physical, chemical, biological, radiological, ergonomic, and behavioral (Breeding, 2011).

Safety Hazards

Safety hazards are commonly occurring in many occupational settings. They are unsafe conditions that increase the risk for injuries, illnesses and even death (OSHA, n.d.-a). Some examples of these hazards are spills on floors that can cause workers to slip and fall, tripping hazards, such as power cords or clutter, moving parts in machinery, electrical hazards, and confined spaces. For prevention tips about slips, trips, and falls in work settings, review the Canadian Centre for Occupational Health and Safety (CCOHS, 2018a) website at: https://www.ccohs.ca/oshanswers/safety_haz/falls.html. For information about working in confined spaces, hazards, and hazard control, review the Canadian Centre for Occupational Health and Safety (CCOHS, 2018b) website at: https://www.ccohs.ca/oshanswers/hsprograms/confinedspace_intro.html.

Biological Hazards

Biological hazards include infectious microbiologic agents, such as bacteria and viruses, blood and other body fluids, biologic allergens, plants, insect bites, molds, and other biohazardous materials. An estimated 190 biologic agents pose health risks in the workplace. These hazards pose various health risks, including infectious, allergenic, toxic, and carcinogenic conditions. Employees that work in agricultural, medical, health, and laboratory settings are likely to have the highest levels of risk for these hazards; however, exposures are not restricted to these settings.

Physical Hazards

Physical hazards in the work environment include ionizing and nonionizing radiation, exposure to sunlight and ultraviolet radiation, hot and cold temperatures, and loud noise.

Ionizing radiation

Ionizing radiation refers to "particles, charged or uncharged, that are energetic enough to knock electrons out of the material that the radiation is passing through" (Plog & Quinlan, 2012, p. 261). Producers or sources of ionizing radiation are the sun, radioactive materials, radiation-producing machines, the cosmos, and nuclear reactors. Radioactive materials are unstable forms of elements that emit ionizing radiation as they decay. Some examples of radioactive elements are: plutonium, uranium, curium, actinium, and thorium (Helmenstine, 2017). Radioactive materials may be naturally occurring, extracted by people, or artificially produced. Some types of machines can produce radiation when operated, and may be referred to as radiation-producing machines (RPMs). Examples of these machines are x-ray machines, linear accelerators, and electron microscopes. Nuclear reactors may be used to produce power or conduct research. Nuclear reactors produce ionizing radiation from several sources: fuel rods, neutron production, activation, and fission fragments. Some above ground nuclear weapon testing was conducted prior to the Limited Test Ban Treaty (1963), contributing to the presence of radioactive substances in our environment.

Human health effects of radiation

Ionizing radiation can cause chemical changes in cells and damage them. Some cells may die or become abnormal, either temporarily or permanently. By damaging the genetic material (DNA) contained in the body's cells, radiation can cause cancer (Environmental Protection Agency [EPA], 2018)." For more information about the health effects of radiation, a brief summary is provided by the Centers for Disease Control and Prevention (CDC, 2015) at: https://www.cdc.gov/nceh/radiation/health.html.

Health effects of radiation may be classified as deterministic effects or stochastic effects. Deterministic effects are those that occur for everyone when the exposure reaches a certain threshold level. That threshold level may vary by individual. Stochastic effects are those in which the risk of developing a particular condition or disease increases with an increase in exposure to the agent, but where only a fraction of those exposed developed the health effect (Plog & Quinlan, 2012, p. 274)." For example, leukemia is a stochastic effect of extensive exposure to x-rays by clinicians who do not use protective equipment.

Nonionizing radiation

Non-ionizing radiation is electromagnetic radiation that is lower energy radiation, and has a lower frequency. Nonionizing radiation often generates heat; for example, a microwave heats food and water quickly. Examples of non-ionizing radiation are microwaves, radio waves, infrared radiation from heat lamps, and extremely low frequency (ELF) radiation. Electromagnetic fields associated with electric power lines and other sources have been the focus of epidemiological studies in occupationally and community-based settings.

Potential health effects of nonionizing radiation

Exposure to extremely low frequency (ELF) electric and magnetic fields, such as from power lines, appliances, and electrical substations, has been shown, among children, to be associated with a higher risk of health problems, such as leukemia (NIEHS, 2018). The International Agency for Research on Cancer (IARC), a component of the World Health Organization, classified extremely low frequency electromagnetic fields as "possibly carcinogenic to humans" primarily based on studies of childhood leukemia (National Cancer Institute [NCI], 2016). Exposure to static magnetic fields has been shown to be associated with nausea, metallic taste in the mouth, dizziness, flashes of light in the eyes when the head is moved, and effects on the circadian rhythm (Plog & Quinlan, 2012, p. 294).

Thermal Stress

Thermal stress includes excessively high temperatures and cold stress. These exposures may occur for people who work outdoors, or work near ovens, freezers, or other environments with temperature extremes.

Heat stress and heat-related health problems

People who are exposed to heat while working may experience heat-related illnesses (OSHA, n.d.-b). Some common symptoms of heat stress are elevated body temperature and heart rate, and increased sweating. There are at least six different types of heat-related disorders, including heat stroke, heat exhaustion, dehydration, heat syncope, heat cramps, and heat rash. Heat stroke is the most serious heat-related illness. If it is not addressed, it can lead to seizures or becoming unconscious and in more severe cases, permanent disability and death. Heat exhaustion is a heat-related illness that is milder than heat stroke. Heat cramps are muscle cramps that occur from the losses of fluid and electrolytes from sweating.

Cold stress

The body does not have the same types of physiological adaptive mechanisms for cold stress as it does for heat stress (sweating). One response to cold from the body is shivering; however, this is not a great protective mechanism but indicates that a person may have hypothermia. Hypothermia can progress and cause central nervous system depression, organ failure, and death.

Ergonomic Hazards

Ergonomics has been defined as the "scientific study of people at work (NIOSH, 2018d)." A more detailed definition of ergonomics is "the scientific discipline concerned with the understanding of interactions among humans and other elements of a system, and the profession that applies theory, principles, data and methods to design in order to optimize human well-being and overall system performance" (International Ergonomics Association, 2018). The goals of ergonomics are to make work safe, prevent injuries to soft tissue, and prevent "musculoskeletal disorders (MSDs) caused by sudden or sustained exposure to force, vibration, repetitive motion, and awkward posture" (NIOSH, 2018d), and optimize the well-being of workers.

Strategies applied in ergonomics

Occupational health and safety workers often work to design or redesign work spaces, tasks, displays, lighting, tools, and equipment to meet the needs of employees' physical capabilities and limitations (NIOSH, 2018). This may occur in industrial settings and office-based settings. In some cases, this may involve matching people with the tasks and roles that are a good fit. This may consider both human capacity for mental workload and physical workload. Efforts may include engineering approaches, administrative approaches, and protective equipment. Watch the following brief video on "Workplace Ergonomics" (Montana State Fund, 2014): https://www.youtube.com/watch?v=QeDUCXfzI6U.

Chemical and Dust Hazards

"Chemical hazards are present when a worker is exposed to any chemical preparation in the workplace in any form," solid, liquid or gas (OSHA, n.d.-a). Some examples of hazardous chemicals are pesticides, cleaning products, asbestos, particulate matter, vapors, fumes, and solvents. For information about specific chemical profiles, review the Canadian Centre for Occupational Health and Safety (CCOHS, 2018c) website at: https://www.ccohs.ca/oshanswers/chemicals/chem_profiles/. Another source of chemical information is the OSHA occupational chemical database: https://www.osha.gov/chemicaldata/.

Industrial toxicology and toxins. Industrial toxicology focuses on harmful properties of substances that are encountered in the workplace. Some of these toxins may also be encountered in homes and in the community. "A toxic effect is any reversible or irreversible harmful effect on the body as a result of contact with a substance via the respiratory tract, skin, eye, mouth, or other route" (Plog & Quinlan, 2012, p. 123). Toxicity refers to the capacity of a substance to cause harm. It is not really a "property" of a substance but a manifestation of it. Toxicity generally depends on the quantity or dose of the substance. Some substances, such as some minerals and vitamins are important to health in certain quantities, yet can be toxic if larger amounts than necessary are taken.

Routes of entry into the body

The route of entry of a substance into the body can affect whether a harmful effect occurs. Substances may enter the body through the skin, respiratory tract, gastrointestinal tract, injection, or multiple routes. Inhalation is a common route of entry for industrial exposures. Smaller particles are more likely to reach the alveoli; and some gases and vapors may be absorbed into the bloodstream from the lungs. Skin absorption is a second possible route of entry for substances. Absorption can vary based on the type and properties of the substance, environmental temperature, skin pH, presence of perspiration, area of the body and thickness of the skin, and presence of skin damage, such as abrasion dermatitis. Ingestion is believed to be a relatively uncommon route of entry in the workplace; however, this can occur when workers eat or smoke in areas where substances are in use or if proper hand washing is not done. For example, in a study of pesticide protective behaviors, consistent glove use was observed among 39% of farm workers, and hand washing before eating occurred among only 17% of workers (Walton, et al., 2016). These behaviors are likely to result in inadvertent ingestion of toxic pesticides. Injection is a route of entry in some industries, such as health services, which can result in transmission of blood-borne pathogens and infection.

Effects of exposure to air and other contaminants

The effects of exposure to air contaminants or air pollution can be classified as irritants, allergens, systemic toxins, or site-specific or organ-specific toxins (Plog & Quinlan, 2012, p. 129). Some toxic substances can selectively target or affect specific organs in the body, such as the central nervous system, cardiovascular system, and respiratory system, while others may affect multiple organs. For example, evidence is growing to show an association between exposure to some types of pesticides and development of Parkinson's disease (Brouwer et al., 2017).

However, pesticides are also known to affect other organs and systems of the body. For example, acute illnesses related to pesticide exposures may resemble acute upper respiratory track illnesses, conjunctivitis, and gastrointestinal illnesses (Alarcon et al., 2005). Symptoms of pesticide poisoning vary with the specific type(s) of pesticide exposures, and may include coughing, shortness of breath, nausea, vomiting, dizziness, muscular weakness, muscle twitching, tingling sensations, headaches, and eye, nose, throat and skin irritation (Alarcon et al., 2005; EPA, 2008; NIOSH, 2007; Sanborn et al., 2007). High severity acute pesticide-related illnesses may include seizures, pulmonary edema, and damage to the kidneys and central nervous system (Alarcon et al., 2005; EPA, 2008). In addition, there is growing evidence that pesticide exposure is associated with chronic health effects such as asthma (Hoppin et al., 2008), cancer, damage to the liver, central nervous system dysfunction, immune system problems, and reproductive problems (Baldi et al., 2003; Cooper & Jones, 2008; EPA, 2008; Kamel & Hoppin, 2004; Kamel et al., 2005; Landrigan et al., 2005; Landrigan et al., 1999; NIOSH, 2007, Sanborn et al., 2007; Silver, 2006). Exposure to pesticides during childhood has been linked to an increased risk of leukemia, Hodgkin lymphoma, and renal, hepatic, soft tissue, bone and brain tumors (Belson, Kingsley, & Holmes, 2007; Carozza, Li, Elgethum, & Whitworth, 2008; Shim, Mlynarek, & van Wijngaarden, 2009). Prenatal pesticide exposure is associated with a number of health problems in their exposed children, including: neurologic abnormalities, autism (Colborn, 2006), attention deficit disorder/attention deficit hyperactivity disorder (ADD/ADHD) (Colborn, 2006), birth defects, altered fetal growth, fetal death, elevated blood pressure, brain and nervous system cancers (TEDE, 2007), leukemias, lymphomas, and Ewing's sarcoma (Buka, Koranteng, & Osornio Vargas, 2007; Colborn, 1995; Grandjean, Harari, Barr, & Debes, 2006; Roberts et al., 2007; Sanborn et al., 2007; Shim, Mlynarek, & van Wijngaarden, 2009; Sanborn et al., 2007; Shirangi, Fritschi, Holman, & Bower, 2009).

The effects that toxins have on the body are likely to depend on the point of exposure or entry into the body. Some gases and vapors can act as asphyxiants, reducing the body's access to oxygen. Some chemicals can burn the skin and mucous membranes, such as strong acids and bases. One example of a highly toxic acid is hydrogen sulfide (H2S). The health effects of H2S generally result from inhalation and vary based on the quantity and duration of exposure. Examples of symptoms and effects at lower exposure levels are nausea, headache, fatigue, loss of appetite, airway problems, and dizziness; higher exposure levels can lead to staggering, collapse, unconsciousness, and death (OSHA, n.d.-c).

Read about the health effects and control strategies at this OSHA website: https://www.osha.gov/hydrogen-sulfide.

Table 1. List of Five Sets of Exposure Guidelines

Acronym	Guideline Name	Source
PEL	Permissible Exposure Limit	Occupational Safety and Health Administration (OSHA); United States; Legal exposure limits
TLV®	Threshold Value Limit®	American Conference of Governmental Industrial Hygienists (ACGIH®); United States
STEL	Short-term exposure limit	American Conference of Governmental Industrial Hygienists (ACGIH®); United States; for some gases and vapors
REL	Recommended Exposure Limit	National Institute for Occupational Safety and Health (NIOSH); United States
MAK	Maximum Concentrations Values in the Workplace	DFG (German Research Foundation) Commission for the Investigation of Health Hazards of Chemical Compounds in the Work Area (MAK-Commission); Europe

Gases, vapors, and solvents

Everyone can be exposed to potentially harmful chemicals. These exposures occur at work, in our homes, and in our communities. Many hazardous chemicals are commonly used in homes, such as air fresheners, scented and other cleaning products, or having clothes dry cleaned with solvents. And, thousands of chemicals and chemical compounds are in use in work settings. These substances may occur in the form of gases, vapors, fumes, dusts or mists. "A gas is a formless liquid that completely fills its container and exerts an equal pressure in all directions" (Plog & Quinlan, 2012, p. 150). A vapor is a substance that is liquid at normal temperature and pressure yet some of, the vapor part is diffused or suspended in the air. A solvent is a liquid in which a solute, which may have been a solid, gas, or liquid, is dissolved or suspended in the solvent. A solvent may also be described as a medium for a reaction. Common examples of solvents are water, nail polish remover, and turpentine.

Particulate matter

Particulate matter (PM), also known as particle pollution (Environmental Protection Agency [EPA], 2017), is a "mixture of solid particles and liquid droplets found in the air (EPA, 2018)." Inhalation is the most important exposure route for most particulate matter. After being inhaled, the particles can affect the heart and lungs and cause serious health effects (EPA, 2017). One relatively new PM concern is nanotechnology and the production of engineered nanoparticles (ENPs) that are very small in at least two dimensions. The types of PM are dusts, mists, fumes, biologic agents, and smoke. Several examples of the most widely used and pervasive PM types are: asbestos, cotton, diesel exhaust, lead, pesticides, and wood dust. Engineered nanoparticles may be introducing relatively new health risks.

Routes of exposure for particulate matter

Inhalation is the most important exposure route for most PM. Once particles enter the respiratory tract, they may directly damage the lung, persist in the lung tissue and cause chronic health problems, be dissolved and absorbed by the body to cause systemic effects, or may be cleared from the lungs and swallowed, and then be absorbed by the digestive tract. It is also possible that some particles may be transported from the nasal mucosa to the central nervous system. Other routes of exposure for some types of PM are ingestion and skin contact. Skin contact with some particulates can cause burns or cancer.

Leaf blowers and particulate matter

One example of a common home and occupational hazard occurs in lawn care, the use of leaf blowers. Leaf blowers blast air at high speeds, sending many contaminants and particulates in the air, such as fungi, insecticides, herbicides, spores, heavy metals, and other particulate matter (PM). One leaf blower used for an hour sweeps up about five pounds of PM into the air that takes hours to settle. This contamination poses many health hazards, including the risk for allergic reactions, infections such as fungal lung infections, and toxic effects.

Biological reactions to particulate matter

Exposure to PM can induce biological responses ranging from acute to chronic, local to systemic, and mild to life threatening (Plog & Quinlan, 2012, p. 172). Some examples of biological reactions from inhaled PM are: irritation of the airways, breathing difficulties, pulmonary edema, bronchitis, allergic sensitization, fibrosis or scarring of lung tissue, emphysema, systemic toxicity, lymphatic toxicity, oncogenesis, infection, and metal fume fever. Workers may also experience adverse health effects from other routes of exposure. Pneumoconioses are a group of interstitial lung diseases caused by the inhalation of certain dusts and the lung tissue's reaction to the dust. The common types of pneumoconiosis are asbestosis, silicosis, and coal workers' pneumoconiosis (CWP). These diseases are caused by inhaling particulates, including asbestos fibers, silica dust, and coal mine dust (NIOSH, 2017). For more information about air pollution see the chapter on air in UNIT III: Environmental Health Sciences.

Engineered nanoparticles

Engineered nanoparticles (ENPs) are one type of product from nanotechnology, which involves manipulating matter to form structures that are very small. Nanoparticles need to be intentionally engineered to be ENPs. Nanoparticles have not been used long enough to study and understand the health effects of exposure to these small particles. There is evidence to suggest that some materials that are not highly toxic on the macro-scale may be highly toxic on the nano-scale. Epidemiologic and experimental studies have demonstrated that combustion-derived nanoparticles (CDNP), often found in air pollution, contribute significantly to pulmonary and cardiovascular disease and deaths. It can be expected that ENPs will mirror the adverse health effects associated with CDNP.

Exposure routes and distribution of nanoparticles

Nanoparticle exposure can occur through inhalation, ingestion, and skin contact. Some exposures through the respiratory and digestive tracts may cross into other areas of the body and lead to exposure of other organs and tissues. There is some evidence that several engineered nanoparticles may enter the brain through nasal mucosa and olfactory neuron axons; others may enter the brain through the bloodstream. There is conflicting evidence about whether nanoparticles cross the placental barrier and the impact on the developing fetus.

Work Organization Hazards

Work organization hazards include stressors, such as workload demands, intensity and/or pace, workplace violence, control over work, social relationships and support, and sexual harassment (OSHA, n.d.-a).

Workplace bullying and incivility

Workplace incivility and bullying are occupational health and public health issues. Sometimes the two terms are used interchangeably. Some people distinguish the two with incivility being considered less intense and perhaps the precursor of bullying. Incivility may be considered: "low-intensity deviant behavior with ambiguous intent to harm the target, in violation of workplace norms for mutual respect (Longo, 2017)." Bullying may be defined as "behaviors intended to degrade or humiliate another and that continue over a period of time (Longo, 2017)." Examples of bullying are threatening language or behavior, constant and unreasonable criticism, and deliberate undermining of activities.

Bullying and incivility are common problems in many organizations, including health services organizations. It is a challenge to quantify the problem of bullying; it often goes unreported (Thompson, 2013). However, the literature suggests bullying is fairly common in nursing (Thompson, 2013; Vessey et al., 2009; Wilson, 2016). One large international study (N=2,000) indicated that 80% of participating nurses reported that they witnessed bullying in the workplace (Thompson, 2013b). Of these, 51% were nurse-to-nurse bullying (Thompson, 2013). A survey conducted in 2008, which included every region of the United States and 17 other countries, concluded that 75% of healthcare workers experience violence in forms other than physical violence, such as bullying, intimidation, criticism, and outbursts of anger (Hader, 2008). Of those subjected, 75% experienced criticism from their supervisors, colleagues, and physicians; 51.9% experienced verbal abuse directly from their coworkers (Hader, 2008).

OCCUPATIONAL AND ENVIRONMENTAL REGULATORY AGENCIES AND LAWS

Federal Regulatory Agencies

Several federal agencies oversee occupational health and/or environmental health, including:

- Occupational Safety and Health Administration: created in 1971

- National Institute of Occupational Safety and Health (NIOSH): established by the Occupational Safety and Health Act (OSHAct); it is housed within the Centers for Disease Control and Prevention (CDC)

- Environmental Protection Agency (EPA)

The Occupational Safety and Health Administration (OSHA) was created by the Occupational Safety and Health Act (OSHAct) of 1970. The OSHA is charged with helping employers to achieve health and safety goals by enforcing standards, through education, training and technical assistance, and creating partnerships and consulting with employers, employees, and organizations regarding preventing injuries and illnesses (Plog & Quinlan, 2012).

Occupational Safety and Health Act

The first phrase of the OSHAct is: "To assure safe and healthful working conditions for working men and women; by authorizing enforcement of the standards developed under the Act; by assisting and encouraging the States in their efforts to assure safe and healthful working conditions; by providing for research, information, education, and training in the field of occupational safety and health; and for other purposes (OSHA, 2004). It emphasizes the goal of achieving safe and healthy working conditions.

The OSHAct specifies two duties for employers. One is to provide employees with work settings that are "free from recognized hazards that are causing or are likely to cause death or serious harm to their employees" (Plog & Quinlan, 2012, p. 7). The second duty is that employers must comply with all standards under OSHAct. To learn more about OSHAct, browse through the Act at: https://www.osha.gov/laws-regs/oshact/toc.

Federal Regulations and Governmental Standards for Toxic Substances

Two major federal regulations for toxic substances are the OSHAct and the Toxic Substances Control Act of 1976. The Occupational Safety and Health Administration (OSHA) has adopted Permissible Exposure Limits (PELs) for more than 400 substances (Plog & Quinlan, 2012). This is a very small number out of the approximately 84,000 chemicals that may be in use in businesses, based on the Environmental Protection Agency's inventory (U.S., Government Accounting Office, 2013).

The OSHA has the authority to develop standards that employers must follow to protect the health and safety of workers. However, these standards are developed using a "very extensive and lengthy process that includes substantial public engagement, notice, and comment. The agency must show that a significant risk to workers exists and that there are feasible measures employers can take to protect their workers" (Plog & Quinlan, 2012, p. 810). The stages and steps of "The OSHA Rulemaking Process" are outlined in a one-page online document: https://www.osha.gov/OSHA_FlowChart.pdf

Legal requirements for OSHA standards

There are six legal requirements for OSHA standards:

- "Each standard must substantially reduce a significant risk of material harm" (Plog & Quinlan, 2012, p. 811)

- Technologically feasible: "protective measures being required already exist, can be brought into existence with available technology, or can be created with technology that can reasonably be developed" (Plog & Quinlan, 2012, p. 811)

- Economically feasible: not adversely affect long-term profitability or competitiveness

- Address a significant risk; and standards must protect to a high degree

- Cost-effective measures

- Must have substantial evidence to support the standards

These legal requirements substantially limit the ability to create protective standards and do not adhere to the precautionary principle.

EXPOSURE GUIDELINES

Different governmental agencies and professional organizations have established exposure guidelines for various chemicals or substances. The acronyms, names and source of several of these guidelines are listed in Table 1.

Threshold limit values: The American Congress of Governmental Industrial Hygienists (ACGIH) recommends Threshold Limit Values (TLVs®). These are voluntary "exposure guidelines established for airborne concentrations of many chemical compounds (Plog & Quinlan, 2012, p. 25)." The TLVs are intended to protect most but not all workers from adverse effects if exposed day-after-day. However, this is not indicating that the levels are safe; and they do not consider cancer and reproductive health risks.

European Maximum Concentration Values in the Workplace (MAKs) are more likely than U.S. standards to be based on health effects and are often developed using an approach called no observed adverse effect (NOAEL) of the most sensitive endpoint.

LIMITATIONS OF ENVIRONMENTAL HEALTH AND SAFETY REGULATIONS AND GUIDELINES

In general, environmental and occupational regulations and guidelines are not sufficient for protecting workers, the community, or the environment. As noted above, only about 400 of approximately 84,000 substances or chemicals have established PELs (Plog & Quinlan, 2012; Government Accounting Office, 2013). Additionally, there are substantial limitations for the PELs that do exist that directly relate to the legal requirements and processes for standard development and approval. The requirements for standards to be technically feasible for industry to comply with, economically feasible and cost-effective, and not threaten long-term profitability or competitive structure undermine the ability to protect the health and safety of workers and the community. As a result, adverse health effects can occur from exposure to substances that are at or below the PELs.

The requirement to have substantial evidence to support the standards can be challenging to meet because of limitations in research funding and methodological challenges in conducting occupational and environmental studies. One challenge is that epidemiologic research on health effects of many exposures may take decades of following and monitoring exposed persons to assess long-term health outcomes. Second, there may not be sufficient funding or human resources to complete all the studies that are needed to assess the health and safety of all potentially harmful exposures. Third, epidemiologic investigations are complex because people are often exposed to many toxic exposures during their lifetime; therefore, it may be difficult to find true unexposed control groups that have not been exposed to toxins with similar health effects of the exposure being studied.

Several factors can affect the response to a toxic exposure, including age, body size, other exposures, overall health status, and the timing of an exposure in a lifespan. Very young children, whose systems are immature, are more vulnerable to exposures and the adverse effects of environmental hazards. Children are especially vulnerable to the adverse effects of environmental hazards because of their developmental stages, higher metabolic rates, immature organ systems, and brains that are not fully developed. Because of their potential for a longer remaining life expectancy than for adults, there is greater potential for children to develop environmentally triggered diseases over their lifespan. Yet, many environmental and occupational studies are based on effects among healthy adult males. Therefore, legally acceptable levels of toxins may be released into communities and the environment, exposing more vulnerable populations.

USE OF STANDARDS AND GUIDELINES BY OCCUPATIONAL HEALTH PROFESSIONALS

Occupational health and safety professionals are responsible for promoting safe and healthful working conditions that protect workers, the community, and the environment. Environmental and occupational standards are not sufficient for meeting this obligation. Therefore, occupational health and safety professionals should consider PELs and TLVs® as minimally acceptable protections. Nurses apply evidence-based guidelines, including the European standards, and supplement these guidelines with published scientific literature on the health effects of environmental and occupational exposures. Using all available information, the Precautionary Principle should be applied.

INTRODUCTION TO THE OCCUPATIONAL HEALTH AND SAFETY TEAM

In a specific workplace, there may be multiple types of occupational health professionals that collaborate to promote health and safety. However, in some workplaces, multiple roles are handled by the same person. Four major occupational health roles are: occupational health nurse, occupational and environmental physician, industrial hygienist, and safety professional.

Occupational Health Nurse

Occupational health nursing "focuses on the promotion, protection, and restoration of workers' health within the context of a safe and healthy work environment (Plog & Quinlan, 2012, p. 4)." Occupational health nurses work to prevent work-related injuries and illnesses, prevent disabilities, and help workers optimize their health status. The occupational health nurse (OHN) may be involved in providing direct care services, however, the major focus should be on primary prevention. Another OHN role is to use a case management approach to help injured workers navigate the care delivery system and return to work appropriately and on a timely basis; this is considered to be tertiary prevention. The OHN often serves in multiple roles, clinician, educator, manager, and consultant.

Nurses' roles in environmental health

Nurses have a history of promoting environmental health, going back to early landmark efforts of Florence Nightingale and Lilian Wald. In addition, nurses are increasingly being called to take action to apply environmental health concepts to all areas of nursing practice, including occupational health, through the professional Scope and Standards of Practice for Nursing (American Nurses Association [ANA], 2021, ANA, 2010; ANA, 2007). There are several sets of standards of practice for nursing that are important to environmental health; one that focuses specifically on environmental health is the ANA's Principles of Environmental Health for Nursing Practice with Implementation Strategies (ANA, 2007).

Occupational and Environmental Health Physician

The primary goal of an occupational and environmental health or medical physician is to prevent occupational illness. To effectively participate in the process of creating a safe and healthy work environment, the occupational medicine physician must understand the jobs, work processes, and materials used in the organization, the potential hazards and risks, and strategies to reduce risks. When occupational injuries or illnesses occur, the occupational medicine physician may be involved with working with the employee to restore health. Occupational physicians may also conduct occupational health histories of employees, be involved in preplacement physical examinations, perform fitness for duty (FFD) evaluations, and conduct return-to-work evaluations.

The occupational medicine physician may work in a range of settings, such as within an occupational health and safety department of an organization or corporate medical department, in a multispecialty group practice or hospital-based program, freestanding occupational health clinic, consulting firm, academic occupational medicine department, environmental agency, government agency, union, or other settings.

Industrial Hygienist

"Industrial hygienists are occupational health professionals who are concerned primarily with the control of environmental stresses or occupational health hazards that arise as a result of or during the course of work" (Plog & Quinlan, 2012, p. 3). This definition highlights the important role that industrial hygienists have in protecting workers and the health of the community. Industrial hygienists consider effects of hazards or exposures quite broadly, focusing on life, health, pain or discomfort, and effects on the aging process. They often need to be generalists, having a broad scope of knowledge and skills.

Industrial hygienists may work as part of a team that may include physicians, nurses, safety professionals, toxicologists, epidemiologists, educators and/or other professionals. In addition, industrial hygienists may supervise occupational safety and health technologists, also called industrial hygiene technicians, who may function in more limited technical areas.

Safety Professional

A safety professional is defined as "a person engaged in the prevention of accidents, incidents, and events that harm people, property, or the environment" (Plog & Quinlan, 2012, p. 728). Although safety in an organization generally requires a multidisciplinary effort involving several members of the occupational health and safety team, the safety professional specifically focuses on identifying and evaluating potential hazards in the workplace and making recommendations for administrative and engineering controls to eliminate or reduce the risk posed by hazards. The discipline applies knowledge of "physics, chemistry, biology, physiology, statistics, mathematics, computer science, engineering mechanics, industrial processes, business, communication, and psychology" (Plog & Quinlan, 2012, p. 726).

GREENING OF INDUSTRIES

A major emphasis in occupational health and industrial hygiene is primary prevention, which involves implementing health promotion and health protection measures in the workplace to prevent diseases and injuries from occurring. By implementing effective evidence-based health promotion activities and keeping people healthier, occupational health professionals can reduce absenteeism at work, help keep people out of the hospital, and reduce the excessive environmental waste associated with hospital-based services. In addition, the implementation of "green" or environmental sustainability practices or initiatives in businesses or industries is consistent with a primary prevention approach.

Environmental sustainability involves a wide range of interventions or strategies, including:

- Implement healthy landscaping without use of pesticides, minimizing water use, and avoiding use of motorized equipment, such as leaf blowers or lawn mowers

- Provide access to public transportation, safe walking and bicycle paths and other alternatives

- Provide a connection with nature

- Use eco-friendly building materials

- Reduce use, reuse, reduce use, and rot or compost

- Conserve energy and water

- Work toward carbon neutrality

- Minimally use toxic chemicals; substitute for healthier alternatives

- Provide access to and promote purchase and consumption of healthy, organically and sustainably grown, and local foods

The benefits to individuals and society of going green are immense, and include:

- Protecting infants from reproductive abnormalities and developmental damage

- Preventing human cancers, infertility, and other health problems

- Reducing the need for landfills

- Reducing organizational costs and clean-up costs for society

- Reducing emissions of dioxins and other toxins into the atmosphere

- Other benefits

Environmental sustainability is healthier, often cost effective, and is consistent with the health professionals' ethical principle of "First Do No Harm."

Greening of Health Care

Some health services organizations are working on "green" or environmentally friendly initiatives. Some organizations have launched green teams and developed sustainability departments. The Preface of the book Greening Health Care (Gerwig, 2015) briefly describes an exemplar hospital that is environmentally sustainable in terms of size, healthy landscaping, access to public transportation, connection with nature, eco-friendly building materials, recycling, conservation of energy and water, carbon neutrality, minimal use of toxic chemicals, and other strategies. These strategies are more in line with "health" than many or most sick care organizations. In addition, in the Preface the author mentions that "the best thing we can do for the environment is to reduce our own health risks, or if we are healthy to stay that way (Gerwig, 2015, p. ix). It is true that most health problems are preventable; and if we change the focus of health services to a greater emphasis on evidence-based strategies to promote health, that should lead to a decrease in the need for sick care services that are financially costly, burdensome to patients and their families, and generally do significant harm to the environment. Any type of industry can implement wellness initiatives that may benefit the employees and the bottom line of the company, while helping to reduce use of sick care services.

REFERENCES

Alarcon, W.A., Calvert, G.M., Blondell, J.M., Mehler, L.N., Sievert, J., Propect, M., et al. (2005). Acute illnesses associated with pesticides exposure at schools. *Journal of the American Medical Association, 294*(4), 455-465.

American Industrial Hygiene Association. (2018). *Discover industrial hygiene.* https://www.aiha.org/about-ih/Pages/default.aspx

American Nurses Association (ANA). (2021). *Nursing: Scope and standards of practice* (4th ed.). American Nurses Association.

American Nurses Association. (2010). *Nursing: Scope and standards of practice* (2nd ed.). American Nurses Association.

American Nurses Association. (2007). *ANA's principles of environmental health for nursing practice with implementation strategies.* American Nurses Association.

Baldi, I., Lebailly, P., Mohammed-Brahim, B., Letenneur, L., Dartiques, J., & Brochard, P. (2003). Neurodegenerative diseases and exposure to pesticides in the elderly. *American Journal of Epidemiology, 157*(5), 409-414.

Belson, M., Kingsley, B., & Holmes, A. (2007). Risk factors for acute leukemia in children: a review. *Environmental Health Perspectives, 115*(1), 138-145.

Breeding, D. C. (2011). *What is hazardous? Occupational Health and Safety.* https://ohsonline.com/articles/2011/07/01/what-is-hazardous.aspx

Brouwer, M., Huss, A., van der Mark, M., Nijssen, P. C. G., Mullerners, W. M., Sas, A. M. G., ... Vermeulen, R. C. H. (2017). Environmental exposures to pesticides and the risk of Parkinson's disease in the Netherlands. *Environment International, 107,* 1100-10. doi: 10.1016/j.envint.2017.07.001.

Buka, I., Koranteng, S., & Osornio Vargas, A.R. (2007). Trends in childhood cancer incidence: review of environmental linkages. *Pediatric Clinics of North America, 54,* 177-203.

Bureau of Labor Statistics. (2017). *Injuries, illnesses, and fatalities.* United States Department of Labor. https://www.bls.gov/iif/

Canadian Centre for Occupational Health and Safety. (2018a). *Prevention of slips, trips and falls.* OSH Answers Fact Sheets. https://www.ccohs.ca/oshanswers/safety_haz/falls.html

Canadian Centre for Occupational Health and Safety. (2018b). *Confined space -- introduction.* OSH Answers Fact Sheets. https://www.ccohs.ca/oshanswers/hsprograms/confinedspace_intro.html

Canadian Centre for Occupational Health and Safety. (2018c) *Chemical profiles.* OSH Answers Fact Sheets. https://www.ccohs.ca/oshanswers/chemicals/chem_profiles/.

Carozza, S. E., Li, B., Elgethun, K., & Whitworth, R. (2008). Risk of childhood cancers associated with residence in agriculturally intense areas in the United States. *Environmental Health Perspectives, 116*(4), 559-565.

Centers for Disease Control and Prevention. (2015). *Health effects of radiation.* https://www.cdc.gov/nceh/radiation/health.html

Colborn, T. (2006). A case for revisiting the safety of pesticides: a closer look at neurodevelopment. *Environmental Health Perspectives, 114*(1), 10-17.

Colborn, T. (1995). Pesticides — how research has succeeded and failed to translate science into policy: endocrinological effects on wildlife. *Environmental Health Perspectives, 103*(S6), 81-85.

Cooper, G. S., & Jones, S. (2008). Pentachlorophenol and cancer risk: focusing the lens on specific chlorophenols and contaminants. *Environmental Health Perspectives, 116*(8), 1001-1008.

Environmental Protection Agency. (2018). *Particulate matter (PM) basics.* https://www.epa.gov/pm-pollution/particulate-matter-pm-basics#PM

Environmental Protection Agency. (2017). *Particulate matter (PM) pollution.* https://www.epa.gov/pm-pollution

Environmental Protection Agency. (2008). *An introduction to indoor air quality; pollutants and sources of indoor air pollution.* http://www.epa.gov/iaq/pesticid.html#Health%20Effects.

Grandjean, P., Harari, R., Barr, D. B., & Debes, F. (2006). Pesticide exposure and stunting as independent predictors of neurobehavioral deficits in Ecuadorian school children. *Pediatrics, 117,* e546-e556.

Hader, R. (2008). Workplace violence survey 2008: unsettling findings. Nursing Management, 39(7), 13-19. doi: 10.1097/01.NUMA.0000326561.54414.58

Helmenstine, T. (2017). *List of radioactive elements.* https://www.thoughtco.com/list-of-radioactive-elements-608644

Hoppin, J. A., Umbach, D. M., London, S. J., Hennengerger, P. K., Kullman, G. J., Alavnia, M. C. R., et al. (2008). Pesticides and atopic and nonatopic asthma among farm women in the Agricultural Health Study. American *Journal of Respiratory and Critical Care Medicine, 117,* 11-18.

International Ergonomics Association. (2018). *Definition and domains of ergonomics.* https://www.iea.cc/whats/index.html

Kamel, F., Engel, L. S., Gladen, B. C. Hoppin, J. A., Alavanjz, M. C. R., & Sandler, D. P. (2005). Neurologic symptoms in licensed private pesticide applicators in the Agricultural Health Study. *Environmental Health Perspectives, 113*(7), 877-882.

Kamel, F., & Hoppin, J. A. (2004). Association of pesticide exposure with neurologic dysfunction and disease. *Environmental Health Perspectives, 112*(9), 950-958.

Krieble, D., Tickner, J., Epstein, P., Lemons, J., Levins, R., Loechler, E. L., ...Stoto. M. (2001). The precautionary principle in environmental science. *Environmental Health*

Perspectives, 109(9), 871-6. https://www.ncbi.nlm.nih.gov/pmc/articles/PMC1240435/

Landrigan, P. J., Sonawane, B., Butler, R. N., Trasande, L., Callan, R., & Droller, D. (2005). Early environmental origins of neurodegenerative disease in later life. *Environmental Health Perspectives, 113*(9), 1230-1233.

Landrigan, P. J., Claudio, L., Markowitz, S. B., Berkowitz, G. S., Brenner, B. L., Romero, H., ... & Wolff, M. S. (1999). Pesticides and inner-city children: exposures, risks, and prevention. *Environmental Health Perspectives, 107*(3), 431-437.

Longo, J. (2017). Cognitive rehearsal. *American Nurse Today, 12*(8). https://www.americannursetoday.com/cognitive-rehearsal/

National Cancer Institute. (2016). *Electromagnetic fields and cancer.* https://www.cancer.gov/about-cancer/causes-prevention/risk/radiation/electromagnetic-fields-fact-sheet

National Institute for Occupational Safety and Health. (2018a). *Hierarchy of controls.* https://www.cdc.gov/niosh/topics/hierarchy/default.html

National Institute for Occupational Safety and Health. (2018b). *Noise and hearing loss prevention.* https://www.cdc.gov/niosh/topics/noise/default.html

National Institute of Environmental Health Sciences. (2018c). *Electric and magnetic fields.* https://www.niehs.nih.gov/health/topics/agents/emf/index.cfm

National Institute for Occupational Safety and Health. (2018d). *Ergonomics and musculoskeletal disorders.* https://www.cdc.gov/niosh/topics/ergonomics/default.html

National Institute of Occupational Safety and Health. (2017). *Pneumoconioses.* https://www.cdc.gov/niosh/topics/pneumoconioses/default.html

National Institute for Occupational Safety and Health (2014). *National occupational research agenda.* https://www.cdc.gov/niosh/docs/96-115/diseas.html

National Institute for Occupational Safety and Health. (2007). *Reducing pesticide exposure at schools, NIOSH fact sheet.* Department of Health and Human Services, Centers for Disease Control and Prevention. https://www.cdc.gov/niosh/docs/2007-150/default.html.

Occupational Safety and Health Administration. (2004). *Public Law 91-596. 84 STAT. 1590. 91st Congress, S.2193. December 29, 1970 as amended through January 1, 2004. (1). An Act.* https://www.osha.gov/laws-regs/oshact/section_1

Occupational Safety and Health Administration. (n.d.-a). *Safety hazards.* https://www.osha.gov/dte/grant_materials/fy10/sh-20839-10/circle_chart.pdf

Occupational Safety and Health Administration. (n.d.-b). *Working in outdoor and indoor heat environments.* https://www.osha.gov/SLTC/heatstress/

Occupational Safety and Health Administration. (n.d.-c). *Hydrogen sulfide.* https://www.osha.gov/SLTC/hydrogensulfide/hazards.html

Plog, B. A., & Quinlan, P. J. (2012). *Fundamentals of industrial hygiene.* National Safety Council.

Roberts, E. M., English, P. B., Grether, J. K., Windham, G. C., Somberg, L., & Wolff, C. (2007). Maternal residence near agricultural pesticide applications and autism spectrum disorders among children in the California Central Valley. *Environmental Health Perspectives, 115*(10), 1482-1489.

Sacramento Metropolitan Air Quality Management District. (2018). *Air quality information for the Sacramento region. Overall health effects.* http://www.sparetheair.com/health.cfm?page=healthoverall

Sanborn, M., Kerr, K.J., Sanin, L.H., Cole, D.C., Bassil, K.K., & Vakil, C. (2007). Non-cancer health effects of pesticides. *Canadian Family Physician, 53,* 1713-1720.

Shim, Y. K., Mlynarek, S. P., & van Wijngaarden, E. (2009). Parental exposure to pesticides and childhood brain cancer: US Atlantic coast childhood brain cancer study. *Environmental Health Perspectives, 117*(6), 1002-1006.

Shirangi, A., Fritschi, L., Holman, C. D. J., & Bower. C. (2009). Birth defects in offspring of female veterinarians. *Journal of Occupational and Environmental Medicine, 51*(5), 525-533.

Sifferlin, A., (2017, October 19). *Here's how many people die from pollution around the world.* Time Health. http://time.com/4989641/water-air-pollution-deaths/

Silver, L. B. (2011, February). *Pesticides, practice prevention.* Learning and Developmental Disabilities Initiative. https://www.healthandenvironment.org/uploads-old/pesticides.pdf

Thompson, R. (2013). Strategies for eliminating nurse-to-nurse bullying. *Med-Surg Matters, 22*(2), 18-19.

U.S. Department of Human Services. (2016). *Asbestos and your health. Health Effects of Asbestos | Asbestos | ATSDR* (cdc.gov)

U.S. Department of Labor. (n.d.). *Business case for safety and health.* https://www.osha.gov/dcsp/products/topics/businesscase/costs.html

U.S. Government Accountability Office (GAO). (2013). *Toxic substances: EPA has increased efforts to assess and control chemicals but could strengthen its approach.* GAO.

University of Wisconsin. (2018). *The triple bottom line.* https://sustain.wisconsin.edu/sustainability/triple-bottom-line/

Vessey, J. A., Demarco, R. F., Gaffney, D.A., & Budin, W. C. (2009). Bullying of staff registered nurses in the workplace: A preliminary study for developing personal and organizational strategies for the transformation of hostile to healthy workplace environments. *Journal of Professional Nursing, 25(5),* 299-306. doi: 10.1016/j.profnurs.2009.01.022

Walton, A. L., LePrevost, C., Wong, B., Linnan, L., Sanchez-Birkhead, A., & Mooney, K. (2016). Observed and self-reported pesticide protective behaviors of Latino migrant and seasonal farmworkers. *Environmental Research, 147,* 275-83. doi: 10.1016/j.envres.2016.02.020.

Wilson, J. L. (2016). An exploration of bullying behaviors in nursing: A review of literature. *British Journal of Nursing, 25(6),* 303-306.

HEALTHY FOOD IN HOSPITALS

Janet Knott, DNP, RN, CNE
Assistant Teaching Professor
The Pennsylvania State University
College of Nursing

Jennifer J. Wasco, DNP, RN
Assistant Professor of Nursing
University of Pittsburgh
School of Nursing

HISTORICAL INSIGHT TO HOSPITAL FOOD

Cultures, religion, and medicine have historically been linked to the earliest known archaic hospitals where monks, soldiers, porters' wives and then nurses prepared the food. Food for the sick in the 1700s consisted of the three Bs; bread, beef, and beer, although alcohol in diets declined in the 1800s. Fruits and vegetables, other than potatoes, were hardly ever a food option whereas the food for the sick traditionally depended on the donations and generosity of family and friends.

The practice of nurses preparing and serving food to the sick was called "Invalid Cookery," in which a few hours were spent training the nurses to prepare the food. Clinical nursing duties in the nutritional care of their patients is clearly defined as Duty #10 in the Lady Probationers Handbook as…."to be competent to cook gruel, arrow bread, egg flip, puddings and drinks for the sick" … (Englert, Crocker & Stotts, 1986, p.522). Several prestigious "Cookery Schools" started in the 1870s which had a significant impact on the nutrition content taught in schools of nursing. In 1893 the Women's Hospital of Philadelphia, the first nurse training school in the county included instruction in foods and methods of cookery (Englert et al., 1986). Student nurses were assigned to work in the kitchen for a month to learn dishwashing, cleaning and the art of preparing food for the sick. It is believed that the word "dietitian" most likely originated during this time, although the exact origin is unknown.

In the 1900s, the development of nutritional science diets was more carefully considered and the health profession began to recognize the importance of providing special diets specific to patients with certain diseases. During this time in 1901, Adelaide Nutting, the Superintendent of Nurses at John Hopkins Hospital, voiced the need to implement a separate program in dietetics. Shortly thereafter, the Department of Public Charities in New York City implemented a dietetic program which sparked the formation of the American Dietetic Association (ADA)

and the establishment of the profession of dietetics in 1917 (Englert et al., 1986).

During the early period of dietetics, nursing curriculum related to nutrition evolved from the Diet Kitchen Course comprising approximately 15 hours in the topics of food, its source, composition and usage in the body, diet in diseases and infant feeding and expanded to approximately 100 hours of content over a three-year period. In 1949, the National League for Nursing (NLN) recognized the importance of nutrition by introducing a nursing achievement test in "Diet Therapy and Applied Nutrition" (Englert et al., 1986). The didactic areas related to nutrition were broken down into three separate sections of food, nutrition and diet therapy. In addition at this time, nurses willingly released their duties of food service preparation to the dietary department. Soon after the directors of nursing schools then invited the dietitian to teach the nutrition-related learning activities. To differentiate the roles, the dietitian's role was to plan and order the patient's meals and the nutritional well-being of the patient was the responsibility of the nurse.

In the 1960s the nursing curriculum changed from the medical to the conceptual model in which the content of nutrition was taught as a continuous "thread" through the curriculum. This curricula change prompted the State Boards of Nursing to eliminate the specific number of required hours in nutrition. Approximately 10% of the State Board Nursing exam consisted of nutrition-related questions in 1972, and was decreased to only 5% in 1982, currently it is difficult to determine the exact percentage dedicated to nutrition since this topic meshes with other subjects in the National Council Licensure Examination (Englert et al., 1986). Currently nursing program curriculum vary, making it difficult to standardize nutrition content into curriculum though five major strategies are employed:

1) Nutrition is taught as a separate subject;

2) Nutrition is included as an integral part of nursing courses;

3) Nutrition is covered in patient-oriented situations, conferences or during studies of special patients;

4) Nutrition is taught as a science course for nurses;

5) Nutrition is taught as a combination of strategies (Englert et al., 1986, p. 527).

If optimal nursing care is to be provided to all patients, then the importance of nutrition should be examined.

NUTRITIONAL INSIGHTS CENTERED AROUND ETHICS

Hospitals are fortunate to have a variety of members on a healthcare team; each member has a unique role in nutrition care for patients. Physicians hold the ultimate responsibility for meeting the patients' healthcare needs, including nutrition, since they are responsible for prescribing the diet order. Physicians perform comprehensive nutrition assessments, order diet counseling and review data on food intake. Not all facilities employ dietitians, and it may be possible if a dietitian is employed by a facility, they may not be able to complete a patient consult without a specific order or trigger to provide nutritional assessment and medical nutrition therapy. Nurses spend a majority of their time with the patients and are on the frontline ready to assess and identify patients' nutritional needs, although they are not permitted to order a patient's diet without consulting with a physician first. Nurses are busy with many responsibilities centered around medication administration and providing essential patient maintenance, however most often it is the nurse who evaluates the patient's nutritional deficiencies that places the patient at risk for inadequate energy to heal, maintain an immune system and skin integrity, absorb/use medications appropriately and support organ function. There is an increase in the risk of malnutrition in adult hospitalized patients, foremost it has been established that nutritional education for nurses must improve (Boarz et al., 2013; Tappenden et al., 2013). Patient nutrition education is a vital piece of healthcare, nutrition education is to be initiated by the physician and dietitian then reinforced by the nurse, although in reality this may not happen due to various reasons, including time constraints, shortened length of stay and knowledge deficit. Tappenden et al., (2013) offers the following recommendations to drive nutritional improvement:

1) Create an institutional culture where all stakeholders value nutrition;

2) Redefine healthcare clinicians' roles to include nutritional care;

3) Recognize and diagnose all malnourished patients and those at risk;

4) Rapidly implement comprehensive nutrition interventions and continued monitoring;

5) Communicate nutritional care plans; and

6) Develop a comprehensive discharge nutrition care and education plan (p. 147).

The transformation of hospitals evolved from financial incentives for keeping beds filled to present incentives for preventing readmissions and promoting wellness. In the United States, healthcare delivery driven by policy is steering the focus on cost, quality, and transparency of care. These changes have promoted the return to re-examining the role of nutrition as a critical component to patient recovery and wellness. Hospitals have a moral obligation to provide a variety of healthy foods since many leading causes of death including obesity, diabetes, heart disease, and cancer, are diet related. Also, it is clear that healthcare workers are aware that foods high in fats and sugars are considered damaging to health and result in increased morbidity and mortality rates. Simply put, serving unhealthy food to patients, staff and visitors is unethical. In a sustainable hospital the fundamental science of providing healthy foods to patients, staff and visitors is embraced by role modeling contagious healthy behaviors such as banning sugar-sweetened beverages, and minimizing the availability of candies, chips, fries, refined grains and cured/preserved meats. Providing wholesome nutrition in hospitals is morally sound, and hospitals should offer food that is beneficial to the planet such as serving dairy products and meats without antibiotics, offering meatless alternatives or meatless days, and choosing food grown by local farmers. By making these simple menu changes, it can have a positive impact on human health and the environment which is good for all.

THE CONNECTION BETWEEN FOOD, HEALTH AND THE ENVIRONMENT

According to the World Health Organization (WHO, 2018), by the year 2020, chronic diseases will account for almost 75% of all deaths worldwide. In the United States, the majority of the nation's 3.3 trillion health care dollars are spent on managing chronic diseases such as diabetes, obesity and heart disease (Center for Disease Control, 2018). Poor eating patterns can be held accountable for these trends. While efforts have been employed to change food consumption patterns in the United States such as banning trans fats (Assaf, 2014) or taxing sugar-sweetened beverages (Mariner and Annas, 2013), these types of initiatives are not holding ground, and the number of food-related diseases is continuing to rise. Additionally, the over-consumption of foods in the United States is not only impacting the health of its people but also the health of our planet. This cycle of activity does not provide a sustainable, healthy environment in which one can live.

According to the United States Department of Agriculture (USDA, 2014), there is strong evidence that new dietary patterns, such as eating more plant-based meals and reducing the consumption of red meat can reduce not only the incidence of chronic disease but also decrease the footprint of food consumption on the environment. Healthcare organizations have responded to this evidence and are actively promoting healthy, environmentally friendly, nutritional offerings for patients, employees, and communities (Healthier Hospitals Initiative, 2012). Hospital systems are incorporating innovative environmental nutrition concepts into daily operations with the goal of providing optimal care to the communities in which they serve.

The traditional discipline of nutrition focuses on the biochemical components of food such as calories, vitamins, and fats and individual food consumption, while the relatively new discipline of environmental nutrition addresses social, political, economic and environmental factors in defining healthy foods (Sabate, Harwatt, & Soret, 2016). Leveraging both nutritional approaches is necessary to promote positive, healthy behaviors. Understanding the intersection of the food supply, health and the physical environment otherwise known as the health-environment-diet trilemma is of great importance for public and environmental health (Sabate et al., 2016). Shifting to healthier diets can reduce diet-related diseases and improve environmental outcomes. The impact of food systems from farm to processing, storage, consumption, and waste is impacting climate change, which is known to have effects on human health. Identifying ways of reducing food waste should be a priority of all healthcare systems. Hospitals can get support from such organizations such as Practice Green Health's program called The Healthy Hospital's Initiative (HHI). The organization provides tools for hospitals to reach sustainable goals around healthier food, the reduction of waste, ideas for less energy consumption and smarter purchasing power.

One suggestion from HHI to reduce the carbon footprint is for hospitals to explore new procurement methods for securing food by partnering with local farmers. Leveraging sustainable-local resources reduces the number of greenhouse gases from vehicle transport as food can travel up to 1,500 miles to reach its final destination (Xuereb, 2006). However, hospital operations need to be aware that some barriers will need to be addressed when considering this option, such as the reliability of supply, the timing of supply, and geographic locations subject to seasonal changes. Despite the challenges, incorporating environmentally-supported concepts must be considered.

Additionally, modifications of food sources may relieve some of the food production burdens on the environment, whereas approximately 14.5% of the worlds greenhouse gas emissions (GHG) is from farming of livestock (Stoll-Kleemann and Schmidt, 2017). Trends are

shifting toward plant-based meals to reduce the environmental burden of meat-based meals, and they offer similar or better nutritional value and have shown to improve health (Evans, Magee, Dickman, Sutter, & Sutter, 2017). In June of 2017, the American Medical Association passed a Healthy Food Options in Hospitals resolution that calls on hospitals to improve the health of patients,

> ### On-Trend: Hospital Based Farmer's Markets
>
> Hospitals are becoming more innovative in the promotion of healthy foods. One such approach is establishing hospital-based farmers's markets for patients, visitors, employees and the community. The benefit of having on the ground farmer's markets can serve a variety of purposes from the basic provision of healthier foods to leveraging new methods in which to provide nutritional educational opportunities.
>
> Interested in establishing a hospital-based farmers market at your hospital? Visit Health Care Without Harm for a step-by-step guide on how to host a farmer's market.

staff, and visitors. Additionally, August 2018, California State Bill 1138 mandated that all hospital systems must offer at least one plant-based option at every meal. With each small initiative, hospitals can pledge to rethink food leveraging to the environmental nutrition approach which can encourage people to live healthy lives, plus maintain planetary survival.

THE ROLE OF HOSPITALS AND HEALTH PROFESSIONALS IN HEALTHIER FOOD

There is a remarkable opportunity for all healthcare providers to educate patients and communities about sustainable eating to achieve optimal health and wellness. With a focus on environmental nutrition and dietary trends, the first ingredient is education. As nutrition and food service-lines are infusing new concepts and ideas into menu choices, there is often a lack of support from other disciplines due to a knowledge deficit for the changes. Therefore, establishing a baseline understanding of nutrition, sustainability, and the environment should be provided to all stakeholders. Steps can also be taken to improve personal awareness by participating in educational programs to learn about plant-based nutritional approaches and in turn apply the knowledge gained to patient care (Evan et al., 2017). Establishing a partnership between the healthcare providers and nutritional services is critical to close communication gaps, clarify roles, and foster effective use of resources and knowledge for continuous improvement in achieving patient health and wellness. It is anticipated with a better understanding of sustainable food practices, support for these new initiatives will increase.

Health care providers can also engage in research to further examine the impact of food production on the health of patients and the planet and advocating for public policies that promote better sustainable farming practices. Finally, health care facilities should consider joining organizations that support plant-based diets such as the Nurses Nutrition Network or Practice Green Health to obtain step-by-step guides on how to move the dial on sustainable food practices. For more about the environmental impacts of food and food production please go to the food and agriculture chapter in Unit V: Sustainable Communities.

REFERENCES

Assaf, R.R. (2014). Overview of local, state, and national government legislation restricting trans fats. *Clinical Therapeutics, 36*(3):328–332.

Bloomfield, J., & Pegram, A. (2012). Improving nutrition and hydration in hospital: The nurse's responsibility. *Nursing Standard (through 2013), 26*(34), 52-6; quiz 58. http://ezaccess.libraries.psu.edu/login?url=https://search-proquest-com.ezaccess.libraries.psu.edu/docview/1011173022?accountid=1315

Boaz, M., Rychani, L., Barami, K., Houri, Z., Yosef, R., Siag, A., . . .Leibovitz, E. (2013). Nurses and nutrition: A survey of knowledge and attitudes regarding nutrition assessment and care of hospitalized elderly patients. *The Journal of Continuing Education in Nursing, 44*(8), 357-64. http://dx.doi.org.ezaccess.libraries.psu.edu/10.3928/00220124-20130603-89

Centers for Disease Control (CDC). (2018). *Health and Economic Cost of Chronic Diseases.* https://www.cdc.gov/chronicdisease/about/costs/index.htm

DiMaria-Ghalili, R. A., Gilbert, K., Lord, L., Neal, T., Richardson, D., Tyler, R., ... & American Society for Parenteral and Enteral Nutrition. (2016). Standards of nutrition care practice and professional performance for nutrition support and generalist nurses. *Nutrition in Clinical Practice, 31*,527-547. doi:10.1177/0884533616653835

Englert D. M., Crocker, K. S., & Stotts, N. A. (1986). Nutrition in schools of nursing in the United States: Part 1, The evolution of nutrition education in schools of nursing. *Journal of Parenteral and Enteral Nutrition, 10*(5), 522-527.

Evans, J., Magee, A., Dickman, K., Sutter, R., & Sutter, C. (2017). A plant-based nutrition program. *AJN American Journal of Nursing, 117*(3), 56–61.

Healthier Hospitals Initiative, 2012. *Healthier Foods Challenge: How to Guide.* http://healthierhospitals.org/sites/default/files/IMCE/public_files/hhi-howto-foods-final.pdf

Jefferies, D., Johnson, M., & Langdon, R. (2015). Nutritional care programme. *International Journal of Nursing Practice, 21*, 286-296. doi:10.1111/ijn.12269

Mariner, W. K., & Annas, G. J. (2013) Limiting "sugary drinks" to reduce obesity—who decides? *New England Journal of Medicine, 368*(19),1763–1765.

Reed, D. (2014). Healthy eating for healthy nurses: Nutrition basics to promote health for nurses and patients. *Online Journal of Issues in Nursing, 19*(3), 62-70. http://ezaccess.libraries.psu.edu/login?url=https://search-proquest-com.ezaccess.libraries.psu.edu/docview/1710043962?accountid=13158

Sabaté, J., Harwatt, H., & Soret, S. (2016). Environmental Nutrition: A New Frontier for Public Health. *American Journal of Public Health, 106*(5), 815–821. https://ezproxy.chatham.edu:4393/10.2105/AJPH.2016.303046

Stoll-Kleemann, S., & Schmidt, U. (2017). Reducing meat consumption in developed and transition countries to counter climate change and biodiversity loss: a review of influence factors. *Regional Environmental Change, 17*(5), 1261–1277.

Tappenden, K. A., Quatrara, B., Parkhurst, M. L., Malone, A. M., Fanjiang, G., & Ziegler, T. R. (2013). Critical Role of Nutrition in Improving Quality of Care: An Interdisciplinary Call to Action to Address Adult Hospital Malnutrition. *MEDSURG Nursing, 22*(3), 147–165. http://ezaccess.libraries.psu.edu/login?url=http://search.ebscohost.com/login.aspx?direct=true&db=a9h&AN=88291445&site=ehost-live&scope=site

United States Department of Agriculture (USDA). (2012). *Census of agriculture. United States. 2014.* http://www.agcensus.usda.gov/Publications/2012

World Health Organization, 2018. *The global burden of chronic diseases.* http://www.who.int/nutrition/topics/2_background/en/

Xuereb, M. (2006). Home-grown hurrah. *Alternatives Journal (AJ) - Canada's Environmental Voice, 32*(3), 18–20.

CONCERNS OF CLEANING PRODUCTS ON OUR HEALTH AND SAFER STRATEGIES

Kathryn P. Jackman-Murphy Ed.D, MSN, RN, CHSE
Director, RN/BSN Program
Charter Oak State College

From the very beginning of our journey to become a nurse, the importance of cleanliness in the prevention of the transmission of diseases began with handwashing and keeping our patient's care area clean. In this effort to protect our families and patients from illness by cleaning our homes and workplace, we also may be exposed to potentially toxic substances. Cleaning products, including those we use to disinfect our hands, have been associated with a variety of health effects, including headache, irritation of the airway (mouth, nose, throat), skin and eye irritation, and even death related to accidental ingestion.

HOW TO CHOOSE PRODUCTS FOR CLEANING OUR HOMES

It is critically important that cleaning products remain in their original packaging with the original label, including warning symbols, and are properly stored and sealed appropriately. If a product is transferred to another container, it should be labeled with the ingredients and the dilution/concentration, if appropriate. This will help users know the chemicals inside, as well as the hazards associated with using the product. Another important consideration is the prevalence of concentrated products which should be only diluted according to the manufacturer's instructions. At times, products may be used at a stronger concentration with the thought "less is more" or "the stronger the better" and expose the user to a higher exposure to chemicals. The Environmental Protection Agency (EPA) recommends using a hazardous materials identification system which uses pictograms, hazard statements, and signal words to communicate hazard information (EPA.gov (a), nd).

At the very least, product labels that use the words "Caution", "Warning", "Danger" or "Poison" should be avoided at all cost. The Ecology Center (EC) goes a step further by recommending purchasing products that require no warning signal words (Ecology Center, 2019). The word "Danger" on a label, signifies a highly toxic product, where just a few drops may be lethal. "Warning" on a label denotes a moderately toxic product, from which a lethal dose can be the result of a teaspoon to a tablespoon. Labels with the word "Caution" have a lower toxicity, with lethal dose coming from an ounce to a pint and have a varying degree of safety. The EC also recommends avoiding products labeled as flammable, which likely contain volatile organic compounds (VOCs), many of which are linked to health effects such as cancer. Products that contain the word "corrosive" should be avoided as they may cause permanent damage to eyes and skin with exposure (Ecology Center, 2019).

The Environmental Working Group (EWG) suggests avoiding antibacterial cleaners, air fresheners, and drain cleaners (EWG (a), 2019). Per the EWG, antibacterial cleaners contain pesticides and do not provide added protection against illness. Air fresheners contain undisclosed and often untested chemicals such as fragrances. Drain cleaners often contain harmful chemicals which can be hazardous if misused, or poisoning due to swallowing, inhaling, or touching the chemicals. Children are more at risk to the effects of even small amounts of certain drugs and chemicals (Mayo Clinic, 2019). It is suggested to look for a safer product, especially if the label for the product you are considering requires multiple pieces of personal protective equipment (EPA (a), nd).

EWG's Guide to Healthy Cleaning (EWG(a), 2019) is an excellent resource to review cleaning products for environmental and health concerns. EWG rates each product with a score from A (few or no known suspected hazards to health or the environment with good ingredient disclosure) to F (potentially significant hazards to health or the environment or poor ingredient disclosure). Consumers can review the list of ingredients, label information, warnings and directions, as well as information for health concerns including asthma and respiratory, skin allergies and irritation, developmental and reproductive toxicity, cancer, and environmental concerns for each of over 2,500 products.

For example, some hand soap/sanitizer may include triclosan which is linked to endocrine disruption, allergies and immunotoxicity, skin, eye, or lung irritation, organ system toxicity and suspected to be an environmental toxin (EWG (a), 2019). A simple safer strategy would be to avoid products with triclosan. The EWG site enables the savvy consumer to be able to review a product, compare information with other products and find safer alternatives all while in the product aisle. For example, the EWG suggests avoiding products that contain ammonia, 2-butoxyelthanol, chlorine bleach, ethanolamines, "active ingredients" such as ADBAC, benzalkonium chloride, and ingredients with names including "monium chloride" or triclosan. EWG provides a wallet-friendly resource that can be taken shopping as you evaluate available products for cleaning: https://static.ewg.org/ewg-tip-sheets/EWG-Cleaners-WalletGuide.pdf. Another resource for the comparison of cleaning products, the ingredients and effects, and a safer alternative. is Clean Water Action's (2019) Green Cleaning Guide; This resource can be found at https://www.cleanwateraction.org/features/green-cleaning-guide.

There are many safer, less hazardous cleaning product lines available such as Seventh Generation and Mrs. Meyers, but these may also be costly and out of reach for some households.

The EWG and Clean Water Actions websites offer recipes for safer home-made cleaning products using a few simple inexpensive ingredients, such as vinegar, castile soap, baking soda, hydrogen peroxide, lemon juice, and washing soda. For example, white vinegar can be used as a deodorizer and fabric softener, as well as used to clean windows, microwaves, and toilets, cut grease and make chrome shine—all for a few pennies! A soft scrub for bathroom surfaces can be made from making a paste from baking soda and a bit of liquid soap. Utilizing green cleaning practices can improve indoor air quality, reduce health risks associated with exposure for ourselves, our families and animals. Creating your own cleaning supplies and reusing dispensing containers such as spray bottles will also help minimize plastic waste entering the waste stream. Women's Voices for the Earth (2019) is another resource for cleaning recipes. Link to the resource: https://www.womensvoices.org/take-action-with-womens-voices/green-cleaning-parties/green-cleaning-recipes/.

HAND SOAP

As nurses we promote hand washing to prevent the transmission of diseases. It is very possible that there are toxic chemicals in the very products we are using to protect our health.

For example, hand soap may contain chemicals linked to irritation, cancer, endocrine disruption, organ system toxicity, and neurotoxicity. Reading the list of ingredients on product labels will help identify the safety of a product. In the healthcare environment, it is vitally important that nurses have a seat at the table on committees that evaluate products prior to purchasing to help identify safer products for use not only by patients, but the community and members of the healthcare team.

LAUNDRY PRODUCTS

We protect our families from everyday dirt and grime by keeping everything in our homes clean, including our clothing. It seems impossible that something we use every day to help protect our families, maybe harmful to them and/or the environment. For example, manufacturers of laundry detergents may use phosphates to prevent dirt from resettling on fabrics and as a water softener. As the

waste water enters streams and rivers, these phosphates feed algae, causing an "algae bloom," an overgrowth of algae which chokes out other plants and marine life (EPA, 2019). Reading labels for the phosphate content is a start in choosing a safer laundry detergent.

Laundry pods are one of the newest laundry products on the market. Many are colorful with attractive designs. Laundry pods have been linked to over 56,000 calls to poison control centers due to exposure or ingestion by children and adults with dementia (Consumer Reports, 2019). It is anticipated that incidences of unintentional child poisoning may increase with the current trend of concentrated products, attractive packaging, and convenient forms such as laundry pods (Schwebel, Evans, Hoeffler, Marlenga, Nguyen, Jovanov, Meltzer, & Sheares, 2017). There are safer alternatives for laundry, including homemade liquid and powder laundry detergents utilizing a few simple ingredients such as borax or washing soda: https://thefrugalgirls.com/2010/08/homemade-liquid-laundry-detergent.html.

Drying clothes outside on a clothesline or drying rack has many benefits including no need for dryer sheets (think of the fragrances!), less wear and tear to clothing from the dryer tumble, conserving energy and resources, and having that "clean, outdoor fresh" smell. Another benefit to drying clothes outside is that sunlight can help bleach and disinfect clothing.

A clothes dryer is recognized as the second highest user of electricity in a household behind a central air conditioner or heat pump (Oasis Energy, 2017) and utilizes approximately six percent of an average home's energy use (National Park Service, 2018). It is estimated that a small load of laundry costs $0.36 to dry (The Simple Dollar, 2019), which can add to a significant amount of money over a year and multiple loads of laundry—let alone the cost and maintenance of a dryer. An Energy Use Calculator can be helpful in assessing the energy usage of household appliances and calculate the cost of usage of each appliance. One energy calculator is available at: https://oasisenergy.com/appliance-electricity-usage. According to the EPA, if all clothes washers and dryers in the U.S. were Energy Star certified, more than 19 billion pounds of carbon pollution would be prevented and more than $4 billion would be saved in energy costs (EPA (b), nd.).

FRAGRANCES

Clean homes should have no odor. Marketing and advertising has convinced us that a clean home smells like "Mountain Air" or a "Spring Meadow." As discussed earlier in this text, the word "fragrance" often is a combination of many ingredients, but are not listed specifically on the label making it difficult for the consumer to choose products. According to the Environmental Working Group's Campaign for Safe Cosmetics (2019), fragrances are linked to health problems such as cancer, reproductive and developmental toxicity, allergies and sensitivities. A safer solution would be to read labels and avoid a product that gives no information other than the word "fragrance."

Essential oils, such as camphor, peppermint, wintergreen, and lavender may be used with caution to add a natural scent, but may not be the safest solution. Essential oils are unregulated and it is difficult to know the specific ingredients of each product. Essential oils should be stored away from children due to the concern of skin irritation, absorption through the skin or ingestion, allergic reactions, and poisoning (Poison Control, 2019). For example, the Poison Control organization cites a case of a 22-month old who was admitted with a seizure and respiratory depression which was linked with an ingestion of camphor which had been placed in the home for roach control. Camphor may also be used as a moth repellent and found in some skin preparations used to relieve pain, irritation, and itching. It is recommended to contact Poison Control immediately for an ingestion of an essential oil or a product containing an essential oil.

As nurses keep our homes and places of work clean to maintain the health and safety of our patients, our communities, and our families. We can build on this effort by evaluating each product we use not only for appropriateness for the task at hand, but also for safety. As well, we need to be part of the decision in the choices of the products utilized in our everyday life, at home, our community and our place of work.

REFERENCES

Campaign for Safe Cosmetics. (2019). *Fragrance.* http://www.safecosmetics.org/get-the-facts/chemicals-of-concern/fragrance/

Clean Water Action. (2019). *Green Cleaning Guide.* https://www.cleanwateraction.org/features/green-cleaning-guide

Consumer Reports (2019). *Tide beats Persil in Consumer Reports' laundry detergent tests.* https://www.consumerreports.org/laundry-detergents/tide-beats-persil-best-laundry-detergents-in-consumer-reports-tests/

The Ecology Center (2019). *Cleaning label signal words.* https://www.ecocenter.org/cleaning-label-signal-words

Environmental Working Group. (2019a). *EWG's guide to healthy cleaning.* https://www.ewg.org/guides/cleaners

Environmental Working Group. (2019b). *EWG's Skin Deep cosmetics database: Triclosan.* https://www.ewg.org/skindeep/ingredient/706623/TRICLOSAN/

Mayo Clinic (2019). *Poisoning: First aid.* https://www.mayoclinic.org/first-aid/first-aid-poisoning/basics/art-20056657

National Park Service. (2018). *Laundry practices and water conservation.* https://www.nps.gov/articles/laundry.htm

Oasis Energy. (2017). *Appliance electricity usage.* https://oasisenergy.com/appliance-electricity-usage/

Poison Control. (2019). *Essential oils: Poisonous when misused.* https://www.poison.org/articles/2014-jun/essential-oils

Schwebel, D. C., Evans, W. D., Hoeffler, S. E., Marlenga, B. L., Nguyen, S. P., Jovanov, E., Meltzer, D.O., & Sheares, B. J. (2017). Unintentional child poisoning risk: A review of causal factors and prevention studies. *Children's Health Care, 46*(2), 109–130. https://doi.org/10.1080/02739615.2015.1124775

Sheares, B. J. (2017). Unintentional child poisoning risk: A review of causal factors and prevention studies. *Children's Health Care, 46*(2), 109–130. https://doi.org/10.1080/02739615.2015.1124775

The Simple Dollar. (2019). *How much do you really save by air-drying your clothes?* https://www.thesimpledollar.com/how-much-do-you-really-save-by-air-drying-your-clothes

US Environmental Protection Agency (EPA). (2019). *Nutrient pollution: Sources and solutions.* https://www.epa.gov/nutrientpollution/sources-and-solutions

US Environmental Protection Agency (EPA)(n.d.a). *How to properly label a cleaning product container.* https://www.epa.gov/sites/production/files/2013-08/documents/fact_sheet_how_to_properly_label_a_cleaning_product_container1.pdf

US Environmental Protection Agency (EPA) (n.d.b). *Energy Star: Certified products: Clothes washers.* https://www.energystar.gov/products/appliances/clothes_washers

Women's Voices for the Earth. (2019). *Green cleaning recipes.* https://www.womensvoices.org/take-action-with-womens-voices/green-cleaning-parties/green-cleaning-recipes/

ENVIRONMENTAL HEALTH LITERACY

Barbara J. Polivka, PhD, RN, FAAN
Associate Dean of Research
University of Kansas
School of Nursing

The goal of Environmental Health Literacy (EHL) is for individuals, families, and communities to understand and "act on health-related information about environmental hazards" (Hoover, 2019, pg. 5). To prevent illnesses and injuries from environmental exposures, it is important that the risks related to environmental factors are known and that individuals, families and communities are aware of approaches that can address, reduce, and eliminate these risks and the environmental exposures (Finn & O'Fallon, 2017). EHL draws from the disciplines of health communication, health literacy, risk communication, and participatory communication (Hoover, 2019). Health communication is focused on developing clear, understandable information so that individuals/families/ communities can make evidenced-based decisions about their health. Health literacy addresses the ability to understand basic health information. EHL extends the ideas of health communication and health literacy to include an understanding of the science related to environmental hazards and the importance of working collaboratively to address hazards. The purpose of risk communication is to provide individuals with "information they need to make informed, independent judgements about risks to health, safety, and the environment" (Morgan, Fischhoff, Bostrom & Atman, 2002). The information must be accurate, understandable, and from trustworthy sources. In risk communication, those creating communication initiatives must know the purpose of the communication, the knowledge level of the audience, and the social/cultural factors that may influence how the communication is interpreted. Participatory communication, on the other hand, involves multidirectional discussions with community members, stakeholders, scientists and others that is collaborative, culturally appropriate and goal oriented (Hoover, 2019). EHL combines these approaches to enable individuals, families, and communities to understand the health impacts of environmental hazards and identify actions steps to address those hazards.

ENVIRONMENTAL HEALTH LITERACY EXAMPLES

EHL has historical roots in natural and human-made disasters such as Hurricane Katrina, Love Canal, the Chernobyl and Fukushima nuclear accidents, and the Deepwater Horizon oil spill. News stories broadcast on television, radio, and via social media provided information about these environmental disasters and increased the public's knowledge and awareness of the risks of environmental hazards (Finn & O'Fallon 2017).

The critical need for safe drinking water has highlighted when lead was found to be present in the Flint, Michigan water supply. In 2014, the city of Flint stopped taking water from Lake Huron, and instead took water from the Flint River. The city failed to implement the appropriate required corrosion-control treatments required by the Environmental Protection Agency (EPA). These and other failures resulted in very high concentrations of lead in water of about one-quarter of the homes. Blood lead concentrations in children increased, especially in the communities where most residents live below the poverty-line (Bellinger, 2016; Butler, Schammeli, & Benson, 2016). Although mistrust of government officials and academics who did not respond to requests for information was high, many community residents continued to actively seek out information about lead levels and their water and the health impacts of these high lead levels until the problem was addressed (Carrera, Kye, Bailey, et al, 2019; McQuaid, 2016). The short video "Without these whistleblowers, we may never have known the full extent of the Flint Water Crises" highlights the persistent efforts of a Flint, Michigan mother and a scientist from Virginia Tech University to expose the high lead levels in the Flint water https://www.youtube.com/watch?v=loQo6PBmZi0.

Water quality is also an issue for American Indian/Alaskan Native communities. Members of the Apsáalooke (Crow Indian) tribe noticed that stomach and lung cancers were occurring at higher rates for tribal members living on or near the reservation than for those living further away. A working group, the Crow Environmental Health Steering Committee, was formed to address the problem. This committee included a county commissioner, a construction manager, and tribal members. Partnerships were formed with a local community college and a state university to test the well water. The committee began an educational campaign on how to decontaminate wells contaminated with bacteria. In addition, the committee determined that if children were better educated regarding environmental hazards, they could be agents of change. A hands-on educational program was developed for school-aged Apsáalooke children to increase their EHL regarding water quality and its health impacts. Children were involved in testing well-water and in reporting results back to their community (Simmonds, Margetts, & Rudd, 2019).

Youth were also involved in an EHL and leadership skills training in California. The focus of this effort was on exposure to endocrine disrupting chemicals in products used by Latina girls. The Health and Environmental Research in Make-up of Salinas Adolescents (HERMOSA) study included 15 youth who collected data from 100 adolescent Latinas that included interviews and urine samples. The 15 youth provided education to the community about endocrine disrupting chemicals in cosmetics and distributed low-chemical replacement products. Participants learned about the results of the study in a community forum, and additional information about endocrine disrupting chemicals was provided. Findings of the study were also presented in the media and social media. The 15 youth investigators indicated they learned a great deal about research and about chemicals they could be exposed to in their beauty products (Madrigal, Minkler, Parra, et al., 2016).

ENVIRONMENTAL HEALTH LITERACY AND NURSING'S ROLE

Brown, Clark, Zimmerman, Valenti, and Miller (2019) identified five stages of EHL awareness that are important for health professionals, including nurses.

- Level 1. Knowledge and understanding about the effects of environmental exposures on human health.

- Level 2. Communicating and providing information to patients about their environmental exposure risks and referring to experts when needed.

- Level 3. Communicating and engaging with community groups about environmental risks and collaboratively strategizing about how to address those risks.

- Level 4. Participating in professional organizations and advocating for environmental health issues. Serving on committees of professional organizations that are addressing environmental health issues or starting such a committee can help to increase nurses EHL as well as impact the policies of the professional organization.

- Level 5. Advocating for environmental health issues at work and/or with legislative or regulatory bodies. In healthcare institutions nurses can work to make the environment safer for patients and for workers. Nurses can inform policy makers about environmental hazards and become a member of an advisory or regulatory board to advocate for EHL.

There are many ways in which nurses can communicate environmental health information. For example, brochures and fact sheets can be prepared as can lectures. Studies concerning communication of environmental information have shown that: (1) those who were well-informed about the topic were more likely to accept the knowledge, (2) those participating in classroom-type lectures were more likely to retain the information than those given brochures, and (3) booklets tend to result in more knowledge retained than fact sheets (Lewis, Yost, etc. 2010). Digital communication strategies have shown potential in increasing EHL. Blogging, smartphone applications, and use of other social media platforms can impact environmental health awareness and knowledge. Smartphone notifications of poor air quality days are a common example of alerting residents to environmental exposures. Caution is needed to assure that the digital information provided is accurate, clear, timely, easily obtainable, interesting, visual, and interactive when possible (Kreps, Wrights, & Burke-Garcia, 2019).

CONCLUSION

Environmental health literacy combines the understanding of the link between environmental exposures and the health impacts of those exposures (Finn & O'Fallon, 2017). Nurses have a dual responsibility to learn about the potential and actual environmental exposures of their patients, co-workers, the community, and themselves. Becoming literate in environmental health is a responsibility of all nurses, as is providing effective communication about environmental risks to patients, families, and communities and working with these constituents to effectively address environmental hazards. Environmental health literacy, a growing discipline, combines strategies from health communication, health literacy, risk communication, and participatory communication to assure individuals, families, and communities understand the risks of environmental exposures and develop and implement effective strategies to eliminate environmental health risks.

REFERENCES

Bellinger, D. C. (2016). Lead contamination in Flint—an abject failure to protect public health. *New England Journal of Medicine, 374*(12), 1101-1103.

Brown, P., Clark, S., Zimmerman, E., Valenti, M., & Miller, M.D. (2019). Health professionals' environmental health literacy. In S. Finn & L. O'Fallon (Eds), *Environmental health literacy* (pp. 195-230). Springer.

Butler, L. J., Scammell, M. K., & Benson, E. B. (2016). The Flint, Michigan, water crisis: a case study in regulatory failure and environmental injustice. *Environmental Justice, 9*(4), 93-97.

Carrera, J. S., Key, K., Bailey, S., Hamm, J. A., Cuthbertson, C. A., Lewis, E. Y., ... & Robinson, D. E. (2019). Community science as a pathway for resilience in response to a public health crisis in Flint, Michigan. *Social Sciences, 8*(3), 94.

Finn, S., & O'Fallon, L. (2015). The emergence of environmental health literacy—from its roots to its future potential. *Environmental Health Perspectives, 125*(4), 495-501.

Hoover, A. G. (2019). Defining environmental health literacy. In S. Finn & L. O'Fallon (Eds), *Environmental health literacy* (pp. 3-18). Springer.

Kreps, G. L., Wright, K., & Burke-Garcia, A. (2019). The use of digital communication channels to enhance environmental health literacy. In S. Finn & L. O'Fallon (Eds), *Environmental health literacy* (pp. 265-283). Springer.

Madrigal, D. S., Minkler, M., Parra, K. L., Mundo, C., Gonzalez, J. E. C., Jimenez, R., ... & Harley, K. G. (2016). Improving Latino youths' environmental health literacy and leadership skills through participatory research on chemical exposures in cosmetics: The HERMOSA study. *International Quarterly of Community Health Education, 36*(4), 231-240.

McQuaid, J. (2016). *Without these whistleblowers, we may never have known the full extent of the Flint water crisis.* Smithsonian Magazine. https://www.Smithsonian.com

Morgan, M.G., Fischhoff, B., Bostrom, A. & Atman, C.J. (2002). *Risk Communication: A Mental Models Approach.* Cambridge University Press.

Simonds, V. W., Margetts, M., & Rudd, R. E. (2019). Expanding environmental health literacy—A focus on water quality and Tribal Lands. *Journal of Health Communication, 24*(3), 236-243.

ENVIRONMENTAL NURSING IN LATIN AMERICA

Doriam Camacho Rodriguez, DNS, MBA, RN
Dean, Faculty of Nursing
Cooperative University of Colombia campus Santa Marta

Translated by:
Adelita G. Cantu, PhD, RN
Associate Professor
University of Texas Health San Antonio
School of Nursing

Since the origins of care, health was directly related to the environment because man had to learn to protect himself from extreme changes in climate, to use plants to treat diseases, to make stone tools and later from other materials, to hunt and fish, and to use the byproducts of animals (1) in short, he learned to use the resources of nature for his survival; however, as a consequence of human actions, problems have been generated such as global warming, greenhouse effect, desertification, acid rain, depletion of natural resources, disappearance of species and the accumulation of toxic and radioactive waste in soil, water and air, generating environmental risk factors that affect the health of human beings (1).

An aggravating factor is that in the last 100 years the population of the earth has quadrupled to 7 billion people, of which most have been concentrated in urban areas, with the Latin American and Caribbean Region being the most urbanized in the world, with 77% of the population living in cities, a figure that is expected to reach 85% by 2030. Cities can offer better opportunities and working conditions, but generate unplanned and unchecked growth, road insecurity and the streets, housing deficit, aging, inefficient public services infrastructure, increasing inequalities in access to health goods and services (2), greater energy consumption and greater transport needs and therefore greater emission of gases into the atmosphere.

On the other hand, in America, there are diverse ecosystems and large reserves, which are vulnerable to deforestation, the conversion of natural habitat for agricultural or livestock use or urban expansion; the alteration of surface waters through the construction of dams, irrigation, and diversion of the current; as well as the loss of biodiversity that can result from overexploitation for fishing or the introduction of invasive species (2).

Latin America is one of the regions with the highest risk of diseases of environmental origin, considering the susceptibility related to social and environmental determinants. According to the World Health Organization in the Region (except Chile) per capita deaths attributable to the environment are related in their order to noncommunicable diseases, injuries and in a smaller proportion due to infections, parasites and neonatal and nutritional diseases (3). This region, like the rest of the world, has been subject to numerous extreme natural events and disasters, related to the effects of climate change, which aggravate the health situation of the most vulnerable populations.

WHAT CAN WE DO IN NURSING TO HELP MINIMIZE THIS PROBLEM?

Nursing professional practice involves the inclusion of ethics and environmental bioethics in the actions performed in each of the performance areas. Several authors in Latin America have made reference to the importance of resorting to the ethics of care, in such a way that resources are used in an organized manner, so that the environment can recover and continue to be self-sufficient. (4) Some of the reflections in relation to the subject are:

- Nursing, by adopting ecosystemic actions in its daily work, advocates for integral attention to the human being and, therefore, has the opportunity to put into practice environmental, ecological, physical, psychological, spiritual and social actions, creating thus possibilities of a complete and interactive attention (5).

- Quality of life and health are closely related to aspects of the ecosystem (6).

- The environmental issue should be part of the debates on education, because this debate favors the reflection of people about what is ecologically healthy, for which nursing should integrate environmental education into its work (7)

- Nursing should be strengthened as a discipline to respond to the needs of nursing research and care education, in line with the trends of globalization in the contemporary world, as well as the drastic impacts on human and environmental health (8).

- The nurse can be an environmental educator and act in this space, favoring reflection on the actions that affect the environment and the risk to the community (9).

- It is necessary to take up the legacy of Florence Nightingale as a way of valuing the environmental dimension as essential for the health assistance process, both in terms of promoting health and quality of life, and minimizing the environmental impact from the health work process. The ethical reflection and the educational approach are fundamental in this process. (10)

- Nursing commitment to globalization is and its impact on individual and collective health is to reflect on its effects on care, with the intention of contributing to health for all; analyzes the importance of recognizing plurality as a way of producing knowledge in nursing and health, as well as the necessary union between reason and emotion. Finally, Do Prado discusses the challenges of education for the construction of an ethical subject, capable of printing the transformations that nursing care requires and desires for Latin America. (11).

- The nursing professional is an important actor in the promotion of health, especially in the environmental health of children and for this it requires interventions aimed at promoting behaviors that favor the environment and that minimize the risk of exposure to environmental risk factors (12)

As was done by the International Council of Nurses (ICN) and the American Nurses Association, in Latin America, some of the associations or colleges of nursing professionals included in their codes of ethics the issue of environmental health, as follows:

- Argentina, Brazil, Uruguay and Paraguay: the Declaration of Ethical Principles, article 7 establishes that the nursing professional has the responsibility of maintaining the natural environment and protecting it from contamination, degradation, destruction and abandonment(13).

- Colombia: the Code of Ethics of Nursing, article 27 states that the nursing professional should refrain from promoting the use of products that he knows hurt human beings or the environment (14).

- Chile: The Code of Ethics of the Nurses' Association of Chile, in section 7.1, establishes that the nursing professional should be informed about the studies and action plans to detect the harmful consequences that the environment exerts on men, as well as the plans for the conservation of natural resources (15).

- Costa Rica: the Code of Ethics and Professional Ethics in its article 29 that the nursing professional must support the health authorities to detect the harmful effects of the environment on human health, as well as in the planning of activities that favor conservation and environmental sustainability and that therefore contribute to the improvement of the quality of health and, in Article 32, establishes that within its competences is education about healthy environments (16).

- Mexico: The Code of Conduct for Nursing, article: 28 establishes that the nurse has the social duty to seek a balance between human development and the conservation of natural resources and the environment, taking into account the rights of future generations (17).

- Peru: The Code of Ethics and Deontology, article 16, determines that the nursing professional must share the responsibility to maintain the natural environment and protect it against contamination, impoverishment, degradation and destruction (18).

It is important to identify that through the Nursing Codes, environmental care and the prevention of environmental risk factors are encouraged, since nursing professionals are in a unique position to interact with the community in the identification of members. potentially linked to environmental exposure (14). Nursing as a historical and ideologically based profession based on welfare principles, teaches a way to rethink the care culture (15). There is a direct connection between nursing actions and environmental health in health care agencies. However, in the daily practice of nursing the environmental impact of procedures such as the administration of a medication, the change of a bandage, or the initiation of an intravenous route are generally not considered; for example, the final destination of the wrappers that represent the by-products of their work is an almost subliminal activity in their professional role, since their approach as a nurse is more frequent in other priorities (16).

What have we researched in Latin America on Nursing and the environment?

In Latin America there are few publications made by nurses in relation to the topic of environmental health. When reviewing the literature, studies with a qualitative approach were found, mostly conducted in Brazil. See tables below for findings.

EDUCATION ABOUT HEALTH AND ENVIRONMENT

The training of nursing professionals aware of the importance of the environment has been established within the guidelines for accreditation of programs under the ARCUSUR model, that programs should guide content on Ecology and health (24).

Title	Objective	Materials & Methods	Results	Conclusions
Nursing and environmental health: possibilities for action to promote health (17)	Understand the meaning of the participation of the members of the Subcommittee of the Rio Salgado Basin Committee	Qualitative research involving 18 members of the Subcommittee of the River Salgado Basin Committee Salgado River Basin - Brazil	The categories were generated: the participation of social conscience, information, communication in the search for solutions that represent the community.	Nursing should include in its practice comprehensive strategies that contribute to improving the quality of life of human beings and the sustainability of natural and social biota
Environmental awareness in Nursing: the reconstruction of a better world with the contribution of students (18)	Identify how words and drawings issued by students in learning scenarios contribute to the formation of a strengthening of environmental awareness to the nursing profession.	Qualitative research, in which 41 graduate students in nursing from a Brazilian Institution of Higher Education participated. A semi-structured survey and the production of free drawings were used. Data analysis was carried out under the modality of thematic analysis	Three thematic units emerged: the humanization of theory and practice allows the formation of an environmental awareness; the experience-skill articulated with the pedagogical practices promote the sustainability of the environment; and socially apprehended and worked as a learning environment-environment of care strengthens nursing students.	A sustainable mentality and culture can be created in the students, in a formative environment that educates in values, so that they become social agents that promote the commitment of the conservation and protection of the planet.
Interface between health and the environment in health professional training	Know the conception of academics from the health area on the health and environment interface, and how it is expressed in their academic experience.	Qualitative, descriptive-exploratory study, carried out with 24 professors from the health area of a public University. The information was collected through a semi-structured interview and the data was analyzed through content analysis.	The categories that emerged were health, environment and poverty, vague notions about health and the environment.	91/5000 It is necessary to include the subject in the training of professionals in the area of health.
Perception of nursing teachers on environmental issues: subsidies for nursing training (19)	Know the perception of nursing teachers about current environmental problems in order to obtain subsidies for reflection on nursing professional training	Qualitative study in which 6 nurse teachers from a University of Brazil participated. A semi-structured survey was used to collect the information, which was closed by saturation of the sample. The data analysis was performed using the content analysis technique.	The categories of analysis that emerged were: the environment as a space of interaction and place for human existence, the current environmental problems: impacts on human life, and environmental responsibility: intertwining between the individual and professional spheres.	In the perception fostered by the teaching nurses there is appropriation of extended and systemic discourses.

The environmental problem in view of community health workers (20)	Know what community health agents think about the problematic environment.	Qualitative study, in which 13 community health agents participated through a semi-structured survey. The data was analyzed through content analysis	Four categories were created: Conception of the environment: convergence between the natural and social environment; The environmental problem: between the impact and the need for education; Environmental responsibility: commitment to health promotion and Training: the need to overcome gaps.	There is a need to address environmental education to strengthen the competencies of community health agents in terms of health promotion, in order to help individuals and the community to deal with socio-environmental situations and to work on the prevention of diseases through exposure to environmental problems.
Mitigate consequences of global warming and greenhouse effect: reflections for health training (21)	Reflect on community knowledge regarding the measures adopted by the effects of global warming, by assuming the role of social responsibility as a health training institution.	Ethnographic qualitative study. The key informants were 20 families, which corresponded to the 20 most vulnerable neighborhoods in the city of Valledupar - Colombia. The "snowball" sampling technique was used. The information analysis was carried out through data triangulation and descriptive validity, and adopted intercultural health education as an epistemic stance.	Three categories were established in a pre-established way: knowledge that people have about climate change and warming, self-care adopted by families in situations of increased temperature and characteristics of collective work in the community.	There is ignorance and lack of commitment of people with the care of life and health of self and of the collective, for which it is the responsibility of the University to train nursing professionals highly sensitive to the effects of global warming and with critical capacity and social conscience to assume a competitive role
Health and environment (in) visibilities and (dis) continuity in nursing professional training (22)	Know the perception of teaching nurses about the relationship between health and the environment and how the subject is approached in nursing professional training.	Qualitative study with an exploratory descriptive approach, in which 17 nurse nurses from the Federal University of Rio Grande do Sul participated. The information was collected through a semi-structured interview and the data were analyzed through content analysis.	Two categories of analysis emerged: health and the environment interface: different areas, and thematic approaches in the professional training of nurses: contexts and challenges.	The participants realize that there is an intrinsic relationship between health and the environment, which is polarized, on the one hand, in a perception that it is linked to a cause and, on the other hand, in the complex perspective of ethics collective
Relationship between attitudes and environmental behaviors in Nursing	Identify the relationship between attitudes and behaviors environmental studies in Nursing students of a	Descriptive study of a cross section in which 190 Nursing students participated. Attitudes and environmental behaviors and their	100% of the attitudes and 46.7% of the behaviors were rated as adequate and a relationship was found between environmental attitudes and age ($\rho = 0.021$), as well as	Although most students have positive environmental attitudes, these are not always reflected in their behavior, making it necessary to improve the training of

students (23)	colombian university	relationship with sociodemographic variables. The statistical correlation was analyzed using the correlation coefficient of Spearman	between environmental behavior and age ($\rho = 0.001$) and, environmental behaviors sex ($\rho = 0.012$).	professionals to promote the reduction of morbidity and mortality from diseases caused as a result of modifiable environmental factors

ENFERMERÍA AMBIENTAL EN AMÉRICA LATINA
Doriam Camacho Rodriguez, DNS, MBA, RN
Dean, Faculty of Nursing
Cooperative University of Colombia campus Santa Marta

Desde los orígenes del cuidado, éste estuvo directamente relacionado con el medio ambiente porque el hombre tuvo que aprender a protegerse de los cambios extremos del clima, a utilizar las plantas para tratar las enfermedades, a elaborar herramientas de piedra y posteriormente de otros materiales, a cazar y pescar, y a utilizar los subproductos de los animales (1) en fin, aprendió a utilizar los recursos de la naturaleza para su supervivencia; no obstante, como consecuencia de las acciones humanas, se han generado problemáticas como calentamiento global, efecto invernadero, desertificación, lluvias ácidas, agotamiento de recursos naturales, desaparición de especies y la acumulación de residuos tóxicos y radioactivos en los suelos, agua y aire, generando factores de riesgo ambientales que afectan la salud de los seres humanos (2).

Un factor agravante es que en los últimos 100 años la población de la tierra se ha cuadruplicado a 7 billones de personas, de las cuales la mayoría se han concentrado en zonas urbanas, siendo la Región de América Latina y el Caribe la más urbanizada del mundo, con el 77% de la población viviendo en las ciudades, una cifra que se espera que alcance el 85% en 2030. Las ciudades pueden ofrecer mejores oportunidades y condiciones de trabajo, pero generan crecimiento no planificado y sin control, inseguridad vial y en las calles, déficit de vivienda, envejecimiento, infraestructura de servicios públicos ineficiente, el aumento de las desigualdades en el acceso a bienes y servicios de salud (3), mayor consumo de energía y mayores necesidades de transporte y por ende mayor emisión de gases a la atmósfera.

Por otra parte, en América, existen diversos ecosistemas y grandes reservas, las cuales son vulnerables debido a la deforestación, la conversión del hábitat natural para uso agrícola o ganadero o la expansión urbana; la alteración de las aguas superficiales a través de la construcción de presas, el riego, y la desviación de la corriente; así como la pérdida de la biodiversidad que se puede producir por la sobreexplotación para pesca o la introducción de especies invasoras (3).

Latinoamérica es una de las regiones con mayor riesgo de enfermedades de origen ambiental, considerando la susceptibilidad relacionada con los determinantes sociales y ambientales. Según la Organización mundial de la salud en la Región (excepto Chile) las muertes per cápita

atribuibles al medio ambiente están relacionadas en su orden con enfermedades no transmisibles, por heridas y en menor proporción por infecciones, parásitos y enfermedades neonatales y nutricionales(4). Esta región, al igual que el resto del mundo, ha sido objeto de numerosos eventos naturales extremos y desastres, relacionados con los efectos del cambio climático, los cuales agravan la situación de salud de las poblaciones más vulnerables.

¿QUÉ PODEMOS HACER EN DESDE ENFERMERÍA PARA CONTRIBUIR A MINIMIZAR ESTA PROBLEMÁTICA?

El ejercicio profesional de Enfermería implica la inclusión de la ética y la bioética ambiental en las acciones que realiza en cada una de las áreas de desempeño. Son varios los autores que en Latinoamérica han hecho relación a la importancia de recurrir a la ética del cuidado, de tal forma que se utilicen los recursos de forma organizada, para que el medio ambiente pueda recuperarse y continúe siendo autosuficiente. (5) Algunas de las reflexiones en relación al tema son:

- La enfermería, al adoptar acciones ecosistémicas en su quehacer cotidiano, aboga por la atención integral al ser humano y, por lo tanto, tiene la oportunidad de poner en práctica acciones de naturaleza ambiental, ecológica, física, psicológica, espiritual y social, creando así posibilidades de una atención completa e interactiva (6).

- La calidad de vida y la salud tienen una relación estrecha con los aspectos del ecosistema (7).

- La cuestión ambiental debe formar parte de los debates sobre la educación, porque este debate favorece la reflexión de las personas sobre lo que es ecológicamente sano, por lo cual enfermería debe integrar en su quehacer la educación ambiental (8)

- Enfermería debe fortalecerse como disciplina para responder a las necesidades de educación investigación y cuidado en Enfermería, acorde con las tendencias de la globalización en el mundo contemporáneo, así como los drásticos impactos en la salud humana y ambiental (9).

- El enfermero puede ser un educador ambiental y actuar es este espacio, favoreciendo la reflexión sobre las acciones que afectan al medio ambiente y el riesgo para la comunidad (10).

- Es necesario retomar el legado de Florence Nightingale como forma de valorizar la dimensión ambiental como indispensable para el proceso de asistencia a la salud, tanto en lo que se refiere a la promoción de la salud y de la calidad de vida, como la minimización del impacto ambiental proveniente del proceso de trabajo de la salud. La reflexión ética y el abordaje educativo son fundamentales en ese proceso. (11)

- El compromiso de Enfermería frente a la globalización es y su impacto sobre la salud individual y colectiva es reflexionar acerca de sus efectos en el cuidado, con la intención de contribuir en la salud para todos; analiza la importancia de reconocer la pluralidad como camino de producción del conocimiento en Enfermería y salud, así como la necesaria unión entre razón y emoción. Finalmente, discute los desafíos de la educación para la construcción de un sujeto ético, capaz de imprimir las transformaciones que el cuidado de enfermería requiere y desea para América Latina (12).

- El profesional de Enfermería es un actor importante en la promoción de la salud, sobre todo en la salud ambiental infantil y para ello requiere realizar intervenciones dirigidas a promover comportamientos que favorezcan el medio ambiente y que minimicen el riesgo de exposición a factores de riesgo ambiental.

Tal y como lo hicieron el Consejo internacional de enfermeras (CIE) y la Asociación Americana de Enfermeras, en Latinoamérica, algunas de las asociaciones o colegios de profesionales de Enfermería incluyeron en sus códigos de ética el tema de salud ambiental, así:

Argentina, Brasil, Uruguay y Paraguay: la Declaración de Principios Éticos, artículo 7 establece que el profesional de Enfermería tiene la responsabilidad de mantener el medio ambiente natural y protegerlo de la contaminación, la degradación, destrucción y abandono(13).

Colombia: el Código deontológico de Enfermería, artículo 27 señala que el profesional de Enfermería se debe abstener de promover la utilización de productos que sepa que hacen daño a los seres humanos o al medio ambiente (14).

Chile: el Código de ética Colegio de Enfermeras de Chile, en el numeral 7.1 establece que el profesional de enfermería debe informarse acerca de los estudios y planes de acción conducentes a detectar las consecuencias nocivas que el medio ambiente ejerce sobre el hombre, así como los planes de conservación de los recursos naturales (15).

Costa Rica: el Código de ética y moral profesional en su artículo 29 que el profesional de enfermería debe apoyar a las autoridades sanitarias a detectar los efectos nocivos del medio ambiente sobre la salud humana, así como en la planificación de actividades que favorezcan la conservación y sostenibilidad del ambiente y que por ende contribuyan al mejoramiento de la calidad de la salud y, en el artículo 32, establece que dentro de sus competencias está la educación sobre ambientes saludables (16).

México: el Código de conducta para la enfermería, artículo: 28 establece que la Enfermera tiene el deber social de buscar un equilibrio entre el desarrollo humano y la conservación de los recursos naturales y el medio ambiente, teniendo en cuenta los derechos de las generaciones futuras (17).

Perú: el Código de ética y deontología, artículo 16 determina que el profesional de Enfermería debe compartir la responsabilidad de mantener el medioambiente natural y protegerlo contra la contaminación, el empobrecimiento, la degradación y la destrucción (18).

Es importante identificar que a través de los Códigos de Enfermería se fomenta el cuidado del medio ambiente y la prevención de los factores de riesgo ambiental, ya que los profesionales de Enfermería están en una posición única para interactuar con la comunidad en la identificación de los miembros potencialmente vinculados a exposición ambiental (14). Enfermería como profesión histórica e ideológicamente fundamentado en los principios de bienestar, enseña una manera de replantear la cultura de cuidado (15). Hay una conexión directa entre las acciones de enfermería y la salud del medio ambiente en las agencias de cuidado de la salud. Sin embargo, en la práctica diaria de enfermería generalmente no se considera el impacto ambiental de procedimientos como la administración de un medicamento, el cambio de un vendaje, o iniciar una vía intravenosa; por ejemplo, el destino final de los envoltorios que representan los subproductos de su trabajo es una actividad casi subliminal en su rol profesional, ya que su enfoque como enfermera es más frecuente en otras prioridades (16).

¿QUÉ HEMOS INVESTIGADO EN LATINOAMÉRICA SOBRE ENFERMERÍA Y MEDIO AMBIENTE?

En Latinoamérica son escasas las publicaciones realizadas por enfermeras en relación al tema de salud ambiental. Al revisar la literatura se encontraron estudios con enfoque cualitativo, en su mayoría realizados en Brasil:

Título	Objetivo	Materiales y métodos	Resultados	Conclusiones
Enfermería y salud ambiental: posibilidades de actuación para la promoción de la salud (17)	Comprender el significado de la participación de los miembros de la Subcomisión del Comité de Cuenca de Río Salgado	Investigación cualitativa en la que participaron 18 miembros de la Subcomisión del Comité de Cuenca de Río Salgado Cuenca del Río Salgado – Brasil	Se generaron las categorías: la participación de la conciencia social, información, comunicación en la búsqueda de soluciones que representan a la comunidad.	Enfermería debe incluir en su práctica estrategias integrales que contribuyan a mejorar la calidad de vida de los seres humanos y la sostenibilidad de la biota natural y social
Sensibilización ambiental en Enfermería: la reconstrucción de un mundo mejor con la contribución de los estudiantes(18)	Identificar cómo las palabras y dibujos emitidos por los estudiantes en escenarios de aprendizaje contribuyen a la formación de un fortalecimiento de la conciencia ambiental a la profesión de enfermería.	Investigación de tipo cualitativo, en el que participaron 41 estudiantes de posgrado en enfermería de una Institución Brasileña de Educación Superior. Se utilizó una encuesta semi-estructurada y la elaboración de dibujos libres. Se realizó análisis de datos bajo la modalidad de análisis temático	Surgieron tres unidades temáticas: la humanización de la teoría y la práctica permite formar una conciencia ambiental; la experiencia-habilidad articuladas con las prácticas pedagógicas promueven la sostenibilidad del medio ambiente; y lo social aprehendido y trabajado como escenario de aprendizaje-ambiente de cuidado fortalece a los estudiantes de enfermería.	Se puede crear una mentalidad y cultura sostenible en los estudiantes, en un entorno formativo que eduque en valores, para que ellos se conviertan en agentes sociales que promuevan el compromiso de la conservación y protección del planeta.
Interfaz entre salud y medio ambiente en la formación profesional en salud	Conocer la concepción de académicos del área de la salud sobre la interfaz salud y medio ambiente, y cómo se expresa en su vivencia académica.	Estudio cualitativo, descriptivo-exploratorio, realizado con 24 profesores del área de la salud de una Universidad pública. La información se recolectó por medio de una entrevista semi-estructurada y los datos se analizaron por medio de análisis de contenido.	Las categorías que emergieron fueron salud, medio ambiente y pobreza, nociones vagas sobre salud y medio ambiente.	Es necesario incluir la temática en la formación de los profesionales del área de la salud.
Percepción de los docentes de enfermería sobre la problemática ambiental: subsidios para la formación en Enfermería(19)	Conocer la percepción de los docentes de enfermería sobre los problemas ambientales actuales con el fin de obtener subsidios para la reflexión sobre la formación profesional en enfermería	Estudio cualitativo en el que participaron 6 Enfermeros docentes de una Universidad de Brasil. Se utilizó una encuesta semi-estructurada para la recolección de la información, la cual se cerró por saturación de la muestra. El análisis de datos se realizó mediante la técnica de análisis de contenido.	Las categorías de análisis que surgieron fueron: el medioambiente como espacio de interacción y lugar para la existencia humana, los actuales problemas ambientales: impactos sobre la vida humana, y la responsabilidad ambiental: entrelazamiento entre las esferas individuales y profesionales.	En la percepción fomentada por los Enfermeros docentes existe apropiación de discursos ampliados y sistémicos.
El problema ambiental a la vista de los agentes de salud comunitaria (20)	con el objetivo de conocer lo que los agentes de salud comunitaria piensan del entorno problemático.	Estudio cualitativo, en el cual participaron 13 agentes de salud comunitaria a través de una encuesta semi-estructurada. Los datos se analizaron a través de análisis de contenido	Se crearon 4 categorías: Concepción del ambiente: convergencia entre el medio natural y el social; El problema ambiental: entre el impacto y la necesidad de educación; Responsabilidad medioambiental: compromiso con la promoción de la salud y Formación: la necesidad de superar brechas.	Existe la necesidad de abordar la educación ambiental para fortalecer las competencias de los agentes comunitarios de salud en cuanto a promoción de la salud, para poder ayudar a los individuos y a la comunidad a enfrentar las situaciones socio-ambientales y a trabajar en la prevención de enfermedades por exposición a los problemas ambientales.

Mitigar consecuencias del calentamiento global y efecto invernadero: reflexiones para la formación en salud (21)	Reflexionar sobre el conocimiento comunitario frente a las medidas que adoptan los efectos del calentamiento global, al asumir el rol de la responsabilidad social como institución formadora de salud.	Estudio cualitativo etnográfico. Los informantes clave fueron 20 familias, las cuales correspondían a los 20 barrios más vulnerables de la ciudad de Valledupar - Colombia. Se utilizó la técnica de muestreo "bola de nieve". El análisis de la información se realizó mediante triangulación de datos y validez descriptiva, y adoptaron la educación sanitaria intercultural como postura epistémica.	Se constituyeron de forma pre-establecida tres categorías: conocimiento que tienen las personas sobre el cambio climático y el calentamiento, autocuidado que adoptan las familias en situaciones de aumento de la temperatura y características de trabajo colectivo en la comunidad.	Existe desconocimiento y falta de compromiso de las personas con el cuidado de la vida y la salud de sí mismo y del colectivo, por lo cual es responsabilidad de la Universidad formar profesionales de enfermería altamente sensibles a los efectos del calentamiento global y con capacidad crítica y conciencia social para asumir un rol competitivo
Salud y ambiente (in) visibilidades y (des) continuidad en la formación profesional en enfermería (22)	Conocer la percepción de enfermeros docentes sobre la relación salud y ambiente y como se da el abordaje del tema en la formación profesional en enfermería.	Estudio cualitativo con enfoque descriptivo exploratorio, en el que participaron 17 enfermeros docentes de cursos de Enfermería de la Universidad Federal de Río Grande do Sul. La información fue recolectada mediante una entrevista semi-estructurada y los datos fueron analizados mediante análisis de contenido.	Surgieron dos categorías de análisis: la salud y la interfaz medio ambiente: áreas distintas, y enfoques temáticos en la formación profesional de las enfermeras: contextos y desafíos.	Los participantes se dan cuenta de que hay una relación intrínseca entre la salud y el medio ambiente, que se polariza, por un lado, en una percepción de que está vinculado a una causa y, por otra parte, en la perspectiva compleja de la ética colectiva
Relación entre actitudes y comportamientos ambientales en Estudiantes de enfermería(23)	Identificar la relación entre actitudes y comportamientos ambientales en estudiantes de Enfermería de una universidad colombiana	Estudio descriptivo de corte transversal en el que participaron 190 estudiantes de Enfermería. Se analizaron las actitudes y comportamientos ambientales y su relación con las variables sociodemográficas. Se analizó la correlación estadística utilizando el coeficiente de correlación de Spearman. R	El 100% de las actitudes y el 46,7% de los comportamientos fueron calificados como adecuados y se encontró relación entre entre las actitudes ambientales y edad ($\rho = 0,021$), así como entre comportamientos ambientales y edad ($\rho = 0,001$) y, comportamientos ambientales sexo ($\rho = 0,012$).	Aunque la mayoría de estudiantes tiene actitudes ambientales positivas, éstas no siempre se ven reflejadas en su comportamiento, haciéndose necesario mejorar la formación de los profesionales para favorecer la disminución de la morbilidad y mortalidad por enfermedades causadas como consecuencia de factores ambientales modificables

REFERENCES/REFERENCIAS BIBLIOGRÁFICAS

1. Berdayes Martínez D et al. Bases conceptuales de Enfermería. Ciencias médicas, editor. La Habana; 2008. p. 194.

2. Pan American Health Organization; World Health Organization. Health in the Americas [Internet]. 2012 [cited 2015 Oct 8]. p. 229. Available from: http://www1.paho.org/saludenlasamericas/docs/hia-2012-summary-print.pdf

3. Pruss-Ustin, A. Wolf, J. Corvalán, C. Bos, R. Neira M. Preventing disease through healthy environments [Internet]. World Health Organization, editor. France; 2016. 10-92 p. Available from: http://apps.who.int/iris/bitstream/handle/10665/204585/9789241565196_eng.pdf?sequence=1

4. Freitas LV, Joventino ES, Ximenes LB, Vieira NFC, Moreira RVO. The ethics of nursing care for environmental crises. Online Brazilian J Nurs [Internet]. 2012 [cited 2016 Dec 4];11(3):893–906. Available from: http://www.gnresearch.org/doi/10.5935/1676-4285.20120060

5. Zamberlan C, Medeiros AC de, Dei Svaldi J, Siqueira HCH. Ambiente, saúde e enfermagem no contexto ecossistêmico. Rev Bras Enferm [Internet]. 2013 Aug

[cited 2016 May 10];66(4):603–6. Available from: http://www.scielo.br/scielo.php?script=sci_arttext&pid=S0034-71672013000400021&lng=pt&nrm=iso&tlng=pt

6. Zamberlan C, Calvetti A, Deisvaldi J, De Siqueira HCH. Calidad de vida, salud y enfermería en la perspectiva ecosistémica. Enfermería Glob [Internet]. 2010 [cited 2018 Dec 14];(20):0–0. Available from: http://scielo.isciii.es/scielo.php?script=sci_arttext&pid=S1695-61412010000300018

7. Eveline Pinheir Eveline Pinheiro Beser o Beserra, Maria Dalva Santos Alves MDSA, Patrícia Neyva da Costa Pinheir Patrícia Neyva da Costa Pinheiro NFCV. Educação ambiental e enfermagem: uma integração necessária Educação ambiental e enfermagem: uma integração necessária. Rev Bras Enferm, Brasília. 2010;63(5):848–52.

8. Silva AL da. Nursing in the era of globalisation: challenges for the 21st century. Rev Lat Am Enfermagem [Internet]. 2008 Aug [cited 2015 Aug 26];16(4):787–90. Available from: http://www.scielo.br/scielo.php?script=sci_arttext&pid=S0104-11692008000400021&lng=en&nrm=iso&tlng=es

9. Beserra EP, Alves MDS. Enfermagem e saúde ambiental na escola. Acta Paul Enferm [Internet]. 2012 [cited 2015 Oct 4];25(5):666–72. Available from: http://www.scielo.br/scielo.php?script=sci_arttext&pid=S0103-21002012000500004&lng=en&nrm=iso&tlng=pt

10. Camponogara S. Saúde e meio ambiente na contemporaneidade: o necessário resgate do legado de Florence Nightingale. Esc Anna Nery [Internet]. 2012 Mar [cited 2018 Dec 14];16(1):178–84. Available from: http://www.scielo.br/scielo.php?script=sci_arttext&pid=S1414-81452012000100024&lng=pt&tlng=pt

11. Do Prado M SRK. Salud y globalización: retos futuros para el cuidado de Enfermería. Investig y Educ en Enfermería [Internet]. 2004 [cited 2018 Dec 14];22(2):104–11. Available from: https://www.redalyc.org/articulo.oa?id=105216892014

12. Camacho-Rodríguez D, Evies-Ojeda A. Revisión sistemática de promoción de la salud ambiental infantil. Duazary [Internet]. 2018 Sep 2 [cited 2019 Mar 28];15(3):81–95. Available from: http://revistas.unimagdalena.edu.co/index.php/duazary/article/view/2500

13. Consejo Regional de Enfermería Mercosur. Declaración de Principios Éticos para la Enfermería del MERCOSUR. [Internet]. 2003 p. 5. Available from: http://test.e-legis-ar.msal.gov.ar/leisref/public/showAct.php?id=23255&word=#

14. Barnes G, Fisher B, Postma J, Harnish K, Butterfield P, Hill W. Incorporating environmental health into nursing practice: a case study on indoor air quality. Pediatr Nurs [Internet]. Jan [cited 2016 Mar 12];36(1):33–9, 52; quiz 40. Available from: http://www.ncbi.nlm.nih.gov/pubmed/20361443

15. Carbogim, F. Friedrich, D. Nepomuceno, C. Campos, B. Oliveira, A. Costa W. Enfermagem e Saúde ambiental: o portfólio como mediador na perspectiva histórico-cultural. Rev enferm UFPE line [Internet]. 2014;8(5):1400–4. Available from: http://www.revista.ufpe.br/revistaenfermagem/index.php/revista/article/viewFile/4524/pdf_5139

16. Shaner-McRae, H; McRae, G & Jass V. Environmentally Safe Health Care Agencies: Nursing's Responsibility, Nightingale's Legacy. OJIN Online J Issues Nurs [Internet]. 2007 [cited 2015 Nov 14];12(2). Available from: http://www.nursingworld.org/MainMenuCategories/ANAMarketplace/ANAPeriodicals/OJIN/TableofContents/Volume122007/No2May07/EnvironmentallySafeHealthCareAgencies.html#Shaner

17. Maria do Socor Maria do Socorro Vieira Lopes o Vieira Lopes, Lorena Barbosa Ximenes LBX. Enfermagem e saúde ambiental: Enfermagem e saúde ambiental: Enfermagem e saúde ambiental: possibilidades de atuação para a pr possibilidades de atuação para a promoção da saúde omoção da saúde. Rev Bras Enferm. 2011;64(1):72–7.

18. Silva CM dos SLMD da, Tanji S, Santos NMP, Viana L de O. Consciência ambiental na Enfermagem: Reconstruíndo um mundo melhor com a contribuição dos estudantes. Rev Enferm Ref [Internet]. [cited 2015 Aug 26];serIII(2):35–43. Available from: http://www.scielo.mec.pt/scielo.php?script=sci_arttext&pid=S0874-02832010000400004&lng=pt&nrm=iso&tlng=pt

19. Viero CM, Camponogara S, Sari V, Erthal G. Perception of nurses-professors about environmental problems: grants to the professional training on nursing. Texto & Context - Enferm [Internet]. [cited 2016 May 11];21(4):757–65. Available from: http://www.scielo.br/scielo.php?script=sci_arttext&pid=S0104-07072012000400005&lng=en&nrm=iso&tlng=pt

20. Camponogara S, Erthal G, Viero CM. <b>A problemática ambiental na visão de agentes comunitários

de saúde</b> DOI: 10.4025/
cienccuidsaude.v12i1.18584. Ciência, Cuid e Saúde
[Internet]. 2013 Sep 26 [cited 2016 Dec 4];12(2):233–40.
Available from: http://www.periodicos.uem.br/ojs/
index.php/CiencCuidSaude/article/view/18584

21. Sánchez Sanabria M, Socarrás Vega M, Herrera FE,
Marín Picón LT, Noriega Galindo DA. Mitigar
consecuencias del calentamiento global y efecto
invernadero: Reflexiones para la formación en salud. Hacia
la Promoción la Salud [Internet]. [cited 2015 Aug
26];18(2):110–22. Available from: http://www.scielo.org.co/
s c i e l o . p h p ?
script=sci_arttext&pid=S0121-75772013000200009&lng=
es&nrm=iso&tlng=es

22. Peres RR, Camponogara S, Costa VZ da, Terra MG,
Nietsche EA. Health and environment: (in) visibilities and
(dis) continuation in nursing professional training. Esc
Anna Nery - Rev Enferm [Internet]. 2016 [cited 2016 Mar
19];20(1):25–32. Available from: http://www.scielo.br/
s c i e l o . p h p ?
script=sci_arttext&pid=S1414-81452016000100025&lng=
en&nrm=iso&tlng=pt

23. Esperanza D, Rodríguez C, Esperanza N, Carvajal J.
Relación entre actitudes y comportamientos ambientales
en estudiantes de Enfermería. [cited 2018 Feb 3]; Available
from: http://www.scielo.org.co/pdf/luaz/n43/n43a15.pdf

24. MERCOSUR - RANA. Criterios de calidad para la
acreditación ARCU-SUR Enfermería [Internet]. 2015
[cited 2018 Sep 10]. Available from: http://
edu.mercosur.int/arcusur/images/pdf/rana/3-
Enfermeria_Maio_2015.pdf

NEONATAL RISK EXPOSURE AND NICU ENVIRONMENT

Sarah Bakke, BSN, RNC-NIC
NICU Nurse
Nemours Alfred I duPont Hospital for Children
Wilmington, DE

Jennifer O'Malley, BSN, RNC-NIC
NICU Nurse
Nemours Alfred I duPont Hospital for Children
Wilmington, DE

Kathi Randall, MSN, RNC, CNS, NNP-BC
NICU Nurse Consultant
Synapse Care Solutions, Inc.

INTRODUCTION

In the United States, over 300,000 neonates are hospitalized in the neonatal intensive care unit (NICU) each year. Studies of newborn cord blood have confirmed that developing fetuses are exposed to nearly 300 different toxic chemicals through the placenta (Environmental Working Group, 2001). However after delivery, term and preterm neonates remain vulnerable to ongoing chemical exposures due to a multitude of physiologic and environmental risk factors; found both at home and in the hospital.

NICU POPULATION RISK

The neonatal period is defined as the first 30 days of life and is marked by rapid growth and development; physically, neurologically, and physiologically. Depending on the gestational age at birth, neonates in the NICU may have immature organ function which makes them particularly vulnerable to the adverse effects of exposure to harmful chemicals or toxicants. Harmful exposures can have long term effects on learning, behavior, and future health (Hagan, Shaw, and Duncan, 2017). Physiologic factors placing the term or even more so the preterm neonate at increased risk for environmental exposures include:

- **Increased growth velocity**: Growth velocity is highest from 0 to 9 months of life. This high growth velocity is characterized by rapid cell division, particularly in the tissues of the blood, epithelium, and lungs. This rapid cell division makes the neonate highly vulnerable to carcinogens (ATSDR, 2016).

- **Increased skin surface area to body weight ratio**: The neonate's ratio of skin surface area to body weight is roughly three times higher than in the adult. Therefore, dermal exposure and transdermal absorption of any toxicant through the skin results in a larger dose per unit of body weight (Guzelian et al., 1992).

- **Increased skin permeability**: Increased skin permeability results in higher rates of absorption of topical chemicals. Even in the term neonate, the stratum corneum, which provides the important barrier function of the skin, is 30% thinner than that of the adult. The degree of thickness of this protective keratinized layer of skin depends upon the level of prematurity, with the most premature neonates having the most permeable skin (Telofski, Morello, Correa, & Stamatas, 2012).

- **Increased perfusion of epidermis**: Neonates have greater perfusion and hydration of their epidermis than older children and adults. This creates greater absorption of hydrophilic toxins such as phenolic compounds found in some disinfectants (Clemens & Neumann, 1989).

- **Increased respiratory rate**: Neonates have respiratory rates 2-3 times higher than the average adult. Premature neonates suffering from respiratory distress syndrome (RDS) may have respiratory rates in excess of 100 breaths per minute. Inhalation exposure can be amplified for premature neonates being cared for in incubators where air-borne toxicants cannot disperse as readily as in an open room. In addition, early exposure to air-borne contaminants has been linked to increased incidence and severity of asthma (ATSDR, 2016).

- **Immature hepatic glucuronidation and renal clearance**: Through glucuronidation, the body increases the water solubility of chemicals allowing for elimination through the urine or feces. Renal clearance is the process of plasma filtration by the kidneys that allows toxins to be eliminated in the urine. Both vital metabolic processes are immature in the neonate resulting in a decreased ability to clear toxins (Ku & Smith, 2015).

COMMON TOXICANTS IN THE NICU
Heavy Metals

Lead, mercury, arsenic and cadmium are all potent neurotoxins and are known to cause developmental delays and other chronic conditions in neonates and growing children. These heavy metals can be transferred from the mother to the fetus through the placenta or to the newborn or infant through human milk. Methylmercury is a well know neurological teratogen, and neonates are highly vulnerable to its adverse effects and even short-term exposure can cause developmental delays and neonatal seizures. In some populations methylmercury has been detected in human milk which can extend a neonate's exposure even after delivery (Falck, Mooney, Kapoor, White, Bearer, El Metwally, 2015).

Volatile Organic Compounds (VOC)

Volatile Organic Compounds are chemical compounds released into the air from solid objects, such as plastic PVC products or building materials, such as plywood and household paint. According to the American Lung Association, breathing VOCs can irritate the eyes, nose or throat, and can cause respiratory distress, damage to the central nervous system, and has been linked to some cancers. Exposure to inhaled VOCs has also been linked to increased urinary biomarkers for oxidative stress and systemic inflammation (Icahn School of Medicine at Mount Sinai, 2019). VOCs may be present in the NICU and can exert a negative effect on staff, visitors, and our tiny patients. Remodeling projects in the NICU, even simple ones like a new coat of paint, should strive to use building materials, paint, and furniture with low or no-VOC's whenever possible.

Phthalates

Phthalates are a group of chemicals known as plasticizers that are commonly used in the manufacture of polyvinyl chloride (PVC) products and in fragrance-laden lotions, soaps, and shampoos. The chemical structure of phthalates is similar to endogenous steroid hormones (e.g. estrogen) so when phthalates are present in the bloodstream they can interact with steroid receptor sites on the cell, causing an endocrine disrupting effect. Increased levels of phthalates and phenols have been linked to a multitude of adverse health effects including asthma, attention-deficit hyperactivity disorder, breast cancer, obesity, type II diabetes, low IQ, neurodevelopmental issues, behavioral issues, autism spectrum disorders, altered reproductive development and male fertility issues (LaRocca, Binder, McElrath, & Michels, 2015).

There are various types of phthalates utilized as plasticizers in the manufacture of medical products commonly used in the NICU. Phthalates are a danger to neonates as they easily leach from a solid plastic material into the air, fluids, or food they contact and cause an exposure. This leaching process may be increased in high heat or humidity conditions such as inside neonatal incubators, when intravenous catheters are exposed to body heat, and when using heated humidified respiratory support circuits.

Phthalates are also commonly used in the manufacturing of "fragrances", including the fragrances added to traditional baby skin care products and shampoos to create that familiar "new baby smell". Starting in-utero, neonates can be exposed to phthalates from the products used by their mother, such as cosmetics, personal care products, and perfumes. These early fetal and neonatal exposures have been linked to poor executive functioning, psychological/psychosocial issues such as depression, inattention, and impaired emotional regulation later in life (Falck et al., 2015).

Phenols

Phenols are manufactured chemical compounds used in disinfectants and plastic products. Like phthalates, phenols are endocrine disruptors, and studies are ongoing to determine their association with a number of adverse effects including breast cancer and the early onset of puberty. While bis-phenol A (BPA) has been removed from a wide variety of plastic products, including most plastic baby bottles, other sources of phenolic compounds remain in use in the hospital, in the NICU, and in the home including Triclosan [5-chloro-2-(2,4-dichlorophenoxy)-phenol] (TRCS) which can be found in cleaners, hand sanitizers, toothpaste, and other personal care products.

Polyethylene glycol, 1,4-dioxane and other ethylated surfactants

Products with ingredients that contain the letter "eth"— such as polyethylene, polyethylene glycol (PEG), and SLS (sodium Laureth sulfate) — should heighten ones suspicions to the possible presence of the toxic contaminant 1,4-Dioxane. During the manufacturing process, PEG and its derivatives can become contaminated with 1,4-Dioxane and ethylene oxide, which are known carcinogens and nervous system toxicants.

Sodium laureth sulfate is often added to products to produce the "bubbly and sudsy" properties of soaps, shampoos, and even toothpaste and exposure may be toxic or harmful to adults and children (SkinDeep, 2019). Polyethylene glycol (PEG) is a petroleum-derived ingredient added to body care products to thicken, soften and to act as moisture-carriers in cosmetic creams; and it is used as a laxative in pharmaceuticals (David Suzuki Foundation, 2019).

Although 1,4-Dioxane can be vacuum stripped from PEG and SLS after manufacturing the FDA does not require that product labels include this disclosure which leaves consumers unsure if the product is contaminated with 1,4-Dioxane. It has been estimated by the Environmental

Working Group (EWG) that 57% of all baby soaps are contaminated with 1,4-Dioxane. A study of lactation transfer of chemicals in human milk concluded that 1,4-Dioxane was among the top 3 of 19 different chemicals that posed the highest exposure risks to infants (Lawrence & Lawrence, 2015). 1,4-Dioxane can be transferred through breast milk and has been known to cause miscarriages and stillbirths when combined with other chemical exposure. The Environmental Protection Agency has classified 1, 4-Dioxane as a carcinogen, it can also cause kidney and liver damage and short term irritation to the eyes, nose and throat in adults. No adverse effects have been studied in the neonatal population (Wilbur, 2007).

Parabens

Parabens are often used as preservatives in personal care products; from baby lotions to deodorants. Parabens may appear on a product's label in various combinations (i.e. butylparaben, propylparaben, etc) and may even be disguised as other names, such as benzoic acid or propyl ester. As with phthalates, parabens are potent endocrine disruptors with strong estrogenic effects, as well as neurotoxicant potential. High doses of parabens can cause hyperbilirubinemia and bone abnormalities. (Cuzzolin, 2017). Parabens typically enter the body through the skin and have been detected in blood samples confirming a systemic absorption from topical exposures and have been linked to breast cancer, as well as reproductive toxicity (Sattler, Randall, & Choiniere, 2012). The Center for Disease Control (CDC) found that the blood of over 60% of children surveyed by the National Center for Environmental Health was contaminated with significant levels of parabens. Most governments around the world have not examined the safety of parabens, an exception is Denmark, which has banned parabens in products for children under 3 years of age (Preethi, 2018).

POTENTIAL EXPOSURE SOURCES IN THE NICU

Bathing and Skin Care

Bathing and skin care products for infants, including soaps, shampoos, lotions and creams are used universally whether the infant is in the home and in hospital and are therefore, a significant source for chemical exposures beginning on the first day of life.

Although recent trends have shown cosmetic and skin care companies rebranding and removing parabens and phthalates from their adult products, these chemicals still remain behind in many popular products marketed for newborns and infants. Phthalates are used to help lotions penetrate and soften the skin, and to help fragrances last longer. Baby powder, lotion, and shampoo with added synthetic fragrance have the highest phthalate concentrations and should be a top priority to be removed from the NICU or at a minimum replaced with safer products which are widely available through hospital purchasing contracts worldwide.

Powders are not recommended for daily use in NICU patients and infants for several reasons. The main substance causing a concern is baby powder. First is the fact that talc is used to create talcum powder, which in turn is used in the formulation of baby powder, which naturally contains asbestos. As recently as 2019, brand name baby powders were removed from the shelves for concerns of asbestos contamination (Dyer, 2019). Second, is the potential aspiration of the talc powder "cloud" into the lungs during use causing a pneumonic reaction, which could lead to aspiration and respiratory distress in some infants (Moon et al, 2011). Most powders also contain synthetic fragrances, which has previously been discussed as a concern. Last and certainly not least, there have been a few recent lawsuit settlements to women who alleged their daily use of Johnson's & Johnson's talcum powder was linked to their diagnosis of ovarian cancer (Dyer, 2019).

Diapers and Diaper Care

Every day in the NICU, hundreds if not thousands of diapers are changed, diaper wipes are used and discarded, and dozens of tubes of diaper cream are used. Unfortunately, these common practices also pose many hidden dangers when it comes to exposures to toxic chemicals. Most disposable diapers are made of polypropylene and polyethylene, which are considered to be "safer" plastics. However, when these materials are exposed to heat (like inside a baby's diaper) they can seep a toxic metalloid, known as antimony, into the skin. Another concern with disposable diapers is the presence of dioxins, which have been named "supertoxins" and is a known carcinogen. Dioxins are by-products of the chlorine manufacturing process and are likely present whenever chlorine bleach, bleached paper or products are used. Dioxins can cause skin lesions and affect the liver, reproductive, nervous, immune and endocrine system (WHO, 2016). In the past, commercial diapers used mostly bleached paper pulp, however consumer pressure over the last decade has moved many brands to switch to a non-chlorine bleaching process to whiten materials used in baby diapers. Along with chlorine and plasticizers disposable diapers may also contain dyes and fragrances, which are all well-known skin irritants.

Disposable baby wipes and diaper rash creams are another staple of baby care, and unfortunately can be heavily laden with chemicals. As mentioned before, phthalates and parabens can likely be found in any product that contains added synthetic fragrances or preservatives. These ingredients can be absorbed during topical application and may potentially cause endocrine disruption, and developmental and reproductive toxicity (SkinDeep, 2019).

Some baby wipes contain ethylated surfactants to enhance cleaning of stool from the skin, which creates the opportunity for additional exposure to the contaminant 1,4-dioxane which may be irritating to sensitive skin. In the NICU, many infants already have broken or irritated skin and the use of these added surfactants could make their skin condition worse and may result in additional absorption of these harsh and harmful chemical additives into their bloodstream.

Artificial Nipples and Bottles

In the last decade, BPA has mostly been removed from all plastic bottles and nipples due to enormous consumer pressure and legislative actions by a few US States. Silicone nipples are now recommended instead of rubber, glass bottles are preferred to plastic, and there is a recommendation to also avoid plastic liners for bottles whenever possible. Even though BPA has been removed from the actual bottle itself it may still be found in the lining material of powdered formula cans or the plastic lids on liquid formula bottles. In the NICU, it is standard practice to warm milk or formula, however heating and reusing plastic bottles can cause an increase of chemicals leaching into the milk (EWG, 2019).

Medical Devices and Accessories

Products such as endotracheal tubes, oxygen masks, nasal prongs or cannulas, venous or arterial catheters, enteral feeding tubes, and parenteral nutrition bags are typically manufactured from phthalate treated PVC (Demirel, Coban, Yildirim, Dogan, Sanci, & Ince, 2016). One of these phthalates, Diethylhexyl phthalate (DEHP) is the most common plasticizer for PVC in medical products. Multiple studies have linked the use of DEHP products to increased phthalate and phenol levels in the urine of NICU patients. A European study measured chemicals from products commonly utilized in the pediatric intensive care unit (PICU), and found that the products were leaching a number of harmful or potentially harmful chemicals including DEHP into the body (Malarvannana, Onghenaa, Verstraete, Puffelenc, Jacobs, Vanhorebeek, Verbruggen, Joosten, Van den Berghe, Jorens, & Covaci, 2019).

In the United States, DEHP alternative products are becoming more widely available, however, many NICUs still utilize phthalate containing medical devices. One recent study found that NICU patients requiring respiratory support through plastic circuits had 95-132% higher levels of phthalate biomarkers in their urine compared with neonates not requiring respiratory support (Mount Sinai, 2018). On the positive side, over the last few years, phenols such as BPA plasticizers have been replaced in most polycarbonate plastic products used daily in the hospital such as intravenous administration sets, syringes, and catheters (Duty, Mendonca, Hauser, Calafat, Ye, Meeker, Ackerman, Cullinane, Faller & Ringer, 2013) but they have not been eliminated completely from all products used in the NICU.

Parenteral Nutrition

Total Parenteral Nutrition (TPN) is a life saving measure to provide adequate nutrients, fluid intake, and the metabolic demands of premature and/or ill infants. Not with-standing the benefits of TPN, there are several risks associated with its long-term use as well, such as liver injury, infection, cholestasis and direct hyperbilirubinemia. Most IV catheters, tubing and other TPN associated products are made of products that expose neonates to phthalates, parabens and other toxins (Oznur, Dilara, Turkan, 2019).

Aluminum is a common contaminant in TPN additives, primarily calcium and phosphate. Overall, TPN accounts for almost 90% of aluminum exposure in neonates. Neonates with aluminum exposure are at an increased risk of a learning delay later in life as well as issues associated with cholestasis from accumulation of aluminum in the liver (Fortenberry, Hernandez & Morton, 2017; Popinska, Ksiazyk, Friedman-Gruszczynska, Nowicka, Migdal, & Pietraszek, 2009). Physicians and researchers agree that a decrease in aluminum contamination from TPN additives is desirable but unlikely due to a lack of alternative products (Griffin, 2019).

Formula and Human Milk

Formula fed infants are at risk for chemical exposures through several separate mechanisms. First, powdered formula and liquid formula concentrate must be reconstituted using water which places the neonate at risk for exposure to water-borne toxicants. Therefore, filtered tap water is recommended when reconstituting powdered or liquid formula. If using bottled water, it should always be fluoride free. Canned formula may contain dangerous chemicals, such as BPA or other phenols found in the inner lining metal cans which can leach into the liquid or powders with prolonged contact. It is recommended by the EWG to use liquid, ready-to-feed, formulas in plastic or glass bottles in lieu of canned powdered formulas whenever possible (EWG, 2019). Additionally, studies have found toxic contaminants and heavy metals in formula which may be byproducts of raw materials or from the manufacturing process. The American Academy of Pediatrics and other leading organizations recommend breastfeeding and/or providing human milk whenever possible. However, even an exclusive human milk diet for the neonate may also pose a risk to the neonate for toxicant exposure depending on the maternal chemical body burden and ongoing environmental exposures such as contaminated drinking water. Maternal exposures directly affect which chemicals and/or toxins are transferred via human milk to the neonate (Lawrence & Lawrence 2015).

Disinfectants and Antiseptics

Hospital policies are highly focused on maintaining an aseptic environment, especially in the NICU environment. Topical antiseptics are used in every health care setting, but they are not without risk such as chemical burns, systemic absorption, and toxicity. Skin antisepsis prior to skin breaking procedures is widely practiced, and protocols vary regarding gestational age guidelines for the type of antiseptic agent utilized. Products of concern in the NICU are betadine (povidone-Iodine) and chlorhexidine (CHG).

Premature neonates and those with non-intact skin are particularly at risk to toxic exposure as studies have found CHG detected in the blood of preterm infants two to three days following topical application (Chapman, Aucott, Gilmore, Advani, Clarke, & Milstone, 2013). While it is known that some systemic absorption of CHG occurs, it is not known what level of serum concentration may cause harm in neonates. Several in vivo, in vitro, and animal studies have raised concerns regarding cytotoxic and neurotoxic effects, as well as disruptions in thyroid function (Chapman, Aucott, & Milstone, 2012). Betadine (povidone-Iodine) is also known to cause thyroid dysfunction and reproductive toxicity. Topical application in neonates less than 32 weeks should be avoided and excess iodine should be removed promptly from the skin of any neonate post-procedure to minimize cutaneous injury and systemic absorption (Williams, Watson, Day, Soe, Somisetty, Jackson, Velten, & Boelen, 2017).

A concern related to topical and surface disinfectants is the noxious scent. The olfactory system of the neonate has been shown to aid in promoting oral feeding, pain reduction and maternal-infant bonding (Van et al, 2017). The sense of smell is developed in utero around 8 week's gestation and is recognized by neonates around 24 week's gestation. This leads us to determine that infants, especially premature infants, have a higher risk of repeated and chronic exposure to noxious scents which have harmful, unintended consequences (Lipchock et al, 2011). All noxious stimuli, including scents, can lead to neurodevelopmental issues later in life (Santos et al, 2015).

Air Quality

Air quality is yet another potential source for chemical exposures, especially for air pollutants, such as VOCs and airborne particles. Neonates may be exposed to several VOCs in the NICU environment and specifically within the microenvironment of the incubator. Studies have found elevated levels of the VOC cyclohexane in unused incubators raising the concern for exposure through inhalation. Airborne particulate matter (PM) including airborne particles are concerning in the NICU as inhalation of these particles has been associated with adverse health effects including increased mortality and respiratory morbidity (Bhangar et al, 2016). While studies have shown that exposure is increased with higher temperatures and humidity in incubators, more research is needed to determine if this is consistent in all types of incubators and what other factors contribute to issues with air quality such as combined medication exposure, maturation of toxins, and do infants on supplemental oxygen have less of an exposure risk than those not (Brion, 2008).

STRATEGIES FOR PROMOTING A SAFER NICU ENVIRONMENT

Demand for "Greener" Practices and Supporting Parents

Just as consumer pressure over the last decade has pushed the cosmetic and household industry to remove potentially harmful ingredients from the products they make, patients have also begun to express their preferences and expectations for "greener" products in the hospital and in the NICU environment.

One in five consumers report preferring alternatives to traditional medicine, and twelve percent report that they would prefer natural remedies over prescription medications (Samueli Institute, 2010). Over the last decade we have all seen an increasing demand for complementary and alternative health products and practices by all patient populations, and in the NICU we have seen some practices such as probiotics, acupuncture and aromatherapy increase in use too. Despite this trend, families with preferences for "organic" products, foods and clothing are often labeled by NICU staff as "difficult", "uneducated", or "hippies". These attitudes and names create a barrier to open communication, family-centered care, and collaboration. It is recognized that the purchasing practices in hospitals may be slow to change, but it is the hope of the authors that NICU policies of the future will allow for families to provide alternative, and potentially safer, products for their infant; especially when the hospital does not have access to them or they are not yet part of the standard of care.

Essential Oils

Essential oils are highly concentrated volatile compounds distilled from the bark, flowers, leaves and roots of plants and provide aromatic scent with many known therapeutic benefits. Studies have proven that neonatal massage is beneficial to neonates, especially those in the NICU. Massages can be done with sunflower or grapeseed oil and may at times include diluted essential oils for term infants.

There is limited research on the use of essential oils in the premature neonatal population. However, evidence is beginning to accumulate for term infants. A clinical trial is underway in Kentucky to investigate the use of aromatherapy patches of lavender and chamomile to calm infants with Neonatal Abstinence Syndrome (NAS) and their pilot data showed a reduction in the length of stay as well as the amount of pharmaceutical intervention required. In this study, the aromatherapy patches were placed in the infant's environment, not on the skin (Daniel, 2017). A randomized control trial from a NICU in Iran showed positive results for pain control during venipuncture blood sampling when term infants were exposed to 8 hours of the scent of lavender at night and then again at the time of blood draw (Razaghi, Hoseini, Aemmi, Mohebbi, & Boskabadi, 2015). Of importance to note is that both studies, although both small samples, also showed no negative reactions to the use of scent for these populations.

Creating Safer NICUs for Babies

In this chapter the authors have discussed the primary sources of exposure in the NICU, the potential health effects of these harmful chemicals, as well as the unique developmental characteristics that make neonates additionally vulnerable to these exposures. We have shared that skin care products made for babies, diapers, feeding systems, medical devices, and accessories, TPN, infant formula, human milk, disinfectants, antiseptics and poor air quality all carry a significant risk of chemical and/or toxin exposure to neonates in the NICU and even after discharge to home. While not all products used in the NICU have safer alternatives, many do.

Hospitals, and NICU nurses in particular, should be diligent in adopting the "Precautionary Principle" (i.e.

better safe, than sorry) in their purchasing practices and when choosing equipment and products for the NICU. NICU nurses need to become strong advocates for purchasing policies that limit, if not eliminate the ongoing use of any product that could potentially be harmful or contribute to long-term detrimental health effects in NICU patients. For example, disposable diapers and skin wipes that are fragrance, chlorine, and dye free should be made available for purchase by special order for the NICU or through existing group purchasing organization contracts. Skin care and bathing products currently in use in the NICU can be easily evaluated at the EWG's SkinDeep® Cosmetic Database (www.ewg.org/skindeep) and many non-toxic alternatives are widely available to hospitals worldwide.

Some medical grade equipment (ventilators, monitors, beds, etc.) do not yet have "healthier" alternatives due to product necessity, availability, cost, and safety, however, it is vital that nurses become a significant voice on purchasing committees, not only to evaluate products for patient safety and efficacy of "greener" products, but also to advocate for the development of safer alternative products directly with manufacturers and vendors when not yet available. A recurrent theme in all literature related to creating more sustainable hospital environments, including NICUs, is cost. Although this may be an initial deterrent, the main barrier to implementation is the overall lack of knowledge about alternative products and the potential health benefits of sustainable, eco-friendly, non-toxic products in the NICU. Awareness and continuing education are key to advancing these initiatives and create more green, sustainable NICUs in the future and safer environments for our tiniest patients, their families, and staff.

REFERENCES

Agency for Toxic Substances & Disease Research (ATSDR). (2016). *Principles of pediatric environmental health.* Environmental Health and Medicine Education. https://www.atsdr.cdc.gov/csem/csem.asp?csem=27&po=9

Bhangar, S., Brooks, B., Firek, B., Licina, D., Tang, X., Morowitz, M. J., Banfield, J.F., Nazaroff, W. W. (2016). Pilot study of sources and concentrations of size-resolved airborne particles in a neonatal intensive care unit. *Building and Environment, 106,* 10-19. doi:10.1016/j.buildenv.2016.06.020

Brion, L. P. (2008). Volatile organic compounds in the air of neonatal incubators. *Journal of Perinatology, 28*(8), 521–522. doi: 10.1038/jp.2008.91

Chapman, A. K., Aucott, S. W., & Milstone, A. M. (2012). Safety of chlorhexidine gluconate used for skin antisepsis in the preterm infant. *Journal of Perinatology: Official Journal of the California Perinatal Association, 32*(1), 4-9. Doi:10.1038/jp.2011.148

Chapman, A. K., Aucott, S. W., Gilmore, M. M., Advani, S., Clarke, W., & Milstone, A. M. (2013). Absorption and tolerability of aqueous chlorhexidine gluconate used for skin antisepsis prior to catheter insertion in preterm neonates. *Journal of Perinatology : Official Journal of the California Perinatal Association, 33*(10), 768-771. Doi:10.1038/jp.2013.61

Clemens, P.C., & Neumann, R.S. (1989). The Wolff-Chaikoff effect: hypothyroidism due to iodine application. *Archives of Dermatology, 125,* 705.

Cuzzolin, L. (2017). Neonates exposed to excipients: Concern about safety. *Journal of Pediatric and Neonatal Individualized Medicine, 7.* Doi:10.7363/070112

Daniel, J. (2017). *The effect of aromatherapy on neonatal abstinence syndrome and salivary cortisol levels.* https://clinicaltrials.gov/ct2/show/NCT03097484

David Suzuki Foundation (2019). *The Dirty Dozen: PEG contaminants and their contaminants.* https://davidsuzuki.org/queen-of-green/dirty-dozen-peg-compounds-contaminants/

Demirel, A., Coban, A., Yildirim, S., Dogan, C., Sanci, R., & Ince, Z. (2016). Hidden toxicity in neonatal intensive care units: phthalate exposure in very low birth weight infants. *Journal of Clinical Research in Pediatric Endocrinology, 8*(3), p. 298-304.

Duty, S.M., Mendonca, K., Hauser, R., Calafat, A.M., Ye, X., Meeker, J.D., Ackerman, R., Cullinane, J., Faller, J., & Ringer, S.. (2013). Potential sources of bisphenol A in the neonatal intensive care unit. *Pediatrics, 131*(3):483-439.

Dyer, O. (2019). California jury awards $29m to woman who said Johnson & Johnson talc caused mesothelioma *BMJ, 364.* doi:10.1136/bmj.l1215

Dyer, O. (2019). Johnson & Johnson recalls its Baby Powder after FDA finds asbestos in sample *BMJ, 367.* doi:10.1136/bmj.l6118

Environmental Working Group. (2015). *Body burden: The pollution in newborns.* https://www.ewg.org/research/body-burden-pollution-newborns

Environmental Working Group (2019). *Guide to baby-safe bottles & formula.* EWG.org/Research/EWG;s-guide-baby-safe-bottles-and-formula

Environmental Working Group. (2019). *Skin Deep® cosmetics database.* https://www.ewg.org/skindeep/

Falck, A. J., Mooney, S., Kapoor, S. S., White, K. M., Bearer, C., & El Metwally, D. (2015). Developmental exposure to environmental toxicants. *Pediatric Clinics of North America, 62*(5), 1173-1197.

Fortenberry, M., Hernandez, L., & Morton, J. (2017). Evaluating Differences in Aluminum Exposure through Parenteral Nutrition in Neonatal Morbidities. *Nutrients, 9*(11), 1249. Doi:10.3390/nu9111249

Griffin, I. J. (2019, June 17). *Parenteral nutrition in preterm infants.* https://www.uptodate.com/contents/parenteral-nutrition-in-premature-infants

Guzelian, P.S., Henry, C.J., & Olin, S.S. (Ed.). (1992). *Similarities and differences between children and adults: implications for risk assessment.* ILSI Press.

Hagan, J.F., Shaw, J.S. & Duncan, P.M. (2017). *Bright futures: Guidelines for health supervision of infants, children and adolescents* (4th ed.). American Academy of Pediatrics.

Icahn School of Medicine at Mount Sinai. (2019). *Air quality in the NICU* [Blog]. http://labs.icahn.mssm.edu/stroustruplab/air-quality-in-the-nicu/

Ku, L. C., & Smith, P. B. (2015). Dosing in neonates: special considerations in physiology and trial design. *Pediatric Research, 77*(1-1), 2–9. Doi:10.1038/pr.2014.143

LaRocca, J., Binder, A., McElrath, T., & Michels, K. (2015). First-trimester urine concentrations of phthalate metabolites and phenols and placenta miRNA expression in a cohort of U.S. women. *Environmental Health Perspectives, 124*(3), p. 380-387, doi: 10.1289/ehp.1408409

Lawrence, R. A., & Lawrence, R. M. (2015). *Breastfeeding: A guide for the medical professional.* https://www.clinicalkey.com/nursing/#!/content/book/3-s2.0-B9780323357760000127?scrollTo=#hl0002771

Lipchock, S.V., Reed, D.R. & Mennella, J.A. (2011). The gustatory and olfactory systems during infancy: implications for development of feeding behaviors in the high-risk neonate. *Clinics in Perinatology, 38*(4), 627-641. doi:10.1016/j.clp.2011.08.008

Malarvannana, G., Onghenaa, M., Verstraete, S., Puffelenc, E., Jacobs, A., Vanhorebeek, I., Verbruggen, S., Joosten, K., Van den Berghe, G., Jorens, P., & Covaci, A. (2019). Phthalate and alternative plasticizers in indwelling medical devices in pediatric intensive care units. *Journal of Hazardous Materials, 363*(5), p. 64-72.

Moon, M.C., Park, J.D., Choi, B.S., Park, S.Y., Kim, D.W., Chung, Y.H., Hisanaga, N., & Yu, I.J. (2011). Risk assessment of baby powder exposure through Inhalation. *Toxicological Research, 27*(3), 137-141. doi:10.5487/TR.2011.27.3.137

Mount Sinai. (2018, September 26). *Mount Sinai researchers identify respiratory support as source of exposure to phthalates in neonatal intensive care units* [Press Release]. https://www.mountsinai.org/about/newsroom/2018/mount-sinai-researchers-identify-respiratory-support-as-source-of-exposure-to-phthalates-in-neonatal-intensive-care-units

Oznur, B., Dilara, K., & Turkan, K. (2019). Enteral and parenteral feeding of neonate. *Journal of Neonatal Nursing, 25*(3), 107-110.

Popinska, K., Ksiazyk, J., Friedman-Gruszczynska, J., Nowicka, E., Migdal, A., & Pietraszek, E. (2010). Aluminum concentration in serum of children on long-term parenteral nutrition and in parenteral nutrition solution components. *E-SPEN, the European E-Journal of Clinical Nutrition and Metabolism, 5*(1). Doi:10.1016/j.eclnm.2009.10.010

Preethi. (2018, February 28). *The Suspicious Seven — 7 deadly villains hiding in your baby's skin and hair care products.* http://krya.in/blogk/2016/05/the-suspicious-seven-7-deadly-villains-hiding-in-your-babys-skin-and-hair-care-products/

Razaghi, N., Hoseini, A. S., Aemmi, S. Z., Mohebbi, T., & Boskabadi, H. (2015, April 01). *The Effect of lavender scent on pain of blood sampling in term neonates.* https://doaj.org/article/d961e868c8704a85b21d3d68c2ff9ad0

Samueli Institute (2010). https://ssihi.uci.edu/

Santos, J., Pearce, S.E., & Stroustroup, A. (2015). Impact of hospital-based environmental exposures on neurodevelopmental outcomes in preterm infants. *Current Opinion in Pediatrics, 27*(2), p. 254-260.

Sattler, B., Randall, K.S., & Choiniere, D. (2012). Reducing hazardous chemical exposures in the neonatal intensive care unit: a new role for nurses. *Critical Care Nursing Quarterly, 35*(1), p. 102-112.

Stroustrup, A., Bragg, J. B., Busgang, S. A., Andra, S. S., Curtin, P., Spear, E. A., ... Gennings, C. (2018). Sources of clinically significant neonatal intensive care unit phthalate exposure. *Journal of Exposure Science & Environmental Epidemiology.* doi: 10.1038/s41370-018-0069-2

Telofski, L., Morello, A., Correa, M., & Stamatas, G. (2012). The infant skin barrier: can we preserve, protect, and enhance the barrier? *Dermatology Research and Practice, 2012.* doi:10.1155/2012/198789

Van, H. C., Guinand, N., Damis, E., Mansbach, A. L., Poncet, A., Hummel, T., & Landis, B. N. (2017). Olfactory stimulation may promote oral feeding in immature newborn: a randomized controlled trial. *European Archives of Oto-Rhino-Laryngology, 275*(1), 125–129. doi: 10.1007/s00405-017-4796-0

Wilbur, S. (2007). *HEALTH ADVISORY.* https://www.ncbi.nlm.nih.gov/books/NBK153666/

Williams, F. L. R., Watson, J., Day, C., Soe, A., Somisetty, S. K., Jackson, L., Velten, E & Boelen, A. (2017). Thyroid dysfunction in preterm neonates exposed to iodine. *Journal of Perinatal Medicine, 45*(1), 135.

World Health Org (WHO). (2016, October 4). *Dioxins and their effects on human health.* https://www.who.int/en/news-room/fact-sheets/detail/dioxins-and-their-effects-on-human-health

Unit V:
Sustainable Communities

WHAT ARE SUSTAINABLE COMMUNITIES?

The term "sustainable communities" refers to a goal to ensure survivable communities globally. Sustainable communities use resources to meet current needs while considering the needs of future generations. Elements of sustainability include safe and healthy housing, transportation that reduces harmful exposures to the environment and provides opportunities for all citizens to engage in community life, access to healthy and affordable foods, smart growth, and social and economic opportunities all supported by involved community members.

For more than 25 years, civic groups, local communities and non-governmental organizations have worked to advance sustainable living. The Institute for Sustainable Communities has partners in the United States, China, Vietnam, Thailand, Bangladesh and India. There are videos online that show the work of sustainable cities, towns and neighborhoods.

Since 2009, the US Federal Government has a program entitled the Partnership for Sustainable Communities that is composed of three federal agencies: the U.S. Department of Housing and Urban Development (HUD), U.S. Department of Transportation (DOT), and the U.S. Environmental Protection Agency (EPA). The goal of the partnership is to protect the environment while improving access to affordable housing, increasing transportation options and lowering transportation costs. According to their website, the "Partnership for Sustainable Communities (PSC) works to coordinate federal housing, transportation, water, and other infrastructure investments to make neighborhoods more prosperous, allow people to live closer to jobs, save households time and money, and reduce pollution. The partnership agencies incorporate six principles of livability into federal funding programs, policies, and future legislative proposals" (PSC, 2016).

Successful projects sponsored by the partnership include Bridgeport, CT, Greenville, SC and Milwaukee, WI. In addition, other examples of communities that have developed programs for sustainable communities include those supported by the Making a Visible Difference in Communities program of the EPA, as well as Smart Growth initiatives.

INTRODUCTION

Unit V includes a discussion about Green Buildings, which is a topic that many nurses are likely to know about as a result of the current efforts to build environmentally responsible workplaces. The Green Cleaning in Homes chapter provides information and resources to inform nurses about healthier choices for cleaning products. Unit V also addresses transportation concerns, Brownfields in communities, and antibiotic use in agriculture. These topics impact the health and well being of community residents. The chapter, Environmental Justice, builds upon the issue of health disparities related to the social determinants of health. While communities work to foster social and economic health and well-being, hazardous exposures impact community citizens differently. This chapter addresses both the development of the environmental justice movement, the federal and state mandates developed in response to this movement and efforts by community members to address injustice and work toward healthy sustainable communities.

ECOLOGY, ECOSYSTEMS, AND WATERSHEDS
Adelita G. Cantu, PhD, RN
University of Texas Health San Antonio
School of Nursing

The word **Ecology** originated in the late 19th century and was first called oecology from the Greek oikos that meant 'house' + –logy. The Oxford English Dictionary defines ecology as the branch of biology that deals with the relations of organisms to one another and to their physical surroundings. An additional definition is the political movement that seeks to protect the environment, especially from pollution (OED, 2015).

Ecology refers to the study of any living thing in relation to its environment. Darwin, around the year 1859, classified the "web of life" and acknowledged the immense complex set of interrelationships that existed between organisms and their environment (Sattler, 2009). Similarly, **ecosystem** describes the active communities of microorganisms, plants, and animals, along with the lifeless environment in which they live (Allender, 2014). Rainforests are Earth's oldest living ecosystems that cover only 6% of the earth's surface but end up housing more than ½ of the earth's plant and animal life (SRL, 2014). According to the Environmental Protection Agency (EPA), **watersheds** are lands where the water that is found under it and drains to the same spot. The well-known scientist geographer, John Wesley Powell described a watershed as "that area of land, a bounded hydrologic system, within which all living things are inextricably linked by their common water course and where, as humans settled, simple logic demanded that they become part of a community." A watershed describes an area of land that contains a common set of streams and rivers that all drain into a single larger body of water, such as a larger river, a lake or an ocean. For example, the Mississippi River watershed is an enormous watershed (mbgnet, 2002).

There is a simplified version of the several different levels of ecologic systems that exist and are mentioned above. This simplified version is broken down into two levels, the microsystem and the macrosystem. The microsystem can be thought of as the environment that is directly surrounding the individual, for instance their family and household. On the other hand, the macrosystem is the broader framework, in which the microsystem is embedded. The macrosystem consists of one's culture, their traditions, customs, societal norms, governmental agencies, schools, organizations, economic policies and the physical environment (Sattler, 2009). The relationship between Commoner's Law and these ecological systems can be compared as "everything is connected to everything else and everything must go somewhere." Ecosystems help regulate water, gases, waste recycling, nutrient cycling, and biology as well as provide recreational and cultural opportunities for human use. The scientific analysis of **ecosystems** is critical to understanding of environmental health impacts on human health; this synergistic relationship among human beings and the environment has impacts along the human development continuum.

Further, a **watershed** can provide several ecosystem services like "nutrient cycling, carbon storage, erosion/sedimentation control, increased biodiversity, soil formation, wildlife movement corridors, water storage, water filtration, flood control, food, timber, recreation, and reduced vulnerability to invasive species, the effects of climate change, and other natural disasters". Rainforests provide food, water, and oxygen to the rest of the world, and its temperate and tropical rainforests have a dramatic relationship with climate change since it helps regulate earth's temperature and its weather patterns (The Nature Conservancy, 20015).

An increase in human demands, like home heating and cooling, causes an increase in the use of fossil fuels, like natural gas, oil, and coal. Burning fossil fuels releases toxic chemicals that create air pollution and contribute to global warming (Allender, 2014). Global warming then has impacts on ecosystems and watersheds throughout the world; thus the delicate balance within ecosystems and watersheds with the resultant weather and environmental impacts continues to impact climate change and its consequences of poor water quality, air pollution and drought.

REFERENCES

Allender, J. (2014). Environmental Health and Safety. In *Community and public health nursing: Promoting the public's health* (8th ed., p. 286). Wolters Kluwer/Lippincott Williams & Wilkins Health.

Maurer, F., Smith, C., & Sattler, B. (2009). Environmental Health Risks: At Home, at Work, and in the Community. In F. A. Maurer & C. M. Smith (Eds) *Community health for families and populations* (4th ed., p. 242). Saunders/Elsevier.

Missouri Botanical Garden. (2002). What is a Watershed. http://www.mbgnet.net/fresh/rivers/shed.htm

Protect & Save Rainforests | The Nature Conservancy. (n.d.). http://www.nature.org/ourinitiatives/urgentissues/rainforests/

US Environmental Protection Agency. (n.d.). *Benefits of healthy watersheds.* http://water.epa.gov/polwaste/nps/watershed/benefits.cfm

US Environmental Protection Agency. (n.d.). *What is a watershed?.* http://water.epa.gov/type/watersheds/whatis.cfm

GREEN CLEANING, DISINFECTING, AND SANITIZING IN HOMES

Kate Lawler, EdD, MSN, RN, ANP-BC
Professor
Immaculata University

Ruth McDermott-Levy, PhD, MPH, RN, FAAN
Professor
Co-Director, Mid-Atlantic Center for Children's Health and the Environment
Villanova University
M. Louise Fitzpatrick College of Nursing

WHY GREEN CLEANING IS RECOMMENDED IN HOMES

Exposure to potentially toxic substances is often a result of common household activities. The Environmental Protection Agency (EPA) found levels of common pollutants to be 2 to 5 times higher inside homes than outside, regardless of the home's location (EPA, n.d.a.). Health effects from chemical exposures include eye, nose and throat irritation, headaches, nausea, contact dermatitis, and central nervous system dysfunction. Inhalation of respiratory irritants is a common trigger of asthma symptoms. Many toxic chemical cleaning products are not only more expensive than more natural methods, they also end up in the water systems after rinsing, and in landfills after disposal of unused products. Some cleaning chemicals are known or suspected to cause cancer in humans (EPA, 2012).

One way to avoid the exposures to potentially toxic chemicals is to read labels carefully. Non-toxic commercial products are available to the consumer who is willing to do some research. The market is full of products that claim to be "all natural", "safe for the environment" or "biodegradable", but these terms are not subject to guidelines for their use. When looking for environmentally safe products, the Environmental Protection Agency has an on-line resource for their Safer Choice Program. This program was developed from the earlier, ``Design for the Environment" (DfE) program. Products with the Safer Choice designation have been evaluated for human health and environmental risks, including risk to fish. This is a voluntary program for companies that make cleaning products to participate and demonstrate that their products meet the EPA Safer Choice Standard (EPA, n.d.b.). Consumers can check if specific products that have been approved have the EPA's "Safer Choice" label by checking the EPA Search Safer Choice Products website at: https://www.epa.gov/saferchoice/products. Look for the Safer Choice label when purchasing cleaning products.

Manufacturers are not required to list the content of cleaning products; however, household products should carry the following warnings if applicable:

- Caution – slightly toxic

- Warning – moderately toxic

- Danger – highly toxic

- Poison–use precautions to avoid exposure (Findley & Formicelli, 2009).

Reading the product labels and using the product as directed is the first step in reducing health risks to the user and those in the home. Sprays, especially aerosols, can linger in the air for hours or days. If used on a regular basis, the result is chronic inhalation of chemical substances. This is important to consider in light of the increasing popularity and frequent (often continuous) use of air "freshening" and scenting candles, sprays, plug-ins, etc. A clean home will be odorless; however, many American consumers have become fond of scenting their home. There are effective ways to ensure that your home has a pleasant scent without using expensive commercial scenting products, for example using flowers or essential oils.

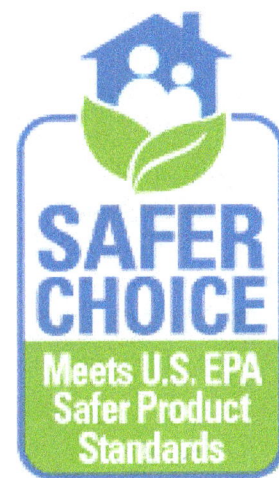

epa.gov/saferchoice

Reprint of EPA Safer Choice Label (2021), reproduced as part of public domain.

SAFER CLEANING PRACTICES IN HOMES

The COVID-19 pandemic highlighted the importance of handwashing and keeping our homes and workplaces clean to reduce the environmental risk of a pathogen such as the SARS-CoV-2 virus. However, when selecting products and cleaning methods we must consider what is the purpose of our cleaning and understand commonly used terms. To reduce exposure of family members to chemicals in the home, greener cleaning products can easily be made from common household ingredients. Many of these cleaning substances have been used effectively for years, but have fallen out of favor due to the successful marketing of "new and improved" methods.

Cleaning, disinfecting, and sanitizing are frequently used interchangeably, but they have very different meanings. *Cleaning* involves removing the dirt and debris on surfaces or objects (CDC, n.d.a.). Soap or a detergent can be used to clean. If everyone in the household is healthy and does not have an infectious disease, general cleaning is appropriate using soap or a detergent. According to the

CDC, cleaning frequently used surfaces removes most pathogens, such as viruses (CDC, 2021). If someone within the home has an infectious disease such a strep throat or the seasonal flu, disinfecting may be needed. Before disinfecting, cleaning of the area or object must occur, then *disinfecting* is done to kill pathogens, such as bacteria. Safer disinfectants have hydrogen peroxide or alcohol as the active ingredient (EPA, n.d.b.). Avoid products with ammonia or bleach and NEVER combine bleach and ammonia; as together, these chemicals create a toxic gas. When using a disinfectant, be sure to follow the instructions and leave on the surface or object for the time directed on the label (CDC, n.d.). *Sanitizing* is done to reduce the overall number of pathogens. Sanitizing is typically reserved for areas where many people come together and there is a risk of infections such as a restaurant or clinic. Examples of sanitizing are using a dishwashing machine or antibacterial wipes (CDC, n.d.).

Some people prefer to use fewer chemicals within their homes to reduce exposure of family members to chemicals., These home recipes that have been used effectively for years, but have fallen out of favor due to the successful marketing of more convenient manufactured products. It is important to note that many of these home recipes have not been tested and often people do not follow the recipe and make their own adaptations. Thus, this is a challenging area to study for safety and efficacy. Nevertheless, we are sharing some common techniques of green cleaning in the home. These products are only recommended for cleaning and no for disinfecting or sanitizing. This is an area for further nursing research.

CLEANING BASICS

One strategy for keeping the home clean is to reduce clutter, which in turn reduces dust. In addition, some houseplants are effective at removing toxins from the air. Through photosynthesis, houseplants use carbon dioxide and emit oxygen and can remove a significant amount of toxic chemicals from the air. Recommended plants include English Ivy, ferns, and rubber plants (Leader, 2013).

Avoid using "antibacterial" soaps and cleaners as they are unnecessary for cleanliness and can be harmful. Many antibacterial products contain triclosan, which has been associated with endocrine system disruption, environmental pollution, and the increasing emergence of drug-resistant strains of bacteria. In addition, antibacterial soaps offer no additional health benefits over washing with soap and water (U.S. Food and Drug Administration, 2013).

Basic cleaning ingredients include the following:

- Distilled water (for mixing ingredients – works better than tap water)

- Baking soda (abrasive)

- Liquid dish soap (non-toxic formula)

- White vinegar (deodorizer, disinfectant)

- Hydrogen peroxide (disinfectant, whitener)

- Lemons (disinfectant, deodorizer, degreaser)

- Spray bottle

- Essential oils (optional, for scenting). Suggestions: lavender, lemongrass, lemon, lime, orange, cinnamon, clove, pine, rose, tea tree.

- Cotton rags (recommended over commercial products that are often made from plastics) (D a d d , 2011; Findley & Formichelli, 2009)

Other helpful items for specific purposes include the following: activated charcoal (deodorant), raw potatoes, (to remove rust from cookware), isopropyl "rubbing" alcohol (disinfectant), and newspapers (use for window washing instead of paper towels).

RECIPES FOR HOME-MADE CLEANING PRODUCTS
(adapted from Dadd, 2011 and Findley & Formicelli, 2009)

All-purpose Cleaner:
1 part white vinegar
2 parts liquid soap
4 parts water
2-3 drops of essential oil (optional) for scenting

Mix ingredients in a spray bottle. This mixture can be used as a basic cleaner for kitchen and bath surfaces, as well as a window cleaner.

Disinfectant:
White vinegar **or**
Hydrogen peroxide
(do not mix)

Wipe with straight white vinegar, followed by hydrogen peroxide for particularly messy clean-ups, for example after handling raw meat. For best results, use hydrogen peroxide from a bottle that has been open for less than six months.

Abrasive Scrub:
Baking soda
Liquid soap

Place baking soda in a dish. Add soap until it makes a paste; dilute with a small amount of water if desired for a looser mixture. Apply to a sponge or brush and scrub.

CLEANING A HOME, SPECIAL TOPICS
(adapted from Dadd, 2011 and Findley & Formicelli, 2009)

KITCHEN
Oven:

2 cups hot water
1 tablespoon liquid soap
1 teaspoon baking soda

First, remove as much soil as possible by scrubbing with crumpled aluminum foil or newspaper. Mix ingredients, apply to soiled areas, let stand for 20 minutes and wipe off. Repeat a needed.

Drain (with garbage disposal) Opener:

1 quart hot water
1 tablespoon of liquid soap

Boil water, then add soap. Pour directly into the drain.

Grill Cleaner:

Crumple aluminum foil into a ball and use as a scrub.

Rusty Cookware:

Cut a raw potato in half. Dip the cut end in salt or baking soda and use as a scrub.

BATHROOM

Toilet Bowl Cleaner:

1 cup vinegar
¼ cup baking soda

Mix ingredients and let sit for 15 minutes to a few hours in the toilet bowl (Overnight is another suggested method). Scrub and flush.

Drain Opener:

1 cup vinegar
½ cup baking soda

Combine the ingredients and pour into the drain. Let sit for 15-20 minutes. Rinse with hot water. Repeat if necessary or leave the mixture to sit overnight.

Mold/Mildew Remover:

2 parts water
1 part hydrogen peroxide

Mix ingredients and spray affected area. Let stand for 10-15 minutes and wipe clean. (Note: hydrogen peroxide may bleach surfaces such as wallpaper, linens or clothing.)

Mirror cleaner:

Use all-purpose cleaner, above. Or half vinegar and half water.

Tub and tile cleaner:

Use abrasive scrub, above.

LIVING AREAS
Dusting/Furniture Polish:
Lemon or pine essential oil
Liquid beeswax

Mix the ingredients and apply a small amount to a lint-free cotton cloth and wipe surfaces.

Windows:

Use the all-purpose cleaner, above. Wipe with newspapers.

Air Freshening:

Baking soda is a traditional and effective odor eliminator. Place an open box in areas where odors accumulate. Some ideas for home scenting include:

- Add essential oils to an aromatherapy infuser. Alternately, mix an essential oil with water in a spray bottle and spritz the air or surfaces. (Try a small amount first to make sure the oils do not stain fabrics.)

- Decorate with fresh or dried flowers, herbs, or citrus

- Simmer aromatics (e.g., citrus fruits or cinnamon) to combat cooking odors.

- Soy candles with essential oils are available commercially.

- Remember to bring in some fresh air from time to time. Even in winter, on milder days briefly open a window a few inches.

CLEANING CLOTHING
Washing:

In general, washing machines clean clothing in cold water as effectively as in hot or warm water. Hot water is needed only for heavily soiled items (such as diapers) or greasy items.

1 bar natural soap, shaved
1 cup borax* or baking soda
1 cup washing soda

Combine the ingredients and store. If a liquid detergent is desired, use liquid (e.g., castile) soap and heat the ingredients in enough water to cover and mix.

*Note: While borax is commonly recommended as a laundry booster, and is safe for the environment, the

Environmental Working Group (EWG) rates borax as "high concern" for developmental and reproductive toxicity and is best avoided, particularly by women and children (EWG, 2011; EGW, 2014).

Fabric softener:

Add distilled white vinegar or baking soda to the rinse cycle.

Drying:

Clothes dryers are the second-largest users of home appliance energy, after refrigerators (Steingraber, 2011). They are also a leading cause of home fires. Keep in mind that the purpose of a clothes dryer is to evaporate water; wet clothing would dry anyway if exposed to air. The sun has been the traditional "solar dryer" since humans began wearing clothing. A brief time spent outdoors can save energy and money and leave your clothing smelling fresh. (Be careful of pollen if allergies are a problem for your family members.) Indoor drying systems can be used in inclement or cold weather. Heavy clothing, such as jeans and towels, can be dried in the drier for 10-15 minutes to remove wrinkles, and then air dried.

DRY CLEANING

The standard cleaning solvent used in commercial dry cleaning facilities is tetrachlorethylene (perchloroethylene), or "perc". The Environmental Protection Agency (EPA) classifies perc as "likely to be carcinogenic" (EPA, 2012). While the EPA does not recommend that consumers avoid wearing clothing that has been dry cleaned with perc, the solvent is a highly toxic environmental contaminant. Consumers can look for dry cleaner facilities that use less toxic methods, such as liquid silicone ("D5"), liquid CO2, or Professional Wet Cleaning (PWC). If clothing is dry cleaned with perc, remove the plastic and air out the clothing prior to bringing it into the home. When purchasing clothing, consider buying garments that can be machine or hand washed.

INTEGRATED PEST MANAGEMENT

Integrated Pest Management (IPM) is an environmentally sensitive approach to pest control. IPM uses knowledge of the behavior and life cycles of pests to achieve the least possible hazard to people, property, and the environment (EPA, 2014). Pests need a place to live, food, and water. The first step in the home setting is to avoid keeping food in open containers and to keep surfaces free of food and soil. In addition, cracks and holes where pests enter the home should be repaired. Fix areas where there are water leaks, such as pipes and faucets.

Avoid using insect sprays and foggers; in general, enclosed traps expose family members to fewer chemicals. Be sure to handle any traps according to the directions and keep out of the reach of children. For crawling insects, food-grade diatomaceous earth, a non-toxic fine powder, can be applied to surfaces where these pests are found, such as in cracks and crevices, in garbage cans, or in drains. But keep this powder away from pets, children, and food. When seeking a pest management company, select a company that uses integrated pest management.

RESOURCES

* Guides to product safety: Environmental Working Group
* Toxic substances information: Agency for Toxic Substances and Disease Registry
* Pediatric environmental hazards: Children's Environmental Health Network
* Green Seal of Approval
* Health indoor living information: Healthy House Institute
* Alternatives to pesticides: Pesticide Action Network
* Information/advocacy on cold-washing and air-drying laundry: Project Laundry List
* Information/advocacy on protecting families from toxic chemicals: Safer Chemicals, Healthy Families
* Information/advocacy for safer products for women: Women's Voices for the Earth

REFERENCES

Center for Disease Control and Prevention (n.d.) *How to clean and disinfect schools to heap stop the spread of flu.* https://www.cdc.gov/flu/school/cleaning.htm

Center for Disease Control and Prevention (2021). *Cleaning and disinfecting your home: Every day and when someone is sick.* https://www.cdc.gov/coronavirus/2019-ncov/prevent-getting-sick/disinfecting-your-home.html

Dadd, D. (2011). *Toxic free.* Jeremy P. Tarcher/Penguin.

Environmental Working Group (EWG). (2011). *Borax: Not the green alternative it's cracked up to be.* http://www.ewg.org/enviroblog/2011/02/borax-not-green-alternative-its-cracked-be

Environmental Working Group (EWG). (2014). *EWG's guide to healthy cleaning.* http://www.ewg.org/guides/cleaners/

2507-20MuleTeamBoraxNaturalLaundryBoosterMultiPurposeHouseholdCleaner

Findley, M. & Formichelli, L. (2009). *The Complete idiot's guide to green cleaning* (2nd ed.). Penguin.

Leader, D. (2013). *Ten houseplants that may purify indoor air.* http://copd.about.com/od/livingwithcopd/tp/10-Houseplants-That-May-Purify-Indoor-Air.htm

Steingraber, S. (2011). *Raising Elijah.* Perseus.

U.S. Environmental Protection Agency (EPA). (2012). *EPA releases final health assessment for tetrachloroethylene (perc): Public health protections remain in place.* https://yosemite.epa.gov/opa/admpress.nsf/0/e99fd55271ce029f852579a000624956

U.S. Environmental Protection Agency (EPA). (n.d.a.). *Volatile organic compounds' impact on indoor air quality.* https://www.epa.gov/indoor-air-quality-iaq/volatile-organic-compounds-impact-indoor-air-quality

U.S. Environmental Protection Agency (n.d.b). *Learn about the Safer Choice Label.* https://www.epa.gov/saferchoice/learn-about-safer-choice-label

U.S. Environmental Protection Agency (EPA). (2014). *Integrated pest management principles.* http://www.epa.gov/pesticides/factsheets/ipm.htm

U.S. Food and Drug Administration (FDA). (2013). *Triclosan: What consumers should know.* http://www.fda.gov/ForConsumers/ucm205999.htm

TRANSPORTATION AND HEALTH IMPLICATIONS
Lillian Mood, RN, MPH, FAAN
Retired, South Carolina Department of Health and
Environmental Control
Columbia, SC

In addressing health issues, transportation is almost always part of the problem or part of the solution. That is so whether improving air quality, getting children immunized, providing early prenatal care, utilizing appropriate preventive and primary care services, or responding to an emergency. Transportation can be defined broadly as the means of moving people and goods to desired destinations. Transportation includes public transit options of rail and bus; individual automobile use and shared rides; bicycling and walking.

The health benefits of active transportation that includes biking and walking as part of a pattern of regular exercise are well known in preventing obesity and numerous chronic diseases, and in promoting health and quality of life. In fact, Maizlish and colleagues (2013) found that physical activity was increased from four to 22 minutes a day, the risk of cardiovascular disease and diabetes was decreased by 14%.

Public transit carries with it exercise benefits because transit riders walk or bike to transit stops. In addition, public transit lessens the health effects of air and water pollution, the risk of injury and deaths from automobile accidents, the stresses of driving in congested traffic and driver road rage. An often overlooked benefit of transit is its role in developing a sense of community among regular riders, reducing social isolation as a risk to health.

Adequate, available, affordable public transit provides access to health care, to jobs, to education, to grocery stores, to religious and social gatherings, all of which are essential components of healthy living. Without alternatives to driving individual cars, some of the most vulnerable segments of the population—the poor, persons with disabilities, the elderly—are even more likely to be unable to meet basic requirements for daily living, much less to have productive roles in society. Not having to own a car or reduced use of an automobile lessens stress on family budgets.

Public transportation helps alleviate environmental, energy, and economic problems. As documented in the American Public Transportation Association's 2014 Fact Book: "Public transportation plays an important role in reducing the nation's energy use and greenhouse gas emissions. Due to the combined reduction in private passenger vehicle miles, reduced automobile congestion and reduced travel distances due to the proximity created by public transportation, more than 4 billion gallons of gasoline are saved and 37 million metric tons of carbon dioxide emissions are avoided" (APTA, 2014, p.21).

"According to the US Environmental Protection Agency's Greenhouse Gas Calculator, it would require 7.2 million acres of new pine or fir forests per year to match the annual carbon dioxide reductions provided by public transportation. Priced at $3.60 per gallon, the 4 billion gallons of gasoline saved annually saves the US consumer $14.4 billion per year" (APTA, 2014, p.21).

"Transit's impact on reducing congestion has also resulted in significant savings for drivers and their communities. Without transit, drivers would have used 450 million more gallons of gasoline because of added roadway congestion during 2011. Drivers would have been stuck in traffic an additional 865 million hours if there were no transit. Overall, the costs of congestion to drivers would have been an additional $20.8 billion if there had been no transit service" (APTA 2014 Fact Book, p. 21-22).

Opportunities for improving health through transportation include:

3. Policies that support adequate funding for public transit as well as safe roads.

4. Built community design/modification that includes:

    • cross streets,

    • eliminating single entrance/exit neighborhoods,

    • safe spaces for walking and biking for children and adults, i.e. bike lanes/paths, sidewalks, to shops, restaurants, work, and entertainment.

    • mixed used neighborhoods to increase ease of access to shopping and services

5. Applying proven strategies for rural transit, e.g., van pools, park and rides, flexible routes.

6. Use of existing and additional rail lines for passenger as well as freight service.

7. Programs that assist first time riders, especially the elderly.

8. Collaborative efforts with schools and employers to encourage, facilitate and provide incentives for transit use.

REFERENCES

American Public Transportation Association. (2014). *2014 Public transportation fact book*. http://www.apta.com/

resources/statistics/Documents/FactBook/2014-APTA-Fact-Book.pdf

Maizlish, N., Woodcock, J., Co, S., Ostro, B., Fanai, A., & Fairley, D. (2013). Health co-benefits and transportation-related reductions in greenhouse gas emissions in the San Francisco Bay area. *American Journal of Public Health, 103*(4), 703–709. doi: 10.2105/AJPH.2012.300939.

BROWNFIELDS AND NURSING IMPLICATIONS
Robyn Gilden, PhD, RN
Director, Environmental Health Certificate Program
Associate Professor, Family and Community Health
University of Maryland
School of Nursing

In this chapter we will learn what brownfields are and what the nursing implications should be related to them. This will include nursing education, practice, policy/advocacy, and research.

DEFINITION OF A BROWNFIELD

Brownfields can be defined in a variety of ways, but the term typically refers to urban industrial or commercial facilities that are abandoned or underutilized due, in part, to environmental contamination or fear of contamination. There have been special efforts in recent years to target brownfields for cleanup and reuse for several reasons, including the potential to revitalize distressed communities, increase tax dollars, and provide new jobs.

AUTHORIZING LEGISLATION AND ENVIRONMENTAL PROTECTION AGENCY (EPA) MISSION

In January, 2002, Public Law 107-118 (H.R. 2869): "Small Business Liability Relief and Brownfields Revitalization Act" was enacted:

"To provide certain relief for small businesses from liability under the Comprehensive Environmental Response, Compensation, and Liability Act of 1980, and to amend such Act to promote the cleanup and reuse of brownfields, to provide financial assistance for brownfields revitalization, to enhance State response programs, and for other purposes" (GPO, 2002). EPA's Brownfields Initiative empowers States, communities, and other stakeholders in economic development to work together in a timely manner to prevent, assess, safely clean up, and sustainably reuse brownfields.

WHY IS THE BROWNFIELDS ISSUE IMPORTANT?

In recent years, many manufacturing plants and military bases have closed or relocated. Often, new development on these "brownfield" sites is made difficult by real or perceived environmental contamination. Through the Brownfields Cleanup and Redevelopment Program, EPA helps states, tribes, communities, and other organizations to:

- environmentally assess existing properties,
- prevent further contamination,
- safely clean up polluted properties, and
- design plans to re-use them.

EPA's investment in the Brownfields Program has resulted in many accomplishments, including leveraging more than $14 billion in brownfields cleanup and redevelopment funding from the private and public sectors and leveraging approximately 60,917 jobs. The momentum generated by the Program is leaving an enduring legacy. The Brownfields Program and its partners have provided guidance and incentives to support economic revitalization, and empower communities to address the brownfields in their midst. EPA's Brownfield Program continues to look to the future by expanding the types of properties it addresses, forming new partnerships, and undertaking new initiatives to help revitalize communities across the nation (EPA, 2015).

To view the brownfields and other related sites in your area, go to Clean-ups in my Community. You have a choice of mapping cleanups across the USA, mapping or listing cleanups for a ZIP code or city, or creating a table of cleanups or grants.

STATE EXAMPLE: MARYLAND

As indicated above, EPA does not regulate the Brownfields program alone, but delegate's authority to the States. States take a wide range of approaches and use an assortment of tools. Some States specifically address brownfields through their voluntary cleanup programs, others supplement their voluntary program activities, and still others have separate brownfields cleanup and redevelopment programs.

In Maryland, this program is called the Brownfields Redevelopment Initiative (MD Department of the Environment, 2015). Brownfields are included in Voluntary Cleanup Program and the goals are:

1. Encourage the investigation of eligible properties with known or perceived contamination;

2. Protect public health and the environment where cleanup projects are being performed or need to be performed;

3. Accelerate cleanup of eligible properties; and

4. Provide predictability and finality to the cleanup of eligible properties (MD Code, 1997).

WHY NURSES?

So what can nurses bring to the very technical world of hazardous waste cleanup, like brownfields? There are actually a lot of important roles that we are uniquely trained to do. We can:

- Enhance community connections / facilitate dialog

- Identify populations at risk

- Improve community education and risk communication

- Expand the multidisciplinary nature of your environmental health (EH) work

- Assist with translating science into policy

- Enlist undergraduate and graduate students for data collection.

CHALLENGES OF COMMUNITY INVOLVEMENT AT BROWNFIELD CLEANUPS

One of my former roles was providing community outreach and technical assistance to residents with hazardous waste sites in their midst. Through the six plus years I worked for the US EPA funded Hazardous Substances Research Center (the only regional center that had a school of nursing conducting the outreach), I learned some important lessons.

Including all stakeholders: It was often difficult to know who the stakeholders were, when first interacting with a community. I was often approached by a small group of concerned citizens or someone from the local government. This is not a comprehensive list, but you need to make sure to include:

- Community members

- Local businesses

- Representatives from local, state and federal government

- Local and state health department

- Department of Environment

- Health care providers

- Religious leaders

- Schools

- Financial institutions

- Developers

- Contractors

- Youth

- Responsible party(s)

Multiple agendas: I learned very early, there were often multiple agendas and they were not always obvious. Mostly citizens were concerned about health and then property values or effect on business. Then there would be other hidden agendas, like avoiding liability.

Who's in charge: One of my major tasks was trying to help the community understand the roadmap of who was in charge of the decision-making authority. Depending on the type of site and what city and state it is in, who is in charge can change. It is possible for EPA or State Department of Environment to have the lead. Also involved will be potentially responsible parties and their contractors, EPA's contractors, other consultants, Agency for Toxic Substances and Disease Registry (ATSDR), State Health Department, Local Health Department, and other local officials.

Agency responsibilities and limitations: Closely tied to who is in charge, is what each organization is allowed to do by the regulations that govern them. EPA and state departments are directed and limited by their legislative mandates. There are some things they have to do and some processes are set by the regulations. Some things they have no control over. For example, they cannot address property values or zoning; this is a local level issue. That is why it is important to have a large group of stakeholders at the table, so if an issue does not fall under one agency, it probably does fall under another.

POLICY GAPS

After introducing the brownfields definition, legislation, program and implementation, some policy gaps have been identified for future advocacy:

- Environmental justice in permitting process: Need to consider the cumulative impacts already in the community before siting new facilities.

- No program exists to address community-wide elevations of background contaminants

- No program exists to address multimedia problems

- No program exists to address school siting. Some sites do not have coverage under current regulations; schools are one of these. They often fall through the cracks and a school can build without any testing or cleanup.

ADDITIONAL RESOURCES

National Library of Medicine

- MEDLINEplus

- TOXNET

Agency for Toxic Substances and Disease Registry

- ToxFAQs

- Toxicological Profiles

Environmental Protection Agency

- Envirofacts

- IRIS

- Tools and Technical Information

- Brownfield Training Conference Newsletter emails

REFERENCES

Maryland Code (1997). *Voluntary cleanup program.* http://www.lexisnexis.com/hottopics/mdcode/

Maryland Department of the Environment (2015). *Brownfields Redevelopment Initiative.* http://www.mde.state.md.us/programs/Land/MarylandBrownfieldVCP/Pages/programs/landprograms/errp_brownfields/bf_info/index.aspx

US Environmental Protection Agency (2015). *Brownfield and land revitalization basic information.* http://www.epa.gov/brownfields/basic_info.htm

U.S. Government Printing Office (2002). *Public Law 107-118 (H.R. 2869): "Small Business Liability Relief and Brownfields Revitalization Act".* http://www.gpo.gov/fdsys/pkg/PLAW-107publ118/html/PLAW-107publ118.htm

HEALTH IMPLICATIONS OF FOOD AND AGRICULTURE
Barbara Sattler, RN, DrPH, FAAN
Professor Emeritus
University of San Francisco

INTRODUCTION

In Michael Pollan's best-selling book The Omnivore's Dilemma, he characterizes the American people as collectively suffering from a "food disorder" (Pollan, 2006). In the context of Pollan's critique of the American diet, we are suffering from an abundance of food choices but a lack of understanding about how our food is grown and raised, processed and transported, marketed and ultimately shows up on our plate, or too often eaten from a to-go container.

We further lack an understanding about the abiding relationship between our health and what we eat. As a result, we have both an epidemic of obesity and a crisis of chronic diseases. This chapter is not about human nutrition but rather about some of the public health implications of how we grow and raise our food. Having said that, there is a growing understanding of "food as medicine" which explicitly recognizes the benefits of healthy foods generally and of specific foods in terms of their ability to ward off chronic diseases and address specific health effects, including diabetes and cardiovascular diseases.

As nurses, we encourage people to eat a "healthy diet" but what do we really know about how healthy our food is - for the immediate consumer of the food, for those that farmed and harvested it, for those involved in its slaughter and processing, and equally importantly for the ecosystem that supports it all along the way. On average food products in the US travel 1,500 miles from farm to table. (CUESA, n.d.) This reliance on distant food sources alone is a significant contributor to climate change. This chapter will review some of the human and ecological health impacts of our current agricultural practices.

MODERN FARM PRACTICES

For many people who do not live in agricultural areas our image of a "farm" is often some variation on the theme of a beautiful green setting with cows and chickens and corn fields, images that evoke the many "farm toys" and "farm books" that are created for children – the ones with the big red barns. The truth is that most of the food in the US is produced by single-animal or single-crop production and on very large scales.

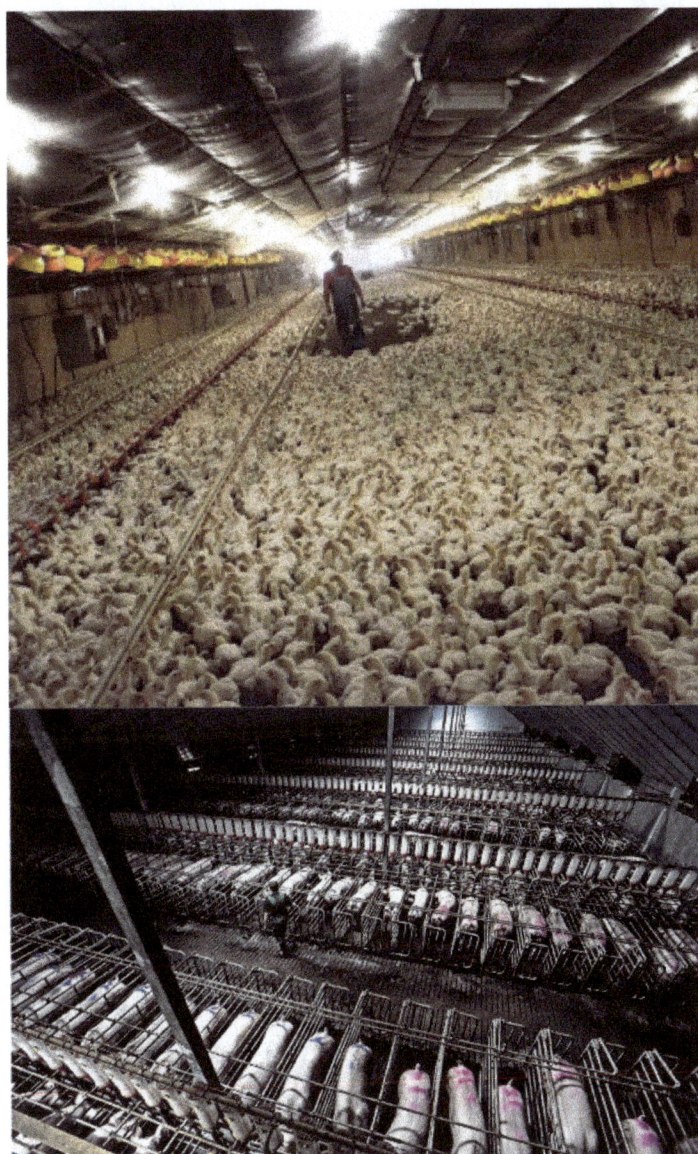

50,000,000,000 animals are raised and slaughtered in factory farms globally each year. (Duda, 2016)

Meat Animals

Confined Animal Feed Operations

In terms of meat animal production, the idealized farm has been replaced by Confined Animal Feeding Operations (CAFOs) which are the type of animal production facilities that are sometimes referred to as factory farms. These facilities house over a thousand large animals like beef cows or hogs, and tens of thousands of chickens. Over 50% of our meat in the US is derived from animals in CAFOs, even though they comprise only 5% of US farms. This gives a sense of the scale of their production (UCS, https://www.organicconsumers.org/sites/default/files/cafos_uncovered.pdf).

There are a great many human and ecological health issues that arise when raising animals this way. There is also the obvious ethical one regarding the inhumane way in which the animals are treated.

The most significant ecological issue is waste management. Animal waste is not regulated in the same way that human waste is. For example, an adult hog can produce 7 pounds of waste a day, which in the case of a 5,000-hog CAFO translates to 245,000 pounds of hog manure a week. In hog production, lagoons are created to hold the combined urine and manure. The contents of these "holding" ponds can leach into the ground and overflow into nearby waterways, particularly when there are extreme rain events – perhaps indicating that hold-nothing ponds might be a better term. These lagoons also produce air pollutants, including volatilized ammonia, and extremely noxious odors that are associated with health risks to the nearby community. Airborne ammonia is also a known respiratory irritant. The farmworkers who work inside the pig barns have increased risk of respiratory disfunction that is associated with gases, microbes, endotoxins, and dust (Charavaryamath and Singh, 2006).

When released into nearby waters, two main components of manure, nitrogen and phosphorus, can cause eutrophication – which acts like aquatic fertilizer and causes the proliferation of certain plants and organisms that rob the waterways of oxygen thus killing the fish and other marine life. Further downstream and into bays and oceans this eutrophication is responsible for dead zones, which have occurred in the Gulf of Mexico and the Chesapeake Bay.

Companies that operate CAFOs have been able to reduce their costs by their "economy of scale" but also through significant public subsidies, including (until very recently) low-cost feed. They have also benefited from taxpayer-supported pollution cleanup programs and technological "fixes" that may be counterproductive to overall human and public health, such as the overuse of antibiotics (Gurian-Sherman, 2008).

When our tax dollars are used to subsidize bad farming processes, then better/good farming practices appear, by comparison, to be less cost effective. But if smaller scale sustainable farms were on a level economic playing field, they would be equally and even more efficient. There is clear evidence that smaller scale, pasture-based production can be profitable and better for the environment. Later in this chapter we will discuss the US Farm Bill that is responsible for setting food production subsidies and many other food-related policies.

Antibiotic Use in Animal Production

No nurse farmer would allow their animal to suffer with an infection for which an antibiotic exists. But the majority of antibiotics used in animal production are not prescribed for infections. Low (non-therapeutic) levels of antibiotics have been found to increase the weight of animals – as much as 5%. Given that farmers and ranchers sell their meat animals by the pound, using antibiotics in the feed of their otherwise healthy animals has become a regular practice.

According to the FDA, more than 20 million pounds of medically important antibiotic drugs were sold for use on livestock farms in 2014 — about 80 percent of all antibiotics sold in the country (Center for Veterinary Medicine, 2015). These antibiotics wind up in the guts of meat animals and they wind up in the manure. This results in manure-related run-off into waterways and manure that may be spread on fields where food crops are grown. The presence of antibiotics in our environments create the conditions for antibiotic-resistant organisms to develop. Community-acquired antibiotic resistant infections are on the rise and a major public health concern. We also know that workers in chicken houses, where non-therapeutic antibiotics are put in the chickens' water, develop antibiotic-resistant organisms in their guts (RuleSean et al, 2008).

Since 2017, the US Department of Agriculture has decreed that medically important antibiotics – those used for treated humans – should not be used to promote animal growth. There are still numbers of antibiotics that are being used, however, and as a result, antibiotic resistant organisms are likely to keep developing.

The former Director-General of the World Health Organization (WHO), Margaret Chan, noted that, "[I]n the absence of urgent corrective and protective actions, the world is heading toward a post-antibiotic era, in which many common infections will no longer have a cure and, once again, kill unabated" (Chan, 2011). WHO released the first-ever report on global antibiotic resistance in 2014, outlining the serious threat antibiotic-resistant bacteria present to public health around the world (WHO, 2014). This is an issue that is extremely important for nurses to track and to engage in policy decisions that aid in the prevention of antibiotic resistant organisms.

HORMONE USE IN ANIMAL PRODUCTION

Beef Cattle

Since the 1950s, the US Food and Drug Administration (FDA) has approved a number of steroid hormone drugs for use in beef cattle and sheep, including natural estrogen, progesterone, testosterone, and their synthetic versions

(US FDA, 2020). The steroids are delivered via a subcutaneous implant. [No steroid hormone implants are approved for growth purposes in dairy cows, veal calves, pigs, or poultry.] Europe has had a non-hormone treated cattle (NHTC) program since 1999 and China limits its acceptance of US meat imports because of hormone usage. Few long-term studies have been done to establish the human health risks.

Dairy Cows

The hormone that is given to dairy cows is bovine somatotropin (bST), also known as bovine growth hormone or recombinant bovine growth hormone (rBGH). It is an animal drug approved by the FDA to increase milk production in dairy cows (US FDA, 2020). Fifteen to 20% of US dairy cows receive rBGH and there is some controversy regarding the potential human health risks associated with this hormone. In their 2015 review article, Malekinejad and Rezebakhch found that "the presence of steroid hormones in dairy products could be counted as an important risk factor for various cancers in humans" (Malekinejad & Rezebakhch, 2015). The FDA does not consider rBGH a health threat to humans. However, the American Cancer Society notes that there have been studies showing strong associations between consuming dairy products from cows that have been given rBGH and certain cancers (prostate, breast, and colorectal) and it must be noted that there have been studies showing little evidence of association (ACS, 2014).

Nevertheless, there is adequate evidence that rBGH can be harmful to the cows that receive it. The health effects that they experience are the following: 50% increase in lameness, 25% increase in mastitis, as well as increased risk for infertility problems, cystic ovaries, fetal loss, and birth defects (Center for Food Safety, n.d.). The increase in mastitis is then associated with increased use of antibiotics.

Regarding rBGH, the following recommendation for Nurse Actions is part of Health Care Without Harm's factsheet on rBGH:

What Nurses Can Do

1. **Educate yourself & other nurses with the Nurse's Toolkit on rBGH.** You'll find scientific studies & other important information from Health Care Without Harm on rBGH. Visit: https://noharm-global.org/documents/nurses-are-concerned-artificial-growth-hormones-dairy-products..

2. **Educate your patients.** Ask them to read the "Know Your Milk" brochure & watch the video from the Oregon Physicians for Social Responsibility's Campaign for Safe Food. Visit: www.oregonpsr.org.

3. **Purchase organic or rBGH-free dairy products** and encourage your family and your patients to do the same. For a list of rBGH-free dairy products in your state from Food and Water Watch, visit: www.foodandwaterwatch.org.

4. **Ask your hospital or health care facility to purchase rBGH-free dairy products** and join other hospitals around the country in doing so. For more information, visit: www.healthyfoodinhealthcare.org.

5. **Start a green team or food committee at your hospital or health care facility** to address these and many other environmental health and healthy food concerns.

The whole factsheet can be found here: https://noharm-uscanada.org/sites/default/files/documents-files/131/Nurses_Concerned_rBGH.pdf

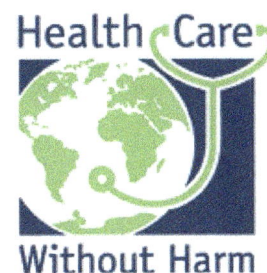

PLANT-BASED FOODS

The first things that we need to know about healthy plant food production – healthy for humans and healthy for whole ecosystems – is what is going on with our soil, seeds, and pollinators, along with water and climate. And then we can move on to other critical topics, like farmworker health and safety, pesticides, and climate.

Soil

"The nation that destroys its soil destroys itself." Franklin Roosevelt

Soil is the organic matter and minerals on the surface of the land on which plants and other life grows. Without soil, we will have no food. And yet, we have been in a steady state of abusing and losing soil, one of nature's most important gifts to us. Each year, an estimated 50 trillion pounds of fertile soil are lost due to erosion. That is 7,500 pounds lost every year for every person on the planet (UNCCD, 2015. This fertile soil either blows away or erodes and runs towards the oceans via creeks, stream, rivers, and lakes.

Soil is so much more than dirt – it's alive. Soil is a living ecosystem—a large community of living organisms linked together through nutrient cycles and energy flows. Every teaspoon of soil is home to billions of microorganisms—

bacteria, fungi, nematodes, insects, and earthworms that each play important roles (UME, 2018).

As we are only recently discovering the importance of the human microbiome, soil scientists have long understood the importance of the microbiome of the soil. And it turns out there is a connection between the two. Clinical interventions to improve our human microbiome with probiotics and prebiotics are showing promise.

Just as we have unwittingly destroyed vital microbes in the human gut through overuse of antibiotics and highly processed foods, we have recklessly devastated soil microbiota essential to plant health through overuse of certain chemical fertilizers, fungicides, herbicides, pesticides, failure to add sufficient organic matter (upon which they feed), and heavy tillage. These soil microorganisms -- particularly bacteria and fungi -- cycle nutrients and water to plants, to our crops, the source of our food, and ultimately our health. Soil bacteria and fungi serve as the "stomachs" of plants. They form symbiotic relationships with plant roots and "digest" nutrients, providing nitrogen, phosphorus, and many other nutrients in a form that plant cells can assimilate. Reintroducing the right bacteria and fungi to facilitate the dark fermentation process in depleted and sterile soils is analogous to eating yogurt (or taking those targeted probiotic)…to restore the right microbiota deep in your digestive tract (Amaranthus and Allen, 2013).

We are now in a place where critical soil microbes that are necessary for healthy soil have been destroyed in many large-scale, single crop (mono-culture) commercial agricultural enterprises. These are the microbes that would otherwise be helping plants to access, conserve, and cycle nutrients and water for plants and, equally importantly, regulate climate. The result is dying soil and crops that are losing their nutrient content.

To shore up the deficits in our soil, the US has become a major importer of synthetic fertilizers. Though only 5% of the world's population, the US uses 12% of the world's synthetic nitrogen fertilizer which is produced by natural gas (fossil fuel) powered ammonia plants in countries like Trinidad and Tobago (Philpott, 2010). Consider the climate change contribution that producing and transporting fertilizers is making to greenhouse gases. In this way, modern industrial farming is extractive – continually taking from the soil and using petrochemical fertilizers and other fossil-fuel related inputs to make up the difference.

In instances where conventional, mono-culture farming continues, the introduction of micro-organisms into the soil has been shown to increase nutrient up-take and reduce water needs. This trend is in play as the bio-fertility (micro-organisms) industry has become a $500 million industry. This is yet another industry that is using energy, water and other resources and transporting product.

[To better learn about the plight of soil on earth, watch Dirt: The Movie, a great documentary available for free on YouTube.]

The following are a set of tips that nurses (and others) can follow to support healthy soil.

Six tips for healthy soil in your garden

1. Test your soil (Google "soil testing" in your city / county).

2. Add organic matter.

3. Incorporate compost to compacted soil to increase air, water and nutrients for plants.

4. Protect topsoil with mulch or cover crops.

5. Don't use potentially harmful chemicals.

6. Rotate the annual vegetable crops.

For a fuller explanation of each of these tips, go to : https://extension.umn.edu/how-manage-soil-and-nutrients-home-gardens/living-soil-healthy-garden

As is often true, once we are clear about the problem, we can work on the solutions. First and foremost, we have discovered that organic farming, no-till (or minimum tilling) farming, cover crops, and rotating crops can help naturally replenish the soil and keep it healthy. We need to be incentivizing these farm practices.

SEEDS

There is something wonderful about the similarity between human and plant embryos - in both, an entire life form begins.

Seeds are host to plant embryos, much like the womb, and every plant, including our food plants begin with a seed.

Seed Basics:

There are 3 types of seeds:

1. Heirloom Seeds or Open-Pollinated Seeds are sometimes known as "true to type" seeds. They come from plants that are naturally pollinated. They will grow into

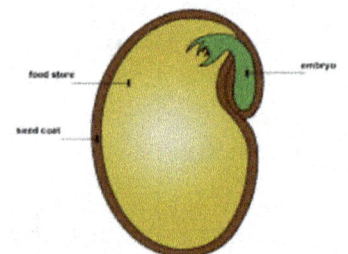

plants from which you can harvest the seeds and grow an identical plant again and again. Most heirlooms have been around a long time – centuries or more.

2. Hybrid Seeds are created by humans by crossing two varieties of the same plant (species). If you harvest the seeds from these plants for next year, there is no guarantee that you will get a plant that looks the same as its parent.

3. Genetically Modified Seeds are created by selecting traits that are expressed in genetic materials from not just other varieties of plants, but even other species (like fish) and inserting them into the genetic makeup of the new plant seed. This is an excellent short (7-minute) video explaining the process of genetic modification. Stick with the video to see the scientific explanation. It is quite an amazing scientific feat.

Another thing you may see on a seed packet is the USDA Certified Organic symbol. Those seeds come from plants that were grown without the use of chemical pesticides or synthetic fertilizers and on soil that does not contain sewage sludge.

One of the things that GMO seeds have been designed to do is resist chemical pesticides. The most commonly sold resistant seeds are designed to resist glyphosate, an herbicide (kills plants) which is sold commercially as Round-up. These seeds are called Round-up Ready and the plants they produce will not be harmed by Round-up applications, but all the other plants that are sprayed in the area will die. There have been multiple negative changes that have occurred because of genetic modification:

- GMO seeds are patented and therefore protected as "intellectual property" causing a whole cascade of legal problems for farmers around the world.

- GMO seeds now dominate several critical crops, including corn and soy.

- GMO seeds are produced by large, multinational corporations versus the local and small-scale seed exchanges that dominated the agricultural landscape up to the mid-20th century.

Over 10,000 years ago, humans started to grow and raise their food. A key element to growing food has always been to save the seeds from current harvests to plant for the following year's crops. Historically there was huge diversity in food crops. Seed exchanges were a common occurrence in agricultural communities, often located in the public libraries. Seed libraries were created to promote community gardening and local food systems. Recently corporations have been lobbying for laws and regulations to render seed exchanges illegal and they have been successful in some cases.

Today, large multinational pharmaceutical/chemical companies dominate the seed industry. Another way of saying this is that these same companies command global food access. Below is a graphic that depicts the global sale (and control) of seeds by corporation and even at the writing of this chapter mergers are being discussed that would create an even smaller number of larger and incredibly influential agricultural corporations (Maisashvili, 2016). It should be noted that these same companies produce both seeds and pesticides, thus cornering the market on large-scale agricultural in-puts.

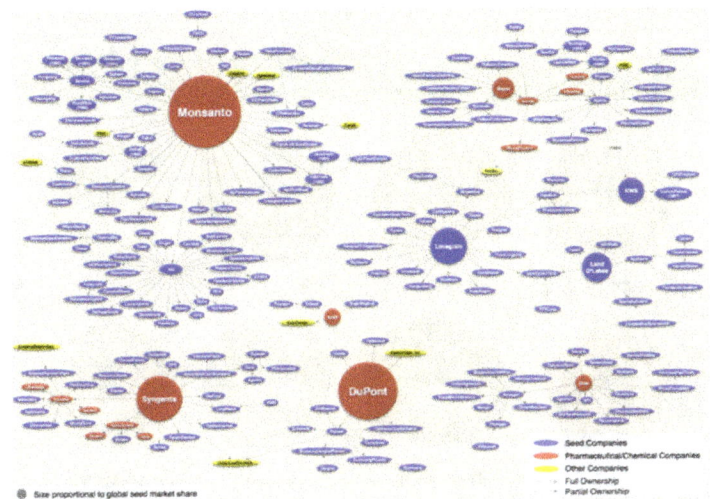

Achieving food / seed sovereignty will require the securing of rights to breed and exchange open-pollinated seeds. Seed sovereignty can be defined as the right "to breed and exchange diverse open-sourced seeds." This is seen as critical to a healthy food system, one that supports agricultural biodiversity and food security.

MONOCULTURE FARMING

Currently, large scale food production requires very specific and consistent size, shape, smell, and shelf-life of plant food products in order to package and sell them either directly to consumers or to food processing corporations. Because of this emphasis on uniformity, we have also lost much in diversity. For example, there are 7,500 varieties of apples in the world, 2,500 of which can be found in the US, but less than 90 varieties are grown commercially in the US. Yet when you go to any given grocery store you are likely to have only a handful of selections. (In the early 19th century, there was an estimated 14,000 apple varieties in North America.) Over time, this has seriously diminished seed diversity.

One reason that seed and plant diversity is important in food production is that if a monoculture crop succumbs to a fungus or bacteria or insect, the whole crop is at risk. Having variety can mean that some crops will be resistant to the threat and thus help to maintain availability of that produce. Having variety also allows us to breed more desirable features in future plants, such as disease resistance.

Another important reason for seed/plant diversity is nutritional content. In their study of the polyphenols (chemicals associated with disease prevention for a wide range of chronic diseases, including cardiovascular diseases and cancer) found in apple skins, Loncaric et al (2020) observed that traditional apple skins had statistically higher levels of polyphenols compared to current commercial apples. The traditional apples (Illustrated left) were recommended as healthier options.

The manner in which we are farming the majority of vegetables is one crop at a time and on a grand scale. There are several elements that go along with large scale production:

1. Annual tilling of the soil, which releases soil into the air, releases carbon into the air (contributing to greenhouse gases), and destroys the soil's natural ecosystem

2. Repeatedly planting annual vegetable crops in the same soil depleting the soil of its minerals and nitrogen such that farmers than have to artificially add these things back using synthetic chemicals to make up for the loss.

3. Reliance on synthetic, often toxic, pesticides that include insecticides, herbicides, and fungicides. (More on agricultural pesticides later in this chapter, as well as under Pesticides in the Hazards A-Z section of the ANHE website.)

POLLINATORS

The third in the trifecta of plant essentials is pollinators. According to the National Park Service, "A pollinator is anything that helps carry pollen from the male part of the flower (stamen) to the female part of the same or another flower (stigma). The movement of pollen must occur for the plant to become fertilized and produce fruits, seeds, and young plants. Some plants are self-pollinating, while others may be fertilized by pollen carried by wind or water. Still, other flowers are pollinated by insects and animals - such as bees, wasps, moths, butterflies, birds, flies and small mammals, including bats" (NPS, 2018). Pollinators are responsible for more than 1,200 crops in the US and more than different 180,000 plants. Together, these plants protect soil from erosion, provide oxygen, support wildlife, and, of course, provide food.

The world's food crops are being threatened because the world of pollinators is being significantly diminished. There are a number of reasons for this crisis, the profligate use of agricultural, lawn, and indoor pesticides (many of which are designed to kill insects); the loss of supportive habitat; mites and viruses and other pathogenic organisms; and our changing climate. In 2018, the Monarch butterflies, those iconic orange, black and white beauties, were reportedly down by 84% in North America. This may foresee the end of Monarch migrations.

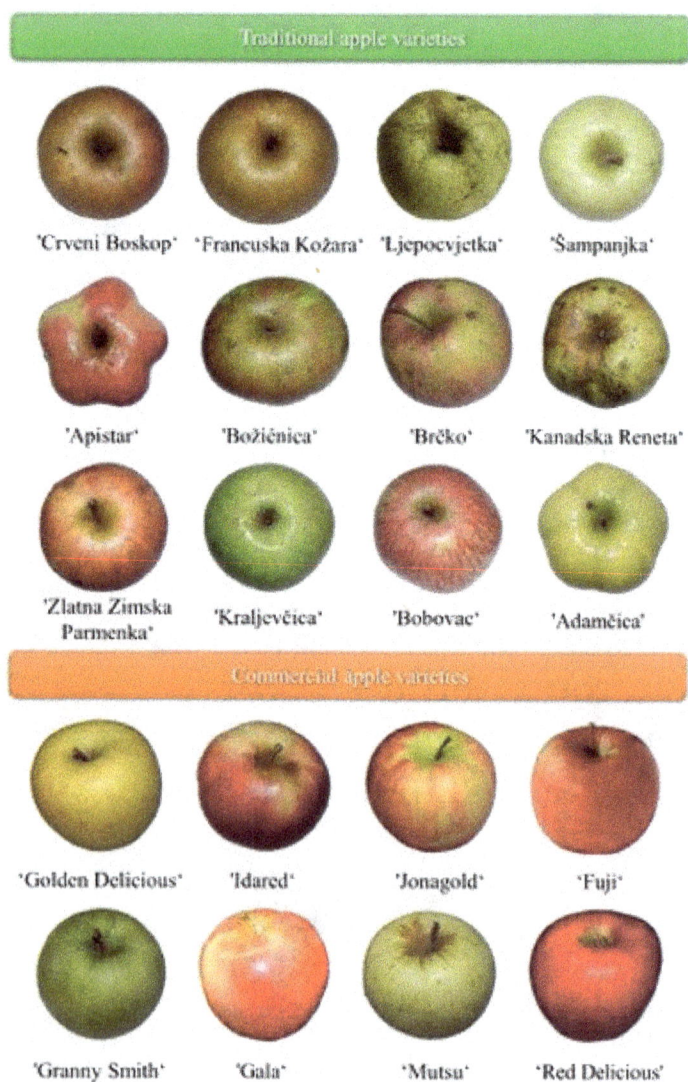

Traditional apple varieties:
'Crveni Boskop' 'Francuska Kožara' 'Ljepocvjetka' 'Šampanjka'
'Apistar' 'Božičnica' 'Brčko' 'Kanadska Reneta'
'Zlatna Zimska Parmenka' 'Kraljevčica' 'Bobovac' 'Adamčica'

Commercial apple varieties:
'Golden Delicious' 'Idared' 'Jonagold' 'Fuji'
'Granny Smith' 'Gala' 'Mutsu' 'Red Delicious'

Apple varieties used in the Loncaric study. Found here: https://www.mdpi.com/2304-8158/9/1/80/htm

Honey bees contribute over $20 billion value to food production in the US (ABF, 2020) and they enable the production of 90 critical food crops; without them we would not have these crops (WHOPS, 2014). Commercial beekeepers transport bee boxes from farm to farm appropriately timing their presence with the plants blossoming seasons.

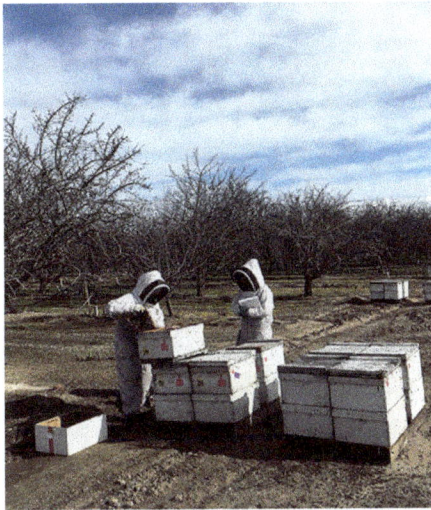

Bee box placement for pollination of almond orchard (USDA ARS) Found here: https://tellus.ars.usda.gov/stories/articles/bolstering-bees-in-a-changing-climate/

Losses experienced in managed honey bee colonies are nearly 40% annually, jeopardizing the solvency of the US beekeeping industry. Causes of colony losses include nutritional stress from lack of pollen and nectar sources, parasitic Varroa mites and the viruses they transmit, and pesticide exposure (including neonicotinoids, which are specifically known to harm bees) (Cox-Foster, retrieved 7/1/20). For wild honey bees and other pollinators, loss of habitat is a serious contributor to their decline. There are also evidence that electric and magnetic frequencies, cell towers, and radio frequencies can compromise bee colony health (Kumar, 2018).

The use of the word crisis when talking about things that significantly threaten our food supply is not hyperbole. The crisis of pollinator decline was raised to high relief and addressed by President Obama when he created the Federal Strategy to Promote the Health of Honey Bees and Other Pollinators. This serious call to action demanded a response by several cabinet level agencies, including the Department of National Security. After all, if pollinator decline persisted, food security is at stake in the US, as well as globally. Elements of the Strategy included new research, public education, public/private partnerships to develop and protect habitat, and land use policies for transportation and energy programs. The programs that were initiated are still underway.

Climate change is also a significant contributor to pollinator decline. Changing weather patterns mean changing plant patterns, causing nutritional stress. Shifts in temperature, droughts, and flooding further destroy pollinator habitat.

PESTICIDES IN AGRICULTURE

Just as many modern industries rely on toxic chemical inputs, so do many of our farms. While pesticides are often successful at combatting their targeted agricultural pests, they are just as often creating human and ecological health risks (Donley, 2019).

The word pesticide is an umbrella term for a category of chemicals that are formulated, produced and applied to harm a biological system. Pesticides are often further categorized by function, for instance, herbicides kill plants, insecticides kill or harm insects, fungicides kill fungus, and so on.

In the US, over a billion pounds of pesticides are used annually and worldwide the number is over 5 billion (Marquez, 2018). Pesticides generally are made up of both an "active ingredient", the chemical specifically formulated to harm an organism and the "inert or other ingredients" which are the chemicals that help to deliver the active ingredient or increase its efficacy. Information regarding these "other" compounds is considered proprietary business information and is most often not publicly available. Many active ingredients in pesticides are petrochemically-derived.

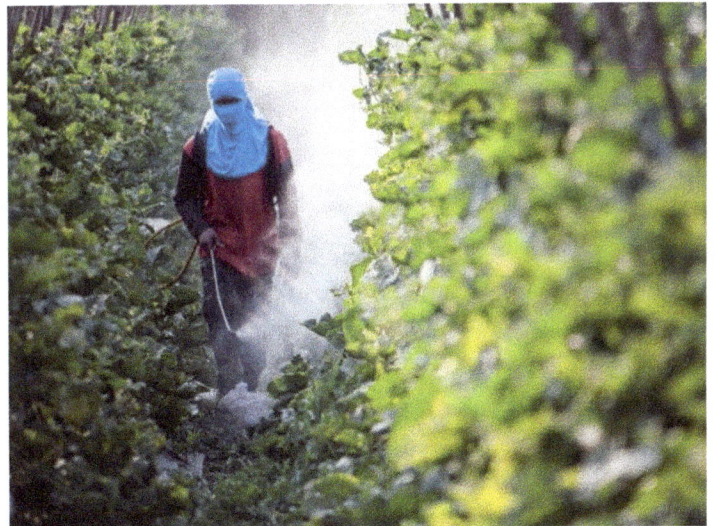

In some instances, pesticides will kill something outright, like the herbicide glyphosate (known widely as Roundup) that kills plants. In other instances, pesticides prevent reproduction, like oral flea medication that is used to control dog and cat fleas. And in other situations, the pesticides harm the neurological system of an insect or rodent. What must be understood is that many of the pesticides that are used in agriculture come with potential human health risks to those who work in the fields, to those who live in agricultural communities, and to those that eat the food products on which the pesticide residues remain.

Pesticides banned in the EU account for more than a quarter of all agricultural pesticide still used in the US, accounting for 322 million pounds a year (Donley, 2019). In the US, pesticides are regulated federally under the Federal Insecticide, Fungicide, and Rodenticide Act (FIFRA). Under FIFRA, a pesticide is defined as "any substance or mixture of substances intended for preventing, destroying, repelling, or mitigating any pest or intended for use as a plant regulator, defoliant, desiccant, or any nitrogen stabilizer." All pesticides must be registered with the Environmental Protection Agency (EPA). (Even the antimicrobial soap that you may have in your bathroom or purse contains a pesticide that must be registered with the US Environmental Protection Agency because the antimicrobial ingredient was formulated to kill microbes.) Here you can find the official EPA summary of FIFRA.

Of the 12 chemicals that were originally targeted for prohibition or elimination by the international treaty, the Stockholm Convention on Persistent Organic Pollutants, 10 of them were pesticides (UNEP, 2001). (An additional 10 chemicals have been added to the list.)

Collectively pesticides have the potential to cause a very long list of health risks including cancer, birth defects and other birth outcomes, reproductive health risks, neurological problems, and many more. Nevertheless, it is important for nurses to be specific when talking about pesticides and health risks because all pesticides do not cause all of the health risks. To be evidence-based, nurses must evaluate the specific evidence for specific pesticides. When asking patients about potential pesticide exposures it is important to get as specific information as possible. The evidence in the literature is substantial and easily accessible.

The US Geological Survey (USGS) monitors ground and surface water for 76 pesticides and seven pesticide breakdown products. A survey found that 90% of streams and 50% of wells tested were positive for at least one pesticide (USGS, n.d.). Contaminated water has one of the greatest impacts on ecological health, creating risks to aquatic life and then by extension to the entire food chain within the natural world.

PESTICIDES IN THE ATMOSPHERE AND WATER

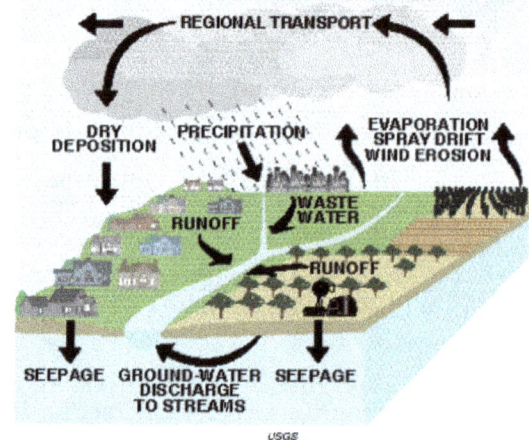

USGS: ca.water.usgs.gov/pnsp/atmos/atmos_1.html

One of the most important laws affecting pesticides and food is the 1994 Food Quality Protection Act (FQPA). The major elements of FQPA are as follows (EPA, n.d.):

- Set "tolerances" (amount of pesticide residues allowed on produce) to achieve "a reasonable certainty of no harm"

- Reassess, over a 10-year period, all pesticide tolerances that were in place when the FQPA was signed, in 1996

- Consider the special susceptibility of children to pesticides by using an additional tenfold (10X) safety factor when setting and reassessing tolerances unless adequate data are available to support a different factor;

- Consider aggregate risk from exposure to a pesticide from multiple sources (food, water, residential and other non-occupational sources) when assessing tolerances

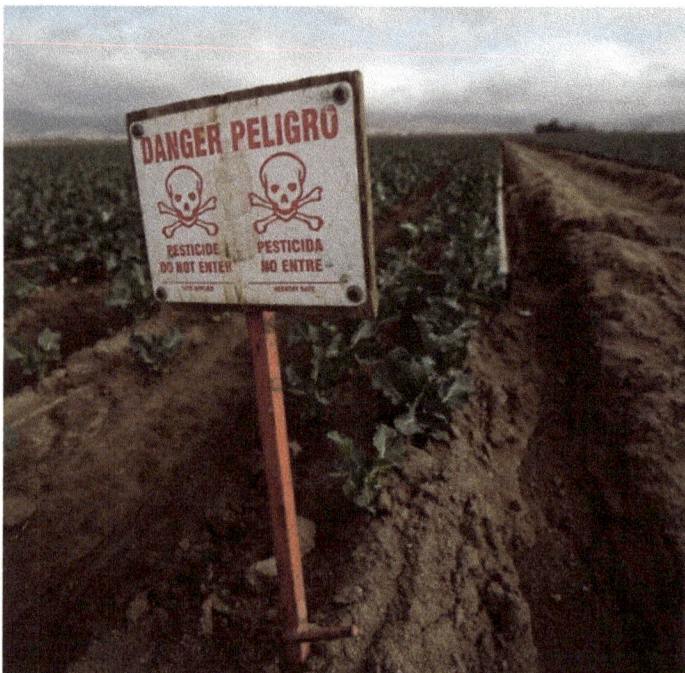

- Consider cumulative exposure to pesticides that have common mechanisms of toxicity

While all of the basic elements are important the last two elements represent the first time that the EPA was required to look at multiple and cumulative exposures, a very important environmental health concept. Despite the codification of pesticide safety, the US has not yet achieved the goal of keeping everyone safe from pesticide-related health risks.

The EPA's Office of Pesticides provides a wide range of information and on their website information can also be found in Spanish and materials for children to learn about pesticides.

USDA CERTIFIED ORGANIC

In order to help the public, choose crops (and meat/poultry) that has been grown without the use of potentially harmful chemicals like pesticides, the US Department of Agriculture (USDA) has a designation of "USDA Certified Organic." Farmers can apply for this designation for their farms and food producers can do the same for their retail products. Farmers must farm organically for 3 years before they can apply for the certification and they must submit an organic farm management plan, as well as pay a fee. In addition to assurances about not using pesticides, farmers commit to other practices as well. For instance, crops that are designated USDA Certified Organic cannot be genetically modified organisms (GMO), the soil in which the crops are grown cannot have been augmented by sewage sludge, and no pesticides or synthetic fertilizers can be used on the crops. Food processors cannot use radiation to control bacteria.

"As for organic meat [and dairy], regulations require that animals are raised in living conditions accommodating their natural behaviors (like the ability to graze on pasture), fed 100% organic feed and forage, and not administered antibiotics or hormones. When it comes to processed, multi-ingredient foods, the USDA organic standards specify additional considerations. Regulations prohibit organically processed foods from containing artificial preservatives, colors, or flavors and require that their ingredients are organic, with some minor exceptions. For example, processed organic foods may contain some approved non-agricultural ingredients, like enzymes in yogurt, pectin in fruit jams, or baking soda in baked goods." (USDA, McAvoy, 2019)

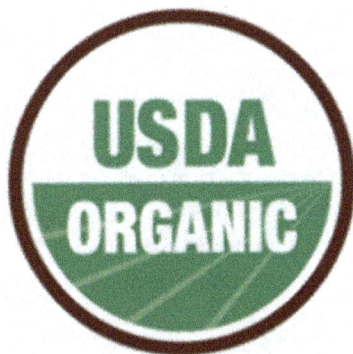

For many small scale, organic farmers who sell their produce via farm stands or farmers' markets, the fees for organic certificate may be prohibitive ($500 - $1,200). When purchasing from such places ask about how the produce was grown. Farmers are often eager to share information about their organic practices.

It should be noted that farmers (and gardeners) can use a pest management approach that avoids toxic chemicals called Integrated Pest Management (IPM), even if they are not certified organic. This approach is multifaceted and considers the type of plants you choose (pest resistant), how to weed/cultivate instead of using herbicides, and many practices to reduce the use of pesticides. The IPM Institute of America provides detailed information on how to enlist IPM strategies.

FARMWORKERS

There are likely over 3 million farmworkers in the US alone, but it is very difficult to know for sure. They are often immigrants, do not speak English or speak it as a second language, are sometime migratory for their work, and, given political concerns are not likely to want to be too visible. On the other, more important hand, they are the ones responsible for feeding us every day and they are treated extremely poorly. Despite the fact that farmworkers feed us, between 45 – 82% of farmworkers can be food insecure, depending on their location and the time of year.

By most measures of social determinants, farmworkers in the United States are considerably more vulnerable than the general population. From the perspective of economics, education, healthcare access, housing, and workplace and environmental exposures, farmworkers' statistics raise significant public health concerns (Sattler, 2019).

Farmworker children are not protected under US child labor laws and can work in the fields early in their childhood. Of children working in the fields, 24% are younger than 14 years old. According to the National Children's Center for Rural and Agricultural Safety and Health, a child dies every 3 days in an agricultural-related accident and 33 children are injured (NCCRASH, 2018). The vast majority (75%) of crop workers lack any form of health insurance. Farmworker families have exposures to pesticides in the fields, in their homes, and in their foods thus experiencing a cumulative impact that is far greater than other populations. They also have a host of other health and safety issues including stress, farm machinery injuries, and sexual harassment.

In this Farmworker Factsheet, many of the important demographics regarding migrant farmworkers are described and here you can read an overview of the housing challenges faced by farmworkers. As nurses, whether we live in a rural, farming community or not, we should be aware of the unfair burden that farmworkers pay in order to grow and raise our food.

CLIMATE CHANGE

Climate change is covered more fully in its own eText chapter but it merits a few words here. As is true for all living organisms, plants have a temperature range in which they can flourish. As things heat up beyond this range, plants will fail. Many of the food crops that have flourished for centuries are now showing signs of stress and newer varieties are being developed that can withstand the heat. But at some point, it may become difficult to find replacements.

Many forests have been destroyed to make way for beef cattle grazing or growing grains to feed beef and other meat animals. This forest destruction means less trees to absorb CO_2 and create O_2. The massive, intentional fires in Brazil in recent years were often implemented to make room for grazing land.

Flooding and droughts have been disastrous for farmers all over the world and is likely to continue until we make inroads into climate change mitigation. Climate change has already resulted in regional famines and climate-related migrations of people.

On the other hand, there is real evidence that some farming practices can actually sequester carbon while producing food crops. This is something we will be hearing more about and we will be seeing policies to support shifting farming practices with carbon as an important metric.

AGRICULTURAL POLICIES

The biggest and most important US policy affecting agriculture is the Farm Bill, which has the second largest federal budget attached to it – second only to the military budget. See here for a very simple primer on the Farm Bill. The Farm Bill also provides subsidies and incentives that help, for the most part, keep the industrial farming model in play. Powerful big ag and pharmaceutical/chemical company interests have overwhelming influence on the Farm Bill, which is reauthorized every 5 years. The last

reauthorization was in 2018. Very little is budgeted in the Farm Bill that will help move the farm industry to more sustainable, less fossil fuel-intensive, carbon sequestering practices. This has been left to the states and some states do provide grant and tax incentive programs for farmers to become more sustainable.

The USDA is the federal agency responsible for food production and every state has a state-level equivalent agency. In some agricultural states, like California, every county also has a County Agriculture Commissioner.

Every state has at least one "land grant" university, usually one of the large state universities, that is required to have a significant focus on agriculture, including agricultural research, education and "extension" (Cooperative Extension Service - translating the science into practice). Each of the land grant universities helps to inform the Cooperative Extension Service which, in turn, works with farmers, ranchers, and consumers. They also support the Master Gardener Programs, non-academic programs that are open to the public.

WHAT'S ON THE HORIZON?

Farming has gone through huge transformations in the last half century and has become large in scale with regional monocultures (i.e., wheat, soy). While this is producing lots of food products, it is also slowly destroying the soil, harming humans, and obliterating whole ecosystems. This is not sustainable.

There are many new small initiatives that are helping to slowly shift our food production to more local/regional, integrated (versus monoculture), and sustainable practices. The demand for "organic" produce has helped to provide an economic incentive for some large-scale conventional farmers to shift away from using pesticides and become certified organic.

Some small-scale farmers are moving beyond organic and are trying to fully integrate sustainability practices with cover crops, no-till practices, rotating crops, inclusion of farm animals in food plant production, and other practices that were once mainstay on traditional family farms – the ones with the red barns.

The terms permaculture, agroecology, biodynamic, and regenerative farming all represent philosophies and approaches to sustainable farming that are designed to counter-balance the predominant industrial food model. As you can see by the definitions that the proponents for these approaches propose, there is much overlap among them.

- **Permaculture**: "The conscious design and maintenance of agriculturally productive systems which have the diversity, stability, and resilience of natural ecosystems. It is the harmonious integration of the landscape with people providing their food, energy, shelter and other material and non-material needs in a sustainable way." Defined by Bill Mollison, the man who coined the word. (Quote found here: https://modernfarmer.com/2016/04/permaculture/)

- **Agroecology**: Is farming that "centers on food production that makes the best use of nature's goods and services while not damaging these resources" by " improving soil and plant quality through available biomass and diversity, rather than battling nature with chemical inputs" and "improv(ing) food yields for balanced nutrition, strengthen(ing) fair market for their produce, enhance(ing) healthy ecosystems, and build(ing) on ancestral knowledge and customs." Definition found here: https://www.agroecologyfund.org/what-is-agroecology

- **Biodynamic: Farming** is a "holistic, ecological, and ethical approach to farming, gardening, food, and nutrition. It is about reverence for the land and for water, for food, animals, and each other. It goes beyond sustainability – it's regenerative agriculture. Biodynamic farming practices clean our air by sequestering carbon in the soil and using no chemical fertilizers, pesticides or herbicides. Animals are treated with compassion and respect and given the freedom to lead happier lives." Definition found here: https://modernfarmer.com/2016/04/permaculture/ [Biodynamics is rooted in the work of philosopher and scientist Dr. Rudolf Steiner, whose 1924 lectures to farmers opened a new way to integrate scientific understanding with a recognition of spirit in nature. (Biodynamics Association, n.d.)]

- **Regenerative**: "(D)escribes farming and grazing practices that, among other benefits, reverse climate change by rebuilding soil organic matter and restoring degraded soil biodiversity – resulting in both carbon drawdown and improving the water cycle". Definition found here: https://regenerationinternational.org/why-regenerative-agriculture/

Regardless of the approach to farming it is clear that we are going to need more farmers in the US. For every young person entering into farming there are 6 farmers over the age of 65. According to the 2017 Census of Agriculture from the US Department of Agriculture (USDA), there were over 321,000 young farmers (under the age of 35) in the US. That count is up from 2012, when there were 208,000, which is encouraging. They are joining the ranks with new knowledge and often more sustainable approaches to food production. While this number is hopeful, they are not even close to replacing the farmers who are 65 and older.

In order to incentivize young farmers, there are programs to pay for their education which will help them avoid tuition debt and increase their economic chances of purchasing farms and ranches. To further support young farmers, places like New York have created programs like the New Farmers Grant Fund Program that provides $50,000 grants to farm projects that advance "sustainable agricultural production practices."

A specific, though smaller trend is the proliferation of urban farms and gardens. (Lots of gardens resulted from COVID's sheltering in place.) Pediatric Nurse, Atiya Wells, started Bliss Meadows Farm in Baltimore City a project "at the intersection of environmental and food justice" that helps to build community and introduce urban children to nature and the growing of food. But this form of farming is not likely to put a significant dent in real food needs. In an article entitled, "The real value of urban farming. (Hint: It's not always the food", Plumer (2016) contends that "Maybe...urban agriculture is most valuable for how it forces us to be more conscientious about the people who feed us: the farmworkers, the truck drivers, the processors and the packagers, the prep cooks, all of whom work for next to nothing and have little time themselves to play in the dirt."

In their 2020 Workshop Proceedings: Innovations in the Food System – Exploring the Future of Food, the National Academy of Science, Engineering and Medicine highlights the thinking of international experts regarding trends in food and agriculture. Some of the topics that are covered include meat alternatives, food packaging, water/land us, food waste, and food access/security. (NAS, 20200

Health Care Without Harm is an international non-profit organization that is helping hospitals to be more sustainable and one of their important programs is bringing healthy foods to health care institutions. They provide excellent resources on how to bring healthy food to health care institutions and for nurses who want to support sustainable agriculture and a sustainable food system, the Health Care Without Harm's Food Program can also provide technical assistance and support. They define a healthy food system as one that conserves and renews natural resources, advances social justice and animal welfare, builds community wealth, and fulfills the food and nutrition needs of all eaters now and in the future (HCWH, n.d.). As an example of their resources is this factsheet on a healthier food purchasing standard.

More information on food and agriculture can be found on ANHE's website here. Also, ANHE sponsors a Food and Agriculture Committee where nurses who have a particular interest in this area meet and work on food/ag issues.

CONCLUSION

This chapter covered some of the agricultural and health basics but the food system is much larger and includes food processing, distribution, marketing, consumption, nutrition, food additives/preservatives, food waste and many more issues which were not covered in this chapter. Also, not covered were food insecurity and the role that poor diets are having on chronic disease risk, really important issues for nurses to consider. All of these components have implications for public health.

As you are eating your next meal perhaps you will think about your food a little differently having read this chapter. The adage, you are what you eat still holds true but in addition, what you choose to eat also is reflected in ecological health and in the health of all those who work in the food system. This is an area where nurses can have a great impact as individuals, as educators, in patient care settings, and in the policy arena. Much work is ahead of us on the public health implications of food and agriculture.

REFERENCES

Amaranthus, M., & Allyn, B. (2013). *HEALTH — Healthy Soil microbes, healthy people: The microbial community in the ground is as important as the one in our guts. Atlantic.* https://www.theatlantic.com/health/archive/2013/06/healthy-soil-microbes-healthy-people/276710/

American Beekeeping Federation. (2020). *Pollinator facts: Honeybees are pollinators.* https://rb.gy/cf05bg

American Cancer Society. (2014). *Recombinant Bovine Growth Hormones.* https://www.cancer.org/cancer/cancer-causes/recombinant-bovine-growth-hormone.html

Center for Food Safety. (n.d.). *About RBGH.* https://www.cancer.org/cancer/cancer-causes/recombinant-bovine-growth-hormone.html

Center for Veterinary Medicine. (2015, December). *SUMMARY REPORT on Antimicrobials Sold or Distributed for Use in Food-Producing Animals.* FDA Department of Health and Human Services. http://www.fda.gov/downloads/ForIndustry/UserFees/AnimalDrugUserFeeActADUFA/UCM476258.pdf

Chan, Margaret. (2011). *World Health Day 2011: Combat drug resistance: no action today means no cure tomorrow. World Health Organization.* http://www.who.int/mediacentre/news/statements/2011/whd_20110407/en/index.html

Charavaryamath, C. & Singh, B. (2006). Pulmonary effects of exposure to pig barn air. *Journal of Occupational Medicine and Toxicology, 1,*10.doi: 10.1186/1745-6673-1-10

Cox-Foster, D. (n.d.). *Bolstering bees in a changing climate.* U.S. Department of Agriculture Agricultural Research Service (ARS). https://tellus.ars.usda.gov/stories/articles/bolstering-bees-in-a-changing-climate/

Center for Urban Education and Sustainable Agriculture (n.d.) *How far does your food travel to get to your plate?* https://cuesa.org/learn/how-far-does-your-food-travel-get-your-plate#:~:text=The%20True%20Cost%20of%20Food,large%20quantities%20of%20fossil%20fuels

Donley, N. (2019). The USA lags behind other agricultural nations in banning harmful pesticides, *Environmental Health, 18*(44). https://ehjournal.biomedcentral.com/articles/10.1186/s12940-019-0488-0

Duda, R. (2016). *Why and how to use your career to end factory farms.* 80,000 Hours. https://80000hours.org/2016/04/new-profile-on-factory-farming/

Gurian-Sherman, D. (2008). *CAFOs uncovered: The untold cost of CAFOs. A report of the Union of Concerned Scientists.* https://www.organicconsumers.org/sites/default/files/cafos_uncovered.pdf

Health Care Without Harm. (n.d.). *Healthy food in health care.* https://noharm-uscanada.org/issues/us-canada/healthy-food-health-care

Kumar, S.S. (2018). Colony Collapse Disorder (CCD) in honey bees caused by EMF radiation. *Bioinformation, 14*(9):, 521–524. doi: 10.6026/97320630014521

Loncaric A, Matanovic K, Ferrer P, Kovac T, Sarkan B, Babojelic MS, and Lores M. (2020). Peel of traditional apple varieties as great source of bioactive compounds: extraction by micro-matrix solid-phase dispersion. *Foods.,9*(1), 80. https://doi.org/10.3390/foods9010080

Maisashvili A. H., Bryant, J.M., Knapek, G., Outlaw, J., and Richardson, J. (2016). *Seed prices, proposed mergers and acquisitions among biotech firms.* Choices. https://www.choicesmagazine.org/choices-magazine/submitted-articles/seed-prices-proposed-mergers-and-acquisitions-among-biotech-firms

Malekinejad, H., & Rezebakhch, A., (2015). Hormones in dairy foods and their impact on public health - A narrative review article. *Iranian Journal of Public Health, 44*(6),742-58.

Marquez, E. (2018). *In the US and in the world, pesticide use is up.* Pesticide Action Network. http://www.panna.org/blog/us-and-world-pesticide-use

National Academy of Science, Engineering, and Medicine. (2020). Workshop proceeding: Innovations in the food system – Exploring the future of food. National Academy Press. https://doi.org/10.17226/25523

National Children's Center for Rural and Agricultural Health and Safety. (2018). *2018 Factsheet childhood agricultural injuries in the US.* https://www.marshfieldresearch.org/Media/Default/NFMC/PDFs/2018%20Child%20Ag%20Injury%20Factsheetpdf.pdf

National Park Service. (2018). *What is a pollinator?* https://www.nps.gov/subjects/pollinators/what-is-a-pollinator.htm

Philpott, T. (2010). *Our other addiction: the tricky geopolitics of nitrogen fertilizer.* Grist. https://grist.org/article/2010-02-11-tracking-u-s-farmers-supply-nitrogen-fertilizer/

Plumer, B. (2016). *The real value of urban farming. (Hint: It's not always the food.)* VOX. https://www.vox.com/2016/5/15/11660304/urban-farming-benefits

Pollan, M. (2006). *The omnivore's dilemma: A natural history of four meals.* Penguin Press.

Rule, A. M., Evans, S. L., & Silbergeld, E. K. (2008). Food animal transport: A potential source of community exposures to health hazards from industrial farming (CAFOs). *Journal of Infection and Public Health, 1*(1), 33-39. https://doi.org/10.1016/j.jiph.2008.08.001

United Nations Convention to Combat Desertification. (2015). *Land Degradation Neutrality: Resilience at Local, National, and Regional Levels.* http://catalogue.unccd.int/858_V2_UNCCD_BRO_.pdf

United Nations. (n.d.). Stockholm Convention Overview. http://www.pops.int/TheConvention/Overview/tabid/3351/Default.aspx

US Environmental Protection Agency (EPA). (n.d.). Laws and Regulations. Summary of the Food Quality Protection Act. https://rb.gy/xgt8ct

US Food and Drug Administration (FDA). (2020a). *Steroid Hormone Implants Used in Food-Producing Animals.* https://www.fda.gov/animal-veterinary/product-safety-information/steroid-hormone-implants-used-growth-food-producing-animals

US Food and Drug Administration. (2020b). *Product Safety Information: Bovine Somatotropin (bST).* https://www.fda.gov/animal-veterinary/product-safety-information/bovine-somatotropin-bst

University of Minnesota Extension. (2018). *Living soil: Healthy garden.* https://extension.umn.edu/how-manage-soil-and-nutrients-home-gardens/living-soil-healthy-garden

White House Office of the Press Secretary. (2014). *Fact sheet: The economic challenge posed by declining pollinator populations.* https://obamawhitehouse.archives.gov/the-press-office/2014/06/20/fact-sheet-economic-challenge-posed-declining-pollinator-populations

World Health Organization. (2014, April). *Antimicrobial resistance: global report on surveillance 2014.* http://www.who.int/drugresistance/documents/surveillancereport/en/

ENVIRONMENTAL JUSTICE

Jeanne Leffers, PhD, RN, FAAN
Professor Emeritus
University of Massachusetts Dartmouth
College of Nursing and Health Sciences

Dorothy Lewis Powell, RN, EdD, FAAN
Professor Emeritus
Duke University
School of Nursing

Adelita G. Cantu, PhD, RN
Associate Professor
University of Texas Health San Antonio
School of Nursing

In order to understand the multifaceted reasons for health disparities, it is essential to consider the inequities in environmental exposures among various population groups. Inequities that are not evenly distributed among populations are considered unfair or unjust. Environmental exposures are considered one of the social determinants of health: circumstances that occur where people live, learn, work, play, and pray that have an impact on health and well-being. Thus, in response to inequities in environmental exposures and health outcomes, nurses and others seek environmental justice.

According to the Environmental Protection Agency (EPA) "Environmental Justice (EJ) is the fair treatment and meaningful involvement of all people regardless of race, color, national origin, or income with respect to the development, implementation, and enforcement of environmental laws, regulations, and policies" (EPA 2019a). Further, this goal will be achieved when everyone enjoys the same degree of protection from environmental and health hazards, and equal access to the decision-making process to have a healthy environment in which to live, learn, and work.

This definition suggests a legal mandate to respond to factors that cause health disparities that are related to environmental policies that fail to address health outcomes caused by environmental hazards. The Environmental Protection Agency's (EPA's) explanation of fair treatment is that "no group of people should bear a disproportionate share of the negative environmental consequences resulting from industrial, governmental and commercial operations or policies" (EPA, 2018). The EPA website further indicates that meaningful involvement means that "people have an opportunity to participate in decisions about activities that may affect their environment and/or health; the public's contribution can

influence the regulatory agency's decision; their concerns will be considered in the decision-making process; and the decision makers seek out and facilitate the involvement of those potentially affected" (EPA, 2018).

In response to the mounting concerns raised by citizens, scholars and activists, the federal government continues to address environmental racism (Mikati et al, 2018). Many communities bear the extra burden of waste, pollution and hazardous exposures. These communities across the globe are the homes to persons of color and those living in poverty. Considered a form of institutionalized racism, environmental racism, "refers to environmental policy, practice or directive that differentially affects or disadvantages (whether intended or unintended) individuals, groups or communities based on race and color" (Bullard, 2002). Environmental racism is defined as "the disproportionate impact of environmental hazards on people of color" (Environmental Justice Network, 2015). (See http://www.ejnet.org/ej/)

HISTORY

Historically, people of color and those living in poverty have borne the greatest burden of exposure to environmental hazards in their communities, homes, workplaces and schools. Such exposures most often come from landfills, garbage dumps, chemical plants, factories, smelters and incinerators that are built in low income and minority communities (Bullard, Johnson & Torres, 2011). Further, the regulations that led to such communities resulted from racist policies such as redlining and siting of transportation routes (Bullard, 2021). The roots of the movement to address this injustice began in the 1960s with several key events. First, the publication of Silent Spring by Rachel Carson (1962) informed the general public of the health hazards associated with pesticides. In addition, during the 1960s Cesar Chavez and farmworkers protested their exposures to harmful pesticides in their agricultural work in fields treated with chemicals hazardous to human health (Skelton and Miller, 2014). The Civil Rights movement led to the Civil Rights Act of 1964 that prohibited the use of federal funds to discriminate based upon race, color or national origin.

Concerns for civil rights and equal opportunity under the law developed during the 1960s. Public concerns for both health and the environment also gained momentum and culminated with the creation of the Environmental Protection Agency in 1970 under President Nixon. The EPA was charged to protect human health and the environment. Legislation such as the Clean Air Act of 1970 and the Clean Water Act of 1972 launched a series of legal mandates for the EPA to regulate and enforce standards to protect health and the environment.

These inequities continue to threaten those living in communities that were unjustly bearing the toxic burdens. Citizens in Warren County, North Carolina began what is known as the environmental justice movement. The dumping of 31,000 gallons of polychlorinated biphenyl (PCB) in 1973 along roadways contaminated large areas of soil. In response to citizen pushback, the state devised a plan to build a landfill for the contaminated soil. The landfill was to be located in Warren County, a largely African American community that lacked both a mayor and a city council. In addition, it was ranked as one of the three poorest communities in terms of gross domestic product. The local African American citizens protested the plans for the landfill fearing that their water would become contaminated by PCBs. (Click on the links below to watch videos)

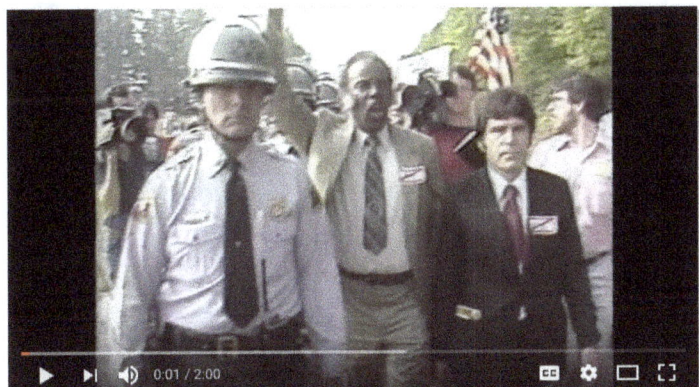

[PCB Protest in Warren County 1982](#)

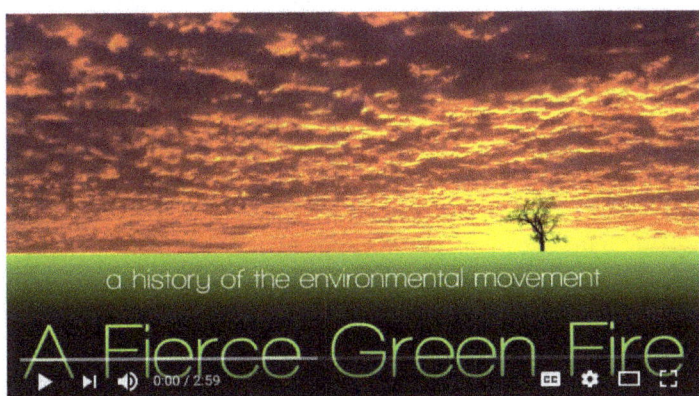

[Robert Bullard - The Genesis of Environmental Justice](#)

Dr. Robert Bullard, currently the Dean of the Barbara Jordan-Mickey Leland School of Public Affairs at Texas Southern University in Houston, Texas, is considered by many to be the "father of environmental justice." He became active in the environmental justice movement in the early 1980s when he actively investigated the siting of municipal waste sites in predominantly black communities in Houston. His scholarship led to his book, Dumping in Dixie: Race, Class and Environmental Quality published in 1990. During the past 25 years of his academic career he has published 18 books and championed topics such as environmental racism, regional equity, environmental justice, climate justice, sustainable development, urban land use, smart growth, industrial facility siting, community reinvestment, housing, and transportation.

FEDERAL AND STATE MANDATES

Federal and state mandates were developed in response to the growing movement to address environmental injustice. President Bill Clinton signed [Executive Order 12898](#), "Federal Actions to Address Environmental Justice in Minority Populations and Low-Income Populations," on Feb 11, 1994. The purpose of the Order was to address the human health and environmental conditions of minority and low-income populations with the goal of achieving environmental protection for all communities. The Order directed the EPA and other federal agencies to develop [environmental justice strategies](#) to help each agency address how their programs create disproportionately high and adverse human health or environmental effects on minority and low-income populations. The Order aims to provide minority and low income communities access to public information and public participation in matters relating to human health and the environment through fair treatment and meaningful involvement (EPA, 2017).

At the Federal level, in February, 2024, the EPA's Office of Environmental Justice (OEJ) will recognize the the 30th anniversary of the signing of EO 12898. The [OEJ webpage](#) offers links to their environmental justice strategic planning grants and resources as well as detailing how the Office's Enforcement and Compliance Assurance goes after pollution problems that impact communities through vigorous civil and criminal enforcement (EPA. 2023a).

STATE AND REGIONAL EPA ENVIRONMENTAL JUSTICE (EJ) OFFICES

The EPA also supports 10 regional offices across the United States where each includes an EJ office (EPA, 2023b). During the past two decades, state legislatures have addressed EJ for their communities. In Massachusetts, for example, an Environmental Justice Policy was signed in 2002 that guides efforts to address inequities and injustices for people of color and low income populations. Their services include links to state policies and initiatives, modules to address smart growth/

smart energy policies, and case studies. The Massachusetts toolkit is available online. In addition, the Massachusetts Environmental Justice site offers tools such as EJ mapping. With EJ mapping, Geographic Information Systems (GIS) tools can be used to map various toxic exposures to communities that meet the criteria for EJ.

An example of an educational module is Brownfields where the viewer can see examples of how former brownfields have been revitalized into useful and beautiful additions to the community. According to the EPA, a brownfield is a property, the expansion, redevelopment, or reuse of which may be complicated by the presence or potential presence of a hazardous substance, pollutant, or contaminant (EPA, 2023c). The Jackson Square case study of a Jamaica Plain neighborhood in Boston, Massachusetts, highlights the development of an 11 acre former urban intersection comprised of brownfields and heavy traffic use into a mixed-income, mixed-use, and sustainable transit-oriented area (Mass.gov, 2019).

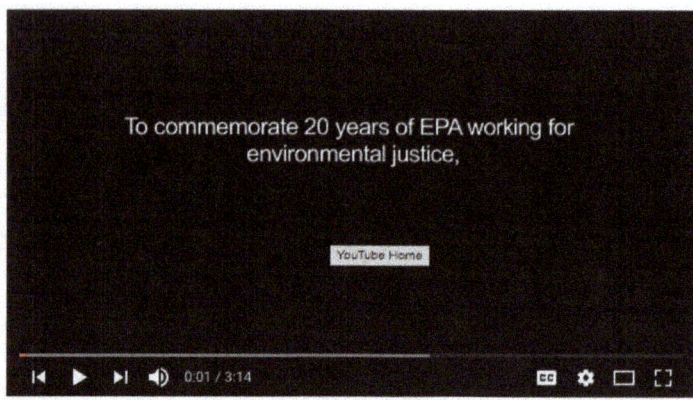

[EPA 20th Anniversary Environmental Justice Video Series: Edith Pestana](#)

RELATIONSHIP TO SOCIAL DETERMINANTS OF HEALTH (SDH)

The EPA's new Office of Environmental Justice and External Civil Rights works with the Office of Land and Emergency Management that has recently released the ["EJ Action Plan: Building Up Environmental Justice in EPA's Land Protection and Cleanup Programs](#)." to bring tools, practices and projects to land pollution and clean up programs such as Superfund sites, Brownfields and otherland pollution (EPA, 2023d).

Environmental justice is essential for the protection of those who live in overburdened communities and to provide legal support to remedy the disparities in their environment. However, an upstream approach is required to more effectively address the needs of EJ communities.

To address the root causes of such disparities, a social determinants of health (SDH) approach must be taken. The World Health Organization defines SDH as "the conditions in which people are born, grow, live, work, and age. These circumstances are shaped by the distribution of money, power and resources at global, national, and local levels" (World Health Organization, 2014b). In response to a charge from EPA to address the impact of social determinants of health upon children's health, the [EPA's Children's Health Protection Advisory Committee (CHPAC)](#) sent a letter to EPA Administrator Gina McCarthy in November 2013 urging EPA to "incorporate SDH in all programs, policies and regulatory efforts across all offices of the Agency."

CASE EXAMPLES OF CITIZENS' ENVIRONMENTAL JUSTICE EFFORTS

As noted earlier, the roots of the EJ movement began with those living in affected communities voicing their concerns to seek equity. Efforts by those living in affected communities provide excellent examples of how to promote environmental justice.

WE-ACT

In 1988, the organization [West Harlem Environmental Action (WE-ACT)](#) was founded in New York City to address environmental justice. WE-ACT was the first environmental justice organization in the city and one of the first in the U.S. run by people of color. Issues of environmental racism led to the siting and environmental exposures from the following: North River Sewage Treatment Plant, 6 out of 7 New York City diesel bus depots in Northern Manhattan, a 24-hour Marine Transfer Station in Manhattan, as well as the practice of using Northern Manhattan communities as New York City's dumping ground.

Currently the organization has grown and serves to inform, educate, train and mobilize residents of North Manhattan on environmental issues that impact their health, lives and community. Recent efforts emphasize citizen participation in public policy and enforcement of environmental regulations. WE-ACT works on the city, state and federal levels to improve policy on environmental health and justice. In 2016, WE-ACT helped to pass the country's first Safe School Water Act, which mandates testing and remediation for lead in all New York State schools. In 2017, WE-ACT was instrumental in passing NYC's Environmental Justice Study Bill and Environmental Justice Policy Bill which provides the city and all New Yorkers more information to identify and address environmental injustices.

Through the years WE-ACT has worked to broaden their efforts to address climate justice, extreme heat and health equity, develop a climate ready plan for northern Manhattan, educate women of color about the toxins in personal care and cosmetic products, promote sustainable public housing,waste justice, improve energy efficiency with green efforts such as decarbonization, electric buses, a move from gas to electricity using renewables such as solar power, while still working to address environmental toxins, asthmas disparities and healthy homes (WE-ACT, 2023).

Jesus People Against Pollution

Jesus People Against Pollution (JPAP) is a grassroots environmental justice organization located in Columbia, Mississippi. The organization was created in response to an explosion in March 1977 at the Reichold Chemical Company. "The explosion wrecked the facility and poisoned the local air, water and land with cancer-causing agents and other dangerous compounds. After the explosion, Reichold abandoned the site and left toxic, deadly substances buried in 55 gallon drums in the earth and around the nearby community and in local landfills" (Earthjustice, 2015). In time, toxic chemicals oozed into the water tables and soil, causing the ground to spontaneously combust, vaporizing into the atmosphere, and leaving offensive odors making many people sick. The community has sustained health problems ranging from nose-bleeds and respiratory problems to cancers and premature deaths. Consistent with the well documented practice of "waste following waste," the Reichold site was compounded further by pesticide spraying, oilfield operations, transportation, nuclear waste and incineration. Advocacy by JPAP played a role in the Reichold site being listed as a Superfund Site in the 1980s; however, it has since been delisted. It is now considered a brownfield site and continues to seek remediation in the form of relocation and life-time environmental/primary health care for impacted residents.

JPAP is a grassroots advocacy organization that has also embraced a mission to "educate and inform impacted communities about the availability of toxicology and environmental health information so that communities can   better understand the relationship between environmental   exposure and disease." Its founder and primary   spokesperson Charlotte Keys, Evangelist and Environmental Justice Advocate, is a national figure frequently speaking in the policy arena and contributing to   the EJ dialogue at relevant federal agencies.   This organization continues to advocate for EJ and collaborates with other environmental justice organizations in their advocacy efforts such as their joint letter to President Joseph Biden in 2022 in opposition to the Senate Energy Independence and Security Act of 2022 (WE-ACT 2013b).

Native Americans and Nuclear Waste

During the 1990s a number of Native American tribes fought legal battles to protect their sacred land from radioactive waste disposal. The Eastern Navajo reservation residents fought to protect their land by filing a suit with the Nuclear Regulatory Commission to block a permit for uranium mining in Church Rock and Crown Point, New Mexico. Likewise, the Western Shoshone tribe in Nevada is fighting Yucca Mountain dumping (University of Michigan, 2015). The Mojave tribe in California and the Skull Valley Goshutes in Idaho are also fighting the construction of radioactive waste dumps on their tribal lands.

Noteworthy recent examples of meaningful involvement not occurring was the indigenous people of   Standing Rock and the Dakota Access Pipeline. Energy   Transfer Partners proposed a new 1,200-mile oil pipeline from the Bakken oil fields to the Midwest, chose a route crossing the Missouri River just yards upstream from the Standing Rock Sioux reservation. The Tribe's principled   resistance to the project captured the attention of the entire world, leading to historic protests at the remote site in North Dakota. The Obama administration vindicated the Tribe's concerns when it blocked the final permits to cross the Missouri River and promised a full environmental review that looked at the Tribe's treaty   rights as well as alternative routes.

Increasingly fracking is occurring on Tribal lands again being challenged by those Native peoples most affected. Most recently construction site at Lithium Nevada near Thacker Pass, has been challenged by the Reno-Sparks Indian Colony (that includes people from the Shoshone, Paiute, and Washoe nations) to cease work at the site that is the location of a massacre of native people by the US Cavalry in 1865. The UN affiliated Indigenous Environmental Network promotes respect for native lands in their efforts to promote health, planetary health and address climate change.

HYDRAULIC FRACTURING (FRACKING) AND ENVIRONMENTAL JUSTICE

A growing concern for environmental justice is for communities throughout the United States that have hydraulic fracturing (fracking) operations. Studies in Pennsylvania and in Texas indicate that poverty is closely correlated with communities where fracking occurs (Bienkowski, 2015). Many citizens of such communities are   taking action to address the concerns in their communities (Carre, 2012) by addressing public policy. New York State has banned fracking and Maryland has a moratorium on fracking, while many cities and counties have enacted legislation to limit fracking. In July 2012, Longmont City Council passed a set of regulations governing fracking within city limits, and in November 2012, voters approved an all-out ban of the practice (Earthjustice, 2019).

OCCUPATIONAL JUSTICE

As noted in our discussion of vulnerable populations, workplace exposures vary by type of occupation, location of work, and biologic, physical (including ergonomic), chemical, noise and radiologic exposures. Further, various population groups are more vulnerable, such as pregnant people, children, adolescents, older adults and those from ethnic and racially marginalized groups. Adverse health effects can occur immediately or many years later. The federal government regulates worker safety primarily through the Occupational Safety and Health Administration (OSHA) within the U.S. Department of Labor.

Other agencies offer guidance and support for education and research to improve workplace safety. One must consider all aspects of a work environment including job stress, opportunities for healthy diet and exercise, violence, and protective equipment, in addition to the specific workplace exposures in any particular occupation. The Centers for Disease Control (CDC) notes in their Immigrant Worker Safety and Health website that, "Immigrant workers face a disproportionate risk for workplace injury and illness. This is due to a confluence of factors including an overrepresentation in the most hazardous industries including construction and agriculture. Additionally, workplace safety interventions often do not reach immigrant worker populations due to barriers created by social, cultural, and economic issues including language, literacy, and marginal economic status. Furthermore, immigrant workers often lack knowledge of their rights to workplace safety and are reluctant to pursue these rights" (CDC, 2014).

Ethnic and racially marginalized groups are more likely to be employed in physically demanding jobs with hazards such as construction, farming, mining and meat packing (Frumkin, 2010). Immigrants are often employed in more hazardous work settings (Panikkar, et al., 2014). Factors such as language proficiency and access to occupational health services contribute to their type of employment. Murray (2003) studies low-income workers and their health risks. She reports that industries such as forestry, fishing, farming, and machine operators are among those with the highest proportion of workers who live in

poverty. She further notes that Black and Latino workers lag behind White workers in both their compensation for their work and job desirability. Arcury and colleagues (2002) looked at the multiple risks of farmworkers from pesticide exposure in farm fields and also in their homes. Study findings indicate that the farmworkers were exposed to pesticides to a great degree in their housing and workplaces. Ahonen and colleagues (2007) note that immigrant workers are not only overrepresented in the most hazardous work conditions but are exposed to the most danger within those jobs.

Although the Environmental Justice movement began in response to communities where residents experienced disproportionate exposures to hazardous chemicals, the federal government recognizes that many people are exposed not only in their homes but also in the workplace. In collaboration with the Department of Health and Human Services (HHS), President Biden developed the Justice40 Initiative at DHHS. The Department of Labor also has programs to promote environmental justice through the Justice40 Initiative to support training and workforce development.

INTERNATIONAL HAZARDOUS WASTE DISPOSAL

In addition to the negative extremes of social determinants of health acting as magnets to environmental justice issues, the rise of economic globalization, liberalized trade rules and the dominance of multinational corporations play key roles in transporting environmental pollution from industrialized to developing countries (Clapp, 2014). Shipping hazardous waste from developed countries to developing countries for disposal is a regular practice. The receiving countries often have inadequate or lax regulations and protocols, inadequate resources, and insufficient training for the safe management and disposal of environmental waste. According to the Basel Action Network the primary motivation for exporting hazardous waste to developing countries is economic. As the deleterious health and environmental impacts of unsound disposal of hazardous waste have become increasingly apparent, governments of industrialized countries have enacted stringent regulations for waste disposal---a costly endeavor. An economist with the World Bank wrote (and later retracted) that "the economic logic behind dumping a load of toxic waste in the lowest wage country is impeccable and we should face up to that" (Lipman, 2011). He further noted, "health-impairing pollution should be done in the country with the lowest cost, which will be the country with the lowest wages." Evidence collected in the late 1980's found that 'the average disposal cost of one ton of hazardous waste in Africa was between US $2.50 to $50.00, while the cost in industrialized countries ranged from US $100 to US $2,000" (Lipman, 2011).

Dumping of waste in developing countries has occurred in some cases with the consent of governments and in other cases as part of an illegal scheme frequently related to strategic motives of the sending country, and corruption of the receiving government (Lipman, 2011). This dumping occurs with little regard for the people who will handle or work with the received toxic waste. Just as the motives for permitting the siting of "dirty industries" in low income, often jobless communities in the U.S. are based on promises of jobs, money and political favor, the same inducements are evident in developing countries.

The Basel Convention on the Control of Trans boundary Movements of Hazardous Waste and their Disposal (Lipman, 2011) is an international treaty that was designed to reduce the movements of hazardous waste between nations and specifically to prevent transfer of hazardous waste from developed to less developed countries (Basel, 2015). It was signed in 1989 and became effective in May, 1992. As of February, 2014, 180 states and the European Union are parties to the Convention. Fourteen (14) of 194 United Nations (UN) member states have not signed, including the United States.

Recently the UN took action to curb the plastic waste crisis by adding plastic to the Basel Convention, a treaty that controls the movement of hazardous waste from one country to another. The amendments require exporters to obtain the consent of receiving countries before shipping most contaminated, mixed, or unrecyclable plastic waste, providing an important tool for countries in the Global South to stop the dumping of unwanted plastic waste into their country.

E-waste is another environmental health problem. E-waste results from the rapid obsolescence of electronic gadgets in response to the high demand for new technology. Electronic equipment contains toxins, including mercury, lead, cadmium, arsenic, beryllium brominated flame retardants, and on burning, dioxins and polycyclic aromatic hydrocarbons (WHO, 2022). The latter are some of the most toxic substances to humans. Early manufacturers gave little thought to their disposal, the level of toxicity in their products, or potential reclamation of non-toxic components of the electronic products.

There is little financial value in recycling outdated electronic waste in the U.S. and other industrialized countries. There are few incentives or government regulations at this time to safely manage the disposal of e-waste in industrialized countries. Many have advocated for humanitarian reasons to send old or refurbished computers and computer parts to resource poor countries. Others have found it considerably cheaper to dispose of e-waste in developing countries. The most common destinations of waste from Europe and the US are the Far East, India, Africa, and China (Greenpeace International, 2009; WHO, 2022). Targeted countries lack the proper infrastructure and regulations/or adherence for disposal of e-waste.

The growing numbers of scrap yards in developing countries seek to harvest parts and precious metals (copper, iron, silicon, nickel and gold) from electronic equipment during recycling and sell them for profit; workers and purchasers are exposed to toxins. In developing countries, children are used in recycling, removing metal and parts by hand. Mislabeling is a common practice in shipping hazardous waste, which is in non-compliance with the requirements of the Basel Convention. Because the U.S. has never signed the Basel Convention, its shipments are not illegal. Additionally, lax maritime and immigration regulations place vulnerable populations at-risk, particularly those who are poor and people of color. The U.S. also sends much of its hazardous waste to prisons in the U.S. to be processed in less regulated environments without the same worker protections and rights afforded in the private sector (Greenpeace, 2015). These are serious environmental justice issues.

Fourteen (14) of 194 United Nations (UN) member states have not signed, including the United States.

Recently the UN took action to curb the plastic waste crisis by adding plastic to the Basel Convention, a treaty that controls the movement of hazardous waste from one country to another. The amendments require exporters to obtain the consent of receiving countries before shipping most contaminated, mixed, or unrecyclable plastic waste, providing an important tool for countries in the Global South to stop the dumping of unwanted plastic waste into their country.

E-waste is another environmental health problem of recent ascent (e-Stewards, 2008). E-waste results from the rapid obsolesce of electronic gadgets in response to the high demand for new technology. Electronic equipment contains toxins, including mercury, lead, cadmium, arsenic, beryllium brominated flame retardants, and on burning, dioxins and polycyclic aromatic hydrocarbons. The latter are some of the most toxic substances to humans. Early manufactures gave little thought to their disposal, the level of toxicity in their products, or potential reclamation of non-toxic components of the electronic products.

There is little financial value in recycling outdated electronic waste in the U.S. and other industrialized countries. There are few incentives or government regulations at this time to safely manage the disposal of e-waste in industrialized countries. Many have advocated for humanitarian reasons to send old or refurbished computers and computer parts to resource poor countries. Others have found it considerably cheaper to dispose of e-waste in developing countries. The most common destinations of waste from Europe and the US are the Far East, India, Africa, and China (Greenpeace International, 2009). Targeted countries lack the proper infrastructure and regulations/or adherence for disposal of e-waste.

The growing numbers of scrap yards in developing countries seek to harvest parts and precious metals (cooper, iron, silicon, nickel and gold) from electronic equipment during recycling and sell them for profit; workers and purchasers are exposed to toxins. In developing countries, children are used in recycling, removing metal and parts by hand. Mislabeling is a common practice in shipping hazardous waste, which is in non-compliance with the requirements of the Basel Convention. Because the U.S. has never signed the Basel Convention, its shipments are not illegal. Additionally, lax maritime and immigration regulations place marginalized populations at-risk, particularly those who are poor and people of color. The U.S. also sends much of its hazardous waste to prisons in the U.S. to be processed in less-regulated environments without the same worker protections and rights afforded in the private sector (Greenpeace, 2015). These are serious environmental justice issues.

In addition to the work to reduce global waste, deal with plastic waste, electrical stewardship the Basel Network works to encourage green ship recycling for the old ships that have reached their ability for safe use (Basel Action Network, 2023).

CLIMATE CHANGE AND ENVIRONMENTAL JUSTICE

In recent years, among the most pressing international environmental threats is climate change. The Center for Progressive Reform provides a thorough overview of international environmental justice and climate change. Their focus upon climate justice seeks to highlight the increased risks that many face through protection of vulnerable populations, seizing federal opportunities and reforming state governance. Global warming and climate change result from the burning of fossil fuels, including coal, gas, and oil for cars and industries. Fossil fuels are primary sources of carbon dioxide that is one of the principal gases responsible for trapping heat in the atmosphere. The release of these gases has increased by one-third since the Industrial Revolution (middle of 19th century). The rate of discharge is expected to double by the end of the 21st century, associated with increasing energy consumption in developing countries. Of significance, the United States is responsible for 25 percent of the world's greenhouse gases, although it only contains 4 percent of the world's population (Center for Progressive Reform, 2019).

"Greenhouse gases will substantially disrupt ecosystems and water supplies across the globe, intensifying dangerous weather patterns and causing a host of other health, environmental, economic, and social problems" (EPA, 2015b). The effects of climate change are most devastating to populations in urban centers and coastal regions and those dependent upon subsistence fishing. Such populations are overwhelmingly people of color and dwell in poor communities. Contributing to already existing health and environmental problems, heavy rains, floods, and hurricanes occurring over a few days can further compound the health challenges of these vulnerable communities. Similarly, rural areas in developing countries experience droughts and excessive heat, limiting hydration for humans and animals and diminishing the production of food for subsistence and as a marketable crop.

Between 2030 and 2050, climate change is expected to cause approximately 250,000 additional deaths per year, from malnutrition, malaria, diarrhea and heat stress (WHO, 2019).

In weather-triggered disasters, people and animals die; homes, crops, and resources are destroyed; and public health infrastructure (hospitals and clinics, roads) are damaged. These catastrophes threaten the health, food security and livelihoods of poor populations across the globe, particularly people of color. Hence, these disparities can be characterized as environmental injustices and/or environmental racism (Environmental Justice Network, 2015).

Recent studies of the disproportionate impact of heat exposure in "heat islands" as well as flooding show that historic discriminatory policies such as redlining contribute to the inequities in neighborhoods exposure to excess heat and flooding. Redlining is a term used to describe the discriminatory policies of the early 1900s in the United States that segregated white neighborhoods and communities from those where people of color could live. While this also contributed to the inequitable siting of hazardous waste areas, siting of polluting power plants and other pollutants that create areas such as "Cancer Alley" in Louisiana, the impacts are also noted in inequitable climate risks. Heat islands are urban areas that suffer higher temperatures than other urban areas of the same city or community due to unshaded areas and roadways as well as high concentration of concrete areas, close proximity of buildings and lack of green space. Areas of cities and communities with high populations of people of color and those living in poverty are noted to be areas identified as heat islands (Hoffman, Shandas, & Pendelton (2020). Further, we see examples of flooding disproportionately impacting racially segregated areas such as the Ninth Ward of New Orleans in 2005 due to Hurricane Katrina and more recent storms in Houston,

Policy debates have prevailed over time to have all nations significantly reduce the use of carbon-based fuels. "Developing countries maintain that they should not have to bear social and economic burdens of controlling greenhouse gas emissions disproportionate to their causal responsibilities, particularly when they have yet to achieve a basic level of development" (International Environmental Justice, 2013).

The The Paris Agreement is a landmark environmental international accord that was adopted by nearly every nation in 2015 to address climate change and its negative impacts. The agreement aims to substantially reduce global greenhouse gas emissions in an effort to limit the global temperature increase in this century to 2 degrees Celsius above pre-industrial levels, while pursuing means to limit the increase to 1.5 degrees. The agreement includes commitments from all major emitting countries to cut their climate altering pollution and to strengthen those commitments over time. The pact provides a pathway for developed nations to assist developing nations in their climate mitigation and adaptation efforts, and it creates a framework for the transparent monitoring, reporting, and ratcheting up of countries' individual and collective climate goals. Under Trump, the United States pulled out of the agreement. However over 30 mayors, 3 governors, 80 university presidents and 100 businesses pledged to uphold the Paris Accord goals (Tabuchi & Fountain, 2017).

On January 20, 2021 President Biden officially brought the US back into the Paris Agreement.

MOVEMENT TO GLOBALIZE ENVIRONMENTAL JUSTICE

Levy & Patz (2015) state that "Climate change-the global climate crisis might be the defining moral issue of the 21st century" p. 311. Not only are millions of people affected by climate change impacts each year, but the human costs contribute to mass migration of populations affected by climate events. Reasons for this migration result from food scarcity, land availability, fresh water availability,

extreme weather events and human health impacts (McMichael, C, Barnett, J. & McMichael, A.J., 2012). While voices note that this is a time of crisis, the concerns for global justice reach back decades.

Robert Bullard, the father of Environmental Justice, noted that "all people and communities are entitled to equal protection of environmental and public health laws and regulations" (Bullard, 1990). The concept of environmental justice applies to communities where there are perceived disadvantage, whether due to race, ethnicity, socioeconomic status, immigration status, lack of land ownership, geographic isolation, formal education, occupational characteristics, political power, gender, or other characteristics, which puts them at disproportionate risk for being exposed to environmental hazards (Claudio, 2007). The movement to globalize environmental justice parallels a series of environmentally-oriented agreements and global conventions. Following is a timeline of early, progressive milestones in the globalization of environmental justice:

1991: Principles of Environmental Justice, a guide for grassroots organizing, was adopted by environmental justice leaders during the First National People of Color Environmental Leadership Summit, Washington, D.C.

1992: The Earth Summit in Rio de Janeiro, Brazil, lacked a focus on environmental justice within the context of human health; human health and urban centers were not considered part of the environment. However, a promising sign was that the Principles of Environmental Justice (1991) had been translated into Portuguese and circulated to local community leaders at the Summit.

2000: The United Nations Summit in New York adapted the eight UN Millennium Development Goals that included one on "Ensuring Environmental Sustainability."

2002: The leadership of the World Summit on Sustainable Development in Johannesburg, South Africa formally recognized the issue of environmental inequity.

Advocates, including grassroots workers for environmental justice, face common concerns around the globe and share a common goal of improving the conditions for vulnerable populations in their nations. Throughout the world, disadvantaged communities typically suffer the highest burdens of environmental degradation. With increased attention to common international environmental justice issues, grassroots and other community-based advocacy groups have begun to communicate across national and continental borders. Such groups share concerns, approaches to advocacy, and educational materials and approaches, and coordinate strategies for addressing common offenses. Several universal concerns and international strategies are highlighted below:

- Rural farm workers across Latin America, South Africa, among others, suffer from the effects of disproportionate exposure to pesticides and other chemical agents as well as the lack of access to health and education services. Members of the Farmworkers Associations of Florida have exchange visits with citrus farmers in Brazil to trade ideas on how to address environmental justice issues. The problems faced are the same across international borders: literacy, lack of government support, the strong influence of chemical industries that produce pesticides, and lack of access to healthcare and housing. http://www.floridafarmworkers.org/

- Global Alliance for Incinerator Alternatives (GAIA), headquartered in the Philippines, aims to coordinate efforts to reduce waste and stop incineration around the world with a particular focus on representing disadvantaged communities in both developed and developing countries. Its approaches include sharing information electronically, coordinating regional meetings, developing joint strategies for community organizing, and hosting international training sessions where skills can be shared. GAIA has members in over 77 countries (Claudio, 2007). http://www.no-burn.org/about

- Poor and disadvantaged communities around the globe face similar problems associated with globalization and the advance of multinational corporations. Diamond, Louisiana is home to more than 130 petrochemical facilities, incinerators, and landfills known as the Chemical Corridor or Cancer Alley. Other similar sites are victims of the "waste follows waste" phenomena (http://www.ejnet.org). See the following site for images of the Vision Project http://www.visionproject.org/images/img_magazine/pdfs/canceralley_louisiana.pdf

- Grassroots organizations such as Concern Citizens of Norco, established in 1990, engaged and confronted leadership of The Shell Corporation, owner of nearby petrochemical facilities in Louisiana, to take responsibility for the pollution and to relocate people to cleaner locations. The group used strategies such as highly visible campaigns at the state, national, and international levels, winning the community relocations and a reduction in Shell's toxic emissions by 30%. The persistent advocacy and community organizing earned Margie Richard, founder of Concern Citizens Norco, the Goldman Environmental Prize (Claudio, 2007).

- Similar cases of multiple toxic waste facilities located in the same area have spread internationally and are generally owned by multinational corporations. The Shell Corporation has multiple toxic waste facilities such as plants, landfills, and incinerators in Texas, South Durban, South Africa, the Philippines, Nigeria, Brazil, Curacao, and Russia. Lessons learned about the strategies used by Concern Citizens Norco have been shared around the globe, linking environmental justice issues internationally.

- One grassroots organization is Friends of the Earth International, described as the largest grassroots environmental network with 70 national members and 5,000 local activist groups who are supported in community organizing and finding common grounds for action.

In 2015 Pope Francis in his encyclical Laudato Si: Care for Our Common Home, wrote, "Climate change is a global problem with grave implications: environmental, social, economic, political and for the distribution of goods. It represents one of the principal challenges facing humanity in our day. Its worst impact will probably be felt by developing countries in coming decades." His Holiness Pope Francis, 2015). This document with its strong focus on justice has fostered greater interest and collaboration globally.

International collaboration and partnering continues to grow. Collaborators share experiences, strategies and educational resources, and engage in collaborative problem solving. Common strategies for class advocacy for environmental justice include the following:

- use of media,

- mediation,

- expert testimony,

- community organizing,

- program development, and

- coalition building (Powell, 1999).

Health professionals must be part of the response to global climate justice (Nicholas & Breakey, 2017; Butterfield, Leffers, & Vasquez, 2021). Organizations such as the Alliance of Nurses for Healthy Environments (ANHE) sponsor a Global Nurses Climate Change Committee to engage nurses globally to take action to address climate change with a focus upon equity and justice. Additionally, ANHE offers a podcast series entitled the Climate Justice Podcast Series. Nurses across the US and beyond collaborate to address climate justice using a global lens.

NURSES AND ENVIRONMENTAL JUSTICE

Nurses became involved in environmental justice largely through their work with communities and concern for social justice. Dorothy Powell, EdD, RN, FAAN, retired and Clinical Professor Emeriti of Duke University was one of the first nurses to become involved in the environmental justice movement. Active in the Civil Rights Movement in Vance County, North Carolina, during her youth, she credits her involvement in environmental justice to the events in Warren County, a neighboring county to Vance County. She became aware of the oil dumping there through the work of her uncle and other community leaders. In 1978, when PCB-laced oil was dumped along the roadways of Warren County, critics claimed that the area was selected because it was rural and a majority of the residents were poor, black and politically unable to determine their fate. However, hundreds of community activists worked alongside environmental groups and civil rights groups to protest the dumping and the plan for a landfill by physically blocking truck access to the landfill. This powerful example led Powell, an African-American nurse, to be professionally swayed by her commitment to equality and justice as a youth and by the discriminatory practices in neighboring Warren County.

The Mississippi Delta Region (219 counties in 7 states) was another example of environmental pollution and environmental injustices. Through a 1994 agreement with the Minority Health Professions Foundation, Howard University Nursing spearheaded a nursing initiative to enhance understanding of environmental health, including environmental justice, among nursing students and practicing nurses in the region. Funding for the work was through the Center for Disease Control and Prevention (CDC) and the Agency for Toxic Substance and Disease Registry (ATSDR). Dr. Powell and nursing colleagues developed a modular curriculum Environmental Health and Nursing: The Mississippi Delta Project (1999), published by ATSDR. Dr. Powell gained recognition as a leader in environmental justice following publication of the modules where she authored the unit on Environmental Justice and was overall project lead. Other modules included: Environmental Health of the MDR (Hansberry & White, 1999); Role of Culture, Race and Economic Development on Environmental Health (Lassister & Mitchem-Davis, 1999); Toxicology: Major Substances Affecting the Delta (Green, Mitchem-Davis, & Richardson, 1999); Assessing Individual, Family and Community Responses to Toxic Substances (Copes & Richardson, 1999); Community Organization,

Empowerment, Partnering and Education (Lassister, 1999). The learning modules include learning objectives, content, learning activities, teaching methods and evaluation as well as appendices and references.

Other nurses have written on the topic to advance professional understanding of environment and social determinants, justice, and environmental justice (Butterfield, 2002; Larrson & Butterfield, 2002; Pope, Synder & Mood, 1995; Nicholas & Breakey, 2017; Butterfield, Leffers & Diaz Vasquez, 2021)). Lillian Mood, RN, MSN, Director of Risk Communication and Community Liaison, Environmental Quality Control, South Carolina Department of Health and Environmental Control chaired an Institute of Medicine committee to study enhancing environmental health content in nursing. The 1995 report, Nursing, Health & Environment, wove environmental justice throughout the curriculum. The report stressed the importance for nurses to understand the disproportionate risk of economically disadvantaged patients for exposure to hazardous environmental pollutants. Because nurses are accessible to members of vulnerable communities, it is important for nurses to bring the concerns of impacted communities to the policy arena and health systems (Pope, Snyder, & Mood, 1995).

Patricia Butterfield, PhD, RN, FAAN, and Julie Postma, PhD, RN, of Washington State University applied an environmental justice lens to rural environmental health (Butterfield & Postma, 2009) through conceptualization of the Translational Environmental Research in Rural Areas (TERRA) Framework. Rural populations are increasingly challenged by confined animal feeding operations (CAFOs), groundwater exposures, agricultural run-off, as well as exposure to specific hazardous waste sites located in their communities. The framework considers macro determinants as well as family level determinants to better understand the environmental health risks experienced by the rural poor.

Laura Anderko, PhD, RN, the Robert and Kathleen Scanlon Chair in Values Based Health Care at Georgetown University, has served on the National Environmental Justice Advisory Committee Research Workgroup, teaches a course on environmental justice, and worked with communities to address health disparities and justice issues. She has served to advance justice issues at not only Georgetown, but for nurses nationally.

Patricia Butterfield, Jeanne Leffers and Maribel Diaz Vasquez (2021) urge nurses globally to learn from the voices of those in the most impacted regions, and strengthen their commitment to indigenous practices and ancestral knowledge. Further nurses must promote equity in all advocacy efforts to address climate change.

The American Nurses Association in 2007 developed the [ANA's Principles Environmental Health for Nursing Practice and Implementation Strategies](#) that address environmental justice, citing concerns for social justice and health disparities. The nine assumptions upon which the principles are grounded include the following: "environmental and social justice is a right of all populations and assumes that disparities in health are not acceptable."

RESOURCES
Websites

Center for Climate Change, Climate Justice and Health, MGH Institute for Health Professions https://www.mghihp.edu/nursing/centers-initiatives/center-climate-change-climate-justice-and-health

Environmental Protection Agency (EPA). (n.d.) *Environmental justice.* https://www.epa.gov/environmentaljustice

Environmental Protection Agency (EPA). (2014). *EPA Plan EJ 2014.* https://www.epa.gov/environmentaljustice/plan-ej-2014

Environmental Protection Agency (EPA). (2014) *EPA Plan EJ 2014 Progress Report.* https://www.epa.gov/sites/production/files/2015-02/documents/plan-ej-progress-report-2014.pdf

National Institutes of Environmental Health Sciences (NIEHS). Environmental Health Disparities and Environmental Justice https://www.niehs.nih.gov/research/supported/translational/justice/index.cfm

NIEHS-Advancing Environmental Justice http://www.niehs.nih.gov/research/supported/assets/docs/a_c/advancing_environmental_justice_508.pdf

NIEHS-Liam O'Fallon, Coordinator for Partnerships for Environmental Health http://www.niehs.nih.gov/research/supported/dert/phb/ofallon/index.cfm

Environmental Justice Network www.ejnet.org/ and http://www.ejnet.org/ej/

Articles and Books

Anderko, L. (2009). Environments and health. *AJN, American Journal of Nursing, 6*(109),74-76. doi: 10.1097/01.NAJ.0000352484.16736.4e

Bullard, R., Johnson, G., & Torres, A. (2011). *Environmental health and racial equity in the United States: Building environmentally just, sustainable, and livable communities.* APHA Press.

Dressel, A., Anderko, L., & Koepsel, B. (August 2013). The Westlawn Partnership for a Healthier Environment: Promoting environmental justice and building community capacity. *Environmental Justice, 6*(4), 127-132. doi:10.1089/env.2013.0024.

Perry, D. (2005). Transcendent pluralism and the influence of nursing testimony on environmental justice legislation. *Policy, Politics and Nursing Practice, 6*(1), 60-71. doi: 10.1177/1527154404272748

Sattler, B. & Lipscomb, J. (2003). *Environmental health and nursing practice.* Springer.

Thomas, V. M. & Graedel, T. E. (2003). Research issues in sustainable consumption: Toward an analytical framework for materials and the environment. *Environmental Science and Technology, 37,* 5383-5388.

REFERENCES

Ahonen, E. Q., Benavides, F. G., & Benach, J. (2007). Immigrant populations, work and health: A systematic review. *Scandinavian Journal of Work, Environment & Health, 33,* (2), 96-104.

Arcury, T. A., Quandt, S. A., & Russell, G. B. (2002). Pesticide safety among farmworkers: perceived risk and perceived control as factors reflecting environmental justice. *Environmental Health Perspectives, 110* (Suppl 2), 233–240.

Basel Action Network (2023). *Safeguarding people and the planet from toxic waste trade.* https://www.ban.org/

Basel Convention. (2015). *Basel Convention: Controlling transboundary movements of hazardous wastes and their disposal.* http://www.basel.int/

Bienkowski, B. (2015). *Poor in Pennsylvania: You're fracked.* Environmental Health News. http://www.environmentalhealthnews.org/ehs/news/2015/may/pennsylvania-fracking-environmental-justice-poor-economics

Bullard, R. D. 1990. *Dumping in Dixie: Race, class, and environmental quality.* Westview.

Bullard, R.D. (2002). *Poverty, pollution and environmental racism: Strategies for building healthy and sustainable communities.* http://archive.is/LHBko. Also http://geotheology.blogspot.com/2007/03/poverty-pollution-and-environmental.html

Butterfield, P. G. (2002). Upstream reflections on environmental health: An abbreviated history and framework for action: Critique and reflection. *Advances in Nursing Science, 25*(1), 32-49.

Butterfield, P., Leffers, J., & Diaz-Vasquez, M. (2021). Nurses pivotal role in global climate action. *BMJ, 373.* https://www.bmj.com/content/373/bmj.n1049

Butterfield, P. & Postma, J. (2009). The TERRA framework: conceptualizing rural environmental health inequities through an environmental justice lens...translational environmental research in rural areas. *Advances in Nursing Science, 32*(2), 107-17.

Carre, N. (2012). Environmental justice and hydraulic fracturing: The ascendancy of grassroots populism in policy determination. *Journal of Social Change, 4*(1), 1–13. https://www.researchgate.net/publication/228333480_Environmental_Justice_and_Hydraulic_Fracturing_The_Ascendancy_of_Grassroots_Populism_in_Policy_Determination

Carson, R. (1962). *Silent spring.* Houghton Mifflin Company.

Center for Progressive Reform [CPR]. (2019). *International environmental justice and climate change.* http://www.progressivereform.org/climatechange.cfm

Clapp, J. (2014). *Toxic exports: The transfer of hazardous waste from rich to poor countries.* Cornell University Press.

Claudio, L. (2007). Standing on principle: The global push for environmental justice. *Environmental Health Perspectives, 115*(10), A500-A503. http://www.ncbi.nlm.nih.gov/pmc/articles/PMC2022674

Copes, & Rcichardson, T. (1999). Assessing Individual, Family and Community Responses to Toxic Substances. In Powell, D. L. (1999). *Howard University Division of Nursing. Environmental health and nursing: The Mississippi Delta Project, a modular curriculum.* U.S Department of Health and Human Services & ATSDR.

e-Stewards. (2008). *What's driving the e-waste crisis?* http://www.e-stewards.org/the-e-waste-crisis/why-does-this-problem-exist/

Earthjustice. (2015). *Clean air ambassador: Charlotte Keys.* http://www.earthjustice.org/50states/charlotte-keys

Earthjustice. (2019). *Fighting fracking across the U.S.* https://earthjustice.org/features/unfracktured-communities

Environmental Justice Network. (2015). *Environmental justice/Environmental racism.* http://www.ejnet.org/ej/

Frumkin, H., (2010). *Environmental health: From global to local.* Wiley.

Green, P. ,Mitchem-Davis, A., & Richardson, T. (1999). Toxicology: Major substances affecting the Delta. In Powell, D. L. (1999). *Howard University Division of Nursing. Environmental health and nursing: The Mississippi Delta Project,* a modular curriculum. U.S Department of Health and Human Services & ATSDR.

Greenpeace International. (24 February, 2009). *Where does e-waste end up?* http://www.greenpeace.org/international/en/campaigns/toxics/electronics/the-e-waste-problem/where-does-e-waste-end-up/

Greenpeace International. (2015). *Greenpeace International E-Waste.* http://www.greenpeace.org/international/en/System-templates/Search-results/?all=e-waste

Hansberry, A. & White, H. (1999). Environmental Health of the Mississippi Delta Region. In Powell, D. L (Ed). *Howard University. Division of Nursing. Environmental health and nursing: The Mississippi Delta Project, a modular curriculum.* U.S Department of Health and Human Services & ATSDR.

Hilgenkamp, K. (2006). *Environmental health: Ecological perspectives.* Jones and Bartlett.

Howard University Division of Nursing. (1999). *Environmental health and nursing: The Mississippi Delta Project, a modular curriculum.* U.S. Department of Health and Human Services & ATSDR.

International Environmental Justice [IEJ]. (2013). *International environmental justice and climate change.* http://www.progressivereform.org/perspintlenvironjustice.cfm

Larsson, L.S, & Butterfield, P. (2002). Mapping the future of environmental health and nursing: Strategies for integrating national competencies into nursing practice. *Public Health Nursing, 19*(4), 301-308.

Lassiter, P. (1999). Community Organization, empowerment, Partnering and Education. In Powell, D. L. (1999). *Howard University Division of Nursing. Environmental health and nursing: The Mississippi Delta Project, a modular curriculum.* U.S Department of Health and Human Services & ATSDR.

Lassiter, P. & Mitchem-Davis, A. (1999). Role of Culture, Race and Economic Development on Environmental Health in Powell, D. L. (1999). Environmental justice. *Howard University Division of Nursing. Environmental health and nursing: The Mississippi Delta Project, a modular curriculum.* U.S Department of Health and Human Services & ATSDR.

Lipman, Z. (2011). *Trade in hazardous waste: Environmental justice versus economic growth.* http://ban.org/library/lipman.html

Mass.gov (2019). *Case studies environmental justice: Jamaica, MA.* https://www.mass.gov/service-details/case-studies-environmental-justice-ej

Mikati, I. Benson, A. F., Luben, T. J., Sacks, J. D. & Richmond-Bryant, J. (2018). Disparities in distribution of particulate matter emission sources by race and poverty status. *AJPH, 108,* 480-485, https://doi.org/10.2105/AJPH.2017.304297

Murray, L. R. (2003). Sick and tired of being sick and tired: scientific evidence, methods, and research implications for racial and ethnic disparities in occupational health. *American Journal of Public Health, 93*(2), 221-226. doi: 10.2105/AJPH.93.2.221

Panikkar, B., Woodin, M. A., Brugge, D., Hyatt, R., Gute, D. M. & Community Partners Immigrant Worker Project. (2014). Characterizing the low wage immigrant workforce: A comparative analysis of the health disparities among selected occupations in Somerville, Massachusetts. *American Journal of Industrial Medicine, 57*(5), 516-526. http://onlinelibrary.wiley.com/doi/10.1002/ajim.22181/abstract

Pope, A., Snyder, M., & Mood, L. (1995). *Nursing, health & the environment.* The Institute of Medicine, National Academies Press.

Powell, D. L. (1999). Environmental justice. Module 5. In Howard University Division of Nursing. *Environmental health and nursing: The Mississippi Delta Project, a modular curriculum.* U.S Department of Health and Human Services & ATSDR.

Powell, D. & Stewert, V. (2001). CHILDREN : The unwitting target of environmental injustices. *Pediatric Clinics of North America, 5*(48) 1291–1305.

Skelton, R. & Miller, V. (2014). *The environmental justice movement.* Natural Resources Defense Council (NRDC). http://www.nrdc.org/ej/history/hej.asp

Tabuchi, H. & Fountain, H. (2017). *Bucking Trump, these cities, states, & companies commit to Paris Accord.* https://www.nytimes.com/2017/06/01/climate/american-cities-climate-standards.html

University of Michigan. (2015). *Environmental justice case study: The Yucca Mountain high-level nuclear waste repository and the Western Shoshone.* http://www.umich.edu/~snre492/kendziuk.html

US Environmental Protection Agency. (EPA) (2017). *Title VI and environmental justice.* https://www.epa.gov/environmentaljustice/title-vi-and-environmental-justice

US Environmental Protection Agency. (EPA). (2018). *Environmental justice: Learn about environmental justice.* https://www.epa.gov/environmentaljustice/learn-about-environmental-justice

US Environmental Protection Agency. (EPA). (2019a). *Environmental justice.* http://www.epa.gov/environmentaljustice/

US Environmental Protection Agency. (EPA). (2019b), *About the Office of Enforcement and Compliance Assurance.* https://www.epa.gov/aboutepa/about-office-enforcement-and-compliance-assurance-oeca#oej.

US Environmental Protection Agency. (EPA). (2019c), *EPA Organization Chart.* https://www.epa.gov/aboutepa/epa-organization-chart

US Environmental Protection Agency. (EPA). (2019d) *Overview of EPA's Brownfields Program.* https://www.epa.gov/brownfields/overview-epas-brownfields-program

US Environmental Protection Agency. (EPA). (2015b). *Future climate change.* https://www.epa.gov/climate-change-science/future-climate-change

WEACT. (2015). *WE ACT for environmental justice.* http://weact.nationbuilder.com

World Health Organization (2019). *Climate change.* https://www.who.int/heli/risks/climate/climatechange/en

World Health Organization. (2019). *Climate change and health.* https://www.who.int/en/news-room/fact-sheets/detail/climate-change-and-health

COMMUNITY SURVEY FOR POPULATION HEALTH
Kathryn P. Jackman-Murphy, Ed.D, RN, CHSE
Director, RN/BSN Program
Charter Oak State College

A Community Survey can be used as a tool for nurses and other disciplines to learn more about the strengths, resources, and gaps in services of a specific community. It can also provide opportunities for nursing students to critically think for the planning of care in meeting critical needs, such as exposure to chemicals of concern, proper nutrition, safety, medical appointments and activity.

A community survey provides a visual overview of a community and looks to explore needs and problems and the community's strengths and resources for the purpose of observing conditions and trends that could affect the health of the population. Conditions and trends in the community that could affect the health of the population are noted and provide background and context for working in and with the specific community.

Community surveys can be part of a more comprehensive community assessment that is a necessary step in planning community interventions. An extensive community assessment examines other factors such as health data, political information and demographics, socioeconomic data, religion, ethnicity, the language spoken in the home, community protective services such as police and fire departments, and other attributes of a community. A comprehensive community assessment requires the gathering of appropriate data from governmental and non-governmental sources. Additionally much can be learned from community forums and interviews with key informants.

This survey is useful for an examination of a community to identify potential and recognized environmental hazards that can negatively impact health as well as factors that improve health of the community members.

Objective: Explore a particular community while thinking critically and identifying potential and actual contributors, particularly environmental impacts to illness and health.

Windshield surveys are systematic observations made from a moving vehicle.

Walking surveys are systematic observations made on foot. For safety-consider completing in pairs.

Alternate clinical assignment: Have the group complete this via city bus and tour area their clinical facility serves.

Keep in mind your safety. It may not be safe to survey particular neighborhoods. Even if there is no real danger, but only a perception of danger, the resulting anxiety can affect the accuracy and completeness of a survey. Please choose another location or consider doing a windshield survey.

WHAT IS THE DEFINITION OF COMMUNITY?

There are many definitions including common and legal definitions. Below are a few:

- Common possession or enjoyment; participation; as, a community of goods.

- A body of people having common rights, privileges, or interests, or living in the same place under the same laws and regulations; as, a community of monks.

- Society at large; a commonwealth or state; political structure; the public, or people in general.

- Common character; likeness. For example a group of local fishermen can be a community

- A group of people living in a particular local area

- A group of people having ethnic or cultural or religious characteristics in common

- Common ownership: "they shared a community of possessions."

To understand the actual hazards that you may have observed during your tour of the community, examine resources such as EPA's Brownfields (https://www.epa.gov/brownfields). In particular look at the Brownfields near you (https://www.epa.gov/brownfields/brownfields-and-land-revitalization-activities-near-you). If the EPA site fails to identify a site on a map of your community, visit your state Department of Environmental Management. For example Rhode Island has a nice explanation of Brownfields at this link: http://www.dem.ri.gov/brownfields/documents/browneng.pdf while Massachusetts offers this map of the sites in the state https://www.mass.gov/doc/map-of-massachusetts-brownfields-sites/download. Another source of information is the EPA Superfund site, https://www.epa.gov/superfund. Superfund is the term used to describe areas on the National Priorities list for clean-up of toxic substances known to cause harm to human health. A site in Anniston, AL is linked here https://cumulis.epa.gov/supercpad/cursites/csitinfo.cfm?id=0400123.

Finally you can access local data for air quality and water quality in your community through your local or state government. By examining the actual pollution in your community and comparing it with your observations you can learn more about "what the eye does not see" and can improve your ability to identify environmental hazards.

Finally discuss: Have you "seen" these areas in the past? Are areas of concern more apparent to you as you are taking part in this activity?

WHAT TO EXAMINE IN A GENERAL COMMUNITY ASSESSMENT SURVEY

The age, nature, and condition of the community's available housing

- Are there safety concerns?

- Can you identify healthy home concerns? Area surrounding the homes?

Infrastructure

- Condition of the roads, streets, bridges and highways?

- Streetscape. The streetscape is the environment created by streets and the sidewalks, buildings, trees, etc. that line them. Are there trees and/or plants? Are there sidewalks? Are building facades and storefronts attractive and welcoming? Are the streets and sidewalks relatively clean and safe for foot traffic? Are there trash cans? Is there outdoor seating?

- Is there significant construction in the area? Is it contributing to the noise, traffic or pollution in the area?

- Municipal waste water system?

Transtation

- Availability of public transportation. How much does it cost? Are the vehicles energy-efficient?

- The amount of activity on the streets at various times of the day, week, or year

- The noise level in various parts of the community

- The amount and movement of traffic at various times of day

- Is there much bicycle traffic? Are there bike lanes? Are there bike racks in many places?

- Where are the gasoline service stations located? Could there be run off of chemicals used at the station?

- What about bus stations and taxi stands? Are the vehicles left to idle? Do they burn gasoline or diesel?

Availability of food sources

- Are there large chain grocery stores vs. small markets where food may be more expensive

- Farmer's market?

- Proximity of stores (consider how one would transport a week's worth of groceries)

- Food bank or food pantry in the community? If so do they offer fresh fruits and vegetables?

- Proximity/availability and healthiness of fast food restaurants

Community Resources

Public Spaces

- The amount, location, condition, and use of public spaces

- Is it 'black top" or green spaces? Are there public parks? Outdoor athletic opportunities?

- Is it safe for children to attend alone?

- Is there good lighting to extend use in the evening?

- Are the parks located near areas of poor air quality? Near highways?

Community organizations

- What evidence is there of organizations in the community?

- Are there service clubs – Lions, Elks, Masons, etc.? Are there other organizations – centered on community issues, the environment, sports or leisure pursuits, socialization, etc.?

- Is there a Senior Center?

Education

- Public schools. Are schools in different neighborhoods in noticeably different states of repair? Are schools well maintained?

- Are schools located near high traffic areas? Highways?

- Higher education. Are there two- and four-year colleges and/or universities in the community? Where are they located? Do they appear to be open to the community, or do they seem self-contained and isolated?

Health Services

- How many hospitals and clinics are there in the community? Where are they located? How big are they? How easy are they to get to?

- What is the availability of other health care providers?

Community and public services

- Are there identifiable community service providers and organizations in the community – mental health centers, food banks, shelters for the unhoused, welfare offices, etc.?

- Are they concentrated in a particular area? Are they easy to reach by public transportation?

Industry

- What kinds of industries exist in the community?

- Can you identify sources of pollution?

- Are the buildings that are boarded up/not in use?

- Do you know what chemicals might be used or produced by the industry?

Environmental quality

- How much usable green space is there, and is it scattered throughout the community?

- Is there smog or haze? Does the air smell of smoke, garbage, car exhaust, chemicals, industrial waste, etc.?

- Does the water in streams, ponds, lakes, etc. seem reasonably clear? Can you identify safe water sources? Is there a water treatment facility? Or does the community depend upon wells for drinking water?

Differences among neighborhoods or areas of the community

- What are the differences among different parts of the community?

- Are schools, stores, public and other buildings, streets, in different areas in good or inferior condition?

- Do some areas seem neglected, while others are clearly maintained? Are there signs of disrepair, trash or abandoned cars?

- Are there vacant lots or places where rodents or other wildlife might hide?

Advertising that you notice

- i.e. fast food, cigarettes, higher education, etc. What messages are the members of the community getting?

- Communication for informational posters or billboards?

The "feel" of the community.

- What is your overall impression of the community?

Safety

- Community safety. Where are police and fire stations located? Are they in good repair?

- Is the community well-lit at night? Are there bars on the windows?

- Do you see signs of drug use or trafficking?

Rural areas

- Agriculture: Are there farms? How large? What are they growing? Are there animals-cows, horses etc.? Are there farm stands-do they offer organic foods? Crops that need migrant workers?

- Access to safe drinking water?

HEALTHY HOMES ASSESSMENT TOOLS
Adelita G. Cantu, PhD, RN
University of Texas Health San Antonio
School of Nursing

Conditions in the places where people live, learn, work, and play affect a wide range of health risks and outcomes. These conditions are known as social determinants of health (SDOH): Social Determinants of Health. It has been noted that we spend approximately 90% of our time indoors, almost 70% of which is in our homes (EPA, 2018). Pollutants in the home are often 2 to 5 times higher than typical outdoor concentrations (EPA, 2018). People who are often most susceptible to the adverse effects of pollution (e.g., the very young, older adults, people with cardiovascular or respiratory disease) tend to spend even more time indoors (EPA, 2018). Indoor concentrations of some pollutants have increased in recent decades due to such factors as energy-efficient building construction (when it lacks sufficient mechanical ventilation to ensure adequate air exchange) and increased use of synthetic building materials, furnishings, personal care products, pesticides, and household cleaners. Thus, the home in which we live is often a contributing factor to many chronic diseases such as asthma, respiratory, and cardiovascular diseases.

To provide guidance in the assessment of home environments, the National Center for Healthy Housing assessed 20 key factors across 54 communities. The study reported that 35 million – 40% – of metropolitan homes in the U.S. have one or more health and safety hazards. The physical conditions of U.S. housing have declined since the U.S. Census' last survey in 2009. That survey found that about 30 million homes (or 35%) had health and safety hazards.

There are common pollutants that are found in the homes. These include combustion byproducts such as carbon monoxide, particulate matter, and environmental tobacco smoke; substances of natural origin such as radon, pet dander, and mold; biological agents such as molds; pesticides, lead, and asbestos, and various volatile organic compounds from a variety of products and materials.

Health effects associated with indoor air pollutants include irritation of the eyes, nose, and throat; headaches, dizziness, and fatigue, and respiratory diseases, heart disease, and cancer. The link between some common indoor air pollutants and health effects is very well established.

- Radon is a known human carcinogen and is the second leading cause of lung cancer (EPA).

- Carbon monoxide is toxic, and short-term exposure to elevated carbon monoxide levels in indoor settings can be lethal (NCBI).

- Numerous indoor air pollutants—dust mites, mold, pet dander, environmental tobacco smoke, cockroach allergens, particulate matter, and others—are "asthma triggers," meaning that some asthmatics might experience asthma attacks following exposure (IOM).

Populations in inadequate housing are more likely to have environmental diseases and injuries. Substantial disparities in housing have remained largely unchanged. Approximately 2.6 million (7.5%) non-Hispanic Blacks and 5.9 million Whites (2.8%) live in substandard housing and are vulnerable to the health effects associated with indoor air pollutants (Jacobs, 2011). Thus, many of the health disparities (asthma, hypertension, cardiovascular disease, cancer) among historically underrepresented populations are exacerbated by their home environment.

There is strong evidence that healthy home environment assessments encourage household behaviors that reduce asthma triggers and exposure to allergens.

The Green & Healthy Homes Initiative (GHHI) was charged in 2008 by the White House Office of Recovery to lead the national efforts to integrate lead hazard control, healthy homes, weatherization, and energy efficiency work. This project later became the Green & Healthy Homes Initiative that addresses the health and energy efficiency needs of a home through a holistic intervention model. The GHHI describes 11 housing hazards including lead, asthma triggers, household injury, asbestos, carbon monoxide, fire, mold and moisture, pests, radon, tobacco smoke, and volatile organic compounds.

There are a wide variety of healthy home assessment guidance and tools that have been created and are being used to identify hazards in the home. Once identified, mitigation strategies can be taken to decrease the negative health impacts to the occupants from these hazards.

Some of the tools and resources include:

CDC in partnership with the Housing and Urban Department (HUD) have developed a Healthy Housing Inspection Manual. The Healthy Housing Inspection Manual takes environmental health professionals and housing managers, specialists, and inspectors through the elements of a holistic home inspection. It is also a useful reference tool for nurses, outreach workers, and others who are interested in preventing illness and injury due to residential health and safety hazards.

[Home Environmental Health and Safety Assessment Tool](#) This tool from the [Alliance of Nurses for Healthy Environments](#) assesses sources of exposure in the home across ten different areas and provides information on the standards of practice if an exposure is found.

[The Healthy Homes Assessment Tool Checklist](#) from [The Yampa Valley Sustainability Council](#) is a tool that can be used to assess sources of exposure in the home as well safety hazards.

These tools are available online and can be used by health professionals, including community health workers to assess homes to ensure that where people live is healthy and sustainable.

REFERENCES

Centers for Disease Control and Prevention and U.S. Department of Housing and Urban Development. (2008). *Healthy housing inspection manual.* US Department of Health and Human Services.

Environmental Protection Agency. (2018). *Indoor Air Quality: What are the trends in indoor air quality and their effects on human health?* https://www.epa.gov/report-environment/indoor-air-quality.

Environmental Protection Agency. (1987). *Total Exposure Assessment Methodology (team) Study Summary and Analysis, Volume 1 Final Report.* https://bit.ly/3fRnl2v.

Environmental Protection Agency, Exposure Factors Handbook (1997, Final Report). *Total Exposure Assessment Methodology (team) Study summary and analysis, volume 1 final report.* https://cfpub.epa.gov/ncea/risk/recordisplay.cfm?deid=12464.

Environmental Protection Agency. (2019). *Health risk of radon.* https://www.epa.gov/radon/health-risk-radon#bier.

Green and Healthy Homes Initiative. (2020). *About us, Our history.* https://www.greenandhealthyhomes.org/about-us/our-history/.

Home Health Hazards. Green and Healthy Homes Initiative. (2020). *Home health hazards.* https://www.greenandhealthyhomes.org/home-and-health/home-health-hazards/.

Institute of Medicine (US) Committee on the Assessment of Asthma and Indoor Air. (2000). *Clearing the air: Asthma and indoor air exposures.* https://pubmed.ncbi.nlm.nih.gov/25077220/.

Jacobs, D. E. (2011). Environmental health disparities in housing. *American Journal of Public Health, 101*(Suppl 1), S115–S122. https://www.ncbi.nlm.nih.gov/pmc/articles/PMC3222490/.

Office of Disease Prevention and Health Promotion. *Social determinants of health.* https://www.healthypeople.gov/2020/topics-objectives/topic/social-determinants-of-health.

Raub, J. A., Mathier-Nolf, M. M., Hampson, N. B., & Thom, S. R. (2000) Carbon monoxide poisoning. *Toxicology, 1*(145), 1-14.https://pubmed.ncbi.nlm.nih.gov/10771127/.

National Center of Healthy Housing. (2018). *State of healthy housing.* https://nchh.org/tools-and-data/data/state-of-healthy-housing/.

National Center of Health Housing. (n.d.). *State of healthy housing executive summary.* https://nchh.org/tools-and-data/data/state-of-healthy-housing/executive-summary/.

THE ROLE OF TREES IN CLIMATE CHANGE MITIGATION: A STORY OF COMMUNITY MITIGATION EFFORTS IN CHAPIN, SOUTH CAROLINA

Lillian Mood, RN, MPH, FAAN Retired,
South Carolina Department of Health and Environmental Control
Columbia, SC

Introduction by Jeanne Leffers, PhD, RN, FAAN
Professor Emeritus
University of Massachusetts Dartmouth
College of Nursing and Health Sciences

INTRODUCTION

Recently there has been a great deal of publicity about the fires not only in parts of the United States but also in the Amazon region of South America. While media reports, as well as climate change scientists, note that the rise in wildfires and extreme weather events are often the result of climate change, deforestation is a distinct cause of rising green house gas (GHG) emissions (Galford et al, 2010). Additionally wildfires contribute to the loss of trees that serve to mitigate climate change by reducing GHG emissions through carbon dioxide absorption.. One strategy to address this has been the efforts to plant trees for their ability to reduce these emissions, particularly in marginalized communities where environmental injustice occurs (Smith et al, 2020; Rudd et al, 2018). Although many people have yet to make the connections between trees, climate change and health (Wolf et al, 2020), one long term environmental health nurse shares her story with us about efforts she led in her community to plant trees. This was an effort that not only addressed climate change but it also brought community members together for a shared goal, involved students who learned about the importance of trees to their community and health and connected young and older community members around a civic issue.

CHAPIN SEQUOIAS

In the January 2014 issue of Readers Digest an article caught my eye titled, "20 REASONS WHY THIS YEAR WILL BE BETTER THAN LAST". The article contained a collection of indicators including one that told of a large scale effort to plant sequoias and redwoods.

I was intrigued. I had thought that sequoias only grew on the west coast of the USA. In exploring the Internet I learned that sequoias will grow in any temperate climate where they get adequate water and drainage. I began to wonder if we could grow sequoias in my small lakeside community in the center of South Carolina.

There were several reasons for my interest. I spent the final third of my 30+ year career as a public health nurse working in the environmental protection programs of the SC Department of Health and Environmental Control. My position, as the first Director of Risk Communication and Community Liaison in Environmental Quality Control, was the brainchild of Lewis Shaw, PE and Deputy Commissioner. He saw the need for a nurse to bridge the divide between his staff of environmental scientists and engineers and the communities who were often alarmed by real or perceived environmental hazards they feared might be affecting their health. After nearly ten years working to strengthen links between health and environment, I retired with a deep commitment to continuing the work of protecting the environment for the benefit of all communities.

And I love trees! I live in a small log cabin by the lake, and my neighbors are very tolerant of my maintaining a lot of trees, with natural leaf cover on the ground—a home in the woods in the midst of a small neighborhood! They are uncomplaining that many of the leaves they rake in their own yards come from my trees. I am grateful!

It was easy to see the link between planting trees and environmental and population health. The article said, "Sequoias can breathe in CO2 faster and more effectively than almost any other species on earth, mitigating the adverse effects of climate change." (David Milarch, cofounder of Archangel Ancient Tree Archive, which locates, clones, and archives tree genetics, Readers Digest, January 2014, p. 82)

Spurred on by the benefits of trees to a healthy community—as carbon absorbers, heat island preventers, noise and light pollution mitigators, and additions of beauty to our quality of life—my next step was to meet with four friends to test the idea of planting sequoias around our community. They had many questions about what would be required for the trees to thrive and I had few answers. So my next stop was with James Bryan owner of Botanica Nursery.

I knew James as an environmental enthusiast but I was unaware of his special affection for sequoias, and that he had several in his lakeside yard—the tallest about 60 feet at 20+ years of age—and some for sale in his nursery! He had answers for many of our questions. Sequoia semper virans are disease resistant, insect resistant, and non-invasive. They require lots of water for the first two years after planting—about 4 gallons, 3 times per week—and will get adequate drainage if planted on a slope in our dense clay soil. He offered to be a source for the trees at a minimal price and offered to plant and teach others to plant and care for them. He also knew a professor in a city about an hour away who was eager to give seedlings he was nurturing to test their adaptation to other communities.

Armed with encouragement from James, the next breakthrough came at my annual physical exam with my geriatric specialist and D.O. primary care provider, Dr. Sarah Schumacher. As always she asked, "What is on your mind these days? What are you into now?" As I told her about my sequoia brainstorm, her eyes lit up! She said I needed to talk with Lisa Maylath who was the faculty sponsor for the Academic Leadership Academy at our local Chapin High School. Dr. Schumacher's son Adam was a sophomore student in the Academy, and they were interested in projects to benefit the community.

Lisa Maylath was also enthusiastic. She and her family had visited Muir Woods and she was struck by how such mammoth trees could grow from something smaller than a mustard seed. And together we began to think of all the life lessons students might learn from a project that planted sequoias in public places representing all aspects of our community—government, education, business, faith, recreation, non-profits, and neighborhoods. The support and approval of Dr. Akil Ross, principal of Chapin High School, was easily obtained when we told him that eagles, the CHS mascot, loved to roost in high places!

We rounded up a group of community volunteers who were willing to support the student efforts and who brought different areas of expertise and community linkages—Garden Club, Chamber of Commerce, Town government, web site design, event planning, Rotary, and community respect and influence. This was especially important because our community was in a period of upheaval after the unexpected election of a mayor who replaced the long-established and familiar leadership.

Together the students and their project sponsor, biology teacher Karen Walton, with the community volunteers, mapped out a way to proceed. We agreed on a project name, Chapin Sequoias Standing Tall, and several project goals:

1. To bring the community together in an effort everyone could be FOR.

2. To develop a unique feature for our community, one that might make us a destination for visitors.

3. To improve the quality of the environment and the beauty of the town.

4. To demonstrate the wisdom of long-term thinking and planning.

We were clearly embarking on an effort that few, if any, of us would live to see to its full maturity. I had an additional unwritten goal, that students would learn how an idea can become a reality through community networking and cooperation, i.e.that they would learn something about how communities work.

The students divided themselves into teams, each with the support of a community volunteer. There were a total of 30 students involved in the project. I expected that students would gravitate toward the web site team, but the most popular group was Planting! The least sought out was Presentation--no surprise to those of us familiar with people's general aversion to public speaking. Altogether team participation was fairly balanced with each student participating in one team.

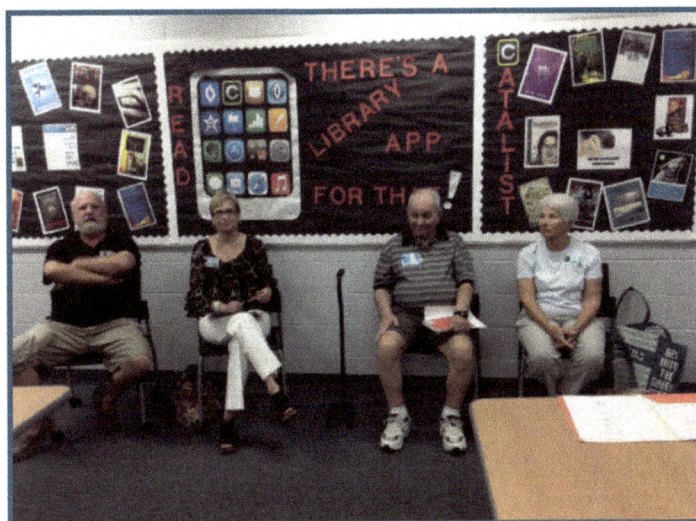

1. Presentation

Speaking to community groups about the project, getting permission to plant in public places, getting sponsors for trees and markers.

2. Planting

Participating in the actual planting of trees.

3. Watering

Watering the trees on campus and developing watering teams in places where new trees did not have access to an irrigation system.

4. Markers

Designing metal numbered markers that identified each tree and linked it to a sponsor. The markers were produced by another group of students in a metal-working class at the nearby Center for Advanced Technology Education (CATE)

5. Website

Developing an accessible computer site Chapin Sequoias informing the public and for tracking the sites where trees were planted, and persons who sponsored trees and markers. chapinsequoiastandingtall.weebly.com

6. Celebration

Planning events to celebrate progress. The first was a student assembly on SC Arbor Day in December of 2014, the key tree-planting time to kick-off the project. The Assembly was festive—the 30 students in the Leadership Academy project team had t-shirts with a tree on the front and a quote from Warren Buffet on the back: "Someone is sitting in the shade today because someone long ago planted a tree." The students formed a circle showing the circumference of a mature sequoia tree. The community volunteers sat in a place of honor, James spoke about sequoia trees, and I described the project origins and plan. The highlight was the unfolding of a 90 foot artistic rendition of a sequoia, painted by a student artist who was also on the wrestling team! It was done on butcher block paper that "grew" before our eyes attached to a lift borrowed from the construction crew doing renovations at the school. At its peak, an eagle rose from the top of the tree!—in reality, an assistant principal dressed in the school mascot costume! Quite a day!

Refreshments followed and sequoia seedlings were available for persons who wanted to purchase them and plant one for themselves.

The project was to be completed in 2 years. At that point the trees would be sufficiently established to survive without intensive watering and care. And the students would be moving into their senior year and onward.

HOW DO WE MEASURE SUCCESS?

1. A total of 41 marked trees were planted at all of the sites planned to represent aspects of the community.

2. An additional nearly 200 trees were bought and planted by individuals who heard of the project and wanted to participate individually. Even though the project has been officially completed for several years, people are still planting trees! Recently a friend, who is also the town attorney, told me that she and her husband celebrated their anniversary by planting two sequoias in honor of their two daughters.

3. Watering teams involved others in the community and "ownership" of the trees and the project grew, e.g., at Crooked Creek Park recreation center a women's tennis group watered on Mondays, an aerobics group on Wednesdays, and after-school middle-schoolers on Fridays. The middle-schoolers loved the trees so much

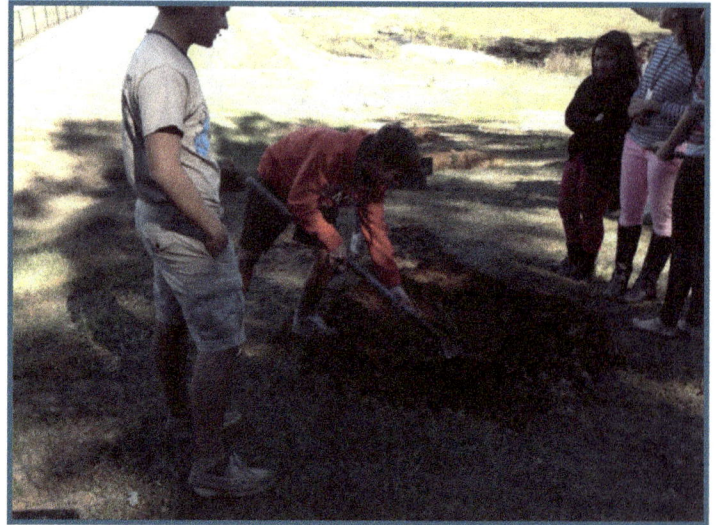

they gave them each a name and made wooden markers separate from the official project markers.

4. Another watering team at a local church watered the trees planted there—the youth group on Sunday evenings, a women's group on Tuesdays, and a men's prayer group on Thursday mornings.

5. A few of the initial plantings did not survive and we learned in replanting to plant first in pots and allow the root system to develop a little rather than putting tubelings directly in to the ground.

6. At the very beginning of the project, the contentious town council was all smiles when Adam's presentation asking permission to plant at Town Hall reminded them that these trees were "for his grandchildren's children." It is possible to find common ground!

7. New connections and friendships were formed that have lasted and carried over into other community initiatives and enriched lives.

And all of us have a story to tell—of community healing and cooperation, of intergenerational friendships, of environmental enhancement, of investing in the future, of Chapin Sequoias Standing Tall.

REFERENCES

Galford, G. L., Melillo, J. M., Kicklighter, D. W., Cronin, T. W., Cerri, C. E., Mustard, J. F., & Cerri, C. C. (2010). Greenhouse gas emissions from alternative futures of deforestation and agricultural management in the southern Amazon. *Proceedings of the National Academy of Sciences of the United States of America, 107*(46), 19649–19654. https://doi.org/10.1073/pnas.1000780107

Rudd, M. A., Moore, A., Rochberg, D., Bianchi-Fossati, L., Brown, M. A., D'Onofrio, D., Furman, C. A., Garcia, J., Jordan, B., Kline, J., Risse, L. M., Yager, P. L., Abbinett, J., Alber, M., Bell, J. E., Bhedwar, C., Cobb, K. M., Cohen, J., Cox, M., Dormer, M., ... Worley, A. N. (2018). Climate research priorities for policy-makers, practitioners, and scientists in Georgia, USA. *Environmental Management, 62*(2), 190–209. https://doi.org/10.1007/s00267-018-1051-4

Smith, P., Calvin, K., Nkem, J., Campbell, D., Cherubini, F., Grassi, G., Korotkov, V., Le Hoang, A., Lwasa, S., McElwee, P., Nkonya, E., Saigusa, N., Soussana, J. F., Taboada, M. A., Manning, F. C., Nampanzira, D., Arias-Navarro, C., Vizzarri, M., House, J., Roe, S., ... Arneth, A. (2020). Which practices co-deliver food security, climate change mitigation and adaptation, and combat land degradation and desertification?. *Global Change Biology, 26*(3), 1532–1575. https://doi.org/10.1111/gcb.14878

Wolf, K. L., Lam, S. T., McKeen, J. K., Richardson, G., van den Bosch, M., & Bardekjian, A. C. (2020). Urban Trees and Human Health: A Scoping Review. *International Journal of Environmental Research and Public Health, 17*(12), 4371. https://doi.org/10.3390/ijerph17124371

NURSE A TREE: NURSE MIGRATION AND SUSTAINABILITY SOLUTIONS

Floro Cubelo, MPH, RN, BSN, CGNC
Senior Lecturer/Head of the Degree Program in Nursing
School of Wellbeing and Culture
Oulu University of Applied Sciences, Oulu Finland

INTRODUCTION

Nurse migration occurs for many reasons. The World Health Organization (n.d.) identified that migration of the healthcare workforce increased during the COVID-19 pandemic and was driven by opportunities in host countries such as educational opportunities, improved working conditions, and increased wages. In 2022, the US noted a 44% increase in applications for nurses from 116 countries compared to 2021 applications (CCNFS, n.d.). In Nordic countries, which include Denmark, Norway, Sweden, Finland, Iceland, the Faroe Islands, Greenland, and Åland Islands, migrating internationally educated nurses (IENs) play a crucial role in meeting existing staffing gaps. These nurses deliver patient care and enhance health outcomes despite the unique challenges they face in assimilating into an unfamiliar work environment. With the increasing impact of the environment and climate crisis on health outcomes, the issue of sustainability and carbon footprint has gained significant importance in the healthcare industry, especially in the context of nurse migration and how it impacts climate change (Cubelo, 2023).

This brief chapter will focus on two key areas that are crucial for promoting sustainable practices among migrating nurses to the Nordic: tree planting and education awareness. A compelling case example that highlights the impact of education awareness is the tree planting campaign. Through this initiative, the engagement and inspiration generated by education awareness efforts influenced various groups and government organizations to replicate the campaign.

The importance of tree growth cannot be underestimated. Trees play a vital role by absorbing carbon dioxide, improving air quality, providing shade, preventing soil erosion, and reducing flood severity (Deng et al., 2013; Gallagher et al., 2015; Janhäll, 2015; Isaifan & Baldauf, 2020). Additionally, all nurses need to stay informed and updated on sustainable healthcare practices, energy-saving techniques, and waste reduction through educational awareness (Cubelo, 2023). However, migrating nurses have an additional consideration, their contribution from air travel to work in the host country and trips home to visit family. This is due to the significant contribution of air travel to greenhouse gas emissions (Klöwer et al., 2021). In fact, flights from the Philippines, a common country of migrating nurses, to Nordic countries have carbon footprints ranging from 647 kg CO_2 – 808 kg CO_2 per one-way flight (Cubelo, 2023). This is not to place blame on migrating nurses who are addressing an important need for the host country and often send remittances to support family back home, but to create awareness and consider solutions.

Educating individuals on sustainable alternatives and promoting the adoption of environmentally preferable practices can reduce the ecological impact of air travel. Prioritizing video conferencing, optimizing travel schedules, and utilizing local resources can help minimize the need for frequent air travel. Promoting environmental responsibility among healthcare professionals can improve their advocacy for sustainable healthcare practices and benefit the planet. Migrating nurses and their host country colleagues can collaborate to reduce the carbon footprint of air travel and promote sustainability through knowledge-sharing and collective action.

One solution that has been piloted has been a tree planting program. The Nurse A Tree (NAT) initiative originated from the ideas and efforts of Filipino Nurses in the Nordic Region. Initially conceptualized by these nurses, the initiative was presented at a conference, where it garnered attention and served as an inspiration for nurses in Ireland. Collaborating with local government officials, the nurses in Ireland worked together to replicate and implement the program. According to the author's estimation, the campaign has facilitated the participation of various local government sectors, non-profit organizations and education sectors from the Philippines, Ireland, Finland, and the United States in planting roughly 100,000 trees. Moving forward, this initiative has the potential to be replicated by other European Member states. In doing so, it is recommended to not only involve nurses but also engage other health professionals in joining the initiative. By broadening the participation to include various health professionals, the impact and reach of the program can be maximized, leading to greater success in reforestation efforts and environmental conservation.

CASE STUDY: IMPACT OF EDUCATIONAL AWARENESS

The NAT project was established in early 2021 with the aim of planting 80,000 trees for nurses in Ireland in partnership with Green Belt, a private forestry group providing professional forestry expertise (Green Belt,

2021). The initiative was inspired by the CleanMed Conference of the Health Care Without Harm Europe, where Floro Cubelo, the President of the Filipino Nurses Association in the Nordic Region, presented his work as a Senior Lecturer/Head of the Degree Programme in Nursing at Oulu University of Applied Sciences. Cubelo's presentation highlighted the role of nurses in promoting sustainable healthcare and inspired the NAT project to plant trees for nurses in Ireland.

The initiative aims to create native woodlands that will help clean the air, enhance wellbeing, and raise awareness of positive climate action. The European Nurse Climate Challenge and Healthcare Without Harm Europe are also collaborating with NAT to promote climate action in healthcare. The trees will be planted on municipal and public lands, as well as with private forest owners, located throughout Ireland, in and close to communities where nurses and their families live and work. The initiative is expected to benefit healthcare in the future by influencing actions taken now and mitigating the effects of respiratory and cardiovascular diseases caused by the environment. Information points will be provided throughout the forest walks to raise awareness of climate action (Green Belt, 2021).

Migrating nurses and host country nurses globally could partner to develop tree planting programs within their region and consider extending the reach back to the migrating nurses' home countries to impact local air quality and climate change. Collaboration with nursing organizations can facilitate this work. Tree planting is an opportunity to highlight nurses' recognition of the impacts of climate change; their role in addressing environmental impacts to the larger community; and the health benefits of the natural environment.

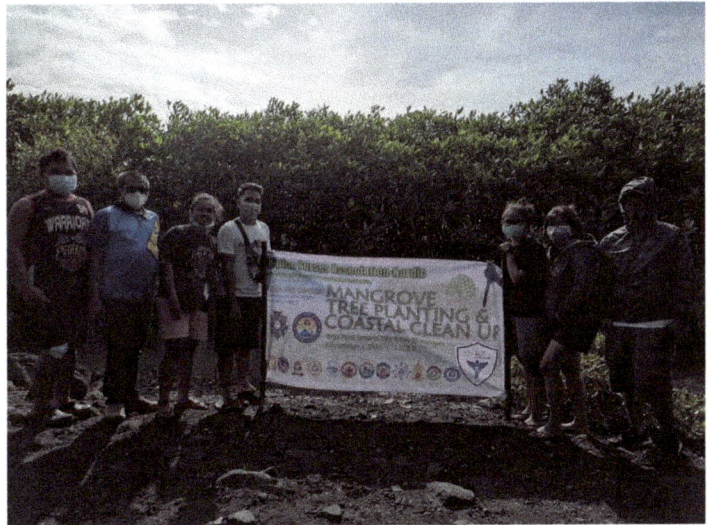

Image 1 FiNAN collaborating with local volunteers and government officials in a tree planting campaign for sustainable healthcare. Used with permission of Floro Cubelo.

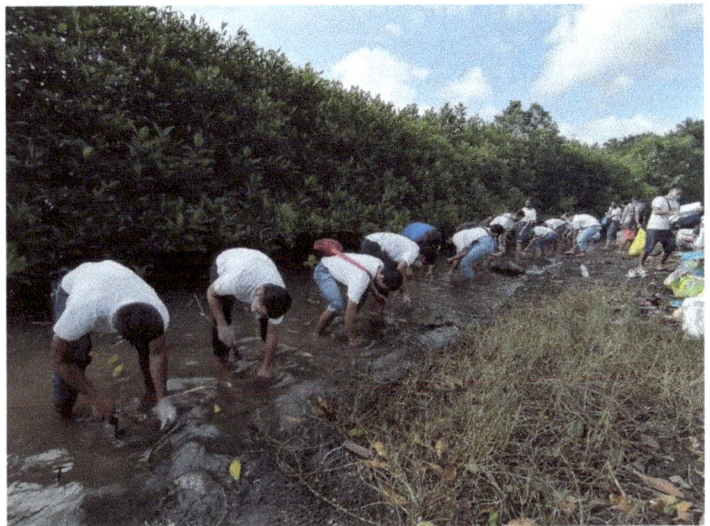

Image 2 Nurse a Tree Campaign Led by Filipino Internationally Educated Nurses in the Nordic Region in Collaboration with local authorities and volunteers in the Philippines. Photo used with permission of Floro Cubelo.

REFERENCES

CGFNS International. (n.d.). CGFNS' *new report highlights nurse migration data to the United States.* https://www.cgfns.org/cgfns-new-report-highlights-nurse-migration-data-to-the-united-states

Cubelo, F. (2023). Internationally educated nurses' role in climate change: sustainability and mitigation practices. *Public Health Nursing.* https://doi.org/10.1111/phn.13185

Deng, X., Zhao, C., & Yan, H. (2013). Systematic modeling of impacts of land use and land cover changes on regional climate: A review. *Advances in Meteorology, 2013,* 1–11. https://doi.org/10.1155/2013/317678

Gallagher, J., Baldauf, R., Fuller, C. H., Kumar, P., Gill, L. W., & McNabola, A. (2015). Passive methods for improving air quality in the built environment: A review of porous and solid barriers. *Atmospheric Environment, 120,* 61–70. https://doi.org/10.1016/j.atmosenv.2015.08.075

Green Belt. (2021). *Nurse A Tree. Planting trees for Ireland's nurses.* Greenbelt.le. https://www.greenbelt.ie/news/nurse-tree-planting-trees-irelands-nurses

Isaifan, R. J., & Baldauf, R. W. (2020). Estimating economic and environmental benefits of urban trees in desert regions. *Urban Forestry & Urban Greening, 8,* 16. https://doi.org/10.3389/fevo.2020.00016

Janhäll, S. (2015). Review on urban vegetation and particle air pollution – Deposition and dispersion. *Atmospheric Environment, 105*, 130–137. https://doi.org/10.1016/j.atmosenv.2015.01.052

Klöwer, M., Allen, M. R., Lee, D. S., Proud, S. R., Gallagher, L., & Skowron, A. (2021). Quantifying aviation's contribution to global warming. *Environmental Research Letters, 16*(10), 104027. https://doi.org/10.1088/1748-9326/ac286e

World Health Organization (n.d.) *Health workforce: Migration.* https://www.who.int/teams/health-workforce/migration

ENGAGING WITH NATURE FOR HEALTH PROMOTION

Maggie Mathison, RN, BSN, PHN
Alliance of Nurses for Healthy Environments

INTRODUCTION

Human beings are living in increasingly urban, man-made environments and have less contact with the living, natural world than at any point in our history. According to the World Health Organization, 54% of the world population lived in an urban area in 2015, and this is likely to increase to 60% in 2030 and 66% in 2050. This societal change has occurred with astonishing rapidity, particularly in the developed world. As Richard Louv, who coined the term "Nature Deficit Disorder," remarks in his book Last Child in the Woods, "In the space of a century, the American experience of nature—culturally influential around the world—has gone from direct utilitarianism to romantic attachment to electronic detachment." (2008, P. 16) Further, our lives are focused on and involved with technology at an unprecedented level. In 2012, for example, the CDC estimated that 98.5% of 12-15 year olds in the United States watched TV daily and 91.1% used the computer daily, outside of school (Herrick, Fakhouri, Carlson, & Fulton, 2014).

In this modern urban, industrialized, and technology-driven human society, there exists unprecedented environmental risk. As detailed in this text, industrial contaminants, pesticides, air pollution, and climate change are growing threats to human health. Health risks arising from a sedentary, indoor lifestyle are also well documented and include obesity and vitamin D deficiency, among others. Nurses and other health professionals have historically focused on identifying and mitigating such risk factors, and treating identified problems. Another critical function of the nursing profession and our healthcare systems is the promotion of health for the individuals and communities they serve. Beyond toxicity and risk, growing evidence exists to show that human contact with nature is a valuable, and perhaps essential, avenue for health and wellbeing.

HEALTH PROMOTION

The World Health Organization defines health promotion as "...the process of enabling people to increase control over, and to improve, their health. It moves beyond a focus on individual behaviour towards a wide range of social and environmental interventions." (World Health Organization, 2018) The American Nurses Association, in a position statement adopted in 1995, calls on the profession to "expand its efforts to design and implement interventions which support promotion of health and prevention of disease/illness and disability."

THE HEALTH-NATURE CONNECTION

The positive health effects of nature seem intuitively known; the walls in office buildings, clinics, and dental suites are frequently adorned with paintings or photographs of flowers, trees, bodies of water, or pastoral views. Many hospitals have an internal television channel which cycles through various natural scenes set to music, meant to help calm anxious and sick patients. Popular culture has chimed in as well- these humorous YouTube videos, providing a play on pharmaceutical advertising, have circulated on social media (warning that some adult language and crude humor is present):

https://www.youtube.com/watch?v=Bf5TgVRGND4

https://www.youtube.com/watch?v=TQ8H4EK2vt4

https://www.youtube.com/watch?v=Bsh_8qxUfDY

Research is accumulating to support this human-nature connection and effects are notable in physiological, psychological, and social domains. Vulnerable populations, including children, the elderly, and low-income communities can be particularly affected by the implementation of efforts to promote health through contact with nature. Organizations and practitioners have begun to use these findings to develop and implement programs and therapies to positively affect health.

Physical Effects

Overweight and obesity are among the primary health risks facing the worldwide population today. In 2016, 39% of adults around the world were overweight, and 13% were obese; these numbers have almost tripled since 1975 (World Health Organization, 2018). Though physical activity in any form has health benefits and can contribute to a healthy weight, exercise in outdoor, natural environments may be particularly associated with consistency and positive effects. Studies have shown that green space is associated with more physical activity and less incidence of overweight and obesity (Coombes, 2009). People who live closer to parks are more likely to exercise regularly than those who live further away from a park (Cohen et al., 2007). Time spent in the outdoors is positively associated with physical activity (Gray, C. et al., 2015), and studies link outdoor natural exercise to greater levels of enjoyment, vitality, and self-esteem (Coon et al., 2011), potentially increasing the likelihood that such exercise routines will be sustained long-term. Some evidence has shown, as well, that diet may improve with active engagement in gardening; Litt et al. (2011) found a 2-fold increase in fruit and vegetable consumption among those participating in community gardening over those who did not.

The practice of Shinrin-Yoku, meaning "taking in the forest atmosphere" and also called forest bathing, originated in Japan in the 1980s and is utilized as a form of Japanese medicine and preventive health care (Hansen, Jones, & Tocchini, 2017). This practice involves being immersed in a forest atmosphere and being mindful of all senses, and has shown numerous measurable physiologic effects. Park, Tsunetsugu, Kasetani, Kagawa, and Miyazaki (2010) found evidence that walking in the forest was associated with lower pulse rate, lower blood pressure, lower sympathetic nerve activity and greater parasympathetic nerve activity than walking in an urban environment. Their studies also measured the stress hormone cortisol and discovered lower concentrations in those exposed to the forest. Li (2010) found that forest bathing is associated with increased natural killer (NK) cells and increased NK cell activity, as well as increased levels of anti-cancer proteins, suggesting enhanced immune functioning resulting from such engagement with nature.

Psychological Effects

Much research into the nature-health connection has focused on brain health, including mental health benefits, attention and cognition effects, and perceptions of wellbeing. Forest bathing, discussed above in regard to physiological effects, has been shown to reduce both acute and chronic stress, with participants reporting lower levels of hostility, depression, and anxiety (Morita et al., 2011). Taking a walk in a natural setting, as compared to an urban setting, can reduce negative affect and rumination, the term used to describe the psychological phenomenon of repeatedly considering and focusing on one's thoughts or problems without resolution, and thought to contribute to depression and anxiety symptoms. (Bratman, Daily, Levy, & Gross, 2015).

Access to nature, whether viewing trees out a window, taking wooded walks, or gardening has demonstrated positive effects on attention and cognition (Lee et al., 2015; Bratman et al., 2015). Symptoms commonly associated with Attention Deficit Hyperactivity Disorder (ADHD), such as impulsivity and inattention, are reduced when people are exposed to nature settings and views, leading some to postulate that nature therapies may be an effective treatment or adjuvant therapy for ADHD and related conditions (Kuo & Faber Taylor, 2004). Commonly experienced symptoms such as inattention, low mood, and poor sense of well-being may be alleviated with nature experiences. This fact, as explained by some researchers

and philosophers, can be explored further and can point to the hypothesis that modern disconnection from the natural world may, in fact, produce such symptoms to begin with. Ecopsychology, which "explores the synergistic relation between personal health and well-being and the health and well-being of our home, the Earth," (https://www.ecopsychology.org/), is a distinct discipline spurring new treatment modalities and research.

Social/Community Effects

Not surprisingly, these beneficial relationships between people and nature seen on individual levels translate more broadly to effects on communities. Green views from the windows of public housing complexes are associated with a stronger sense of community, more feelings of safety, and fewer reports of crimes (Kuo et al., 1998; Kuo & Sullivan, 2001). Living in areas with high proportions of trees and green space may protect against cardio-metabolic illnesses (Hansen, Jones, & Tocchini, 2017) and is associated with overall lower levels of morbidity and mortality (Maas et al., 2009). Urban planners and architects may consider such benefits when designing residences, and public health professionals can advocate for "green design" for health. Cities and counties can promote community access to natural spaces through investing in land conservation and recreation infrastructure.

VULNERABLE POPULATIONS

Children

Children today live indoors much more so than in any previous generation, due to urbanization, parental fears, and electronic use, among other factors. This shift has caused concern among health professionals, educators, psychologists, and child development specialists. Richard

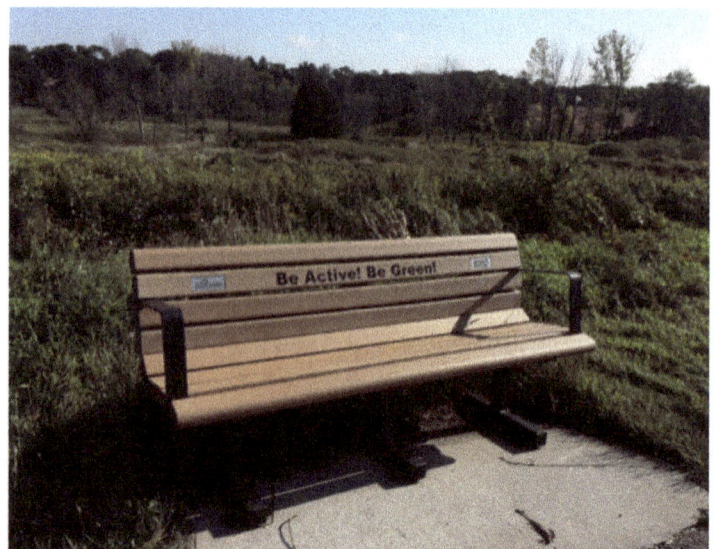

Louv's book Last Child in the Woods (2008) explores this disconnection from nature and addresses what he calls Nature Deficit Disorder, describing the ramifications of human's- in particular children's- alienation from the natural world. Fortunately, the benefits that children can gain from having access to nature, and may in fact need for healthy development, are gaining more attention and support. Research shows that children with more outdoor free time are more active and less sedentary (Gray et. al., 2015), have less stress and show more creative play (Chawla, 2015), and exhibit reduced symptoms of ADHD (Kuo, F., & Faber Taylor, A., 2004).

Recognition of these benefits has spurred trends such as "forest schools" and green schoolyards. One organization, the Children and Nature Network (C&NN), was developed to further the mission to equitably connect children with nature to help them, and natural places, thrive by advocating for policy change, investing in communities, and sharing research and educational resources. Access their website at https://www.childrenandnature.org/. Please view this interview with Cathy Jordan, PhD., consulting research director for the C&NN and associate professor of pediatrics and extension at the University of Minnesota, for a more in depth discussion on children and nature and this organization:

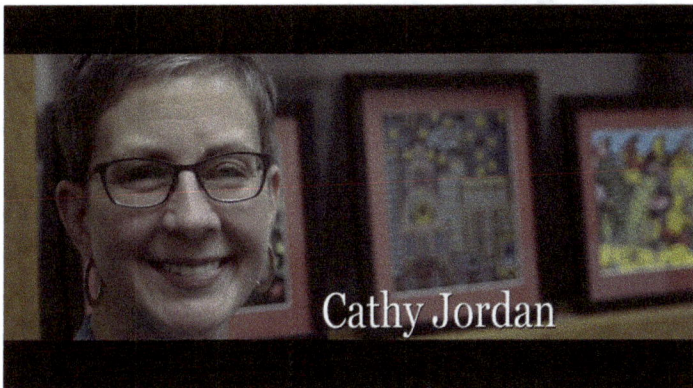
Cathy Jordan

Older Adults

Engaging with and having access to nature can significantly impact the health and wellbeing of people as they age. Studies show that seniors who spend time outdoors in parks, tree-lined streets, or gardens have improved mobility and physical health, less symptoms of depression, a reduction in risk for dementia, and improved social connections (Wolf & Housley, 2016). For those with Alzheimer's, time spent in a garden on a daily basis has shown to reduce agitation and wandering (Day, Carreon, & Stump, 2000). With social isolation and it's associated ill-effects common among older adults accessible common green spaces and community gardens provide opportunities for social interaction and have been shown to increase older people's sense of community belonging (Kweon, Sullivan, & Angel, 1998). Nature Sacred (https://naturesacred.org/) is an organization dedicated to promoting urban nature sanctuaries for health and healing and has an informative section on nature and older populations which can be found here: https://naturesacred.org/nature-seniors/.

Low Income and Disadvantaged Communities

While opportunities to engage with nature have shown benefits for virtually all populations, these effects may be even more pronounced in disadvantaged or low-income communities. A large, observational population study in England found that populations with the most exposure to green space had lower levels of health inequality related to income deprivation than those with less exposure to green spaces (Mitchell & Popham, 2008). This suggests that low-income groups can benefit even more from living with nearby nature than high-income groups. Some cultural groups, such as Native Americans, maintain a spiritual and cultural connection to the land, and this relationship can bolster wellbeing among these communities.

Unfortunately, access to nature and green space is unequal. Low-income and underrepresented neighborhoods often lack safe and maintained parks and trails to utilize. Transportation may be a barrier for such groups to access parks further away, such as National Parks. Research shows that African Americans visit parks less often than Caucasian people, and that this is often the result of lack of access (Weber & Sultana, 2012). Low-income and historically underrepresented people frequently live in urban areas and apartment buildings, where space for outdoor play or gardening is limited or absent.

One initiative being piloted in an urban county in Minnesota, with grant funding from the state, aims to address these disparities using gardening as an avenue for health. This program, called GROW Rx, is a partnership between the county public health department and a local community organization that empowers providers to "prescribe" gardening to their patients to address health concerns. Providers at an urban, Federally Qualified Health Center serving primarily low-income, historically underrepresented, and immigrant patients can write a prescription which will enable the patient to receive a plot in a nearby garden or a small garden box along with soil, plants, and supplies needed to create a garden. The organizers of the project hope to not only promote activity and healthy eating, but to provide a sense of

HOW DOES GROW Rx WORK

Health Practitioners write a prescription for gardening.

The Urban Farm and Garden Alliance fills the prescription with a garden plot or garden box and healthy soil.

Community members receive seeds, plants, tools, and resources tailored to fit their desires for their garden. Continued support and relationships are grown to enhance healthy gardens, healthy communities, and healthy people.

BENEFITS:

Community Asset
- A place for community events and gatherings
- A safe place for children to play outdoors
- A place for the natural environment to thrive within the paved confines of a city.
- Help in "reducing flood risk and moderating climate and pollution, which have knock on benefits for health"[4]
- A more holistic type of neighborhood security, a place where neighbors look out for one another, a community presence on the street.

Physical Activity
- Community gardeners had "significantly lower BMIs" than non gardeners: 1.84 units lower for women, 2.36 units lower for men[3]
- neighbors who worked in the garden "had lower odds of being overweight or obese" than those who did not.[4]
- Gardening may not completely solve the obesity problem in america, but direct and indirect results of gardening could certainly improve the health of many.

Mental Health
- Gardens can be a place of solace and mental healing.
- Mayfield Nurseries' (Hampshire, England) prescription gardening program addresses "depression, anxiety, PTSD or OCD, phobias or agoraphobia" and other mental health ailments.[1]
- One study found that mortality rates were 93% higher in "less green areas" for "deprived groups", but only 43% higher for the same groups in greener neighborhoods.[3]

Neighborhood Support
- Living near a community green space can improve "networks of support and interaction that facilitate bonding, collaboration, problem solving, and community action"[5]
- Cultural or recreational events (think BBQs or sports events) "provide an opportunity for residents to interact with others outside of their family."[5]

*References available upon request

QUESTIONS? WANT TO GET INVOLVED?

Website: urbanfarmandgardenalliance.org/

Email:

Urban Farm & Garden Alliance

This project is partially funded by a $45 million State Innovation Model (SIM) cooperative agreement, awarded to the Minnesota Departments of Health and Human Services in 2013 by The Center for Medicare and Medicaid Innovation (CMMI) to help implement the Minnesota Accountable Health Model

Don't forget to give your plants...

Sunshine, water, and LOVE!

WHAT IS GROW Rx?

Grow Rx is a program with the Urban Farm and Garden Alliance that seeks to address a holistic view of illness and health by prescribing gardening.

WHY PRESCRIBE GARDENING?

Gardening, especially gardening to grow food, can improve both individual and community health. Growing not only yields fresh, nutritious, and organic food but engages neighbors in an activity that connects them to their bodies, to others, and to the earth. These connections can have transformative impacts on physical, emotional, physiological, and spiritual health.

GROW Rx

GROW Rx

By virtue of our numbers, our multifaceted roles, and our trust among the community, nurses are in a strong position to promote health through supporting engagement with nature. As a broader view of health and wellbeing emerges among the healthcare community, and openness to complementary and alternative treatments and prevention modalities increases, nurses can be on the front lines of recommending, implementing, and advocating for nature-based health and healing practices. One example of this synergy is at the University of Minnesota. The Earl Bakken Center for Spirituality and Healing, which supports interprofessional education and research in health and wellbeing, has recently merged with the School of Nursing. The Center counts nature-based therapeutics as a focus area (https://www.csh.umn.edu/education/focus-areas/nature-based-therapeutics) and supports environmentally responsible health care and nature as a path to healing (https://www.csh.umn.edu/education/whole-systems-healing/eco-healing).

Nurses working at the bedside in the hospital environment can consider their patients' view from the window, opening blinds to allow views of greenery when possible, as a view of nature from post-operative patients' rooms has been associated with better outcomes (Ulrich, 1984). Ambulatory clinic nurses can ask patients about their access to nature and the outdoors and provide information on the benefits of and options for incorporating this into their lives. Advanced practice nurses may be in a position to participate in a

agency and empowerment to disadvantaged people through gardening.

Nursing Implications

program such as GROW Rx or other nature prescription opportunities to support their patients' health. Another organization supporting this prescription model is Park Rx America, supporting practitioners in prescribing visits to parks to treat conditions. Their website is https://parkrxamerica.org/.

Public health nurses in the community can assist clients and families to locate and access nearby nature and can educate the community on the health benefits. The American Public Health Association, which includes a public health nursing section, supports the advancement of population health via access to nature. You can access their policy statement, including proposed recommendations and action steps, here: https://www.apha.org/policies-and-advocacy/public-health-policy-statements/policy-database/2014/07/08/09/18/improving-health-and-wellness-through-access-to-nature.

Further research is needed to expand the base of evidence for engaging with nature for health promotion and utilizing nature to treat and heal, and the nursing perspective is welcomed. Nurse researchers Patricia Hansen-Ketchum and Elizabeth Halpenny recommend several areas for further research, including everyday experiences of engaging with nature, especially in rural settings, people's perceptions of barriers, conditions that contribute to disparities in nature engagement, practitioners and policy-makers perceptions of nature-based health promotion, and nature-based interventions in communities, among other areas (2010).

Finally, nurses' voices for advocacy are invaluable. With the knowledge of this intersection between the natural world and human health, nurses can inform patients, other health team members, communities, organizations, and policy-makers. They can use their expertise and the trust from their communities to advocate for incorporating nature-based therapies into treatment plans. They can provide health-related insight to planners, local agencies, and organizations to ensure that the value of green space with regard to health is understood when considering projects and developments. They can bring issues of land conservation, park preservation, and equitable access to natural spaces to candidates and elected officials.

Nurses also have an obligation to consider the health of future generations, and this depends on our current values and decisions. To ensure the protection of human health and the planet's, it will be necessary to create a culture that understands, values, and respects the natural world as irreplaceable and as essential for our own wellbeing. Nurses' voices are needed to create that culture. "In the end we will conserve only what we love; we will love only what we understand; and we will understand only what we are taught." - Baba Dioum, 1968.

REFERENCES

American Nurses Association. (1995). *Promotion and disease prevention*. https://www.nursingworld.org/practice-policy/nursing-excellence/official-position-statements/id/promotion-and-disease-prevention/

Bratman, G. N., Daily, G. C., Levy, B. J., & Gross, J. J. (2015). The benefits of nature experience: Improved affect and cognition. *Landscape and Urban Planning, 138*, 41-50. http://dx.doi.org/10.1016/j.landurbplan.2015.02.005.

Chawla, L. (2015). Benefits of nature contact for children. *Journal of Planning Literature, 30*(4), 433-452. DOI: 10.1177/0885412215595441.

Cohen, D. A., McKenzie, T. L., Sehgal, A., Williamson, S., Golinelli D., & Lurie, N. (2007). Contribution of public parks to physical activity. *American Journal of Public Health, 97*(3), 509-14.

Coombes, E. (2009). The relationship of physical activity and overweight to objectively measured green space accessibility and use. *Social Science and Medicine 2010, 70*(6): 816-22.

Coon, J. T., Boddy, K., Stein, K., Whear, R., Barton, J. & Depledge, M. H. (2011). Does participating in physical activity in outdoor natural environments have a greater effect on physical and mental wellbeing than physical activity indoors? A systematic review. *Environmental Science and Technology, 45*, 1761-1777. http://dx.doi.org/10.1021/es102947t

Day, K., Carreon, D., & Stump, C. (2000). The therapeutic design of environments for people with dementia: A review of the empirical research. *Gerontologist, 40*(4), 397-416.

Gray, C., Gibbons, R., Larouche, R., Hansen Sandseter, E. B., Bienenstock, A., Brussoni, M.,... Tremblay, M. S. (2015). What is the relationship between outdoor time and physical activity, sedentary behaviour, and physical fitness in children? A systematic review. *International Journal of Environmental Research and Public Health, 12*, 6455-6474. http://dx.doi.org/10.3390/ijerph120606455

Hansen, M., Jones, R., & Tocchini, K. (2017). Shinrin-Yoku (Forest Bathing) and nature therapy: A state of the art review. *International Journal of Environmental Research and Public Health, 14*, 851. doi:10.3390/ijerph14080851.

Hansen-Ketchum, P., & Halpenny, E. (2010). Engaging with nature to promote health: bridging research silos to examine the evidence. *Health Promotion International, 26*(1), 100-108. Doi: 10.1093/heapro/daq053.

Herrick, K. A., Fakhouri, T. H. I., Carlson, S. A,, & Fulton, J. E. (2014). *TV watching and computer use in U.S. youth aged 12–15, 2012.* NCHS Data Brief No 157. https://www.cdc.gov/nchs/data/databriefs/db157.pdf

Kuo, F. E. & Faber Taylor, A. (2004). A potential natural treatment for attention-deficit/hyperactivity disorder: Evidence from a national study. *American Journal of Public Health, 94*(9), 1580-86.

Kuo, F. E., Sullivan, W. C., Coley, R. L., & Brunson, L. (1998). Fertile ground for community: Inner-city neighborhood common spaces. *American Journal of Community Psychology, 26*(6), 823-851.

Kuo, F. E, & Sullivan, W. C. (2001). Environment and crime in the inner city- does vegetation reduce crime? *Environment and Behavior, 33*(3), 343-367.

Kweon, B. S., Sullivan W. C., & Angel R. (1998). Green common spaces and the social integration of inner-city older adults. *Environment and Behavior, 30*(6), 832-858.

Lee, K. E., Williams, K. J. H., Sargent, L. D., Williams, N. S. G, & Johnson, K. A. (2015). 40-second green roof views sustain attention: The role of micro-breaks in attention restoration. *Journal of Environmental Psychology, 42,* 182-189. http://dx.doi.org/10.1016/j.envp.2015.04.0030272-4944/

Li, Q. (2010) Effect of forest bathing trips on human immune function. *Environmental Health and Preventive Medicine, 15,* 9-17.

Litt., J. S., Soobader, M., Turbin, M. S., Hale, J., Buchenau, M., & Marshall, J. A. (2011). The influences of social involvement, neighborhood aesthetics and community garden participation on fruit and vegetable consumption. *American Journal of Public Health, 101*(8), 1466-73.

Louv, R. (2008). *Last Child in the Woods: Saving our children from nature-deficit disorder.* Algonquin Books.

Maas, J., Verheij, R. A., de Vries, S., Spreeuwenberg, P., Schellevis, F. G., & Groenewegen, P. P. (2009). Morbidity is related to a green living environment. *Journal of Epidemiology and Community Health, 63*(12), 967-973.

Mitchell, R. & Popham, F. (2008). Effect of exposure to natural environment on health inequalities: An observational population study. *The Lancet, 372,* 1655-1660.

Morita, E., Fukuda, S., Nagano, J., Hamajima, N., Yamamoto, H., Iwai, Y.,...Shirakawa, T. (2007). Psychological effects of forest environments on healthy adults: Shinrin-yoku (forest-air bathing, walking) as a possible method of stress reduction. *Public Health, 121,* 54-63.

Park, B.J., Tsunetsugu, Y., Kasetani, T., Kagawa, T., & Miyazaki, Y. (2010). The physiological effects of Shinrin-yoku (taking in the forest atmosphere or forest bathing): Evidence from field experiments in 24 forests across Japan. *Environmental Health and Preventive Medicine, 15,* 18-26. Doi 10.1007/S12199-009-0086-9.

Ulrich, R. S. (1984). View through a window may influence recovery from surgery. *Science, 224,* 420-421.

Weber, J. & Sultana, S. (2012). Why do so few minority people visit national parks? Visitation and accessibility of "America's best idea." *Annals of the Association of American Geographers,* 1-28. http://dx.doi.org/10.1080/00045608.2012.689.240

Wolf, K. L., & Housley, E. (2016). *The benefits of nearby nature in cities for older adults.* The TKF Foundation. https://naturesacred.org/wp-content/uploads/2011/04/Elder-Briefing_Final_Web.pdf?45ab59

World Health Organization. (2018). *Global health observatory (GHO) data.* http://www.who.int/gho/urban_health/en/

World Health Organization. (2018). *Health promotion.* http://www.who.int/topics/health_promotion/en/

World Health Organization. (2018). *Obesity and overweight.* http://www.who.int/news-room/fact-sheets/detail/obesity-and-overweight

Unit VI:
Climate Change

INTRODUCTION

Climate change is considered our greatest public health threat and our greatest opportunity. Despite the world recovering from and struggling with the impacts of COVD-19, if left unchecked, climate change remains an existential human crisis. Nurses have been on the frontlines of addressing climate change by educating other nurses, patients, communities, and policymakers about our changing climate and consequences for human health. Nurses have also advocated for communities at risk and health protective climate policies at the local, state, national, and international levels. Additionally, nurses are contributing to important climate change and health research. This unit highlights the health impacts of climate change across the lifespan and across populations. Climate change will affect every aspect of nursing care and nurses must be prepared. The first chapter of this unit provides an in-depth overview of climate science, its impacts on human health, and nursing leadership. This unit also includes chapters on climate change and mental health, migration of people, and the impact of climate change on older adults, climate change adaption for children, the effects of climate change on agriculture and farm workers, and inequities within communities of color. As you read these current and important chapters, consider what opportunities you see to influence climate change mitigation and adaptation to support resilient populations.

CLIMATE & HEALTH

Laura Anderko, PhD, RN
Co-Director, Mid-Atlantic Center for Children's Health and the Environment
Villanova University

Stephanie Chalupka, EdD, RN, PHCNS-BC, FAAOHN, FNAP
Professor and Director, MSN Program
Department of Nursing
Worcester State University
Visiting Scientist, Environmental and Occupational Medicine and Epidemiology Program
Department of Environmental Health
Harvard T.H. Chan School of Public Health

"The future depends on what we do in the present"
Mahatma Ghandi

INTRODUCTION

There is growing evidence and concern about the impacts of climate change on health and how to respond to these impacts. As trusted health professionals, nurses have an opportunity to inform others and limit adverse health impacts.

WHAT IS CLIMATE CHANGE?

Climate change is a significant and lasting change in the distribution of weather patterns over periods of time ranging from decades to millions of years. It may be a change in average weather conditions, or in the distribution of weather around the average conditions (i.e., more extreme weather events).

The greenhouse effect is a process caused by greenhouse gases, which occur naturally in the atmosphere. This process plays a crucial role in warming the Earth's surface, making it habitable. However, greenhouse gas emissions (generated by humans) disrupt the natural balance and lead to increased warmth. Greenhouse gases in the atmosphere prevent energy from immediately escaping from the Earth's system. The greenhouse gases then distribute this energy, warming the Earth's surface and lower atmosphere (See Figure 1).

CLIMATE CHANGE AND HEALTH

Human activities are causing environmental changes of epidemic proportions. The earth's temperature is increasing, mainly as a result of human activity such as burning fossil fuel and greenhouse gas emissions. Emissions come from energy production (e.g., coal-fired

Figure 1

Left - Naturally occurring greenhouse gases—carbon dioxide (CO_2), methane (CH_4), and nitrous oxide (N_2O)—normally trap some of the sun's heat, keeping the planet from freezing. Reproduced as part of public domain.

Right - Human activities, such as the burning of fossil fuels, are increasing greenhouse gas levels, leading to an enhanced greenhouse effect. The result is global warming and unprecedented rates of climate change (Will Elder, NPS). Reproduced as part of public domain.

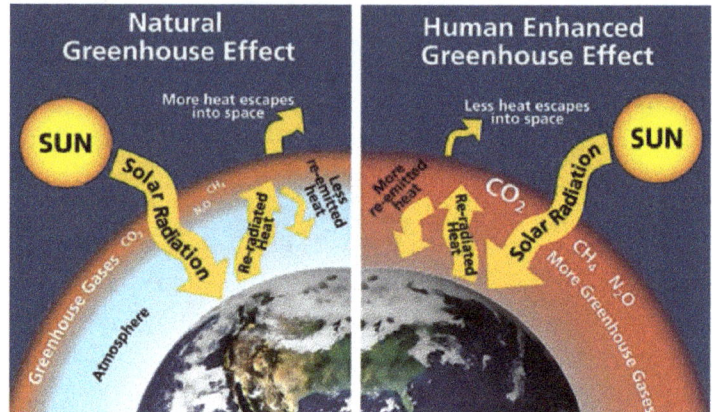

http://www.nps.gov/goga/naturescience/climate-change-causes.htm

power plants), transportation (e.g., automobiles), industry (e.g., hospitals), and agriculture (e.g., fertilizers). These changes are occurring globally at a rate that exceeds what the world has experienced over the last 650,000 years (Parry, Canziani, Palutikof, van der Linden, & Hanson, 2007).

Climate change can be experienced as extreme weather events such as heat waves, melting of snow and ice with rising sea levels, changes in precipitation resulting in flooding and drought, more intense hurricanes and storms, wildfires, as well as poorer air quality. These changes highlight the critical need for us to consider the consequences of these environmental changes on health (See Figure 2). Health impacts can result from direct exposures to climate change through changing weather patterns (e.g., heat waves), or indirectly through changes in water availability, air quality, and resultant changes in agriculture and the economy.

Regional climate changes are on the rise. In some locations, extreme precipitation events are becoming increasingly common such as the Northeast U.S., while in other areas droughts are more frequently experienced such as in the Southwest (Portier & Tart, 2010). The map

Impact of Climate Change on Human Health

Injuries, fatalities, mental health impacts

Asthma, cardiovascular disease

Heat-related illness and death, cardiovascular failure

Malaria, dengue, encephalitis, hantavirus, Rift Valley fever, Lyme disease, chikungunya, West Nile virus

Severe Weather

Air Pollution

Extreme Heat

Changes in Vector Ecology

RISING TEMPERATURES

MORE EXTREME WEATHER

INCREASING CO_2 LEVELS

RISING SEA LEVELS

Environmental Degradation

Increasing Allergens

Forced migration, civil conflict, mental health impacts

Respiratory allergies, asthma

Water and Food Supply Impacts

Water Quality Impacts

Malnutrition, diarrheal disease

Cholera, cryptosporidiosis, campylobacter, leptospirosis, harmful algal blooms

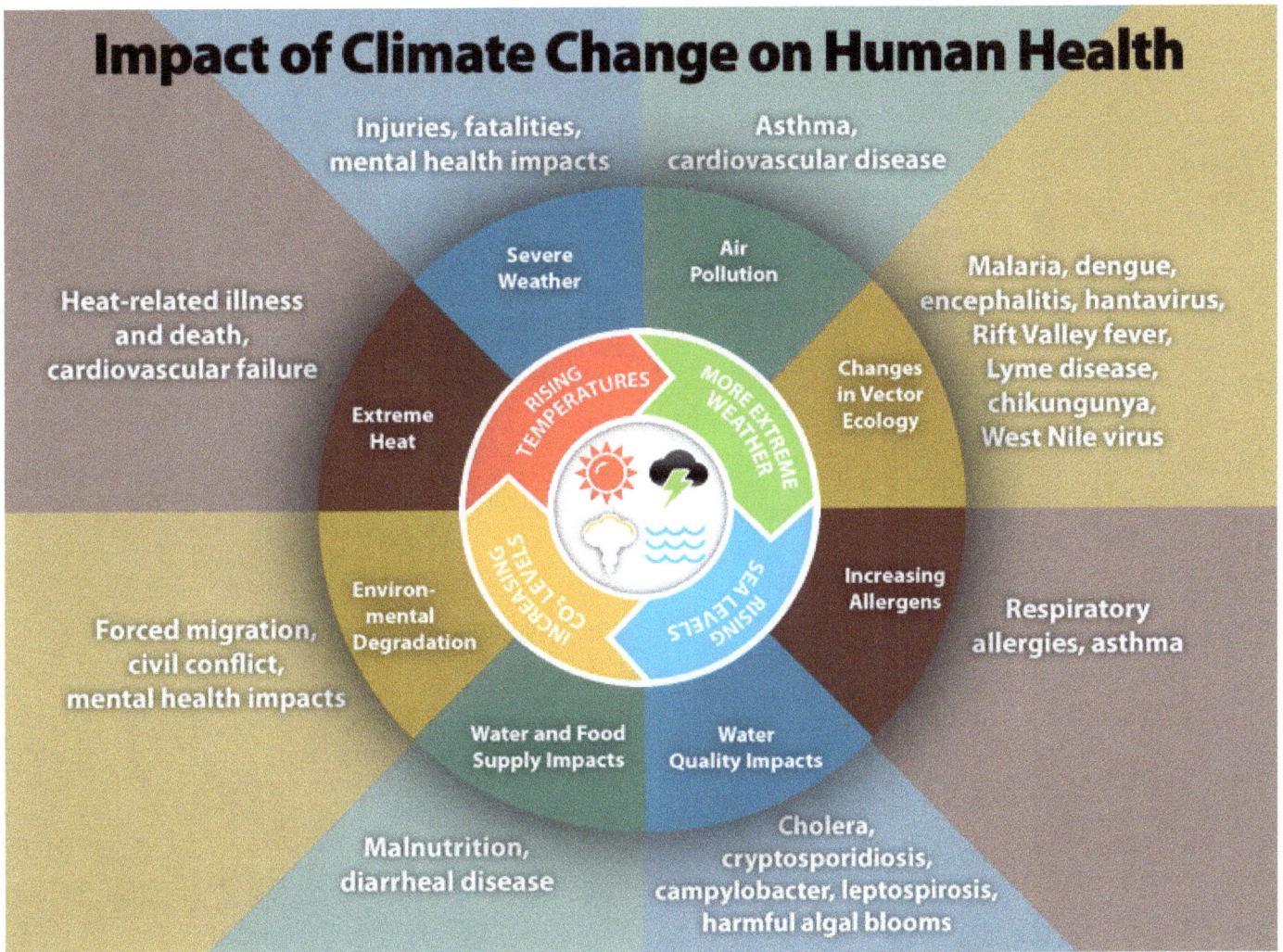

Figure 2: https://www.cdc.gov/climateandhealth/effects/ Reproduced as part of public domain.

from the National Aeronautics and Space Administration (NASA) (see Figure 3) shows a range of extreme weather events in the U.S. and costs associated with them. More data can be found at: https://www.ncdc.noaa.gov/billions/events/US/1980-2018. Health impacts should be considered based on these climate changes, which are regionally determined. These effects will continue to increase with advancing changes in climate.

EXTREME HEAT

Average global temperatures are rising and are expected to continue to increase. The health impact of heat waves is an emerging environmental health concern. Health consequences of this global temperature rise include increasing rates of heat stress and exhaustion, heat cramps, heat stroke, and death. Heatwave events including the 2003 European event with 80,000 victims and the Russian event with approximately 54,000 fatalities have focused attention on the issue. With the anticipated

increase in intensity and frequency of extremely hot weather events the impact on human health is expected

1980-2018* Billion-Dollar Weather and Climate Disasters (CPI-Adjusted)

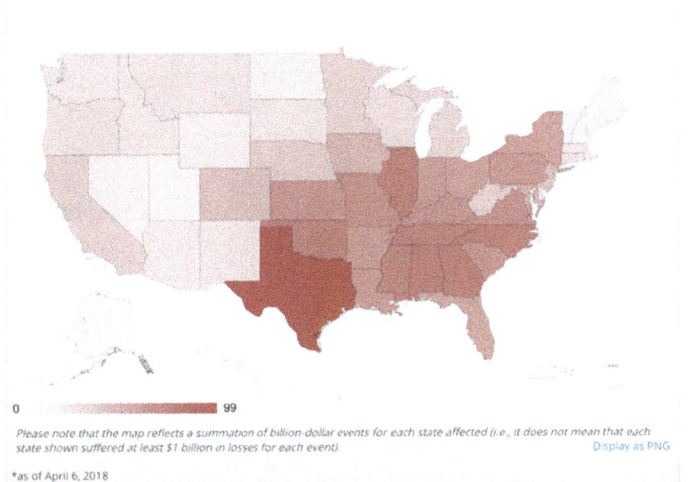

0   99

Please note that the map reflects a summation of billion-dollar events for each state affected (i.e., it does not mean that each state shown suffered at least $1 billion in losses for each event).

Display as PNG

*as of April 6, 2018

Figure 3: Reproduced as part of public domain.

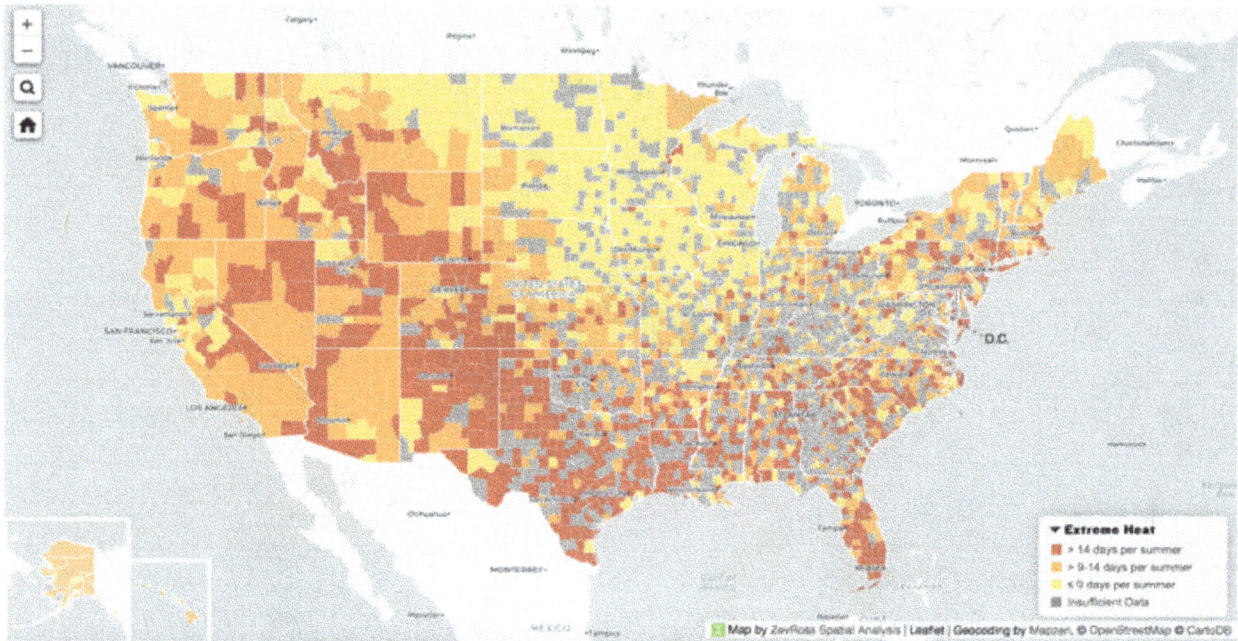

Figure 4: Climate change and health extreme heat map

to increase dramatically (Amengual et al., 2014). Heat–related mortality in U.S. cities is expected to more than double by the mid- to-late 21st century (Stone et al., 2014). In the U.S., extreme heat events already cause more deaths annually than all other extreme weather events combined (Portier and Tart, 2010). Much of the excess mortality from heat waves is concentrated in infants, children, and those with chronic illnesses and those over 65 (Amengual et al., 2014; Portier and Tart, 2010). Those living in urban environments are at added risk because of heat trapping materials used in the construction of roads and buildings (Diffenbach et al., 2017). Figure 4 is an interactive map that indicates extreme heat days by zip code. Visit at: https://www.nrdc.org/climate-change-and-health-extreme-heat#/map.

Additionally, cities lack significant tree cover, exacerbating the high temperatures. Cities frequently experience ambient air temperatures from 1.8–5.4°F (1–3°C) warmer than the surrounding rural and suburban areas. This "urban heat island" also absorbs heat during the daytime and radiates it outward at night, raising nighttime minimum temperatures by 22°F (12°C) (U.S. Environmental Protection Agency (USEPA), 2011a).

WATER SECURITY AND DROUGHT

Water security, or the reliable availability of water for drinking, agriculture, manufacturing, and many other uses, is essential to human health. However, floods and droughts that result from climate change can dramatically impact water availability and surface water quality (Delpla

et al., 2009). In Southern U.S. states, droughts have become a more frequent occurrence; Western states have experienced water shortages worsened by reduced mountain snowpack attributable to global warming (Portier & Tart, 2010).

Figure 5 provides an interactive map from NASA that can be found at: https://www.climate.gov/maps-data/data-snapshots/usdroughtmonitor-weekly-ndmc-2018-05-15?theme=Drought.

Figure 6 shows national trends for Mean Temperature, Maximum Temperature, Minimum Temperature, and Precipitation for each month and season can be accessed using the form online: https://www.ncdc.noaa.gov/temp-and-precip/us-trends/. Reproduced as part of public domain. Maps are available that depict trends for the most

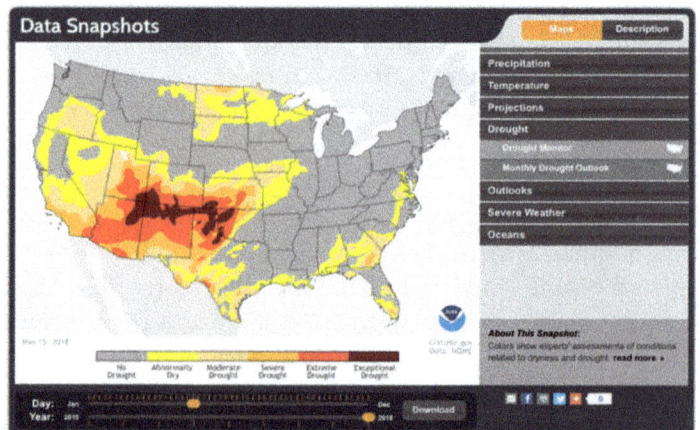

Figure 5: Reproduced as part of public domain.

Average Mean Temperature Trends, April

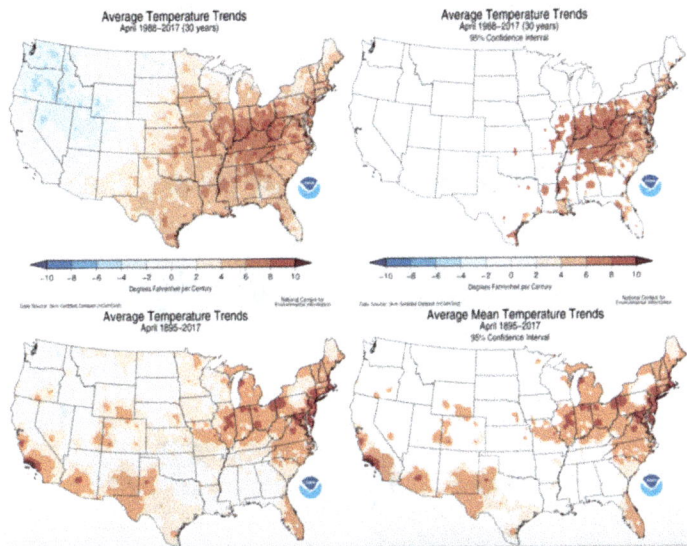

Figure 6

Precipitation and temperature changes affect fresh and marine water quantity and quality primarily through urban, rural, and agricultural runoff. This runoff in turn affects human exposure to water-related illnesses primarily through contamination of drinking water, recreational water, and fish and shellfish.

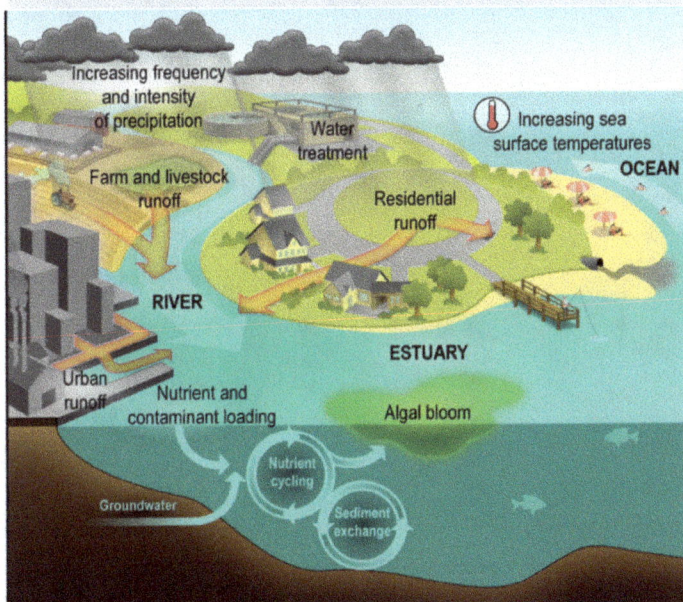

Figure 7: USGCRP (2016). From https:// health2016.globalchange.gov/water-related-illness Reproduced as part of public domain.

recent complete 30-year period and the complete period of record. Each of those maps display the trend regardless of statistical significance as well as trends which exceed 95 percent confidence (trends which are not a result of random chance).

Figure 7 shows links between climate change, water quality and quantity, and water-related illness from: https:// health2016.globalchange.gov/water-related-illness.

INSECT-BORNE DISEASES

Many major infectious disease agents (such as bacteria and viruses) and the vectors or organisms that carry them (e.g. mosquitoes, ticks, and fleas) are highly sensitive to temperature and rainfall. There is potential for climate change to impact the range and incidence of vector borne and zoonotic diseases which are influenced by the ecology of insects and on the life cycles of the disease-causing germs they carry (www.cdc.gov/ncezid). As environmental conditions change, the geographic range of the vectors for illnesses is extended, increasing the potential for infection. For example, as temperature increases, the malaria parasite reproduces at a higher rate and mosquitoes feed more frequently. Changes in climate may make insect-borne diseases harder to control. There are established increases in geographical ranges of deer ticks, for example, that carry Lyme disease. Climate changes have contributed to the emergence of infections carried by mosquitoes like dengue, chikungunya and zika (Asad and Carpenter, 2018).

Figures 8 & 9 from Climate Nexus and the American Public Health Association (APHA) outline Direct and Indirect impacts on disease vectors: https:// climatenexus.org/climate-issues/health/climate-change-and-vector-borne-diseases/

RESPIRATORY DISEASES AND PREMATURE DEATH

It is predicted that health impacts from climate change and ozone pollution in 2020 will result in significant increases in acute respiratory symptoms, asthma-related emergency room visits, weather-related hospital admissions for infants and older adults, lost school days, and premature deaths (Costello et al., 2011). Small changes in temperature (a degree or two) coincide with increasing ground-level ozone and, with it, a significant effect on death rates. An estimated 3,700 deaths annually can be attributed to these small increases in ozone levels (Perera & Sanford, 2011).

Climate change and resulting air pollution poses a serious threat to respiratory health. More than four in ten people live where the air is unhealthy (American Lung Association, 2018). There is now strong evidence linking changes in the seasonal pattern of allergenic pollen and excess death from heat waves. Global warming has caused an earlier onset of the spring pollen season in the Northern Hemisphere and increased the production of allergens (e.g., ragweed) (USGCRP, 2016). Temperature

Direct Climate Change Effects on Disease Vectors

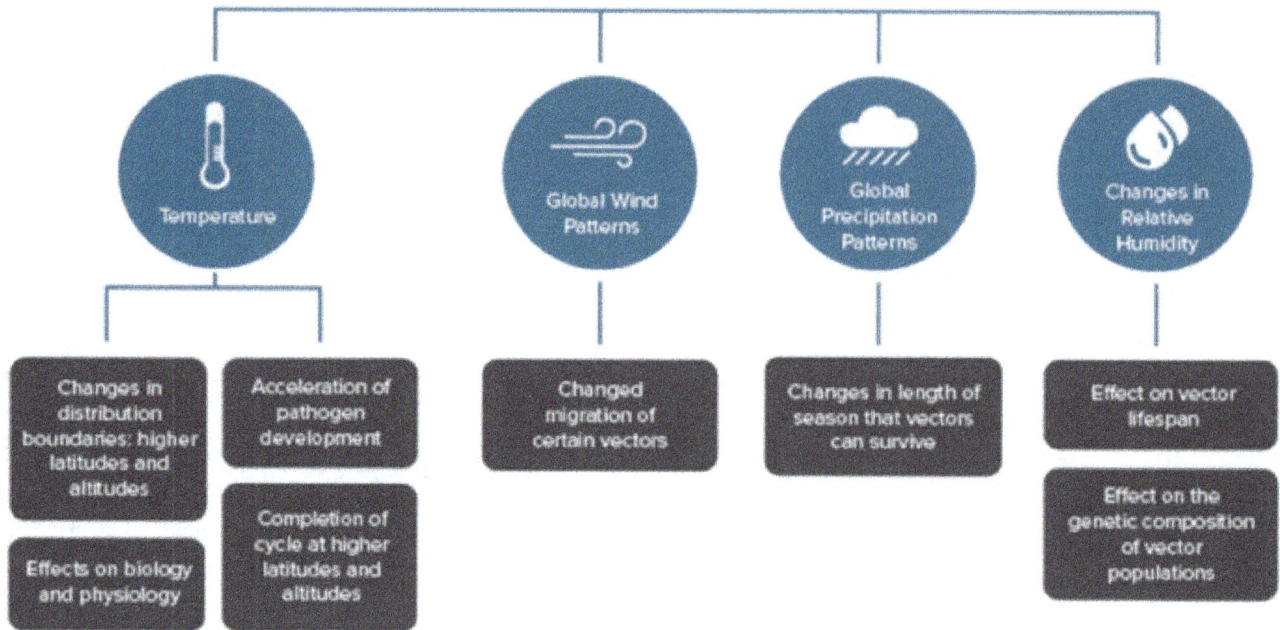

Temperature
- Changes in distribution boundaries: higher latitudes and altitudes
- Effects on biology and physiology
- Acceleration of pathogen development
- Completion of cycle at higher latitudes and altitudes

Global Wind Patterns
- Changed migration of certain vectors

Global Precipitation Patterns
- Changes in length of season that vectors can survive

Changes in Relative Humidity
- Effect on vector lifespan
- Effect on the genetic composition of vector populations

Figure 8: Reproduced as part of public domain.

Indirect Climate Change Effects on Disease Vectors

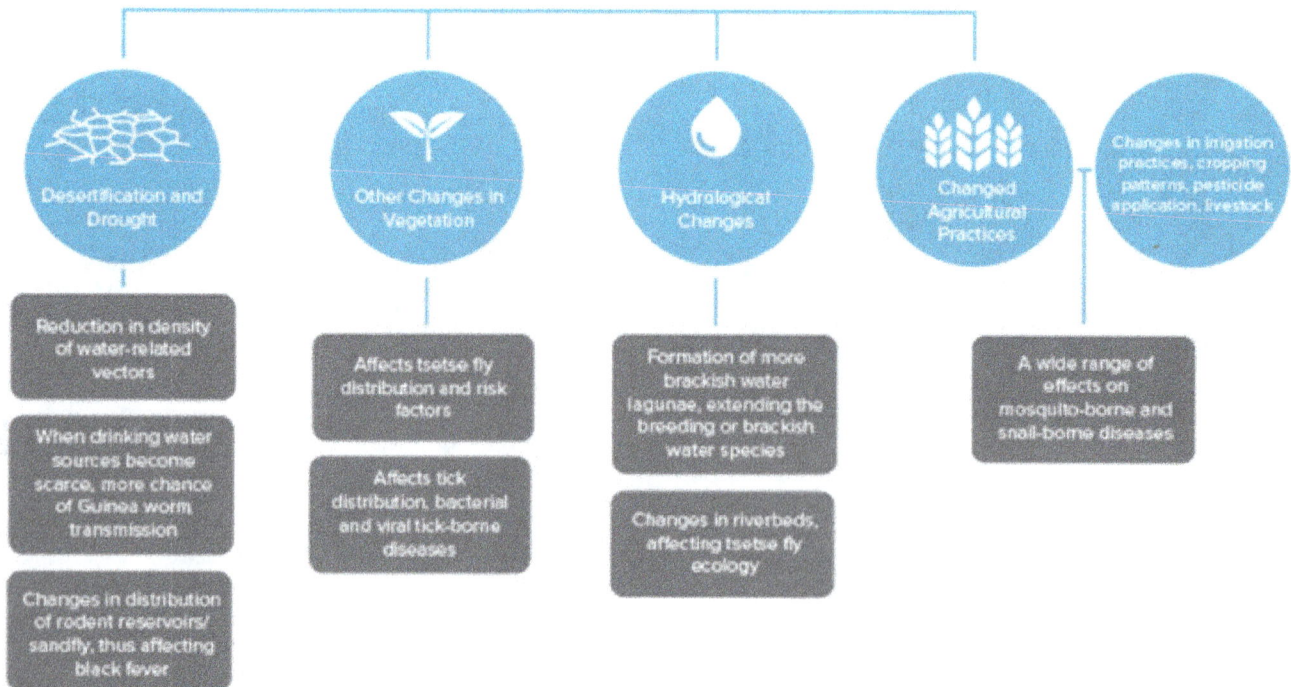

Desertification and Drought
- Reduction in density of water-related vectors
- When drinking water sources become scarce, more chance of Guinea worm transmission
- Changes in distribution of rodent reservoirs/sandfly, thus affecting black fever

Other Changes in Vegetation
- Affects tsetse fly distribution and risk factors
- Affects tick distribution, bacterial and viral tick-borne diseases

Hydrological Changes
- Formation of more brackish water lagunae, extending the breeding or brackish water species
- Changes in riverbeds, affecting tsetse fly ecology

Changed Agricultural Practices
- Changes in irrigation practices, cropping patterns, pesticide application, livestock
- A wide range of effects on mosquito-borne and snail-borne diseases

Figure 9: Reproduced as part of public domain.

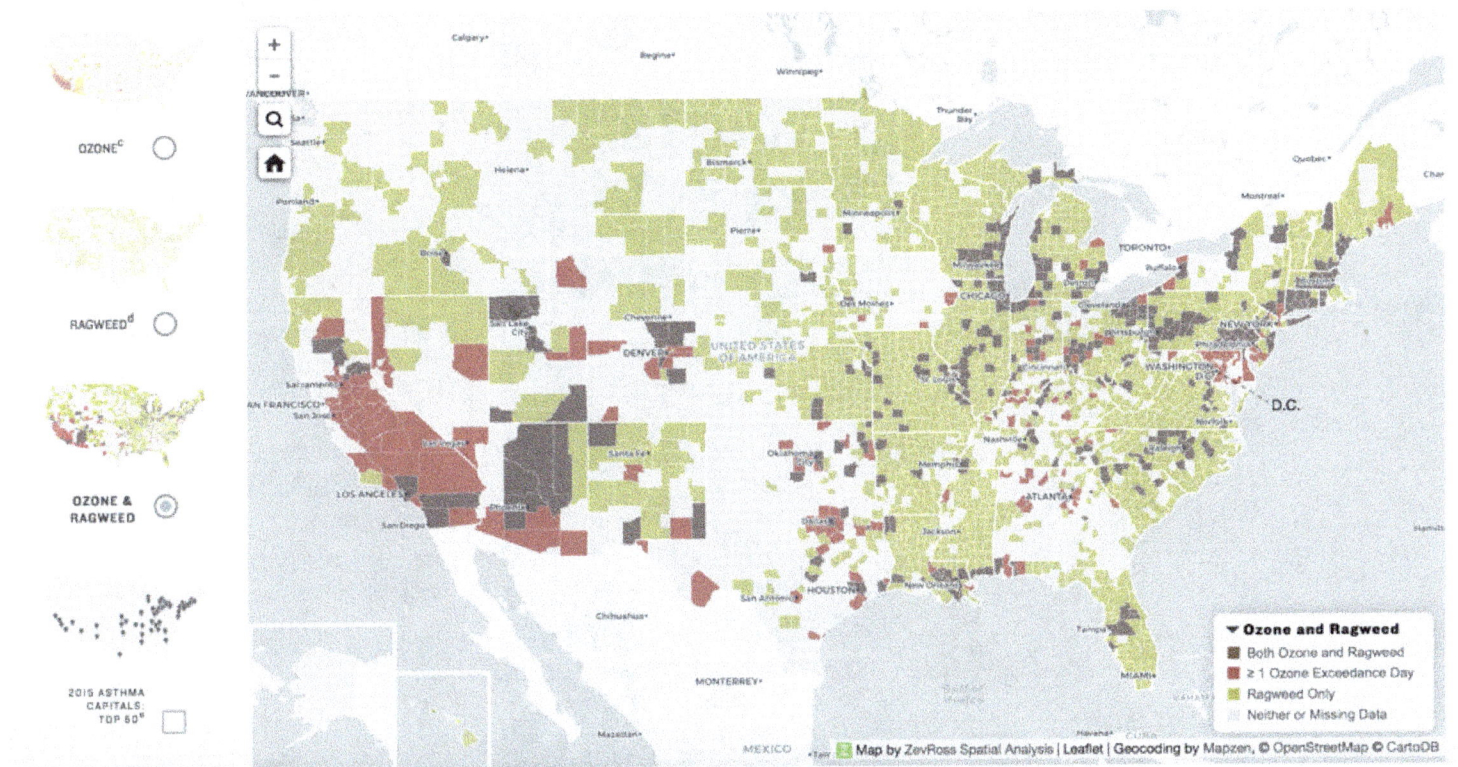

Figure 10: Visit interactive map at: https://www.nrdc.org/climate-change-and-health-air-quality#/map Reproduced as part of public domain.

increases and increased carbon dioxide (CO2) concentrations produce earlier flower blooming, affecting the timing and distribution of allergens such as pollen. It is anticipated that respiratory allergies and asthma will become more common and severe because of increased exposure to pollen, molds, and air pollution as a result of climate change (American Lung Association, 2018; D'Amato et al., 2010). Figure 10 shows ozone and ragweed occurrence in the U.S.

MENTAL HEALTH AND WELLNESS

As climate change increases the frequency and ferocity of weather-related extremes is increasing. As a result, more people are being exposed, or even more tragically, the same people are exposed more with more frequency to personal injury, loss of their homes, income, environmental damage and even loss of lives.

All of this has profound, long-term impacts on mental health and wellness. The changing climate change will bring with it greater numbers who are exposed to extreme events and their sequelae and their subsequent psychological impacts including anxiety, depression, trauma, loss, grief and even suicide (Chalupka, Anderko, & Pennea, 2020; Burke, Sanson, & Van Hoom, 2018; Trombly, Chalupka & Anderko, 2017).

This conceptual design (Figure 11) illustrates the key pathways by which humans are exposed to health threats from climate drivers, and potential resulting mental health and well-being outcomes. The exposure pathways exist within the context of other factors that positively or negatively influence health outcomes (gray side boxes). All of the influencing factors may also be affected by climate change (USGCRP: 2016).

Climate change may affect mental health directly by exposing people to trauma (Berry, Bowen & Kjellstrom, 2010). Adverse psychiatric outcomes are well-documented in the aftermath of natural disasters (Page & Howard, 2010), and can include both acute traumatic stress and more chronic stress-related conditions (such as post-traumatic stress disorder). Extreme heat events, which will become common as global temperatures rise, may be associated with a general increase in aggressive behavior, higher rates of criminal activity, increased suicide rates and child abuse. There will likely be an increase in the overall burden of mental health disorders worldwide as extreme weather conditions and natural disasters can lead to displacement, loss, and social disruption (Berry, Waite, Dear, Capon & Murray, 2018).

Those with mental illness are at special risk from the effects of climate change. Those with mental illness face increased risk of heat related illnesses for several reasons.

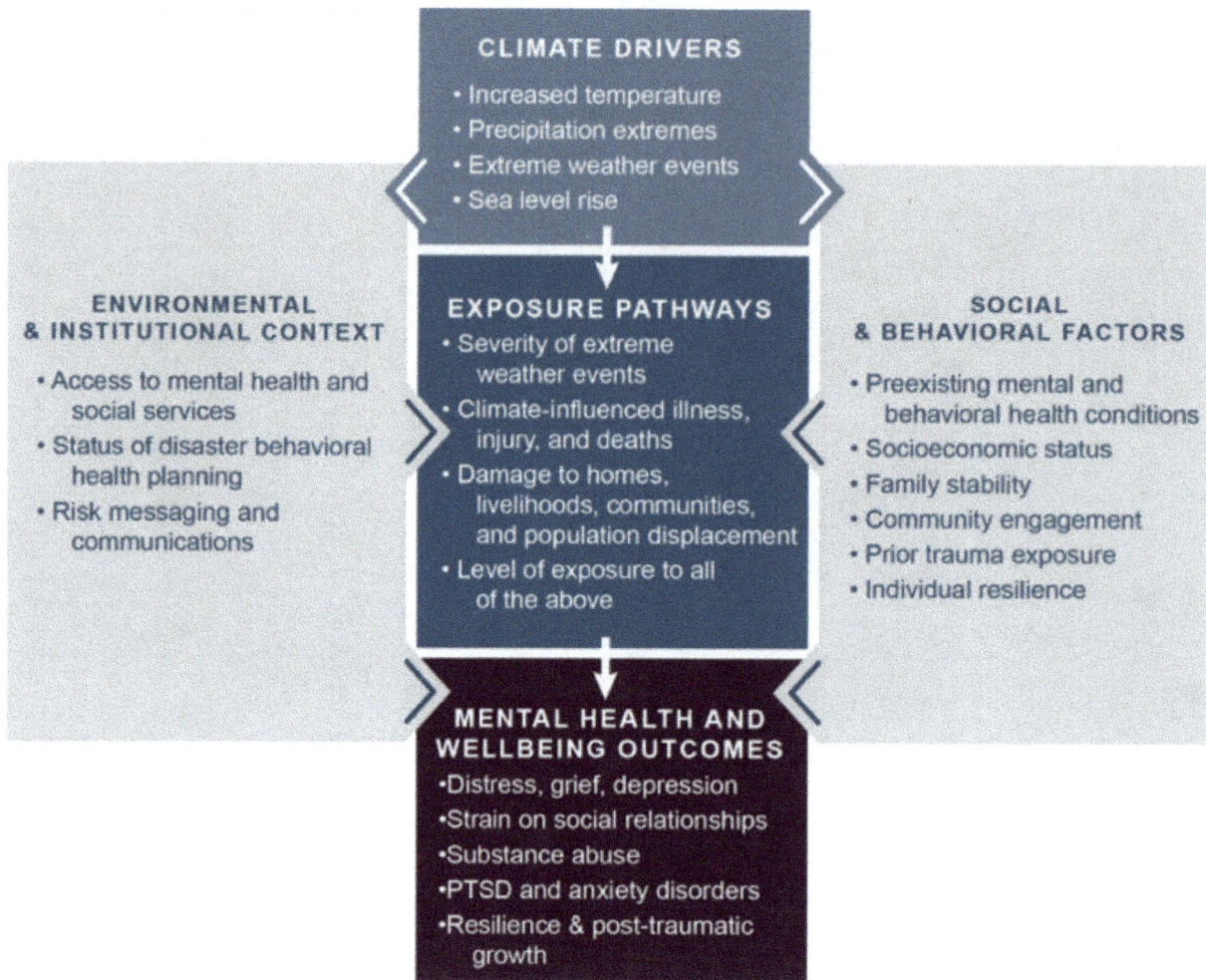

CLIMATE DRIVERS
- Increased temperature
- Precipitation extremes
- Extreme weather events
- Sea level rise

ENVIRONMENTAL & INSTITUTIONAL CONTEXT
- Access to mental health and social services
- Status of disaster behavioral health planning
- Risk messaging and communications

EXPOSURE PATHWAYS
- Severity of extreme weather events
- Climate-influenced illness, injury, and deaths
- Damage to homes, livelihoods, communities, and population displacement
- Level of exposure to all of the above

SOCIAL & BEHAVIORAL FACTORS
- Preexisting mental and behavioral health conditions
- Socioeconomic status
- Family stability
- Community engagement
- Prior trauma exposure
- Individual resilience

MENTAL HEALTH AND WELLBEING OUTCOMES
- Distress, grief, depression
- Strain on social relationships
- Substance abuse
- PTSD and anxiety disorders
- Resilience & post-traumatic growth

Figure 11: Climate Change and Mental Health and Wellness. Reproduced as part of public domain.

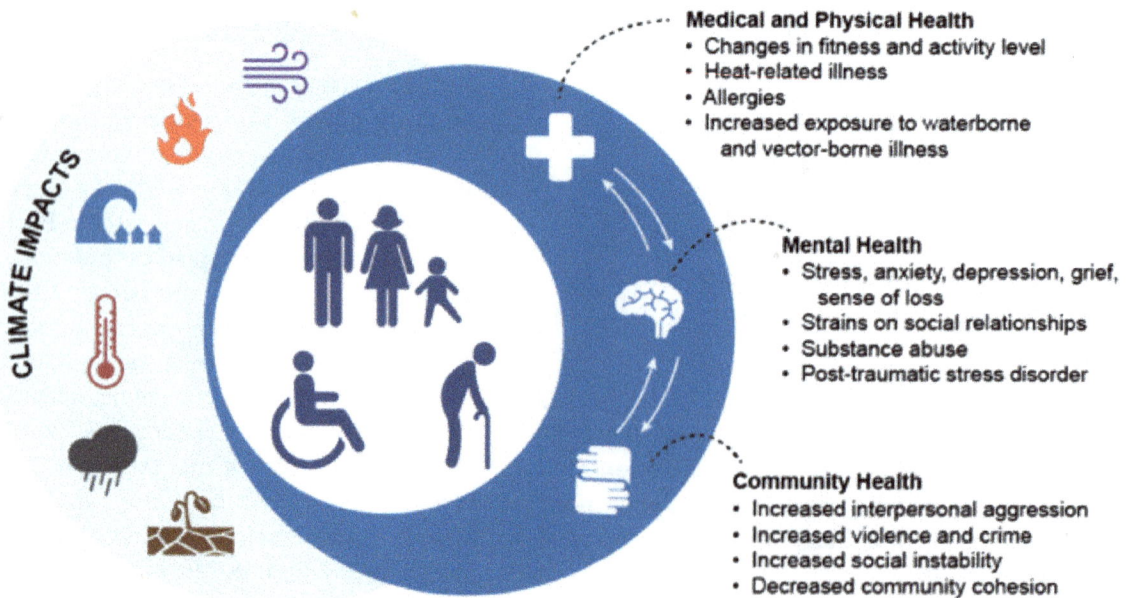

CLIMATE IMPACTS

Medical and Physical Health
- Changes in fitness and activity level
- Heat-related illness
- Allergies
- Increased exposure to waterborne and vector-borne illness

Mental Health
- Stress, anxiety, depression, grief, sense of loss
- Strains on social relationships
- Substance abuse
- Post-traumatic stress disorder

Community Health
- Increased interpersonal aggression
- Increased violence and crime
- Increased social instability
- Decreased community cohesion

Figure 12: U.S. Global Change Research Program, 2016. The Impacts of Climate Change on Human Health in the United States: A Scientific Assessment. Reproduced as part of the public domain.

These include the physical pathology associated with the specific mental illnesses like schizophrenia and accompanying dysfunction of thermoregulation. Psychiatric medications used to treat mental illness (e.g., antipsychotics and anticholinergic medications) have well documented association with heat intolerance (Riley & Kirk, 2017). Finally, the mental impairment accompanying some mental illness may impact an individual's ability to cope with and adapt to extreme weather events (Cusack, de Crespigny, & Athanasos, 2011).

A Public Service Announcement video is available to heighten awareness of heat, stress, and child abuse at: https://www.youtube.com/watch?v=fLm6pdPtl0o#action=share.

Figure 12 outlines mental health impacts from climate change.

FOOD SECURITY

Climate change is associated with seasonal change, with increasing temperatures, periods of drought and flooding resulting in the inability to grow traditional crops. These changes bring with them altered relationships among crops, pests, and pathogens. In addition, it also makes worse declining trends in pollinating insects, increasing ground-level ozone concentrations, and fishery declines especially in areas with limited capacity to adapt to these variations (Burke and Lobell, 2010; Muller et al., 2011; Myers et al., 2017).

It is anticipated that climate change will influence both the quality and the quantity of the food produced as well as its equitable distribution (Myers et al., 2017). Climate change is predicted to worsen malnutrition in the developing world. Extreme weather events and changes in temperature and precipitation patterns can directly damage or destroy crops and other food supplies. This may happen seasonally, but is anticipated to become a chronic problem under changing climate conditions. (Portier and Tart, 2010). It is predicted that by the end of the 21st century one half of the world's population could face severe food shortages due to the impact of rising temperatures on staple food crops. In subtropical and tropical regions, staple food crops could fall by 20-40 percent (Battisti and Naylor, 2009).

Seventy-six percent of the world's population derives most of their daily protein from plants (FAO, 2014). Beyond its influence on yields, rising CO_2 levels are also altering the nutritional composition of crops. Elevated atmospheric CO_2 may widen the disparity in protein intake within countries, with plant-based diets being the most vulnerable (Medek, Schwartz, & Myers, 2017).

Food crops cultivated at elevated CO_2 levels, result in reduced protein content of potatoes, barley, rice, and wheat which are primary sources of dietary protein for many countries. (Myers et al., 2014).

It is predicted that more than 200 million people will fall below thresholds of recommended protein intake, and protein deficiency levels among those already below this threshold will worsen (Medek, Schwartz, & Myers, 2017).

With roughly 83 million people being added to the world's population every year, the upward trend in population size is expected to continue, even assuming that fertility levels will continue to decline (UN, 2017). This population growth combined with the impact of climate change may overwhelm

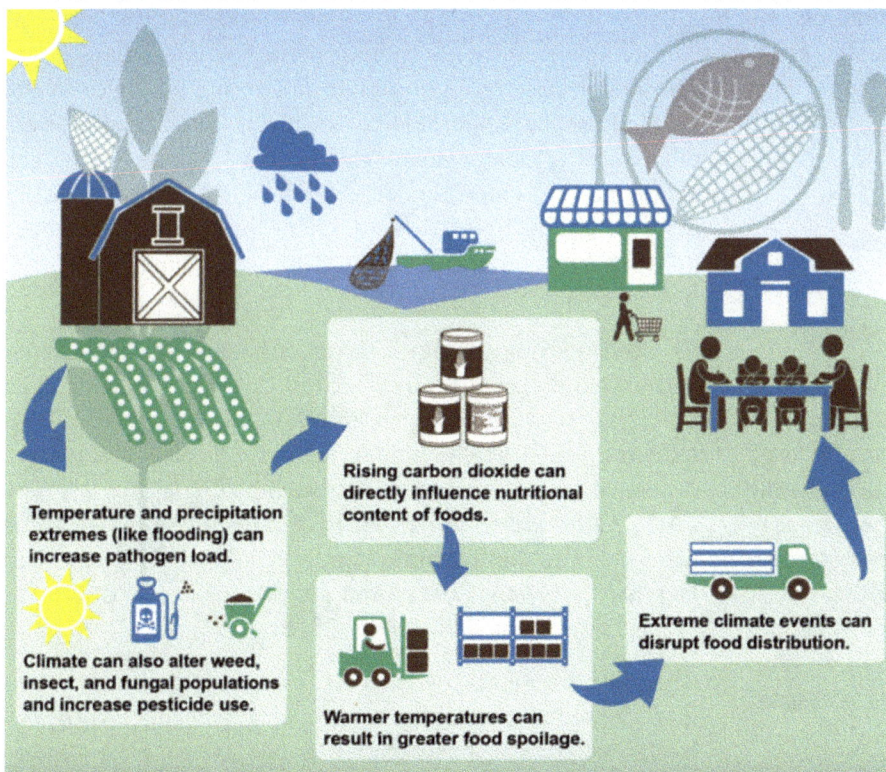

The food system involves a network of interactions with our physical and biological environments as food moves from production to consumption, or from "farm to table." Rising CO_2 and climate change will affect the quality and distribution of food, with subsequent effects on food safety and nutrition.

Temperature and precipitation extremes (like flooding) can increase pathogen load.

Climate can also alter weed, insect, and fungal populations and increase pesticide use.

Rising carbon dioxide can directly influence nutritional content of foods.

Warmer temperatures can result in greater food spoilage.

Extreme climate events can disrupt food distribution.

Figure 13: Reproduced as part of public domain.

global crop production. The capacity to ensure food security and nutritional adequacy in light of the rapidly changing biophysical conditions resulting from man-made climate change will be a major determinant of the next century's global burden of disease (Myers et al., 2017).

Figure 13 provides information on rising CO2 levels and climate change on food safety and security https://health2016.globalchange.gov/food-safety-nutrition-and-distribution.

NATURAL DISASTERS, CLIMATE CHANGE, AND PREPAREDNESS

Extreme weather conditions result in disasters. It has become evident both nationally and globally, that climate change in the form of extreme weather events such as hurricanes, floods, heat waves, droughts, wildfires, and tornados require us to protect our communities through adaptation and preparedness measures to improve resiliency. Many municipalities and states within the U.S. have outlined preparedness and/or adaptation plans to address disasters from extreme weather events. Georgetown Climate Center offers an Adaptation Clearinghouse (http://www.adaptationclearinghouse.org) with policy and adaptation toolkits to assist communities in preparing for extreme weather events.

With the increase in the intensity and frequency of natural disasters there is the threat to public health from fallout of energy sources such as nuclear power. One recent example is the nuclear crisis in the Japan crisis post-tsunami in Fukishima (Eddy and Sase, 2015).

The promotion of sources of energy such as solar and wind would avoid environmental concerns that are present with nuclear energy, as natural disasters increase in the number and severity with climate changes.

A recent study found that wind turbines can actually reduce winds from hurricanes, providing in essence, a protective effect.

Additional benefits of energy sources such as solar and wind are that these are renewable. This means that energy is generated from natural resources that are naturally replenished. Nurses must advocate for clean energy policies that support safe, renewable sources of energy such as wind, solar, geothermal, hydro, tidal, and wave. A comprehensive State Energy and Analysis Tool that can provide a state-level overview of the energy sector and clean energy options can be found at: https://www.eia.gov/state/?sid=US.

For more information about climate preparedness watch the TED Talk: "Let's prepare for climate change" by Vicki Arroyo.

POPULATIONS AT GREATEST RISK

Populations considered most vulnerable to the adverse effects of climate change, lack the ability to adapt to the consequences of climate change. Research shows that up to 20 percent of people exposed to a traumatic event will develop long term psychological dysfunction. Those at greatest risk including the older adults, children, women and the poor who have limited options and resources to adapt to the wide range of climate changes such as heat- and extreme weather events, as well as waterborne, vector-borne, and food-borne illnesses (La Greca et al., 2013; Pietrzak, Fried, Galea, & Norris, 2013). Determinants of vulnerability are outlined in Figure 14 from the Climate and Health assessment.

Women and Children

Women and children are particularly vulnerable to extreme weather events. For example, women and children represented 90 percent of all victims in the 1991 cyclone in Bangladesh (Homer, Hanna & McMichael, 2009). Climate change will increase the risk of infant and maternal mortality, birth complications, and poorer reproductive health, especially in the tropical, developing countries (Rylander, Odlamd & Sandanger, 2013).

Pregnancy and Birth Outcomes

The developing fetus and child are more biologically and psychologically vulnerable to the many direct and indirect effects of global warming. Impacts include increased incidence of infectious disease, heat stress, respiratory disease, pre-term birth, and child abuse. Many of these impacts can affect the health and well-being of children over their lifetime.

While the study of the potential influences on pregnancy and prenatal complications related to climate change is an emerging area of research, there is strong evidence that extreme heat (which leads to poor air quality) can lead to pre-term birth and low birth weight (Zhang, Yu, & Wang, 2017). Other conditions that have been linked to extreme heat include congenital cataracts (Van Zutphen, Lin, Fletcher, & Hwang, 2012) and sudden infant death (Auger, Fraser Smargiassi, & Kosatsky, 2015).

Air pollution increases with extreme heat and may impair lung development indirectly by its association with low birth weight and prematurity. Exposure to air pollution during pregnancy has also been linked to asthma and

EXPOSURE

Exposure is contact between a person and one or more biological, psychosocial, chemical, or physical stressors, including stressors affected by climate change.

SENSITIVITY

Sensitivity is the degree to which people or communities are affected, either adversely or beneficially, by climate variability or change.

ADAPTIVE CAPACITY

Adaptive capacity is the ability of communities, institutions, or people to adjust to potential hazards, to take advantage of opportunities, or to respond to consequences.

VULNERABILITY of Human Health to Climate Change

HEALTH IMPACTS

Injury, acute and chronic illness (including mental health and stress-related illness), developmental issues, and death

Defining the determinants of vulnerability to health impacts associated with climate change, including exposure, sensitivity, and adaptive capacity. (Figure source: adapted from Turner et al. 2003)[4]

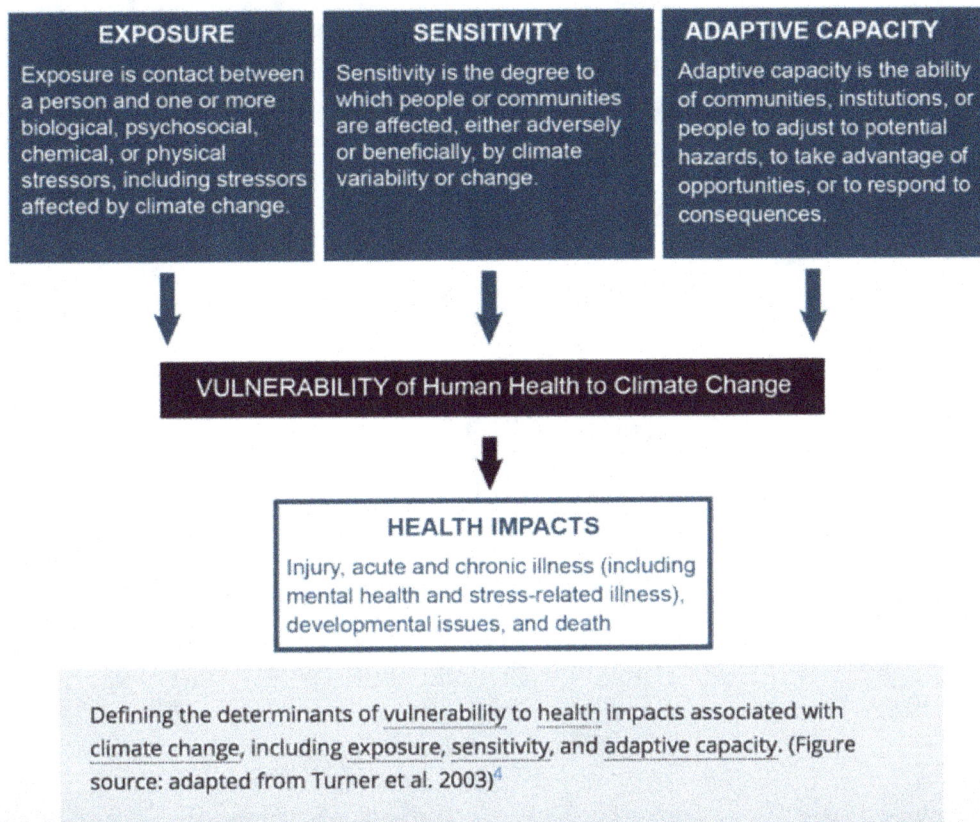

Figure 14: Reproduced as part of the public domain

decreased lung function in infancy and childhood (Korten, Ramsey. & Latzin, 2018).

Pregnant people are less able to regulate the temperature of their bodies. It is theorized that stress from a rising body temperature could also trigger an inflammatory response that constricts a pregnant person's vasculature, making it harder for blood carrying oxygen to reach the placenta which can compromise the fetus. (Kuehn & McCormick, 2017). The dehydration that is associated with overheating may also be significant because it decreases the amount of amniotic fluid which is associated with fetal death. Temperature sensitive proteins in the vessels of the umbilical cord may play a role through vasodilation in the placenta which in turn decreases blood pressure and therefore blood supply to the fetus.

In a study of approximately 60,000 births in California, increased temperatures were significantly associated with preterm birth for all mothers, regardless of maternal racial/ethnic group, maternal age, maternal education, or sex of the infant. An 8.6 percent increase in preterm delivery was associated with a 10°F increase in the weekly average temperature, with greater risks observed for younger mothers, Blacks, and Asians (Basu et al., 2010). Associations between extreme heat and preterm delivery have been supported in subsequent research studies (Carolan-Olah & Frankowska, 2014; Kloog et al., 2015; Schifano, et al., 2016) including a large study of 838,146 births in China (He et al., 2015).

As temperatures continue to increase in many regions of the world, consideration of its impact on birth outcomes is critical (Anderko, Chalupka, & Anderko, 2012; Anderko, Schenk, Hufling, & Chalupka, 2016).

Children

Children are particularly vulnerable to detrimental health impacts from climate change. Children spend more time than adults outdoors, breathe more rapidly than adults, and are still developing their respiratory systems. As temperatures increase, air quality decreases with increased pollution and pollen, increasing asthma attacks and allergies in children. Extreme heat waves increase rates of heat stress and exhaustion, heat stroke and death, especially in infants and children. Children are less able to deal with heat and are more susceptible to dehydration. They are therefore, more vulnerable to heat-related disease and death and will suffer disproportionately as the Earth warms.

As temperatures increase, insects that carry disease such as ticks and mosquitoes expand their range, increasing the risk for diseases such as Lyme Disease, West Nile, and more recently, Zika. As temperatures increase, water security (or the reliable availability of water) for drinking diminishes. Droughts resulting from climate changes can dramatically impact water quality and have also resulted in widespread wildfires across the U.S., adversely impacting air quality from dense smoke that can lead to respiratory and cardiovascular illness in children. Wildfires and other extreme events such as hurricanes have led to depression and post-traumatic stress disorders. Child abuse has been found to increase as much as six-fold during these stressful events when resources are limited to young families (Sheffield & Landrigan, 2011).

Table 1: Summary of information related to health effects and populations most affected by extreme weather events.

Weather	Health Effects	Populations Most Affected
Heat waves	Heat Stress	Extremes of age, athletes, people with respiratory disease
Extreme weather events (rain, hurricane, tornado, flooding)	Injuries, drowning	Coastal, low-lying land dwellers, low socio-economic status (SES)
Droughts, floods, increased mean temperature	Vector, food, and water borne diseases	Multiple populations at risk
Sea-level rise	Injuries, drowning, water and soil salinization, ecosystem and economic disruption	Coastal, low SES
Drought, ecosystem migration	Food and water shortages, malnutrition	Low SES, older adults, children
Extreme weather events, drought	Mass population involvement, international conflict	General population
Increases in ground-level ozone, airborne allergens, and other pollutants	Respiratory disease exacerbations (COPD, asthma, allergic rhinitis, bronchitis)	Older adults, children, those with respiratory disease
Climate change generally; extreme events	Mental health	Young, displaced, agricultural sector, low SES

Source: https://www.cdc.gov/climateandhealth/effects/default.htm

Older Adults

The older adult population of the United States is projected to grow substantially in the coming decades. The number of older adults aged 65 and older is projected to nearly double between 2015 to 2050 from approximately 48 million to 88 million. Nineteen million of the 88 million will be 85 years of age and older. The older adult population is highly varied with respect to their climate-related vulnerabilities due to the diversity of overall physical and mental health, disability status, educational attainment, socioeconomic status, and social support networks (USGCRP, 2016).

Older persons are among the most at risk population facing increased challenges in adapting to climate change, with potentially far-reaching implications for the health of individuals as well as for societal strategies to cope at both the population and policy levels (Pillemer and Filliberto, 2017). Advanced age is one of the most significant risk factors for heat-related death in the U.S. because older adults are less able to regulate extremes in temperatures. Exposure to extreme heat can result in multiple adverse effects in older adults. Extreme heat events are projected to become more frequent, of longer duration, and more intense in the future, particularly in large metropolitan areas and in higher latitudes. (USGCRP, 2016). Older adults, aged 65 and older, represent the majority of deaths associated with extreme weather events (Thacker, M., Lee, R., Sabogal, R., Henderson, A., 2008). For example, in New Orleans, people aged 60 and older comprised 15 percent of the population prior to Hurricane Katrina. However, more than 70 percent of those who died as a result of the hurricane were older adults (Beneson, 2009). Superstorm Sandy also hit older adults particularly hard with approximately half of those who died aged 65 or older (New York Times, 2012).

Extreme high temperatures are associated with an increase in hospital admissions for cardiovascular and respiratory disorders, with older adults among the most impacted. Long-term increases in temperature variability can increase the risk of mortality in susceptible older people (Zanobetti, O' Neil, Gronhand, & Schwartz, 2012). Future climate-related increases in summertime temperatures may increase the risk of death in older people with chronic conditions, particularly those suffering from congestive heart failure and diabetes. (Anderko, Chalupka, & Afzal, 2012; Anderko, Chalupka, Gray, & Kesten 2013; USGCRP, 2016).

Finally, where one lives can be an important determinant of the impact of climate change on the health of older adults. For example, about 20 percent of older adults live in an area in which a hurricane or tropical storm made landfall within the last 10 years. The increasing severity of tropical storms may pose risks for older adults living in coastal areas. For older adults residing in cities, factors such as the urban heat island effect, urban sprawl, and neighborhood safety may also present risks (USEPA, 2016).

Older adults are also more likely to live alone, with limited social contacts and support. Disabilities in one or more areas related to communication (seeing, hearing, or speaking), mental functioning (such as Alzheimer's disease or dementia), and physical functioning (limited or no ability to walk, climb stairs place older adults at risk (Haq, 2017).

Interruptions in medical care and the difficulties associated with transporting patients with their necessary medication, medical records, and any equipment, such as oxygen, can be catastrophic. Extreme events can also cause power outages that can affect electrically-powered medical equipment and elevators, leaving some older adults without treatment or the ability to evacuate. The loss of electricity during a storm can make it difficult to get food, medicine, and other needed services to older adults and those with limited mobility living in multi-story buildings with elevators. As evidenced by the impact of Hurricane Maria, those with disabilities, chronic medical conditions, or living in nursing homes or assisted-living facilities are particularly at risk (Amengual et al., 2014; Anderko, Chalupka, Afzal, 2012; Anderko, Chalupka, Gray & Kesten,. 2013; EPA, 2016).

Finally, older adults are at even greater risk of exposure because they are more likely to reside in risk prone locations such as cities (urban heat islands), coastal or flood-prone areas, isolated rural areas, or areas with increased levels of air pollution or aging and poorly maintained infrastructure (Miranda, Hastings, Aldy, & Schlesinger, 2011).

Underresourced

Those living in poverty are also extremely vulnerable to many of the health effects of climate change. Existing illnesses and challenges in daily life are further complicated by disruptions in access to public services, displacement from homes and the need to migrate with limited transportation options, and increased stress as a result of extreme climate events (Anderko, Chalupka & Afzal, 2012; Anderko, Schenk, Huffling, & Chalupka, 2016).

One study found that as temperatures rise, the economic yield is reduced (Fritze, Blashki, Burke, & Wiseman, 2008). Changes to existing ecosystems can impact livelihoods, such as those who rely on natural resources for their economic well-being (e.g., farmers). Indigenous groups that rely on subsistence living are particularly sensitive to these impacts (Cunsolo Willox et al., 2013; Kjellstrom and McMichael, 2013).

People living in poverty have less capacity to adapt to the challenges brought by climate change. Frequently unable to evacuate in a natural disaster, they are left more exposed to its effects. They also have higher exposure to the dangerous conditions created by poor air quality and extreme heat events.

Those with lower incomes are disproportionately impacted by the extreme weather and natural disasters. They frequently have reduced mobility and access to healthcare although they typically have a greater burden of chronic disease which can be exacerbated by climate. Additionally, financial limitations can hamper their ability to access to buy goods and services that might help them to cope more effectively with the effects of disasters (Bourque and Cunsolo Willox, 2014: USGCRP, 2016).

In addition, many low-income people in the United States are employed in sectors of the economy that are very climate-dependent (e.g., fishing or farming).

Changes to existing ecosystems can impact livelihoods, such as those who rely on natural resources for their economic well-being (e.g., farmers). Indigenous groups that rely on subsistence living are particularly sensitive to these impacts (Cunsolo Willox et al., 2013; Kjellstrom and McMichael, 2013). One study found that as temperatures rise, the economic yield is reduced (Fritze, Blashki, Burke, & Wiseman, 2008).

ADVOCACY: THE CLEAN AIR ACT AND CLIMATE

Clean air, with reductions in carbon pollution, is essential for a healthier climate and public. The health, environmental, and economic impacts of air pollution are significant. Each day, air pollution causes lost days at work and school, as well as reduces agricultural crop and commercial forest yields by billions of dollars each year.

The original Clean Air Act of 1963 was passed and established funding for the study of and cleanup of air pollution. However, there was no comprehensive federal response until Congress passed a much stronger Clean Air Act of 1970. That same year Congress created the Environmental Protection Agency (EPA) and gave it the primary role in carrying out the law.

In 1990, Congress revised and expanded the Clean Air Act, providing EPA broader authority to implement and enforce regulations reducing pollutant emissions.

By reducing air pollution, the Clean Air Act has led to significant improvements in human health and the environment in the United States.

Since 1970,

- The six most commonly found air pollutants have decreased by more than 50 percent,

- Air toxics from large industrial sources, such as chemical plants, petroleum refineries, and paper mills have been reduced by nearly 70 percent,

- Production of most ozone-depleting chemicals have ceased.

At the same time,

- The U.S. gross domestic product (GDP) has tripled

- Energy consumption has increased by 50 percent

- Vehicle use has increased by almost 200 percent (Johnson, 2011, USEPA, 2011b).

The US EPA (2011b) reports that by 2020, the Clean Air Act Amendments will prevent over 230,000 early deaths.

Table 2 presents some additional data related to health benefits of the Clean Air Act.

In 2014, President Obama unveiled the Clean Power Plan (CPP) issued under section III(d) of the Clean Air Act, which established a federal framework to reduce carbon emissions from existing fossil fuel-fired power plants. This was a key component of the Obama's administration strategy for meeting U.S. commitments under the Paris Accord (https://archive.epa.gov/epa/sites/production/files/2015-08/documents/fs-cpp-overview.pdf).

NURSES: OPPORTUNITIES FOR ACTION

Climate change will continue to cause enormous health challenges, which will require a significant response from nurses. According to Dr. Margaret Chan, Director General of the World Health Organization (2007), "We have compelling reasons for doing so. Climate change will affect, in profoundly adverse ways, some of the most fundamental determinants of health: food, air, water."

Nurses have a significant role and professional responsibility to act (Pollitt, P., Sattler, B., Butterfield, P., Anderko, L., Brody, C., Mood, L., ... & Cook, K., 2020). The American Nurses Association has taken a stand on climate and the role of nurses through resolutions introduced in 2008. In 2018, the American Academy of Nursing released its own policy statement on climate change and outlined nurse's professional obligations to address health issues emanating from climate changes (Leffers & Butterfield, 2018).

To be successful, nurses must first become informed about the health implications of climate change in order

Table 2: Health Benefits of the Clean Air Act

The 1990 Clean Air Act Amendments prevents (in cases):		
	2010	**2020**
Asthma Exacerbation	1,700,000	2,400,000
School Loss Days	3,200,000	5,400,000
Lost Work Days	13,000,000	17,000,000
Chronic Bronchitis	54,000	75,000
Emergency Room Visits	86,000	120,000
Heart Disease - Acute Myocardial Infarction	130,000	200,000
Adult Mortality- Particles	160,000	230,000

USEPA: https://www.epa.gov/clean-air-act-overview/benefits-and-costs-clean-air-act-1990-2020-second-prospective-study
Reproduced as part of public domain.

to educate clients, communities and healthcare systems (Sherman, J., Thiel, C., MacNeill, A., Eckelman, R, et al., 2020). to advocate effectively for healthy public policy (Anderko, Schenk, Huffling, & Chalupka, 2016). A list of key resources can be found on the Health Care Without Harm website (with a focus on health care institutions): www.noharm.org and the Alliance of Nurses for Healthy Environments (ANHE) website www.envirn.org which also offers a free online media module series on Health, The Clean Air Act and Health at: https://envirn.org/advancing-clean-air-climate-health-opportunities-for-nurses/.

Nurses have been in the forefront of facing the challenges of climate change and advocating for actions that will reduce health impacts at the individual and societal levels. There are several examples of nurses leading the way.

In 2013, the White House Champion of Change award for Climate Change and Public Health was awarded to two exceptional nurses for their work:

Laura Anderko PhD, RN

https://obamawhitehouse.archives.gov/champions/public-health-and-climate/laura-anderko

and Therese Smith, RN, BSN, MPA

https://obamawhitehouse.archives.gov/champions/public-health-and-climate/therese-smith.

Charlotte Wallace, RN, MS was invited to join President Obama as he outlined climate changes and public health impacts, discussing the role of health professionals in supporting healthy public policy: https://blog.aahs.org/uncategorized/nursing-blog/charlotte-wallace-rn-represents-nursing-at-round-table-with-president-obama

Patricia Butterfield, PhD RN participated on a panel at a White House Summit on Climate Change and Health, discussing the role of climate change In curriculum and best practices in the field. https://news.wsu.edu/2015/04/14/wsu-part-of-white-house-public-health-climate-change-discussion/

Katie Huffling, DNP, RN, CNM, FAAN orchestrated the first White House event dedicated to nurses responding to climate change and health impacts. The summit brought together nurse leaders from national organizations to learn about health impacts and craft a response from the nursing profession on how best to address these needs. https://envirn.org/anhe-white-house-climate-and-health-roundtable/

ADAPTATION

There are a number of strategies to adapt to climate changes and ultimately, build community resiliency and preparedness.

At the Places Where We Practice

- Plan for health risks: asthma, allergies, infectious disease, cardiac and respiratory, heat related events

- Develop disaster preparedness plans: floods, fires and storms

- Incorporate resilience into design, operations, and energy options. The Climate Resilience Toolkit provides a step by step guide and case studies of successful projects within healthcare settings. Available at: https://toolkit.climate.gov. Another resource is Climate Smart Healthcare, a guide for healthcare systems across the world (World Bank, 2017).

At Home

- Prepare for change in temperatures and precipitation

- Cooler buildings, more shade structures

- Adequate water run-off: more permeable surfaces, effective guttering

- Plant trees, manage invasive species

- Garden for food production

- Develop connections and friendships in neighborhoods

- Address depression and anxiety

In our Communities

- Identify at-risk populations and help ensure safety

- Build supportive networks

- Institute early warning systems

- Support sustainable businesses, programs, and organizations

- Work toward Zero Waste

- Address disaster preparedness

In the Policy Arena

- Influence urban planning, city growth plans

- Communicate with elected officials regularly

- Get involved with nursing organizations

Figure 15

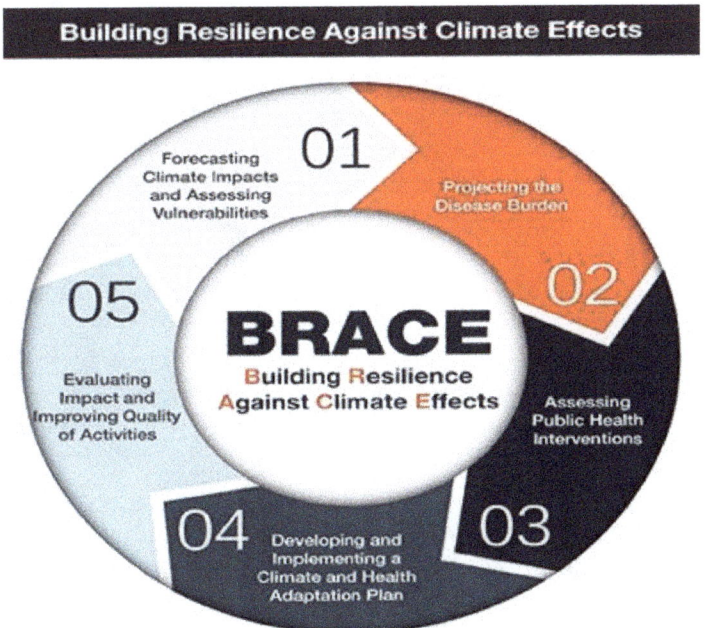

Building Resilience Against Climate Effects

01 Forecasting Climate Impacts and Assessing Vulnerabilities

Projecting the Disease Burden

02 Assessing Public Health Interventions

03 Developing and Implementing a Climate and Health Adaptation Plan

04

05 Evaluating Impact and Improving Quality of Activities

BRACE Building Resilience Against Climate Effects

https://www.cdc.gov/climateandhealth/BRACE.htm
Reproduced as part of public domain.

Building Resilience Against Climate Effects: B.R.A.C.E.

A broader view of "what to do" for health professionals includes the BRACE framework offered by CDC that evaluates population health impacts.

The Climate and Health Program at the Centers for Disease Control and Prevention (CDC) developed the Building Resilience against Climate Effects (BRACE) framework to help communities, health departments, and other health facilities prepare and respond to these changes. The BRACE framework incorporates an assessment of climate change impacts, a vulnerability assessment, the modeling of projected health impacts, an evidence-based evaluation of intervention options, a strategy for implementing interventions, and systematic evaluation of all activities in an iterative framework (see Figure 15).

The vulnerability assessment is critical in various stages as an agency works through the BRACE framework – (i) in Step One, it guides health agencies to assess specific communities and places that are vulnerable to projected climate impacts; (ii) Step Two considers the disease burden of climate change; (iii) Step Three provides knowledge on which specific public health interventions to implement in order to reduce the health burden; (iv) Step Four provides community characteristics (e.g., socioeconomic, environmental, infrastructural) in the development and implementation of a climate and health adaptation plan; and (v) Step Five evaluates the impact and makes improvement.

Implementing steps to reduce greenhouse gas (GHG) emissions is only part of the challenge of addressing climate change. Scientific evidence indicates that even if GHG emissions were to be stabilized at current levels, the earth is already committed to significant warming by the end of the century (Watts et al., 2017; WHO, 2017). Climate change preparedness projects must begin immediately, as we advocate for regulations to reduce GHG emissions. Nurses can play a vital role in local and regional climate adaptation strategies by preparing their communities to be resilient and best cope with the anticipated health impacts of climate change (Anderko, Schenk, Huffling, & Chalupka, 2016; Gould, 2011). Georgetown Climate Center has an Adaptation Clearinghouse with information for local communities and a listing of adaptation plans for each state in the US. Another resource includes a report entitled Adaptation in Action that can be found at: https://bit.ly/2VCpla4.

Effective advocates influence public policy, laws, and budgets by using facts, their relationships, the media, and messaging to educate government officials and the public on the changes they want to bring for a healthier environment. The ANHE website offers reports and information on communicating risks related to climate change along with webinars, podcasts and more at: https://envirn.org/climate-change/.

Tips for advocating effectively include:

- **Know the facts:** To gain and maintain credibility, it is critical that you have the all of the facts on both sides of any issue. Having this information will help you in conversations with government officials, the media, other advocates, and the general public.

- **Use the facts:** Any position you take should be grounded in the facts. It is often helpful to put your facts into one-pagers that you can distribute. Many organizations such as the American Lung Association provide talking points or letters that can guide you.

- **Have a clear and concise message:** Government officials, the press and the general public do not have time for long-winded conversations or documents— you need to get to your point quickly and concisely. And remember to watch out for the jargon and acronyms used in different fields — you want everyone to understand the issues you are raising.

- **Nurture relationships and work collaboratively:** Advocacy is a joint venture- you need to find your allies and work with them. Your chances of success are much greater when there are large numbers of organizations and people on your side. Whenever possible, be sure you and your allies have consistent data and the same messages.

- **Engage the public:** Use the media, social media, petitions, letters, e-mails and other grassroots strategies to engage as many people as you can. Remember numbers speak loudly to elected officials!

- **Make your voice heard!** Advocacy is not the place for being shy. Make sure you spread the word— through meetings with government officials, press conferences, letters, petitions, rallies, and phone calls.

- **Share:** And don't forget to talk about what you are advocating for at dinner parties and social events-- you never know who can become a useful ally.

- **Say thank you:** Remember that everyone is busy and their time is valuable. Keep your meetings short and always say thank you afterwards. When your advocacy is a success, always thank everyone who helped you achieve your victory!

CONCLUSION

Nurses are trusted by society worldwide. They must advise and advocate for a cleaner environment that mitigates climate change through strong clean air and energy policies.

APPENDIX A - CLIMATE CHANGE RESOURCES

- Visit the National Park Services' website to learn more about the difference between global warming and climate change and for further description of the greenhouse gas effect.

- The National Institute of Environmental Health Sciences' website lists the health impacts of climate change, along with strategies to reduce health impacts, and identifies areas for further research.

- The Centers for Disease Control and Prevention's website lists the effects of climate on health and provides fact sheets to use for further education.

- The Intergovernmental Panel on Climate Change works to advance understanding of climate change and impacts by reviewing and assessing current scientific, technical and socio-economic information. View their latest assessment report here.

- The National Climate Assessment, a report developed by over 300 experts and a Federal Advisory Committee, details the impacts of climate change across the differing regions of the United States.

- The U.S. Environmental Protection Agency's website has resources for learning about climate change and the action the EPA is taking to reduce impacts on human health and the environment.

- The World Health Organization's website identifies what is being done on a global level to address the threat of climate change and offers actions to take to advance climate solutions.

- Learn how to apply health promotion interventions in caring for the planet and the systems in which human existence depends at Planetary Health Now!

APPENDIX B INTERNATIONAL NURSING AND HEALTH CLIMATE ORGANIZATIONS AND INITIATIVES

Global Alliance of Nurses for Healthy Environments www.envirn.org

Canadian Association of Nurses for the Environment/ Association d'infirmières et infirmiers pour l'environnement http://www.cnhe-iise.ca/

Center for Climate Change, Climate Justice, and Health https://www.mghihp.edu/climate

Climate and Health Alliance Australia https://www.caha.org.au/

Climate Change and Health Curriculum https://globalhealthcenter.umn.edu/climate-change-and-health-curriculum

Climate Change and Human Health ECHO https://hsc.unm.edu/echo/institute-programs/climate-change/

ECOSERV Lambayeque Peru https://www.ecoservperu.com

GalesActGreen Nigeria: @GalesAct: https://twitter.com/GalesAct?s=08

Global Climate and Health Alliance https://climateandhealthalliance.org/about/

Global Consortium on Climate and Health Education https://www.publichealth.columbia.edu/research/global-consortium-climate-and-health-education

International Council of Nurses https://www.icn.ch/nursing-policy/position-statements

International Council of Nurses collaboration with WHO https://climateandhealthalliance.org/working-group/

Millennial Nurses Network, Santiago, Chile https://portal.alemana.cl/wps/wcm/connect/ingles/home/news/clinica-alemana-presents-its-fourth-sustainability-report

National Student Nurses Association https://www.nsna.org/population-and-global-health-committee.html

Nurses Climate Challenge https://nursesclimatechallenge.org

Nurses Drawdown https://www.nursesdrawdown.org/

NurSuS, UK, Europe http://nursus.eu/about-us/

Universidad Cooperativa de Colombia https://www.ucc.edu.co/Paginas/inicio.aspx

UK Health Alliance on Climate Change http://www.ukhealthalliance.org

UN Climate Justice in Sustainable Development Goals https://www.un.org/sustainabledevelopment/blog/2019/05/climate-justice

REFERENCES

Amengual, A., Homar, V., Romero, R., Brooks, H. E., Ramis, C., Gordaliza, M. & Alonzo, S. (2014). Projections of heat waves with high impact on human health in Europe. *Global and Planetary Change, 1*(19): 71-84. (http:// dx.doi.org/ 10.1016/j.gloplacha.2014.05.006)

American Lung Association. (2018). *State of the Air 2018.* http://www.lung.org/assets/documents/healthy-air/state-of-the-air/sota-2018-full.pdf

Anderko, L., Chalupka, S., Du, M., & Hauptman, M. (2019). Climate changes reproductive and children's health: a review of risks, exposures, and impacts. *Pediatric Research.*

Anderko, L., Chalupka, S., Gray, W. & Kesten, K. (2013). Greening the 'Proclamation for Change': Healing through sustainable health care environments. *American Journal of Nursing, 113*(4):52-59.

Anderko, L. Chalupka, S. M., & Afzal, B. M. (2012). *Climate change and health: Is there a role for the healthcare sector?* Catholic Health Association of the United States. http://www.chausa.org/docs/default-source/general-files/9c161534f9e94b3bb2f34a3cc191e97f1-pdf.pdf?sfvrsn=0

Anderko, L., Schenk, E., Huffling, K., & Chalupka, S. (2016) *Climate change, health and nursing: A call to action.* Alliance of Nurses for Healthy Environments. https://envirn.org/climate-change-health-and-nursing/.

Asad, H. & Carpenter, D. (2018). Effects of climate change on the spread of zika virus: a public health threat. *Reviews on Environmental Health, 33*(1), pp. 31-42. doi:10.1515/reveh-2017-0042

Auger, N., Fraser, W. D., Smargiassi, A., & Kosatsky, T. (2015). Ambient heat and sudden infant death: A case-crossover study spanning 30 years in Montreal, Canada. *Environmental Health Perspectives, 123*(7), 712–716. http://doi.org/10.1289/ehp.1307960

Battisti, D. S., and Naylor, R. L. (2009). Historical warnings of future food insecurity with unprecedented seasonal heat. *Science, 323*(5911), 240–44. doi:10.1126/science.1164363.

Basu, R., Malig, B., & Ostro, B. (2010). High ambient temperature and the risk of preterm delivery. *American Journal of Epidemiology, 172*(10), 1108-17. doi: 10.1093/aje/kwq170.

Benson, W. F. (2009). *CDC's disaster planning goal: Protect vulnerable older adults.* http://www.cdc.gov/aging/pdf/disaster_planning_goal.pdf

Berry, H. L., Bowen, K. & Kjellstrom, T. (2010). Climate change and mental health: A causal pathways framework. *International Journal of Public Health, 55*(2), 23–132. Doi: 10.1007/s00038-009-0112-0

Berry, H., Waite, T. D., Dear, K. B. G., Capon, A. G., & Murray, V. (2018). The case for systems thinking about climate change and mental health. *Nature Climate Change,* 8(4):282-290

Bourque, F., & Cunsolo Willox, A. (2014). Climate change: The next challenge for public mental health? *International Review of Psychiatry, 26,* 415-422. doi:10.3109/09540261.2014.92

Burke, M. & Lobell, D. (2010). Climate effects on food security: An overview. *Climate Change and Food Security Advances in Global Change Research, 37*(1), 13-30, doi: 10.1007/978-90-481-2953-9_2.

Burke, S.E.L., Sanson, A.V., & Van Hoom, J. (2018). The psychological effects of climate change on children. *Current Psychiatry Reports, 20*(5), 35.

Carolan-Olah, M., Frankowska, D. (2014). High environmental temperature and preterm birth: a review of the evidence. *Midwifery, 30*(1), 50-9. doi: 10.1016/j.midw.2013.01.011

Chalupka, S., Anderko, L. & Pennea, E. (2020). Climate Change, climate justice, and children's mental health: A generation at risk, *Environmental Justice, 13*(1).

Chan, M. (September, 2007). *Address to the Regional Committee for the Western Pacific.* World Health Organization. http://www.who.int/dg/ speeches/2007/20070910_korea/en/.

Costello, A., Maslin, M., Montgomery, H., Johnson, A. M., & Ekins, P. (2011). Global health and climate change: Moving from denial and catastrophic fatalism to positive action. *Philosophical Transactions of the Royal Society of London, Series A, Mathematical and Physical Sciences, 369*(1942), 1866-82.

Cunsolo Willox, A., Harper, S., Edge, V., Landman, K., Houle, K., & Ford, J. (2013). The Rigolet Inuit Community Government 'The land enriches the soul': on climatic and environmental change, affect, and emotional health and well-being in Rigolet, Nunatsiavut, Canada. *Emotion Space and Society, 6*(14), 14–24.

Cusack, L., de Crespigny, C., & Athanasos, P. (2011). Heatwaves and their impact on people with alcohol, drug and mental health conditions: A discussion paper on clinical practice considerations. *Journal of Advanced Nursing, 67*(4), 915-22. doi: 10.1111/j.1365-2648.2010.05551.x.

D'Amato, G., Cecchi, L. ,D'Amato, M., & Liccardi, G. (2010). Urban air pollution and climate change as environmental risk factors of respiratory allergy: An update. *Journal of Investigational Allergolology Clinical Immunology, 20*(2): 95-102.

Delpla, I., Jung, A.V., Baures, E., Clement, M., & Thomas, O. (2009). Impacts of climate change on surface water quality in relation to drinking water production. *Environment International, 35*, 1225–1233.

Diffenbaugh, N. S., Singh, D., Mankin, J. S., Horton, D. E., Swain, D. L., Touma, D., ... & Rajaratnam, B. (2017). Quantifying the influence of global warming on unprecedented extreme climate events. *Proceedings of the National Academy of Sciences, 114*(19), 4881-4886.

Fritze, J.G., Blashki, G.A., Burke, S. & Wiseman, J. (2008). Hope, despair and transformation: Climate change and the promotion of mental health and wellbeing. *International Journal of Mental Health Systems, 2*(13). https://doi.org/10.1186/1752-4458-2-13

Food and Agriculture Organization of the United Nations (2014). *Food balance sheets, 1970–2011.* FAO. http://www.fao.org/faostat/en/#data/FBS/visualize

Gould, R. (April 12, 2011). *Climate change and the role of health care professionals: Education, mitigation, and advocacy.* Earth Day Webinar hosted by Practice Greenhealth. http://www.practicegreenhealth.org/private/material/3582.

Haq, G. (2017). Growing old in a changing climate. *Public Policy & Aging Report, 27*(1), 8-12. doi.org/10.1093/ppar/prw027

He, J. R., Liu, Y., Xia, X. Y., Ma, W. J., Lin, H. L., Kan, H. D., ... & Muglia, L. J. (2016). Ambient temperature and the risk of preterm birth in Guangzhou, China (2001–2011). *Environmental Health Perspectives, 124*(7), 1100-1106.

Homer, C. S. E., Hanna, E. & McMichael, A. J. (2009) Climate change threatens the millennium development goal for maternal health. *Midwifery, 25*(6):606-12. doi: 10.1016/j.midw.2009.09.003

Johnson, L (2011, March 1). *Gains from Clean Air Act: Bull Market Without the Bust.* http://switchboard.nrdc.org/blogs/ljohnson/gains_from_clean_air_act_a_bul.html.

Kjellstrom, T., & McMichael, A. J. (2013). Climate change threats to population health and well-being: the imperative of protective solutions that will last. *Global Health Action, 6*, 10.3402/gha.v6i0.20816. http://doi.org/10.3402/gha.v6i0.20816

Knowlton, K. (2008). *Preparing for global warming: A framework for protecting community health and the environment in a warmer world.* http://www.nrdc.org/globalwarming/preparedness.pdf.

Kuehn, L., & McCormick, S. (2017). Heat exposure and maternal health in the face of climate change. *International Journal of Environmental Research and Public Health, 14*(8), 853. http://doi.org/10.3390/ijerph14080853

Kloog, I., Sorek-Hamer, M., Lyapustin, A., Coull, B., Wang, Y., Just, A. C., ... & Broday, D. M. (2015). Estimating daily PM2.5 and PM10 across the complex geo-climate region of Israel using MAIAC satellite-based AOD data. *Atmospheric Environment, 122*, 409-416.

La Greca, A. M., Lai, B. S., Llabre, M. M., Silverman, W. K., Vernberg, E. M., & Prinstein, M. J. (2013). Children's post-disaster trajectories of PTS Symptoms: Predicting chronic distress. *Child and Youth Care Forum, 42*(4), 351-369.

Leffers, J. & Butterfield, P. (2018). Nurses play essential roles in reducing health problems due to climate change. *Nursing Outlook, 66*, 210-213.

Medek, D. E., Schwartz, J. & Myers, S. S. (2017). Estimated effects of future atmospheric CO_2 concentrations on protein intake and the risk of protein deficiency by country and region. *Environmental Health Perspectives, 125*(8). DOI:10.1289/EHP4

Miranda, M. L., Hastings, D.L, Aldy, J.E. & Schlesinger, W.H., (2011). The environmental justice dimensions of climate change. *Environmental Justice, 4*, 17-25. doi:10.1089/env.2009.00

Muller, C., Cramer, W., Hare, W., & Lotze-Campen, H. (2011). Climate change risks for African agriculture. *Proceedings of the National Academy of Sciences, 108*(11), 4313-4315.

Myers, S. S., Smith, M. R., Guth, S., Golden, C. D., Vaitla, B., Mueller, N. D., Dangour, A. D., & Huybers, P. (2017). Climate change and global food systems: potential impacts on food security and undernutrition. *Annual Review of Public Health, 38*, 259–77. https://doi.org/10.1146/annurev-publhealth-031816-044356

Myers, S. S., Zanobetti, A., Kloog, I., Huybers, P., Leakey, A. D., Bloom, A. J., ... & Usui, Y. (2014). Increasing CO_2 threatens human nutrition. *Nature, 510*(7503), 139-142.

New York Times (2012, November 1). *Mapping Hurricane Sandy's deadly toll.* https://archive.nytimes.com/www.nytimes.com/interactive/2012/11/17/nyregion/hurricane-sandy-map.html.

Page, L. A., & Howard, L.M. (2010). The impact of climate change on mental health (But will mental health be discussed at Copenhagen? *Psychological Medicine, 40*, 177–180. doi:10.1017/S0033291709992169.

Parry, M. L., Canziani, O. F., Palutikof, J. P., van der Linden, P. J., Hanson, C. E., (Eds.) (2007). *Climate change 2007: Impacts, adaptation and vulnerability.* Contribution of

Working Group II to the Fourth Assessment Report of the Intergovernmental Panel on Climate Change. Cambridge University Press.

Perera, E. M., & Sanford, T. (2011). *Climate change and your health: Rising temperatures and worsening ozone pollution.* The Union of Concerned Scientists. http://www.ucsusa.org/assets/documents/global_warming/climate-change-and-ozone-pollution.pdf.

Pietrzak, R. H., Van Ness, P. H., Fried, T. R., Galea, S., & Norris, F. H. (2013). Trajectories of posttraumatic stress symptomatology in older persons affected by a large-magnitude disaster. *Journal of Psychiatric Research, 47*(4), 520–526. http://doi.org/10.1016/j.jpsychires.2012.12.005

Pillemer, K., & Filiberto, D. (2017). Mobilizing older people to address climate change. *Public Policy & Aging Report, 27*(1),18–21. https://doi.org/10.1093/ppar/prw030

Pollitt, P., Sattler, B., Butterfield, P., Anderko, L., Brody, C., Mood, L., ... & Cook, K. (2020). Environmental nursing: Leaders reflect on the 50th anniversary of Earth Day. *Public Health Nursing, 37*(4),614-625. https://doi.org/10.1111/phn.12703

Portier, C.J., & Tart, K.T. (eds) (2010). *The Interagency Working Group on Climate Change and Health (IWGCCH): A human health perspective on climate change: Report outlining the research needs on the human health effects of climate change.* Environmental Health Perspectives and National Institute of Environmental Health Sciences.

Reilly T.H., & Kirk M.A. (2007) Atypical antipsychotics and newer antidepressants. *Emergency Medicine Clinics of North America, 25*(2), 477–497

Rylander, C., Odland, J. O., & Sandanger, T. M. (2013) Climate change and the potential effects on maternal and pregnancy outcomes: an assessment of the most vulnerable the mother, fetus, and newborn child. *Global Health Action, 6,* 19538. http://dx.doi.org/10.3402/gha.v6i0.19538

Schifano, P., Asta, F., Dadvand, P., Davoli, M., Basagana, X., & Michelozzi, P. (2016). Heat and air pollution exposure as triggers of delivery: A survival analysis of population-based pregnancy cohorts in Rome and Barcelona. *Environment International, 88,* 153–159. doi: 10.1016/j.envint.2015.12.01

Sheffield, P. E. & Landrigan, P. J. (2011). Global climate change and children's health: Threats and strategies for prevention. *Environmental Health Perspectives, 119*(3), 291–298. doi:10.1289/ehp.1002233

Sherman, J. D., Thiel, C., MacNeill, A., Eckelman, M. J., Dubrow, R., Hopf, H., ... & Bilec, M. M. (2020). The green print: advancement of environmental sustainability in healthcare. *Resources, Conservation and Recycling, 161,* 104882.

Stone, B., Vargo, J., Liu, P., Habeeb, D., DeLucia, A., Trail, A., Hu, Y., & Russell, A. (2014). Avoided heat-related mortality through climate adaptation strategies in three US cities. *PLOS ONE, 9*(6), DOI: 10.1371/journal.pone.0100852

Thacker, M., Lee, R., Sabogal, R., & Henderson, A. (2008). Overview of deaths associated with natural events, United States, 1979-2004. *Disasters, 32,* 303-315. doi:10.1111/j.1467-7717.2008.01041.

Trombly, J., Chalupka, S., & Anderko, L. (2017).Climate Change and Mental Health. *American Journal of Nursing, 114*(4), 44-52. doi: 10.1097/01.NAJ.0000515232.51795.fa

United Nations Department of Social Economic and Social Affairs (2017). *The World Population Prospects: 2017 Revision.* https://www.un.org/development/desa/publications/world-population-prospects-the-2017-revision.html

US Environmental Protection Agency (EPA) (2011a). *Heat Island Impacts.* http://www.epa.gov/heatisld/impacts/index.htm.

US Environmental Protection Agency (EPA), Office of Air and Radiation. (March 2011b). *The Costs and Benefits of the Clean Air Act: Summary Report.* https://www.epa.gov/sites/production/files/2015-07/documents/summaryreport.pdf

US Environmental Protection Agency (USEPA). (2016). *Climate change and the health of older adults. EPA 430-F-16-058.* https://archive.epa.gov/epa/climate-impacts/communicating-vulnerabilities-climate-change-older-adults.html

USGCRP. (2016). *The Impacts of Climate Change on Human Health in the United States: A Scientific Assessment.* Crimmins, A., J. Balbus, J.L. Gamble, C.B. Beard, J.E. Bell, D. Dodgen, R.J. Eisen, N. Fann, M.D. Hawkins, S.C. Herring, L. Jantarasami, D.M. Mills, & S. Saha. M.C. Sarofim, J. Trtanj, and L. Ziska, Eds. U.S. Global Change Research Program, Washington, D.C. http://dx.doi.org/10.7930/J0R49NQX

Van Zutphen, A. R., Lin, S., Fletcher, B. A., & Hwang, S.-A. (2012). A Population-based case-control study of extreme summer temperature and birth defects. *Environmental Health Perspectives, 120*(10), 1443–1449. http://doi.org/10.1289/ehp.1104671

Watts, N., Amann, M., Adger, W. N., Ayeb-Karlsson, S., Bellasova, K., Bouley, T., ... Costello, A. (2017). The Lancet Countdown on health and climate change: From 25 years of inaction to a global transformation for public health. *Lancet, 390*(10107).

World Bank. (2017). *Climate-Smart Healthcare: Low-Carbon and Resilience Strategies for the Health Sector.* World Bank.

World Health Organization (2017). *G7 health ministers.* http://www.who.int/dg/speeches/2017/g7-health-ministers/en/.

World Health Organization (WHO) (2009). *Protecting health from climate change: connecting science, policy and people.* World Health Organization.

Zanobetti, A., O' Neil, M. S., Gronhand, C. J., & Schwartz, J. D. (2012) Summer temperature variability and long-term survival among elderly people with chronic disease. *Proceedings of the National Academy of Sciences, 109*(17), 6608–6613. doi:10.1073/pnas.1113070109

Zhang, Y., Yu, C., & Wang, L. (2017). Temperature exposure during pregnancy and birth outcomes: An updated systematic review of epidemiological evidence. *Environmental Pollution, 225*, 700-712. doi: 10.1016/j.envpol.2017.02.066

CLIMATE CHANGE AND THE HEALTH OF OLDER ADULTS

Stephanie Chalupka, EdD, RN, PHCNS-BC, FAAOHN, FNAP
Professor and Director, Master of Science in Nursing Program
Department of Nursing
Worcester State University
Visiting Scientist, Environmental and Occupational Medicine and Epidemiology Program
Department of Environmental Health
Harvard T.H. Chan School of Public Health

Janna Trombley, MS, RN
Instructor
Department of Nursing,
Worcester State University

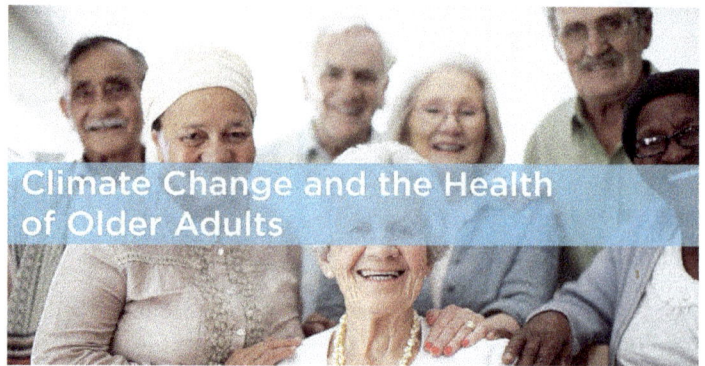

(Image credit: US EPA, 2016) Reproduced as part of public domain.

INTRODUCTION

Climate change will affect everyone but will not affect everyone equally. Some population groups (e.g., children, older adults, those with chronic illness, and the poor) will be more severely impacted because of their unique vulnerabilities. For older adults, climate change is considered to be a "threat multiplier" exacerbating underlying or pre-existing problems (Smyer, 2017). Older adults are a particularly at-risk group due to changes in physiology, age-related mobility limitations, cognition, and restricted access to resources. These factors can increase social vulnerability, limit adaptive capacity, and have significant health implications.

The number of Americans 65 years and older is projected to nearly double from 52 million in 2018 to 95 million by 2060. Those 65 and older will comprise 23% of the US population by 2060 (Population Reference Bureau, 2020). Adults aged 65 and older in the United States are a very diverse population with distinct subpopulations. They can be differentiated by age, socio-economic status, general health, level of disability, race/ethnicity, educational attainment, family/community support, or other characteristics. Therefore, the effects of climate change can be variable depending on health status pre-exposure, social characteristics and psychological well-being (Gamble et al., 2013). Understanding the threats that climate change poses to the health of older adults can help nurses work with older adults, their families, caregivers, community-based organizations, and policymakers to lower the risks and be prepared.

CLIMATE-RELATED FACTORS IMPACTING HEALTH

Heat

Extreme heat and heat waves are projected to increase in frequency, intensity, and duration as a result of climate change (Gamble et al., 2016). The aging adult is particularly at risk due to the adverse health effects related to extreme heat (Gamble et al., 2016). As one ages, the body's thermoregulatory mechanisms can become impaired, thus leading to increased risk of morbidity and mortality from heat related events among older adults (Carnes, Staats, & Willcox, 2014). Adults on multiple medications, specifically medications that impair the body's ability to thermoregulate such as anticholinergics or psychiatric medications, can be even more vulnerable to developing heat related illness (Gamble et al., 2016; McDermott-Levy et al., 2019). There is a well-documented association between increased temperatures and death in adults aged 65 years old or older (Sarofim et al., 2016). There have also been established relationships between increased temperatures and hospitalization for cardiovascular or respiratory conditions among this population (Sarofim et al., 2016; Smyer, 2017).

Extreme Events and Disasters

Older adults are particularly vulnerable to injury, illness, and mortality as a result of climate related disasters (Spurlock et al., 2019). These disasters may include wildfires, floods, and hurricanes. The vulnerability of older adults is largely due to disruptions in access to health services, medications, and safe shelter (McDermott-Levy et al., 2019). Those with impairments in cognition, sensory awareness, or mobility and those who are economically burdened are at even increased risk of poor health outcomes due to difficulty in evacuation and recovery from disaster events (Gamble et al., 2016; Spurlock et al., 2019). In fact, 71% of fatalities associated with Hurricane Katrina in 2004 (Centers for Disease Control and

Prevention [CDC], 2018) and 50% of fatalities associated with Hurricane Sandy in 2012 were among those 65 years old or older (CDC, 2018; Haq & Gutman, 2014; Spurlock et al., 2019). Transportation to safe shelter also increases the risk of delirium among this population (McDermott-Levy & Fick, 2020). Additionally, it has been found that this age group experience symptoms of post-traumatic stress disorder and adjustment disorders at a higher rate than younger adults (Parker et al., 2016). Inability to maintain medication regimens is of particular concern with the older adult population due to increased chronic conditions and functional impairment (McDermott-Levy & Fick, 2020). Due to interruption in health services as a result of disasters, the older adult may be forced to go without medications for an unknown period of time, which can exacerbate these conditions and cause increased morbidity and mortality (Spurlock et al., 2019).

Air Quality

Criteria air pollutants in the United States include ozone, particulate matter, nitrogen dioxide, sulfur dioxide, carbon monoxide, and lead, all of which can be harmful to human health (United States Environmental Protection Agency, 2017). Levels of these criteria pollutants are anticipated to increase as both a direct and indirect result of climate change (Mirsaeidi et al., 2016). Older adults are vulnerable to the impacts of air pollution due to decreased pulmonary function compared to younger individuals (George, Bruzzese, & Matura, 2017). There has been an association found between increased air pollution levels and worsening of chronic conditions such as diabetes, dyslipidemia, cardiovascular, and respiratory illness in older adults, even at levels below the recommended thresholds (Lin, Yan, Liu, Yin, & Kuang, 2017; McDermott-Levy & Fick, 2020). Additionally, exposure to air pollution has been found to be possibly associated with increased risk of dementia among the elderly (Chen et al., 2017; Power et al., 2016). Short-term increases in particulate matter exposure appear to be positively associated with depression related ED attendance risk (Braithwaite et al., 2019). Associations between short- and long-term exposure to ambient air pollution components (specifically fine particulate matter) and depression among older adults have been identified (Buoli et al., 2018; Kioumourtzoglou et al., 2017; Pun, Manjourides, & Suh, 2017).

Older adults will also be exposed to increased levels of allergens due to alterations in the seasonal production of pollen, especially in middle and high latitudes in the United States (Gamble et al., 2013). Additionally, drought and wildfires are anticipated to increase in both frequency and severity, causing increased levels of dust and smoke in the atmosphere, thus exacerbating pre-existing respiratory conditions (Gamble et al., 2013).

Infectious Diseases

Climate change is increasing the geographic range and seasonal distribution of many vector-borne illnesses. Vector-borne diseases, especially those carried by mosquitoes and ticks (e.g., Lyme Disease and West Nile Virus), are projected to become more prevalent as climate change progresses (U.S. Global Change Research Program [USGCRP], 2018). Older adults are more likely to have compromised immune systems, thus putting them at greater risk for the negative sequelae of these diseases (Gamble et al., 2013).

Climate-related extreme rainfall events impact water quality and can cause enteric disease. There are up to 59 million cases of enteric disease attributable to the consumption of contaminated groundwater globally each year. The main pathogens campylobacter, shigella, hepatitis A, giardia, norovirus, and cryptosporidium have also been the cause of several large outbreaks. Exposure to waterborne pathogens in drinking water and recreational water is predicted to continue to increase as the climate changes (Haq, 2017; Hales, 2019). Due to pre-existing medical conditions and lower functioning immune systems, older adults will have a higher risk of acquiring gastrointestinal illnesses, which can lead to increased mortality among this population (Haq & Gutman, 2014; Gamble et al., 2016; USGCRP, 2018).

Food Stress

It is anticipated that climate change will destabilize food systems and compromise food safety, nutrition, production, and distribution (Haq & Gutman, 2014; Ziska et al., 2016). Crop declines could lead to undernutrition, hunger, and higher food prices. More CO_2 in the air could make staple crops like barley and soy less nutritious (Chalupka, Anderko, & Pennea, 2020). Since 2001, the number of food insecure older adults in the United States has doubled to a staggering 5.4 million, and this number is projected to increase due to climate change (Haq & Gutman, 2014; Jih et al., 2018). Climate change will also affect the ability of the older adult to prepare effectively for weather related disasters and they may have difficulty obtaining nutritious food after extreme weather events due to interruptions in the food supply chain (Haq & Gutman, 2014; Ziska et al., 2016).

FACTORS DETERMINING EXPOSURE TO CLIMATE STRESSORS

Many factors impact the degree to which older adults are exposed to climate stressors. These include socioeconomic characteristics, housing, neighborhood infrastructure and available social services. Socioeconomic characteristics including income/available financial resources, educational attainment, access to social and health services can impact the risk for exposure and capacity to adapt. Those living on a fixed income or in poverty, may be at greater risk in extreme heat events due to lack of access to air conditioning or reluctance to use air conditioning because of operating costs. Housing can impact exposure to climate stressors in several ways. Mobile home and manufactured housing residents are disproportionately older adults and lower income. In regions prone to natural hazards, this type of housing is particularly vulnerable to storm related damage (Prasad & Stoler, 2016). Relatively high concentrations of older adults live in areas that are expected to be particularly impacted by climate stressors such as extreme heat events, droughts, hurricanes, wildfires, floods, storm surges, increased airborne allergens, ground level ozone and other air pollutants. These include coastal zones and large urban areas in the Northeast, Midwest, and Southwest United States (USGCRP, 2018)

For older adults living in urban areas, the heat island effect (the city experiences much warmer temperatures than nearby rural areas) can pose additional risks to older adults. For those with limited mobility who reside in multistory buildings with an elevator, a storm-related power outage can make it extremely difficult to get food, medicine, or much needed services (Shih et al., 2018).

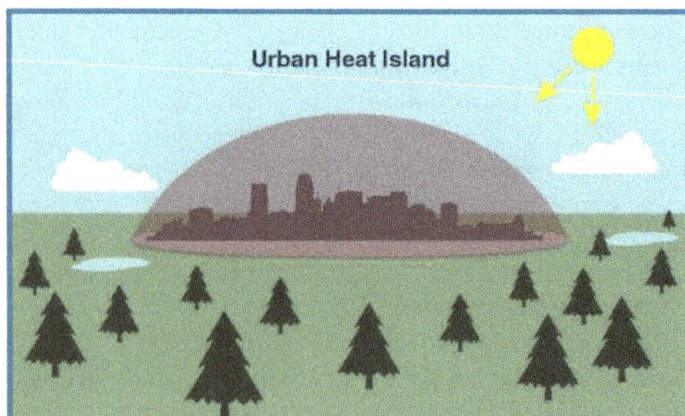

Figure 1. An urban heat island occurs when a city experiences much warmer temperatures than nearby rural areas. The difference in temperature between urban and less-developed rural areas has to do with how well the surfaces in each environment absorb and hold heat. *Image credit: NASA/JPL-Caltech.* Reproduced as part of public domain.

DETERMINANTS OF ADAPTIVE CAPACITY

Adaptive capacity is the capacity to adjust to changes in climate in order to moderate potential damage, take advantage of opportunities, or cope with consequences (Rhoades, Gruber, & Horton, 2018). Several factors impact the ability to which older Americans can adapt to our changing climate. Diminished adaptive capacity places older adults at high risk for experiencing persistent vulnerability in the aftermath of a disaster. Older adults are more likely to be socially isolated. Among Americans age 65 or older, about one-third of Medicare enrollees, or approximately 16 million nationally live alone (Shih et al., 2018). Social isolation is a significant risk factor for death during extreme heat events (National Collaborating Centre for Environmental Health, 2019).

Those with multiple chronic diseases, disabilities and mobility problems, dementia or cognitive impairments, and living in a long-term care facility are among the highest risk group of vulnerable older adults. Even those older adults living in the community can face interruptions in health care continuity as power outages in extreme weather can cripple hospitals and transportation systems and interrupt the delivery of social services when they are most needed.

This persistent vulnerability is seriously exacerbated by a lack of federal and local policies, disaster preparedness education, guidance specific to older adults, tracking systems, and warnings for individuals with sensory impairments (e.g., vision, hearing, and proprioception), compromised ambulation, and chronic conditions (Malik et al, 2018).

Functional limitation/mobility impairments including chronic disease, illness, decreased muscle strength and balance, and cognitive impairment can each significantly decrease the ability of older adults to respond effectively to climate-related stressors and events (Malik et al., 2018). Forty-four percent of people aged 65 and over enrolled in Medicare reported limitations in activities of daily living, instrumental activities of daily living, or were living in a long-term care facility. The prevalence of limitation varies with age and sex with older women reporting more impairment than older men (Federal Interagency Forum on Aging-Related Statistics, 2016). Of Americans 65 and older, about 20 to 25 percent have mild cognitive impairment while about 10 percent have dementia. As the population of older adults is expanding, the number of people affected by dementia is increasing (Langa et al., 2017). These limitations can make responding to climate-related events, evaluation, and recovery is much more challenging for older adults.

Financial resources can also have a powerful impact on adaptive capacity. Limited income or lack of access to transportation can be an impediment to evacuation. Older adults can be more vulnerable to property damage or loss and price-gouging (Federal Emergency Management Agency [FEMA], 2012). In the aftermath of climate-related disasters like hurricanes, tornados and floods, fraudulent contractors frequently prey upon older homeowners. Typically, these contractors request for upfront money but disappear before work is done or do poor quality work leaving the homeowner financially responsible (AARP, 2012; FEMA, 2012). Tools for communication and rapid dissemination of critical information (e.g., internet and social media) for preparation, survivability, and recovery from extreme weather events as well as technology to rapidly identify at risk populations including older adults can support adaptive capacity. Lack of access to, or disruption in, any of these systems can place older adults at greater risk (Gamble et al., 2013).

ADDRESSING THE CHALLENGE: REDUCING VULNERABILITY THROUGH EFFECTIVE ADAPTATION

There is strong evidence that in the absence of effective adaptation, climate change will have a disproportionate impact on older adults due to a wide variety of factors including biological and socioeconomic characteristics, housing, neighborhood infrastructure, and available social services. Effective adaptation measures will be central to addressing the risks associated with climate change faced by older adults. Development of community-based registries to identify location of older adults, particularly those who are homebound, outreach programs targeted towards older adults, and the development of community-based adaptation (e.g., Heat Alert and Response Systems [HARS]) can be effective adaptation strategies to reduce vulnerability of older adults. (See other examples in Table 1). Finally, health care itself is also on the front lines of climate change. Hospitals, health centers, and health care providers must not only reduce their carbon footprint but be ready to respond effectively to climate-related extreme weather events. They must build capacity and resilience to stay operational and serve as community anchors during climate-related disasters. The nurse can be a powerful advocate for coherent policies that address the interface between climate change and older adults. Nurses, as trusted health professionals, have the opportunity to act as critical messengers by communicating the health impacts of climate change, advocating for climate-smart policies at all levels of government, and promoting measures to reduce the vulnerability of older adults and build adaptive capacity.

Table 1

Heat Event Adaptation Strategies
Develop an emergency heat plan to prepare city services for a heat event
Establish cooling centers to reduce heat stress and heat-related deaths and illnesses
Provide emergency notification and well-being checks to protect the most vulnerable
Incorporate heat island reduction strategies - such as green or cool roofs, cool pavements, or increased vegetation and trees - into long-term planning efforts to help lower urban temperatures

REFERENCES

AARP (2012). *Avoiding post-disaster scams.* https://www.aarp.org/money/scams-fraud/info-08-2012/avoiding-post-disaster-scams.html

Braithwaite, I., Zhang, S., Kirkbride, J. B., Osborn, D. P., & Hayes, J. F. (2019). Air pollution (particulate matter) exposure and associations with depression, anxiety, bipolar, psychosis and suicide risk: A systematic review and meta-analysis. *Environmental Health Perspectives, 127*(12), 126002-1-23. doi: 10.1289/EHP4595

Buoli, M., Grassi, S., Caironi, A., Silva Carnevali, G., Mucci, F., Iodice, S., ... Bollati, V. (2018). Is there a link between air pollution and mental disorders? *Environment International, 118,* 154-168. doi: 10.1016/j.envint.2018.05.044

Carnes, B. A., Staats, D., & Willcox, B. J. (2014). Impact of climate change on elder health. *Journals of Gerontology: Biological Sciences, 69*(9), 1087-1091. doi: 10.1093/Gerona/glt159

Chalupka, S., Anderko, L., & Pennea, E. (2020). Climate change, climate justice, and children's mental health: A generation at-risk. *Environmental Justice, 13*(1), https://doi.org/10.1089/env.2019.0034

Centers for Disease Control and Prevention. (2018). *Emergency preparedness & vulnerable populations: Planning for those most at risk.* https://www.cdc.gov/cpr/whatwedo/vulnerable.htm

Chen, H., Kwong, J. C., Copes, R., Hystad, P., van Donkelaar, A., Tu, K., ... Burnett, R. T. (2017). Exposure to ambient air pollution and the incidence of dementia: A population-based cohort study. *Environment International,* 217-277. doi: 10.1016/j.envint.2017.08.020

Federal Emergency Management Agency. (2012). *Scam artists attempt to prey on disaster survivors.* https://www.fema.gov/news-release/2012/12/06/scam-artists-attempt-prey-disaster-survivors

Federal Interagency Forum on Aging-Related Statistics. (2016). *Older Americans 2016: Key indicators of well-being.* https://agingstats.gov/docs/LatestReport/Older-Americans-2016-Key-Indicators-of-WellBeing.pdf

Gamble, J. L., Balbus, J., Berger, M., Bouye, K., Campbell, V., Chief, K., …Wolkin, A. F. (2016). Populations of concern. In *The impacts of climate change on human health in the United States: A scientific assessment (chapter 9).* https://health2016.globalchange.gov/populations-concern

Gamble, J. L., Hurley, B. J., Schultz, P. A., Jaglom, W. S., Krishnan, N., & Harris, M. (2013). Climate change and older Americans: State of the science. *Environmental Health Perspectives, 121*(1), 15-21. doi: 10.1289/ehp.1205223

George, M., Bruzzese, J. M., & Matura, L. A. (2017). Climate change effects on respiratory health: Implications for nursing. *Journal of Nursing Scholarship, 49*(6), 644-652. doi: 10.1111/jnu.12330

Hales, S. (2019) Climate change, extreme rainfall events, drinking water and enteric disease. *Reviews on Environmental Health, 34*(1), 1–3. doi: 10.1515/reveh-2019-2001

Haq, G., & Gutman, G. (2014). Climate gerontology. *Zeitschrift fuer Gerontologie und Geriatrie, 47,* 462-467. doi: 10.1007/s00391-014-0677-y.

Haq, G. (2017). Growing old in a changing climate. *Public Policy & Aging Report, 27*(1), 8-12. doi:10.1093/ppar/prw027

Jih, J., Stijacic-Cenzer, I., Seligman, H.K., Boscardin, J., Nguyen, T.T., & Ritchie, S. (2018). Chronic disease burden predicts food insecurity among older adults. *Public Health Nutrition, 21*(9), 1737-1742. doi: 10.1017/S1368980017004062

Kioumourtzoglou, M. A., Power, M. C., Hart, J. E., Okereke, O. I., Coull, B. A., Laden, F., & Weisskopf, M. G. (2017). The association between air pollution and onset of depression among middle-aged and older women. *American Journal of Epidemiology, 185*(9), 801-809. doi: 10.1093/aje/kww163

Langa, K., Larson, E. B., Crimmins, E. M., Faul, Levine, D. A., Kabeto, M. U. & Weir, D. R. (2017). A comparison of the prevalence of dementia in the United States in 2000 and 2012. *JAMA Internal Medicine, 177*(1), 51-58. doi:10.1001/jamainternmed.2016.6807

Liu, S., Yan, Z., Liu, Y., Yin, Q., & Kuang, L. (2017). Association between air pollution and chronic diseases among the elderly in China. *Natural Hazards, 89,* 79-91. doi: 10.1007/s11069-017-2955-7

Malik, S., Lee, D. C., Doran, K. M., Grudzen, C. R., Worthing, J., Portelli, I., . . . Smith, S. W. (2018). Vulnerability of older adults in disasters: Emergency department utilization by geriatric patients after hurricane sandy. *Disaster Medicine and Public Health Preparedness, 12*(2), 184-193. doi: 10.1017/dmp.2017.44

McDermott-Levy, R., & Fick, D. M. (2020). Advancing gerontological nursing science in climate change. *Research in Gerontological Nursing, 13*(1), 6-12. doi: 10.3928/19404921-20191204-02

McDermott-Levy, R., Kolanowski, A. M., Fick, D .M., & Mann, M. E. (2019). Addressing the health risks of climate change in older adults. *Journal of Gerontological Nursing, 45*(11), 21-29. doi: 10.3928/00989134-20191011-04

Mirsaeidi, M., Motahari, H., Taghizadeh Khamesi, M., Sharifi, A., Campos, M., & Schraufnagel, D. E. (2016). Climate change and respiratory infections. *Annals of the American Thoracic Society, 13*(8), 1223-1230. doi: 10.1513/AnnalsATS.201511-729PS

National Collaborating Centre for Environmental Health (2019). *Extreme heat.* http://www.ncceh.ca/environmental-health-in-canada/health-agency-projects/extreme-heat

Parker, G., Lie, D., Siskind, D. J., Martin-Khan, M., Raphael, B., Crompton, D., & Kisely, S. (2016). Mental health implications for older adults after natural disasters: A systematic review and meta-analysis. *International Psychogeriatrics, 28*(1), 11-20. doi: 10.1017/S1041610215001210

Population Reference Bureau (2020). *Fact sheet: Aging in the United States.* https://www.prb.org/aging-unitedstates-fact-sheet/

Power, M. C., Adar, S. D., Yanosky, J. D., & Weuve, J. (2016). Exposure to air pollution as a potential contributor to cognitive function, cognitive decline, brain imaging, and dementia: A systematic review of epidemiologic research. *NeuroToxicology, 56,* 235-253. doi: 10.1016/j.neuro.2016.06.004

Prasad, S., & Stoler, J. (2016). Mobile home residents and vulnerability in South Florida: Research gaps and challenges. *International Journal of Disaster Risk Science, 7,* 436–439. https://doi.org/10.1007/s13753-016-0101-x

Pun, V. C., Manjourides, J., & Suh, H. (2017). Association of ambient air pollution with depressive and anxiety symptoms in older adults: Results from the NSHAP Study.

Environmental Health Perspectives, 125(3), 342-348. doi: 10.1289/EHP494

Rhoades, J. L., Gruber, J. S., & Horton, B. (2018). Developing an in-depth understanding of elderly adult's vulnerability to climate change. *Gerontologist, 58*(3), 567–577 doi:10.1093/geront/gnw167

Sarofim, M. C., Saha, S., Hawkins, M. D., Mills, D. M., Hess, J., Horton, R., ... St. Juliana, A. (2016). Temperature-related death and illness. In *The impacts of climate change on human health in the United States: A scientific assessment. (chapter 2).* https://health2016.globalchange.gov/temperature-related-death-and-illness

Shih, R. A., Acosta, J. D., Chen, E. K., Carbone, E. G., Xenakis, L., Adamson, D. M., & Chandra, A. (2018). Improving disaster resilience among older adults: Insights from public health departments and aging-in-place efforts. *Rand Health Quarterly, 8*(1), 3.

Smyer, M. A. (2017). Greening gray: Climate action for an aging world. *Public Policy & Aging Report, 27*(1), 4-7.

Spurlock, W. R., Rose, K., Goodwin Veenema, T., Sinha, S. K., Gray-Miceli, D., Hitchman, S., ... Miller, E. T. (2019). American Academy of Nursing on policy position statement: Disaster preparedness for older adults. *Nursing Outlook, 67,* 118-121. doi: 10.1016/j.outlook.2018.12.002

US Environmental Protection Agency. (2015). *Community-based adaptation to a changing climate.* https://www.epa.gov/sites/production/files/2016-09/documents/community-based-adaptation_handout.pdf

US Environmental Protection Agency. (2016). *Communicating vulnerabilities to climate change: older adults.* https://archive.epa.gov/epa/climate-impacts/communicating-vulnerabilities-climate-change-older-adults.html

US Environmental Protection Agency. (2017). *Criteria air pollutants.* https://19january2017snapshot.epa.gov/criteria-air-pollutants_.html

U.S. Global Change Research Program. (2018). *Impacts, risks, and adaptation in the United States: Fourth national climate assessment, Volume II* [Reidmiller, D. R., C. W. Avery, D. R. Easterling, K. E. Kunkel, K. L. M. Lewis, T. K. Maycock, & B.C. Stewart (eds.)]. U.S. Global Change Research Program, Washington, DC, USA, 1515 pp. doi: 10.7930/NCA4.2018.

Ziska, L., Crimmins, A., Auclair, A., DeGrasse, S., Garofalo, J. F., Khan, A. S., ... Walls, I. (2016). Food safety, nutrition, and distribution. In *The impacts of climate change on human health in the United States: A scientific assessment (chapter 7).* https://health2016.globalchange.gov/food-safety-nutrition-and-distribution

CLIMATE CHANGE MITIGATION

Erin Johnson MPH, MSN, RN
Health Promotion Council
Public Health Management Corporation

DEFINITION OF CLIMATE CHANGE MITIGATION

The direct and indirect impacts of climate change on health are well documented. Cardiac and circulatory disease, effects on pregnancy outcomes, respiratory illness, disease vector population patterns, and impacts on safe food and water access are among the health-related concerns associated with climate change (Ghazali et al, 2018). Achieved through policies, programs and individual actions, climate change mitigation generally attempts to reduce human emissions of greenhouse gasses. The United States healthcare sector contributes close to 10% of the nation's greenhouse gas emissions (Eckelman & Sherman, 2016).

In addition to reducing human emissions of greenhouse gasses, climate change mitigation efforts enhance the capacity of carbon reservoirs (such as forests or soil) to absorb carbon-containing greenhouse gases (Drawdown, 2017).

Some examples of climate change mitigation include reducing energy demand, increasing energy efficiency, replacing fossil fuels with lower carbon energy, and reducing the use of fossil fuels in products, processes and as a power source. Mitigation efforts are considered "upstream" determinants of health for current and future generations (Leffers, McDermott-Levy, Nicholas, & Sweeney, 2017 & Butterfield, 2017).

WHY CLIMATE CHANGE MITIGATION?

Prioritization of climate mitigation initiatives, projects, programs and efforts should take the relative potency of greenhouse gases into account – the gases differ in concentration, potency and lifespan, and are variously integrated into our life and industrial processes. Greenhouse gases include carbon dioxide, methane, nitrous oxide, and fluorinated gases. The potency of each gas as a greenhouse or "planet warming" gas depends on how long it remains in the atmosphere and how well it absorbs solar energy. Each of these gases remain in the atmosphere for varying amounts of time – some for just a few years, while others are in the atmosphere for thousands of years. For example, methane is in the atmosphere for a significantly shorter period of time than carbon dioxide, but is far more powerful at trapping heat. Over time, greenhouse gases mix across the entire planet. The Earth and its atmosphere are a closed system, much like a terrarium: greenhouse gases emitted in one place on the planet eventually impact every place on the planet, and similarly gases that are emitted today can impact the climate, biodiversity, population sizes, experiences and survival of many future generations of people, plants, animals and ecosystems (EPA, n.d.).

While the United States healthcare industry is only one of many sources (of direct and indirect) contributors to climate change, it is a significant contributor. Eckelman and Sherman (2016) note that the healthcare industry contributes to acid rain (12%), greenhouse gas emissions (10%), smog formation (10%) criteria air pollutants (9%), stratospheric ozone depletion (1%), and carcinogenic and non-carcinogenic air toxics (1-2%). As a result, the healthcare industry contributes to the burden of disease correlated with fossil fuels pollution and corresponding climate change at the population level. Becoming aware of the connections between health, climate change and fossil fuels extraction and use can help motivate and target efforts to protect human and environmental health: Though climate mitigation, the health of people, communities, and the planet are protected (Schenk, 2019).

WHY NURSES

Nurses can be an enormous asset to mitigation efforts. Effective mitigation efforts are particularly challenging since high-quality policies, strategies, practices and workflows must be developed, implemented and enforced at the systemic level for the most significant impact. As of 2018, there were 2.7 million active registered nurses, the largest group of healthcare professionals (Schenk, 2019). Often working collaboratively, nurses are integrated across all levels of the healthcare system and are present in enormously diverse practice settings. They are intimately involved with the workflow and support of patients in the clinical setting, or in the home. As they go about their work, nurses are able to make gains in efficiency, reducing materials waste and energy use.

Nurses are familiar with the materials and instruments of care, enabling them to be informed participants in decision making about the necessity and utility of specific supplies. They can change how care is clustered, impacting energy consumed by appliances or lighting. Nurses can work together in small groups to conduct environmental projects, analyzing certain practices, products or work flows to determine how to increase efficiencies or reduce environmental impact. Nurses interact with most aspects of the waste stream, enabling them to influence the way in which wastes are segregated, measured and reduced (Schenk, 2019).

A holistic approach to care enables nurses to gain a fluid understanding of which factors impact patient admissions to clinical settings, and subsequent health outcomes upon discharge to home. Through a variety of means, nurses can gather information on how their individual patient is situated in the milieu of family and community life, and how socio-economic factors contribute to environmental health exposures in homes and neighborhoods. For example, a nurse might suspect that the compounded effects of proximity to industrial air pollutants, and a lack of access to prenatal care have put a pregnant woman at greater risk for having a low birthweight baby. Nurses have a great opportunity to provide education, to prevent harm and to care for the well-being of individuals and communities.

For all of these reasons, nurses are uniquely positioned to work individually or collaboratively to initiate and support climate mitigation efforts (Schenk, 2019).

MITIGATION EXAMPLES

Energy efficiency reduces the amount of energy utilized to provide products and services. At the systems level, hospitals and clinics depend on appliances, such as freezers, refrigerators, washers, and dryers to function optimally. Updating older appliances to newer, more efficient appliances can yield great energy efficiency gains (Practice Greenhealth, n.d.). Systems-wide efficiencies can also be achieved through thoughtful changes to lighting (such as passive lighting through design or upgrading fixtures), utilization of window tints to reduce solar heat (and thereby reducing the need for air conditioning), and the installation of green roofs (Practice Greenhealth, n.d.). Hospitals and clinics can work with group purchasing organizations to select products that utilize fewer fossil fuels in the manufacturing and distribution process, and that have a lesser impact on natural systems. Analyzing and considering the entire supply chain of products ordered, from resource extraction, impact on natural systems, to packaging, and distribution can help make decisions about which products to order (McDermott-Levy, Upshall, Moore & Leffers, in review). Working with operating rooms and anesthesia professionals, decisions can similarly be made about which inhaled gases are best for patients and also produce fewer greenhouse gases (Practice Greenhealth, n.d.). Practice settings can work to enhance transportation-related efficiency by creating and utilizing incentive programs to bike to work, to carpool or take public transit (Ghazali, 2018; Schenk, 2019). There are many other small and large steps that organizations and individuals can take to mitigate the most devastating effects of climate change. Most require research, some require changes in policy, purchasing strategies, communications, collaborative strategies or in work flow.

MORE WAYS TO INVOLVED

Organizations like Healthcare Without Harm and Practice Green Health are working hard to address climate impacts in the healthcare setting via materials sourcing, supply chains analyses, changes to workflow, the introduction of metrics, or transportation of goods. Their websites provide tools for institutional-level change and offer resources to stay motivated and informed.

Inspiring and motivating, Project Drawdown "is a world-class research organization that reviews, analyses, and identifies the most viable global climate solutions, and shares these findings with the world." Project Drawdown researches and prioritizes solutions to shift the global climate change conversation from "doom and gloom" defeatism to actionable opportunity and empowerment. The website and accompanying book (called Drawdown) enhance learning and action through a variety of online courses, resources and support and include information on carbon impact, relative costs and savings, the path to adoption and how the proposed solutions work (Drawdown, 2017).

Has your city established an office of sustainability or of climate change? Many municipalities are working to mitigate the impacts of climate change by establishing offices of sustainability or an office specifically dedicated to address climate change. Some cities are creating efforts such as the Philadelphia Climate Collaborative. In other localities, nurses are working alongside governmental officials and corporate leaders to mitigate climate change. For example, in a fascinating and inspiring interview, Beth Schenck (of the Alliance of Nurses for Healthy Environments podcast) spoke to nurse Heidi Ritchie, Director of Policy for Minneapolis about her work on energy and environmental policy at the municipal level. (Schenk, 2019, podcast).

REFERENCES

Butterfield, P.G. (2017). Thinking Upstream. *Advances in Nursing Science, 40*(1), 2–11. doi: 10.1097/ANS.0000000000000161

Climate Collaborative of Greater Philadelphia. https://phillyclimatecollab.com

Eckelman, M. J., & Sherman, J. (2016). Environmental impacts of the US health care system and effects on public health. *PloS One, 11*(6), e0157014.

Environmental Protection Agency (EPA). (2021). *Overview of greenhouse gases.* https://www.epa.gov/ghgemissions/overview-greenhouse-gases

Hawken, P., (Ed.). (2017). *Drawdown: The most comprehensive plan ever proposed to reverse global warming.* Penguin Books. https://www.drawdown.org/solutions

Ghazali, D. A., Guericolas, M., Thys, F., Sarasin, F., González, P.A., & Ghazali, E. C. (2018). Climate change impacts on disaster and emergency medicine focusing on mitigation disruptive effects: An international perspective. *Journal of Environmental Research and Public Health, 15*(7) 1379-1382; doi:10.3390/ijerph15071379

Health Care Without Harm. https://noharm.org

Leffers, J., McDermott-Levy, R., Nicholas, P. K., & Sweeney, C. F. (2017). Mandate for the nursing profession to address climate change through nursing education. *Journal of Nursing Scholarship, 49*(6), 679–687; doi: 10.1111/jnu.12331

Practice Greenhealth. (n.d.) https://practicegreenhealth.org

Schenk, E. C. (2019, April 12). This nurse directs city policy [podcast episode]. *Nurses for Healthy Environments podcast.* https://www.stitcher.com/podcast/alliance-of-nurses-for-healthy-environments/nurses-for-healthy-environments-podcast

Schenk, E. C. (2019). Addressing climate change: We can't afford not to. *Nursing Economic$, 37*(1), 6–8. https://digitalcommons.psjhealth.org/publications/1280

Upshall, A., Moore, C., Leffers, J., McDermott-Levy, R., (in review). Turning up the heat. *Journal of Nurse Practitioners.*

FOOD, AGRICULTURE, AND CLIMATE CHANGE
Cara Cook, MS, RN, AHN-BC
Director of Programs
Alliance of Nurses for Healthy Environments

Without swift action to address climate change, food supply and security is set to be significantly impacted by a warming planet. Yet, industrialized food systems and consumption patterns are a large contributor and driver of climate change. Solutions such as transitioning to more plant-based diets and sustainable food systems are key to addressing climate change.

CLIMATE IMPACTS ON FOOD & AGRICULTURE

According to the Fourth National Climate Assessment, climate change will impact food quality, availability, and supply by affecting crop yields and production. Extreme weather events, such as extreme temperatures, droughts, and floods can reduce crop yields leading to reductions in the amount of food produced and supplied globally impacting access to food (Ebi et al., 2018). Food quality is threatened as higher levels of carbon dioxide concentrations in the atmosphere are shown to lead to reductions in critical nutrients, such as iron, zinc, and protein in crops (Ebi et al., 2018). Further, research draws the connection between hotter temperatures and extreme weather to contamination of food crops with harmful pathogens that cause food-borne illness, such as Salmonella and Campylobacter (Ebi et al., 2018). These are all particularly concerning for areas that already experience challenges to access to quality, nutritional foods. In addition, livelihoods for farmers and those who grow their own food are threatened from the impacts of climate change.

FOOD & AGRICULTURE AS A CONTRIBUTOR TO CLIMATE CHANGE

Climate change is projected to impact food and agriculture. However, our food system itself contributes to worsening climate change. Agriculture, forestry, and other land use contribute 23% of total human-caused greenhouse gas emissions globally, accounting for 13% of carbon dioxide emissions, 44% of methane emissions, and 82% of nitrous oxide emissions (Intergovernmental Panel on Climate Change [IPCC], 2019). Livestock production overall is the source of approximately 14.5% greenhouse gas emissions, mainly from methane emissions because of ruminant animal digestion, manure, production of crops for feed, and deforestation for agriculture use (Center for a Livable Future [CLF], 2015). The Paris Agreement outlines the goal to keep average temperature rise globally to 2 degrees Celsius, however if a business-as-usual scenario is continued agriculture-related emissions will use up almost the entire allowance of greenhouse gas emissions by 2050 (Bajzelj, 2014). Two important areas to consider when looking at food and the agriculture sector's contribution to climate change, and therefore that provide the solutions for addressing agriculture-related emissions, include meat consumption patterns and food waste.

Meat Consumption

When identifying the greenhouse gas footprint of various foods to get an accurate estimate the entire lifecycle including growth, production, transportation, and disposal must be considered. Food ranked as high emitters of

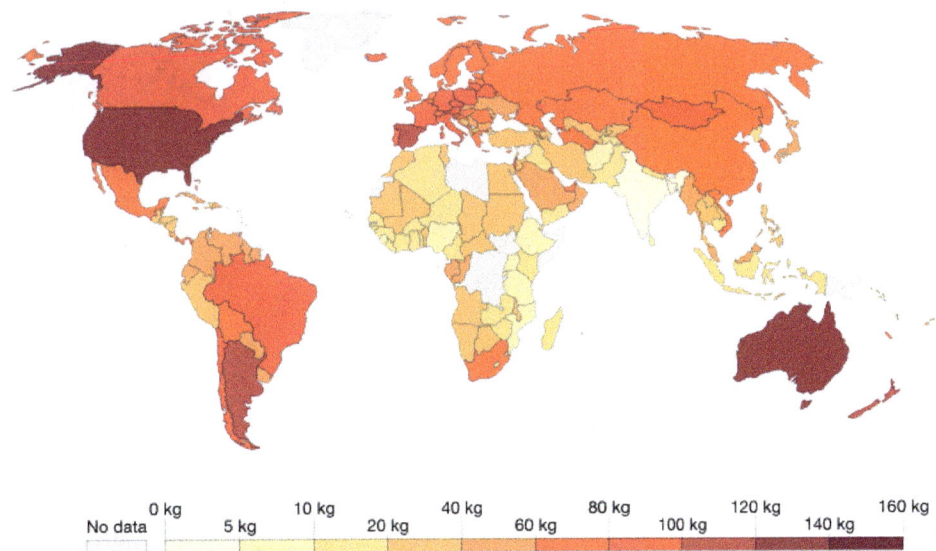

Meat supply per person, 2017
Average total meat supply per person measured in kilograms per year.

Source: UN Food and Agriculture Organization (FAO)
Note: Data excludes fish and other seafood sources. figures do not correct for waste at the household/consumption level so may not directly reflect the quantity of food finally consumed by a given individual.

OurWorldInData.org/meat-production • CC BY

Figure 1: Meat Supply Per Person, 2017. Reprinted from Our World in Data In Our World in Data, n.d., Retrieved April 6, 2021, https://ourworldindata.org/grapher/meat-supply-per-person. Reprinted with permission, Creative Commons BY license.

greenhouse gases, and also more resource-intensive (e.g. water, pesticide, and feed use) foods to produce compared to plant-based protein sources include lamb, beef, cheese, pork, and farmed salmon (Environmental Working Group [EWG], 2011). Higher-income countries have the highest patterns of meat consumption, with Australia and the United States ranked as the top two consumers of meat globally (Ritchie & Roser, 2017). See Figure 1 for a global view of average total meat consumption by country.

Food Waste

Food waste is also a significant contributor to climate change, as much of our food waste goes to the landfill in which it decomposes and releases methane. An estimated 30% of food is wasted globally, meaning if food waste were a country it would be the third largest greenhouse gas emitter (CFL, 2015). The cause of food waste differs by country and is important to note when identifying solutions to address this issue. In high-income countries most of the food waste occurs during consumption and in low to middle-income countries waste occurs due to inadequate transport, storage, or harvesting (Papargyropoulou, Lozano, Steinberger, Wright, & Ujang, 2014).

FOOD AS A CLIMATE SOLUTION

Including solutions to improve food systems and agriculture processes is essential to reduce greenhouse gas emissions and address climate change. There are certainly complexities in food and agriculture climate solutions as these may vary by country and need to account for population growth, food insecurity, and the differing needs of low and high-income countries. The Intergovernmental Panel on Climate Change (IPCC) (2019) released a special report on climate change and land in which they highlight policies that reduce food waste and shift dietary choices have positive impacts such as reducing desertification and land degradation, promoting sustainable land-use, enhancing food security, and reducing emissions.

Additionally, commitments to reduce greenhouse gas emissions from agriculture and food systems must be part of major climate agreements. As part of the Paris Agreement, countries have made commitments, called Intended Nationally Determined Contributions (INDCs) to reduce carbon emissions across sectors. There is an overall lack of commitments to reduce emissions from food waste, dietary patterns, and livestock production among the INDCs put forth thus far

(CFL, 2015). It is estimated that by decreasing meat intake alone by 2050, a reduction in agriculture-related emissions of upwards of 72% could be realized.

Project Drawdown, a research organization that provides an analysis of the top 100 climate solutions globally, has identified 17 solutions relating to food in which reducing food waste and promoting plant-rich diets are among the top five most impactful solutions (Hawken, 2017). Reducing meat and dairy consumption and preventing food waste, through improvements in infrastructure, storage, and processing in low-income countries and changes at the retail and consumer levels in high-income countries are identified as critical to cutting carbon (Hawken, 2017). View the full list of food and agriculture solutions: https://www.drawdown.org/solutions. Nurses Drawdown, a project of the Alliance of Nurses for Healthy Environments and Project Drawdown, identifies action steps that nurses can take to reduce food waste and transition to plant-based diets: https://www.nursesdrawdown.org/food/.

The Food Recovery Hierarchy (figure 2) additionally offers guidance on preventing food waste. Interventions are ranked in terms of environmental and economic

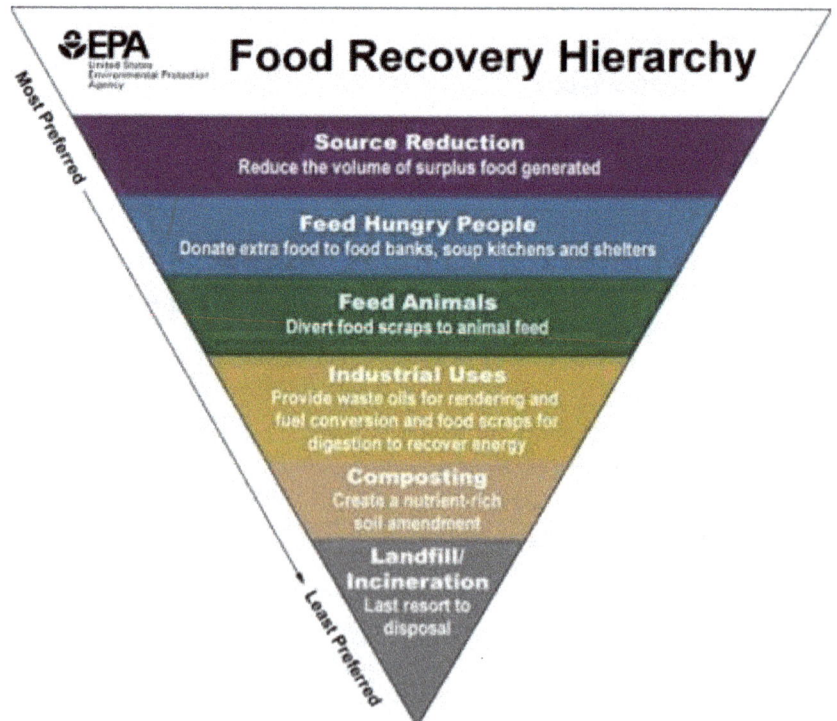

Figure 2: Food Recovery Hierarchy, 2017, Reprinted from the United States Environmental Protection Agency, reproduced as part of the public domain. In U.S. EPA, 2020, Retrieved April 6, 2021, https://www.epa.gov/sustainable-management-food/food-recovery-hierarchy.

benefits with the most preferred, such as reducing food surplus and feeding the hungry, at the top moving down to the least preferred, such as sending food to landfills, at the bottom. The Alliance of Nurses for Healthy Environments' 2020 Student Nurse Committee members developed the Mindless Composting: At Home Starter Guide (https://envirn.org/wp-content/uploads/2020/12/ANHE-Mindless-Composting-Guide.pdf) aimed at raising awareness of the food waste generated and how to implement a composting method at home.

There are numerous campaigns aimed at promoting more plant-based diets and include the Meatless Monday Campaign – eliminating meat one day a week (www.meatlessmonday.com), the Cool Food Pledge – a guidance for facilities and organizations to serve more climate-friendly foods (https://www.wri.org/our-work/project/cool-food-pledge), and the 50by40 (https://50by40.org/) campaign to reduce meat production 50% by 2040. For the health sector Health Care Without Harm (HCWH) has developed various resources to assist hospital and healthcare facilities in reducing meat consumption and serving more sustainable meats. These resources include a "Less Meat, Better Meat" approach that encourages hospitals to reduce the amount of meat served by 20% and with the cost saving purchase more sustainably produced foods (HCWH, 2019) and a "Redefining Protein: Adjusting Diets to Protect Public Health and Conserve Resources" report that summarizes alternative non-meat protein options to guide food purchasing decisions (HCWH, 2017).

National dietary guidelines are another opportunity to promote dietary shifts through the promotion of non-meat protein sources and an emphasis on diets high in fruits and vegetables. The 2015-2020 guidelines in the United States are a step forward in including more options for plant-based proteins, however, these guidelines could be stronger in outlining the health benefits of reducing meat consumption (U.S. Department of Agriculture, 2018). Canada's latest dietary guidelines specifically recommend consuming more plant-based proteins options and the health benefits of such (Health Canada, 2019).

Looking to the solutions present in the agriculture sector and in global food systems provides numerous opportunities for nurses to engage in efforts that promote healthier people through sustainable food systems and curb carbon emissions that contribute to climate change.

REFERENCES

Bajzelj B., Richards, K. S., Allwood, J. M., Smith, P., Dennis, J.S., Curmi, E., & Gilligans, C.A. (2014). Importance of food-demand management for climate mitigation. *Nature Climate Change, 4*(10), 924-929. doi:10.1038/nclimate2353.

Carlsson-Kanyama, A., & Gonzalez, A.D. (2009). Potential contributions of food consumption patterns to climate change. *American Journal of Clinical Nutrition, 89*(suppl), 1740S - 9S.

Ebi, K. L., Balbus, J. M., Luber, G., Bole, A., Crimmins, A., Glass, G., … White-Newsom, J. L., (2018). Human Health. In D. R. Reidmiller, C. W. Avery, D. R. Easterling, K. E. Kunkel, K. L. M. Lewis, T. K. Maycock, & B. C. Stewart (Eds.), *Impacts, risks, and adaptation in the United States: Fourth national climate Assessment, volume II* (pp. 572-603). U.S. Global Change Research Program. doi: 10.7930/NCA4.2018.CH14.

Environmental Working Group. (2011). *Meat eater's guide to climate change and health.* https://www.ewg.org/meateatersguide/.

Health Canada. (2019). *Canada's dietary guidelines for health professionals and policy makers.* https://food-guide.canada.ca/static/assets/pdf/CDG-EN-2018.pdf.

Health Care Without Harm. (2017). *Redefining protein: Adjusting diets to protect public health and conserve resources.* https://noharm-uscanada.org/RedefiningProtein.

Health Care Without Harm. (2019). *Less meat, better meat.* https://noharm-uscanada.org/content/us-canada/less-meat-better-meat.

Intergovernmental Panel on Climate Change. (2019). *IPCC special report on climate change, desertification, land degradation, sustainable land management, food security, and greenhouse gas fluxes in terrestrial ecosystems summary for policymakers (Approved Draft).* https://www.ipcc.ch/site/assets/uploads/2019/08/4.-SPM_Approved_Microsite_FINAL.pdf.

Kim, B., Neff, R., Santo, R., & Vigorito, J. (2015). *The importance of reducing animal product consumption and wasted food in mitigating catastrophic climate change.* https://www.jhsph.edu/research/centers-and-institutes/johns-hopkins-center-for-a-livable-future/_pdf/research/clf_reports/importance-of-reducing-animal-product-consumption-and-wasted-food-in-mitigating-catastrophic-climate-change.pdf.

Papargyropoulou, E., Lozano R., Steinberger J.K., Wright, N., & Ujang Z. (2014). The food waste hierarchy as a framework for the management of food surplus and food waste. *Journal of Clean Production, 76,* 106-115. doi:10.1016/j.jclepro.2014.04.020.

Hawken, P. (2017). *Drawdown: The most comprehensive plan ever proposed to reverse global warming.* Penguin Books.

Ritchie, H., Rosado, P., & Roser, M. (2017). *Meat and seafood production and consumption.* https://ourworldindata.org/meat-and-seafood-production-consumption.

U.S. Department of Agriculture. (2018). *Dietary guidelines for Americans 2015-2020: Dietary guidelines and myplate.* https://www.choosemyplate.gov/dietary-guidelines.

U.S. Environmental Protection Agency. (2017). *Food recovery hierarchy.* https://www.epa.gov/sustainable-management-food/food-recovery-hierarchy.

CLIMATE CHANGE ADAPTATION FOR CHILDREN

Kathryn P. Jackman-Murphy, Ed.D, MSN, RN, CHSE
Director, RN/BSN Program
Charter Oak State College

Ruth McDermott-Levy, PhD, MPH, FAAN
Professor
Co-Director, Mid-Atlantic Center for Children's Health
and the Environment
Villanova University
M. Louise Fitzpatrick College of Nursing

"The life of every child born today will be profoundly affected by climate change." (Watts et al., p.1387)

Climate change, with the rise in the planet's temperature has a negative impact on human health (Martens, 2019). The future for every child will be a planet with more frequent extreme weather events. Nurses are in a unique position to assess health issues related to climate change and provide education for children and their caregivers to help prevent, mitigate, and promote adaptation from the ever-present effects of climate change and promote a healthier life and enhance life expectancy.

Climate change, including extreme weather events such as floods, wildfires, and extreme temperatures, is a threat to children's health (Leffers, 2022). Children are especially vulnerable to the impacts of climate change due to their immature, still-developing organs, including their lungs, brain, liver, and kidneys (American Academy of Pediatrics [AAP], 2019). Additionally, children are dependent on others for food, fluids, shelter, and protection from harm, further increasing their exposure and negative effects on their health from climate change. The developmental milestones /attributes for each child also have an impact on their ability to protect themselves from the harmful effects of climate change. For example, children need support from adults for shelter and nutrition.

EXTREME TEMPERATURES

Climate change leads to periods of extreme heat and cold. Extreme heat is more common; however, periods of extreme cold arise from warming in the Arctic that leads to a weakened jet stream and cold air dipping into regions that are normally warmer (Cohen et al., 2021). Children have increased vulnerability to temperature extremes due to their reliance on others for shelter and their physiology (Leffers, 2022). Children's ability to regulate their body temperature is still developing, thus extreme temperatures place children at greater risk from exposure (O'Lenick et al., 2017).

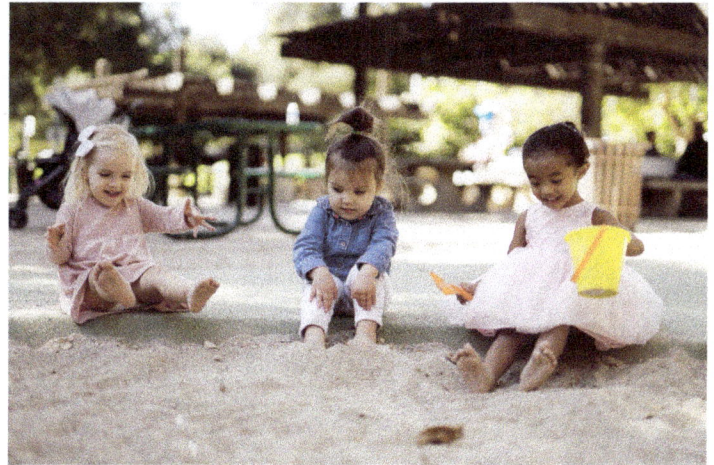
Photo by Fabian Centeno on Unsplash

Children's risk of hypothermia occurs from their greater body surface area-to-mass ratio, meaning that infants and children have less subcutaneous fat for the size of their bodies (AAP, 2019). Children can also experience heat-related illness from extreme heat. They spend more time outdoors, this is especially true during the summer months; thus, increasing their exposure to extreme temperatures (AAP, 2019). Rapid changes in ambient temperature or extreme temperatures can lead to exacerbation of asthma and asthma hospitalizations (McDermott-Levy, Pennea, & Moore, 2023). Anticipatory guidance is necessary when the nurse is working with a child's caregiver to prevent illnesses and harm from extreme weather. The nurse should educate caregiver of the risk to children by extreme temperatures, including:

- Monitoring local weather, particularly during extreme health events.
- Dress the child for weather conditions; layers are good for changing temperatures.
- Be sure the child is acclimated to the temperature.
- Maintain hydration and avoid strenuous activity, especially during the late afternoons and early evenings of very hot days.
- Keep indoors with heat or air conditioning (if able) during extreme temperatures.
- Avoid a supplemental heat source that burns fuels (ie.: coal, diesel, kerosene, wood). This can add to air pollution and the risk of carbon monoxide poisoning.

AIR QUALITY AND WILDFIRES

Air pollution from climate change such as particulate matter (PM), ground-level ozone, and dust from drier conditions and winds can affect children's health. Additionally, climate change has increased the concentration of plant pollen and aeroallergens (Helldén et al., 2021; McDermott-Levy et al., 2023). This is particularly important for children's health as they spend more time outdoors, are more active, and breathe more rapidly than adults; thus, the breathe in more pollution per their body weight (AAP, 2019).

Children with pre-existing respiratory conditions such as asthma or "simple" seasonal allergies may be further impacted because of climate change-related higher heat and carbon dioxide levels which promote plant growth. This increased plant growth will produce more pollen and allergens, prolong allergy seasons, and increase their severity. The allergy season in the United States has increased in length by up to 27 days longer due to increased temperatures (Asthma and Allergy Foundation of America, 2021). Longer and more severe allergy seasons combined with the particulate matter from air pollution can cause an increase in a child's triggers precipitating incidences of asthma exacerbation (George, 2017).

Wildfires also pose a threat to children's health. Children and families across the U.S. have experienced "smoky days" from North American wildfires. Air Quality Index (AQI) has been in the "unhealthy" range hundreds of miles from the site of the fire. Wildfire smoke contains airborne particulates that can place children at risk of acute or future respiratory problems (Holms, Miller, & Balmes, 2021). Nurses must educate caregivers to:

General Air Quality

- Plan outdoor activities using a local air quality source such as AirNow.gov

- Offer the EPA flag program for communities to share the current AQI. https://www.airnow.gov/air-quality-flag-program/

- Share with child's caregivers (school nurse, camp counselor, teacher, babysitter) of the risks to the child's health on poor air quality days.

Aeroallergens

- The Weather Channel provides local pollen counts.

- Plan outdoor activity based on pollen count for sensitive children.

- For children with asthma, plan to have asthma medication with the child.

- When planning to add trees, work with a tree expert to select low-pollen trees.

Wildfires

- Follow directions of local emergency management.

- Limit time and activity outdoors.

- When outdoors, use a correctly fitting respirator (N 95 mask).

- Do not use masks for children under 2 years old.

- If able to stay in the area, while indoors, keep windows and doors closed and keep air conditioning (if available) set to recirculate air. Ideally, air conditioning has a MERV 13 or above air filter (EPA, 2019).

- While in a car, keep windows closed and use the air conditioner set to recirculate. (American Thoracic Society, 2019).

Dust

- Follow warnings from local news.

- Limit outdoor activity when you can see dust in the air.

- Place dust mats at doors to keep dust outside.

- Cover mouth and nose with a mask or wet towel.

- Do not drink water from outdoor open containers (PEHSU, Region 2, n.d.).

- Avoid wearing shoes worn outdoors inside your home.

VECTOR-BORNE DISEASES

There are health benefits to being outdoors. In fact, during the COVID-19 pandemic, families who spent more time outdoors reported better mental health (Hazlehurst et al., 2022). However, as temperatures warm, the geographical range and season for vectors (mosquitos, ticks, and flies) increases (US Global Change Research Program [USGCRP], 2018). Infected vectors carry malaria, dengue fever, Lyme disease, West Nile, and Zika virus. Higher temperatures, increased rainfall and humidity, and flooding provide a favorable habitat for these vectors to breed and multiply (USGCRP, 2018). As previously stated, children spend more time outdoors than adults and consequently are at greater risk of vector-borne illnesses.

Nurses must be aware of the regional risks of vector-borne disease. Such as the types of ticks and mosquitoes in the region. Further, nurses must assess population risk and engage in interventions to decrease risk such as community-wide education and advocacy for evidence-based strategies that reduce exposures to insects that transmit disease and safe and effective vaccines. Other community education can include:

- The insect's habitat, places of exposure, and ways to modify the habitat.

- Safe insect repellent and following manufacturer's directions for proper use.

- Wearing light colored clothing that cover skin and hats in areas of exposure risk.

- Symptoms of insect bite and vector-borne illnesses.

FOOD SECURITY

According to the U.S. Department of Agriculture (n.d.), climate change will disrupt global food security and production leading to diminished food production and availability and increase food prices. Nutritious food plays an integral role in the promotion of the growth, development, and energy needs of children. Elevated carbon dioxide levels associated with climate change have been found to affect the nutritional value of food (Garfield, 2018). Food staples such as potatoes, rice, wheat, and barley had decreased protein levels when grown in elevated carbon dioxide levels (CO_2). There are also concerns that in the presence of high CO_2 levels, minerals such as iron and zinc which are found in cereals and legumes may be lower (Smith, Golden & Myers, 2017). Iron is critical for the creation of hemoglobin. For the developing child, iron deficiency is associated with cognitive and psychological effects and higher blood lead levels (Arcanjo, Arcanjo, & Santos, 2016). Zinc is a vital component for wound healing and immune and metabolic function and deficiencies are associated with diarrhea, infections, hair loss, loss of appetite, and slow growth. (AAP, 2019).

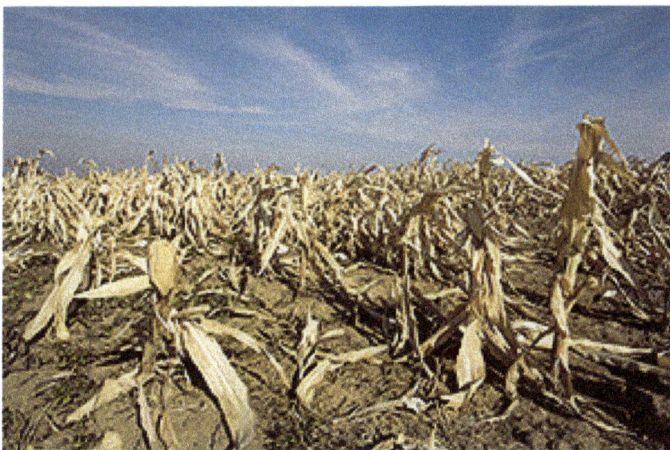

Photo from CDC as part of public domain.

The impact of our changing climate further threatens crop and livestock production due to flooding, droughts, fires, and other extreme weather events. Each of these events may affect crop and livestock yields and worsen the growing conditions resulting in limited supplies of food and increasing costs, further creating barriers towards the availability of affordable, nutritious, life-promoting food (Nissan, Simmons & Downs, 2022). Food insecurity increases in times of weather events when crops may be destroyed and transportation, supply chains, and infrastructure are disrupted, sometimes for extended periods (Oritiz, et. al, 2023). The health effects of malnutrition and infectious disease because of climate change are anticipated to have a disproportionately higher impact on children, resulting in increased morbidity and mortality (Leffers, 2022). Nurses must monitor the evolving science related to food security and nutritional value of food because of climate change. Nurses must also teach families about:

- Decreasing food waste; how to compost food instead of throwing it in trash.

- Transitioning to a more plant-based diet, if able.

- Cooking with cast iron to enhance the amount of iron in food.

- The use of dietary supplements when needed.

- Local sources to access food during times of shortage.

MENTAL HEALTH

Children's mental health is another area that is impacted by climate change. Older children and adolescents are aware of climate change and have more concerns than adults about the impacts of climate change (Crane, Li, Subramanian, Rovit, & Liu, 2022). There can be significant mental health effects from the variety of impacts of climate change including prolonged illness, trauma, or fear for the future. In fact, 51% of adolescents report being anxious about the impact of climate change and 59% were concerned about the impacts of climate change for future generations (American Psychiatric Association, 2022). Further, 68% of young people report feeling sad or afraid of climate change (American Psychiatric Association, 2022a).

Children reported feelings of anger, frustration, depression, grief, anxiety, and powerlessness associated with the climate crisis. Mental health problems related to climate change include post-traumatic stress disorder, anxiety, depression, phobias and panic, cognitive and intellectual disability, and sleep disorders (Sanson, 2021).

Incidences of ecoanxiety, a severe and debilitating worry along with reports of grief connected with ecological loss (current or anticipated) are rising (Wald, 2022). The impact on children's mental health related to climate change can be long lasting, in fact it was found that more children continued to have symptoms of post-traumatic stress disorder much longer, more than two years post-disaster than adults (Wald, 2022). Finally, climate change related disasters were associated with children experiencing exacerbation of schizophrenia and psychosis and exacerbations in acute and chronic mental health disorders such as depression (Crane et al, 2022).

Nurses must teach caregivers that when discussing climate change, the child's developmental stage and their level of understanding must be considered. Also, caregivers should convey an honest yet positive message. Other actions include:

- If interested, participating in climate action can offer the child opportunity to feel empowered, and have a sense of control and confidence (American Psychiatric Association, 2022b; Sanson, 2021).

- Offer honest answers to climate change questions with possible solutions.

- Seek professional support if mental health issues are a concern.

CONCLUSION

The environmental effects of climate change are complex and far-reaching. Children, with their developing bodies and developing pyscho-social health, have unique vulnerabilities to climate change. There are nursing actions related to anticipatory guidance for caregivers and older children to take to maintain health and support climate change adaptation. Additionally, there are resources, such as the Environmental Protection Agency (EPA), Center for Disease Control and Prevention (CDC), the national Pediatric Environmental Health Specialty Units (PEHSU pehsu.net), and American Public Health Association's (APHA) Climate and Health Youth Education Toolkit are accessible to inform nurses in their support of children's adaptation to climate change. The APHA tool kit was developed by the environmental section for health professionals to deliver information to older children in 9-12th grades. There are teaching materials that can guide school nurses and others who work with high school students to educate them about climate change mitigation and adaptation strategies and health-related co-benefits of responding to climate change (Stortstrom, 2023). The toolkit can be accessed at: https://apha.org/Topics-and-Issues/Climate-Change/Education

REFERENCES

American Academy of Pediatrics Council on Environmental Health [AAP]. (2019). *Children's unique vulnerabilities to environmental hazards.* In Etzel, R.A., (Ed.) Pediatric environmental health. (4th ed., pp. 825—852). American Academy of Pediatrics.

American Psychiatric Association. (2022a). *Americans report mental health effects of climate change, worry about future.* https://www.psychiatry.org/News-room/News-Releases/Americans-Report-Mental-Health-Effects-of-Climate

American Psychiatric Association. (2022b). *5 Key things to know about kids and climate change.* https://www.psychiatry.org/News-room/APA-Blogs/5-Key-Things-to-Know-About-Kids-and-Climate-Change

Arcanjo, F. P., Arcanjo, C. P., & Santos, P. R. (2016). Schoolchildren with Learning Difficulties Have Low Iron Status and High Anemia Prevalence. *Journal of Nutrition and Metabolism,* 2016, 7357136. https://doi.org/10.1155/2016/7357136

Asthma and Allergy Foundation of America. (2021). *Extreme allergies and climate change.* https://www.aafa.org/extreme-allergies-and-climate-change/

Cohen, J., Agel, L., Barlow, M., Garfinkel, C. I., & White, I. (2021). Linking Arctic variability and change with extreme winter weather in the United States. *Science, 373*(6559), 1116–1121. https://doi.org/10.1126/science.abi9167

Crane, K., Li, L., Subramanian, P., Rovit, E., & Liu, J. (2022). Climate change and mental health: A review of empirical evidence, mechanisms and implications. *Atmosphere, 13*(12), 2096. MDPI AG. http://dx.doi.org/10.3390/atmos13122096

Environmental Protection Agency (2019). *Wildfire smoke: A guide for public health professionals.* https://www.airnow.gov/sites/default/files/2021-09/wildfire-smoke-guide_0.pdf

Garfield, L. (2018). *Climate change could make your food less nutritious, according to Harvard researchers.* https://www.businessinsider.com/climate-change-food-nutrition-protein-2017-8

George, M., Bruzzese, J. M., & Matura, L. A. (2017). Climate change effects on respiratory health: Implications for nursing. *Journal of Nursing Scholarship: An Official Publication of Sigma Theta Tau International Honor Society of Nursing, 49*(6), 644–652. https://doi.org/10.1111/jnu.12330

Hazlehurst, M. F., Muqueeth, S., Wolf, K. L., Simmons, C., Kroshus, E., & Tandon, P. S. (2022). Park access and mental health among parents and children during the

COVID-19 pandemic. *BMC Public Health, 22*(1), 800. https://doi.org/10.1186/s12889-022-13148-2

Helldén, D., Andersson, C., Nilsson, M., Ebi, K. L., Friberg, P., & Alfvén, T. (2021). Climate change and child health: A scoping review and an expanded conceptual framework. *The Lancet Planetary Health, 5*(3), e164–e175. https://doi.org/10.1016/S2542-5196(20)30274-6

Holm, S. M., Miller, M. D., & Balmes, J. R. (2021). Health effects of wildfire smoke in children and public health tools: a narrative review. *Journal of Exposure Science & Environmental Epidemiology, 31*(1), 1–20. https://doi.org/10.1038/s41370-020-00267-4

Leffers J. M. (2022). Climate change and health of children: Our borrowed future. *Journal of Pediatric Health Care: Official Publication of National Association of Pediatric Nurse Associates & Practitioners, 36*(1), 12–19. https://doi.org/10.1016/j.pedhc.2021.09.002

Martens, D. S. (2019). Early biologic aging and fetal exposure to high and low ambient temperature: A birth cohort study. *Environmental Health Perspectives,* 117001-1-11701-8.

McDermott-Levy, R., Pennea, E., & Moore, C. (2023). Protecting children's health: Asthma and climate change. MCN. *The American Journal of Maternal Child Nursing, 48*(4), 188–194. https://doi.org/10.1097/NMC.0000000000000927

Nissan, H., Simmons, W., & Downs, S. M. (2022). Building climate-sensitive nutrition programmes. *Bulletin of the World Health Organization, 100*(1), 70–77. https://doi.org/10.2471/BLT.21.285589

O'Lenick, C. R., Winquist, A., Chang, H. H., Kramer, M. R., Mulholland, J. A.,Grundstein, A., & Sarnat, S. E. (2017). Evaluation of individual and area-level factors as modifiers of the association between warm-season temperature and pediatric asthma morbidity in Atlanta, GA. *Environmental Research, 156,* 132–144. https://doi.org/10.1016/j.envres.2017.03.021

Ortiz, A. M. D., Chua, P. L. C., Salvador Jr, D., Dyngeland, C., Albao Jr, J. D. G., & Abesamis, R. A. (2023). Impacts of tropical cyclones on food security, health and biodiversity. Bulletin of the World Health Organization, 101(2), 152–154. https://doi-org.nvcc.idm.oclc.org/10.2471/BLT.22.288838

Pediatric Environmental Health Specialty Unit (PEHSU), Region 2 (n.d.). *Saharan dust storms.* https://icahn.mssm.edu/files/ISMMS/Assets/Research/PEHSU/Saharan-Dust-Storms.pdf

Sanson, A., & Bellemo, M. (2021). Children and youth in the climate crisis. *BJPsych Bulletin, 45*(4), 205–209. https://doi.org/10.1192/bjb.2021.16

Smith, M. R., Golden, C. D., & Myers, S. S. (2017). Potential rise in iron deficiency due to future anthropogenic carbon dioxide emissions. *GeoHealth, 1*(6), 248-257. https://doi.org/10.1002/2016GH000018

Stortstrom, M. (2023). *APHA toolkit can help high schoolers make connection on climate, health.* Public Health Newswire. http://publichealthnewswire.org/?p=enviro-toolkit

US Department of Agriculture (n.d.).*Climate change, global food security, and the U.S. food system.* https://www.usda.gov/oce/energy-and-environment/food-security

USGCRP. (2018). *Impacts, risks, and adaptation in the United States: Fourth national climate assessment, Volume II.* U.S. Global Change Research Program. https://doi.org/10.7930/NCA4.2018

Wald, A. (2022). Climate change impacts mental health. In *Environmental Health in Nursing* (pp. 292-303). Alliance of Nurses for Healthy Environments.

Watts, N., Amann, M., Arnell, N., Ayeb-Karlsson, S., Belesova, K., Boykoff, M., Byass, P., Cai, W., Campbell-Lendrum, D., Capstick, S., Chambers, J., Dalin, C., Daly, M., Dasandi, N., Davies, M., Drummond, P., Dubrow, R., Ebi, K. L., Eckelman, M., Ekins, P., … Montgomery, H. (2019). The 2019 report of The Lancet Countdown on health and climate change: ensuring that the health of a child born today is not defined by a changing climate. *Lancet, 394*(10211), 1836–1878. https://doi.org/10.1016/S0140-6736(19)32596-6

CLIMATE CHANGE AND OUTDOOR WORKER HEALTH: THE ROLE OF THE NURSE

Daniel Smith, PhD, AGPCNP-BC, CNE
Weingarten Endowed Assistant Professor
Villanova University
M. Louise Fitzpatrick College of Nursing

Liz Mizelle, PhD, RN-BC, CNE
Assistant Professor
East Carolina University
College of Nursing

Lori Modly, DNP, RN, CPNP-PC
Assistant Clinical Professor
Emory University
Nell Hodgson Woodruff School of Nursing

INTRODUCTION

This chapter will review the connections between climate change and the health of outdoor workers. We will frame the discussion through a recognition that many of the outdoor workers in the United States are immigrant or migrant workers, which further increases susceptibility to both baseline occupational hazards (Moyce & Schenker, 2018; Porru & Baldo, 2022) and climate change-related hazards (Smith et al., 2023). However, a complete and nuanced discussion of the interplay between immigration status, one's job, and climate change is outside this chapter's scope, but we will provide a high-level overview of this interplay. We will use a case study on climate-sensitive diagnoses made with agriculture workers in Southeastern Georgia, USA, highlighting the importance of understanding each worker's unique work history and efforts to combat climate change's impacts on their health. Finally, we will provide nurses with recommended nursing interventions to support the health of outdoor workers in a changing climate.

BACKGROUND

Climate change will disproportionately impact the health of disenfranchised and historically excluded populations (Smith et al., 2023), and of particular interest in this chapter, outdoor workers (Moda et al., 2019). Outdoor workers can be broadly defined as any person whose primary employment causes them to spend most of their working day outside and exposed to various environmental stressors. Examples of such workers include farmworkers, landscapers, and construction workers, but this list is not all-inclusive.

Overall, occupational health risks from climate change can be categorized into 1) amplified existing hazards, 2)

unanticipated or unrecognized hazards, and 3) changes in response to climate change (Keifer, 2016). Outdoor workers are already exposed to environmental stressors, including increased temperatures and other extreme weather events, chemical exposures from the use of fertilizers and pesticides needed to grow crops (Applebaum et al., 2016; Delcour et al., 2015), and air pollution (e.g., wildfire smoke and ozone contamination) (Applebaum et al., 2016). However, those exposures will be more frequent and more severe due to climate change (Applebaum et al., 2016; Smith, Mac, et al., 2022). There will also be unanticipated and unrecognized risks like new insects and parasite risks as vector habitat ranges are expanded (e.g., mosquitos leading to malaria infections, ticks leading to new cases of Lyme's Disease) (Applebaum et al., 2016; Magnavita et al., 2022).

To adapt to climate change, humans are doing a lot of different things, one of those is creating Green Jobs, like installing solar panels. Per definition Green Jobs are those that provide services that benefit the environment or conserve natural resources (Portier et al., 2010). Building new solar power panels and other clean energy plants to combat climate change could increase worker falls and injuries, electrical hazards, and exposure to smoke if the panels are to catch fire on the job site (Portier et al., 2010; White & Doherty, 2017).

Another example of an unanticipated or unrecognized health hazard for outdoor workers due to climate change is the risk of developing chronic kidney disease of unknown etiology (CKDu). CKDu is thought to be the first new chronic condition due to climate change (Glaser et al., 2016; Sorensen & Garcia-Trabanino, 2019). The condition has been heavily described in agricultural workers in Central America but has only recently become of interest to occupational health researchers as a potential threat to outdoor workers in the United States (Smith, Mac, et al., 2022; Smith, Pius, et al., 2022). The etiology of CKDu is complex (Orantes-Navarro et al., 2017); however, the leading hypothesis is that outdoor workers experience frequent heat stress due to a warming climate and dehydration on a daily basis (Smith, Pius, et al., 2022). Over time, this daily acute kidney injury leads to end-stage renal disease, which necessitates the use of renal replacement therapies, such as hemodialysis (Singh et al., 2022; Smith, Mac, et al., 2022).

Wildfires and heat-related illnesses are commonly recognized environmental threats to the health of workers, which will be exacerbated by climate change. Wildfires have always existed to some extent in our world, but they are becoming more common due to climate change (Xu et al., 2020). Exposure to wildfire smoke is known to increase the risk of both cardiovascular and pulmonary disorders, such as chronic obstructive pulmonary disease and asthma (Postma, 2020). Likewise, the rates of heat-related illness are expected to increase for outdoor workers (Smith et al., 2021). As there is no guarantee that workers will be allowed to stop work during periods of heavy wildfire smoke or intense heat, nurses must employ a harm reduction approach to help reduce the burden of disease. This may include increased rest periods for both wildfires and heat-related illnesses (Postma, 2020; Smith et al., 2021), the use of respirators to protect from smoke/air pollution (Navarro, 2020), and ensuring adequate access to water and shade to prevent heat-related illness (Smith et al., 2021).

It is worth noting that a lot of the prevention measures presented in the past paragraph sound good theoretically. However, there are barriers to the implementation of these strategies. Outdoor workers are often at the mercy of their employers in what they can reasonably do to protect themselves during the workday. Consider the Occupational Safety and Health Administration's (OSHA) safety message of "Water. Rest. Shade" for heat-related illness prevention. While it is known that workers need to drink water often and take frequent breaks while working in the heat, this is often not feasible if the person is paid by the piece (i.e., the more you produce, the more you get paid). Piece rate pay has been associated with a greater

risk of developing acute kidney injury at work (Moyce & Schenker, 2018; Smith, Pius, et al., 2022).

Workplace policies and procedures like piece rate pay and employers not being mandated to pay for breaks to protect the health of their employees, are barriers to health-promoting interventions. Similarly, with proper workplace fluid intake, outdoor workers need access to sanitation facilities and built-in time to use said facilities, or else workers may purposefully not drink adequate water during the workday to prevent losing wages while making trips to the sanitation facilities. Furthermore, outside of work, anti-immigrant rhetoric and discrimination negatively impact the health of farmworkers and will likely magnify any climate-related negative health threats. For example, in one Texas-based ethnography, farmworkers reported their employer as the primary source of perceived discrimination, with one worker reporting they were pressured to return to work just a few days after a hospital admission (Snipes et al., 2017). As we center the needs of outdoor workers on protecting their health, it will be essential that nurses be knowledgeable about the multiple levels of power and privilege at play that can impact the health status of outdoor workers in a changing climate.

CASE STUDY

For nurses working with outdoor workers, it is important to remember that each occupation will be impacted uniquely by climate change. Construction workers may not have the same exposure as agricultural workers to increased pesticide and fertilizer use due to climate change. Even within a job sector, the workers may not experience the same environmental exposures. Construction workers may only be exposed to increased temperatures when building the foundation and framing a building and will have access to air conditioning and protection from the environment once they are working on the interior structures of the same building. Other construction workers may not be exposed to any or very little air conditioning during the course of a job, such as those who are working in roadway construction.

To further highlight the differences in hazards experienced by workers, we can examine a case study of the top 20 of the 153 distinct diagnoses made with 1,582 agricultural workers in Southeastern Georgia, USA, during the years 2019 and 2021-2022. Each summer, the Farmworker

Figure 1. Proportions of each of the most frequent diagnoses made in the farms that constitute cluster 1.

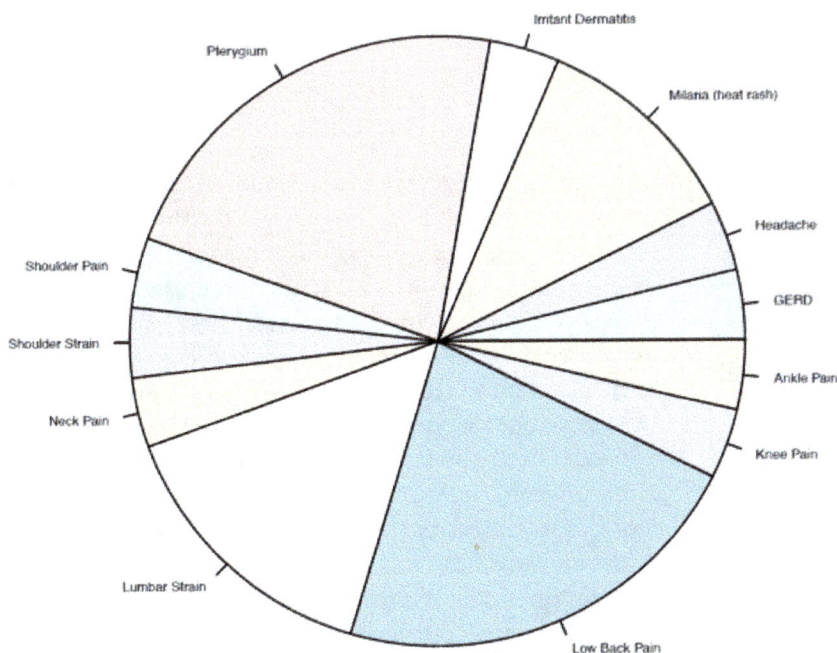

Figure 2. Proportions of each of the most frequent diagnoses made in the farms that constitute cluster 2.

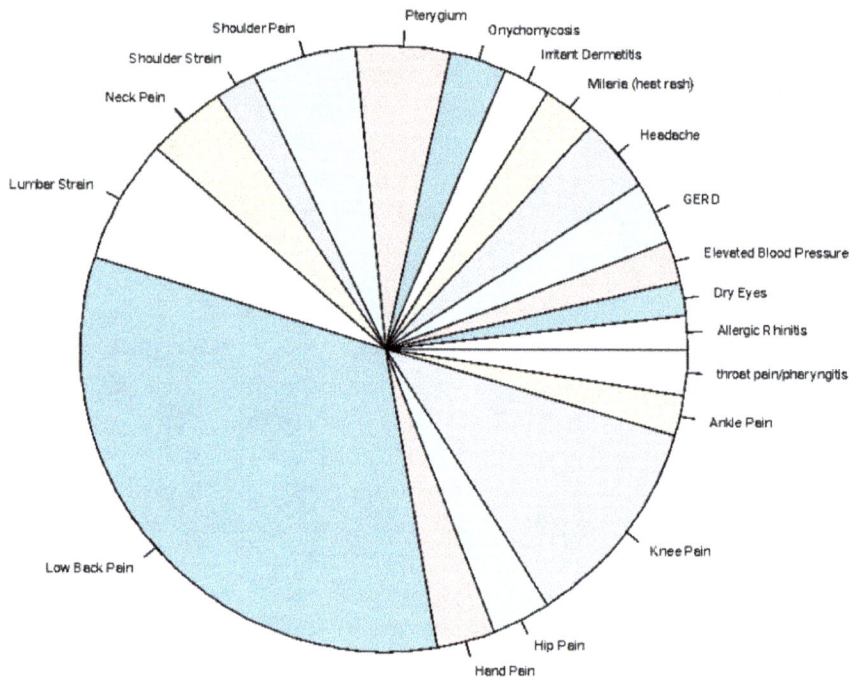

Family Health Program based out of Emory University provides clinical care to farmworkers and their families in conjunction with a local agricultural worker medical clinic. Using cluster analysis to look at differences between the diagnoses made across the farms served by the program, we sought to better understand the rates of any climate-sensitive diagnoses made by the nurse practitioners and nurse practitioner students. We found that most workers were male (93.5%) and had a mean age of 30.45 years (SD +/- 8.39). Cluster analysis showed two clusters of farms: cluster 1, made up of farm A (represented primarily berry harvesters), and cluster 2, made up of farms B, C, D, and E (represented primarily vegetable harvesters). Approximately, 45% of the top diagnoses in cluster 1 (berry harvesters) were musculoskeletal-related and 15% were climate-sensitive diagnoses (e.g., heat rash, pterygium, and sunburn; Figure 1). Pterygiums are characterized by a wedge-shaped overgrowth on the cornea caused by repeated exposure to dust, sand, chemicals, or solar radiation (Solomon, 2006). Within cluster 2 (vegetable harvesters), approximately 33% of diagnoses were climate-sensitive (Figure 2).

As nurses working with disenfranchised populations affected by climate change, analyzing this data reveals a distinct pattern regarding berry farmers and the workplace hazards they encounter. These factors contribute to a higher incidence of climate-sensitive conditions among these workers. From a clinical perspective, it is evident that our prevention efforts should concentrate on addressing conditions like heat rash, pterygium, and sunburn. For instance, berry farmers often face heightened exposure to dust, solar irritation, pesticides, and fertilizers, which are known to increase the likelihood of developing pterygiums. The prevalence of pterygiums is expected to rise due to climate change-induced heat waves and progressively arid and dusty working conditions (Echevarría-Lucas et al., 2021).

The mainstay of pterygium prevention is the use of protective eyewear. However, berry production (and other vegetable production) is dependent on being able to see the color of the fruit/vegetable being harvested. Previously reported barriers to the use of protective eyewear by farmers include visual impairment when wearing the protective glasses (Chatterjee & Agrawal, 2017) and loss of productivity when using the eyewear when workers are paid by the piece (Tovar-Aguilar et al., 2014).

In order to protect the health of outdoor workers due to climate change, nurses and other clinicians must not take a one-size-fits-all approach to occupational health and safety. We must understand the unique hazards experienced by workers from the same occupational sector (i.e., different settings or job duties of construction workers or agriculture workers) AND the differences between occupational sectors (i.e., construction vs. agriculture).

NURSING INTERVENTIONS

In order to address the unique challenges posed by climate change and its impact on the health of outdoor workers, nurses play a crucial role through implementation of various interventions. These interventions can be categorized into four key areas: occupational history, relationship building with employers and advocacy, teaching/promoting evidence-based solutions, and lifelong learning on current environmental and occupational diseases. By focusing on these interventions, nurses can contribute to creating safer work environments, improving the health outcomes of outdoor workers, and mitigating the effects of climate change on occupational health. To effectively meet the health needs of outdoor workers, nurses should do the following:

1. Occupational History

1. Conduct thorough occupational health assessments to gather information about the worker's work history, including past and current job roles, tasks performed, duration of employment, and exposure to occupational hazards.

2. Document any previous work-related injuries or illnesses to identify potential long-term effects or recurring conditions.

3. Collaborate with occupational health specialists and use standardized tools, such as occupational exposure questionnaires, to assess the level of exposure to specific hazards.

4. Utilize electronic health records to maintain a comprehensive record of the worker's occupational history and update it regularly.

2. Relationship building with employers and advocacy

1. Establish collaborative relationships with employers, supervisors, and human resource departments to promote a safe and healthy work environment for employees.

2. Advocate for workplace policies and practices that prioritize employee safety, such as regular breaks, access to clean drinking water, and adequate protective equipment.

3. Offer educational sessions for employers and supervisors to raise awareness about the impact of climate change on occupational health and the importance of preventive measures.

4. Serve as a liaison between workers and employers, facilitating open communication and addressing any concerns related to occupational hazards or health issues.

3. Teaching/Promoting of evidence-based solutions

1. Educate employers and outdoor workers about the potential health risks associated with climate change, including heat-related illnesses, respiratory problems from air pollution, and vector-borne diseases.

2. Provide training on the proper use of personal protective equipment (PPE) and emphasize its importance in minimizing exposure to hazards.

3. Teach strategies for heat illness prevention, such as the importance of hydration, taking regular breaks in shaded areas, and recognizing early signs of heat-related distress.

4. Promote evidence-based guidelines for safe work practices, including proper lifting techniques, ergonomic principles, and the use of engineering controls to minimize exposure to environmental hazards.

4. Lifelong learning on current environmental and occupational diseases.

1. Engage in continuing education programs and professional development opportunities focused on environmental and occupational health.

2. Stay updated on emerging research, guidelines, and best practices related to climate change and its impact on occupational health.

3. Participate in relevant conferences, seminars, and webinars to expand knowledge on environmental and occupational diseases.

4. Collaborate with colleagues, occupational health specialists, and public health agencies to share information and resources regarding environmental and occupational health concerns.

5. Regularly review and update educational materials and resources for patients, incorporating the latest evidence-based information on environmental and occupational disease.

5. Advocacy

1. Advocate for policies that protect outdoor works from the environmental health impacts of climate change at the job site, local, state/regional, and national levels.

CONCLUSION

In conclusion, there are intricate connections between climate change and the health of outdoor workers, with a specific focus on immigrant or migrant workers who are particularly vulnerable to both baseline occupational hazards and climate change-related hazards. By recognizing the unique challenges faced by these populations, nurses can take proactive measures to protect the health and well-being of outdoor workers. Through comprehensive occupational assessments, advocating for safe work environments, promoting evidence-based solutions, and staying informed about environmental and occupational diseases, nurses can contribute significantly to mitigating the adverse impacts of climate change on the health of disenfranchised populations. By collaborating with employers, policymakers, and fellow healthcare professionals, nurses can play a vital role in ensuring that the voices and needs of outdoor workers are heard, and that appropriate preventive measures are implemented to safeguard their health. By taking these steps, nurses can be at the forefront of combating the health effects of climate change and promoting occupational health equity for all.

REFERENCES

Applebaum, K. M., Graham, J., Gray, G. M., LaPuma, P., McCormick, S. A., Northcross, A., & Perry, M. J. (2016). An overview of occupational risks from climate change. *Current Environmental Health Reports, 3*(1), 13–22. https://doi.org/10.1007/s40572-016-0081-4

Chatterjee, S., & Agrawal, D. (2017). Primary prevention of ocular injury in agricultural workers with safety eyewear. *Indian Journal of Ophthalmology, 65*(9), 859. https://doi.org/10.4103/ijo.IJO_334_17

Delcour, I., Spanoghe, P., & Uyttendaele, M. (2015). Literature review: Impact of climate change on pesticide use. *Food Research International, 68*, 7–15. https://doi.org/10.1016/j.foodres.2014.09.030

Echevarría-Lucas, L., Senciales-González, J. M., Medialdea-Hurtado, M. E., & Rodrigo-Comino, J. (2021). Impact of Climate Change on Eye Diseases and Associated Economical Costs. *International Journal of Environmental Research and Public Health, 18*(13), 7197. https://doi.org/10.3390/ijerph18137197

Glaser, J., Lemery, J., Rajagopalan, B., Diaz, H. F., García-Trabanino, R., Taduri, G., Madero, M., Amarasinghe, M., Abraham, G., Anutrakulchai, S., Jha, V., Stenvinkel, P., Roncal-Jimenez, C., Lanaspa, M. A., Correa-Rotter, R., Sheikh-Hamad, D., Burdmann, E. A., Andres-Hernando, A., Milagres, T., … Johnson, R. J. (2016). Climate change and the emergent epidemic of CKD from heat stress in rural communities: The case for heat stress nephropathy. *Clinical Journal of the American Society of Nephrology, 11*(8), 1472–1483. https://doi.org/10.2215/CJN.13841215

Magnavita, N., Capitanelli, I., Ilesanmi, O., & Chirico, F. (2022). Occupational Lyme Disease: A systematic review and meta-analysis. *Diagnostics, 12*(2), 296. https://doi.org/10.3390/diagnostics12020296

Moda, Filho, & Minhas. (2019). Impacts of climate change on outdoor workers and their safety: Some research priorities. *International Journal of Environmental Research and Public Health, 16*(18), 3458. https://doi.org/10.3390/ijerph16183458

Moyce, S. C., & Schenker, M. (2018). Migrant workers and their occupational health and safety. *Annual Review of Public Health, 39*(1), 351–365. https://doi.org/10.1146/annurev-publhealth-040617-013714

Navarro, K. (2020). Working in smoke: Wildfire impacts on the health of firefighters and outdoor workers and mitigation strategies. *Clinics in Chest Medicine, 41*(4), 763–769. https://doi.org/10.1016/j.ccm.2020.08.017

Orantes-Navarro, C. M., Herrera-Valdés, R., Almaguer-López, M., López-Marín, L., Vela-Parada, X. F., Hernandez-Cuchillas, M., & Barba, L. M. (2017). Toward a comprehensive hypothesis of chronic Interstitial nephritis in agricultural communities. *Advances in Chronic Kidney Disease, 24*(2), 101–106. https://doi.org/10.1053/j.ackd.2017.01.001

Porru, S., & Baldo, M. (2022). Occupational health and safety and migrant workers: Has something changed in the last few years? *International Journal of Environmental Research and Public Health, 19*(15), 9535. https://doi.org/10.3390/ijerph19159535

Postma, J. (2020). Protecting outdoor workers from hazards associated with wildfire smoke. *Workplace Health & Safety, 68*(1), 52–52. https://doi.org/10.1177/2165079919888516

Solomon A. S. (2006). Pterygium. *The British Journal of Ophthalmology, 90*(6), 665–666. https://doi.org/10.1136/bjo.2006.091413

Singh, A., Zaita, B. M., Gupta, I., & Kaur, G. (2022). Documenting disease in the undocumented migrants: a case report of chronic kidney disease of unknown origin in a Central American migrant. *Cureus.* https://doi.org/10.7759/cureus.24566

Smith, D. J., Ferranti, E. P., Hertzberg, V. S., & Mac, V. (2021). Knowledge of heat-related illness first aid and self-reported hydration and heat-related illness symptoms in migrant farmworkers. *Workplace Health & Safety, 69*(1), 15–21. https://doi.org/10.1177/2165079920934478

Smith, D. J., Mac, V., Thompson, L. M., Plantinga, L., Kasper, L., & Hertzberg, V. S. (2022). Using occupational histories to assess heat exposure in undocumented workers receiving emergent renal dialysis in Georgia. *Workplace Health & Safety, 70*(5), 251–258. https://doi.org/10.1177/21650799211060695

Smith, D. J., Mizelle, E., Leslie, S. L., Li, G. X., Stone, S., Stauffer, P., Smith, A., Lewis, G., Rodden, E. L., McDermott-Levy, R., & Thompson, L. M. (2023). Intervention studies to reduce the impact of climate change on health in rural communities in the United States: A systematic review.

Environmental Research: Health, 1(3), 032001. https://doi.org/10.1088/2752-5309/acbbe6

Smith, D. J., Pius, L. M., Plantinga, L. C., Thompson, L. M., Mac, V., & Hertzberg, V. S. (2022). Heat Stress and kidney function in farmworkers in the US: A scoping review. *Journal of Agromedicine, 27*(2), 183–192. https://doi.org/10.1080/1059924X.2021.1893883

Snipes, S. A., Cooper, S. P., & Shipp, E. M. (2017). "The only thing I wish I could change is that they treat us like people and not like animals": Injury and discrimination among Latino farmworkers. *Journal of Agromedicine, 22*(1), 36–46. https://doi.org/10.1080/1059924X.2016.1248307

Sorensen, C., & Garcia-Trabanino, R. (2019). A new era of climate medicine - addressing heat-triggered renal disease. *New England Journal of Medicine, 381*(8), 693–696. https://doi.org/10.1056/NEJMp1907859

Tovar-Aguilar, J. A., Monaghan, P. F., Bryant, C. A., Esposito, A., Wade, M., Ruiz, O., & McDermott, R. J. (2014). Improving eye safety in citrus harvest crews through the acceptance of personal protective equipment, community-based participatory research, social marketing, and community health workers. *Journal of Agromedicine, 19*(2), 107–116. https://doi.org/10.1080/1059924X.2014.884397

White, J. R., & Doherty, M. (2017). Hazards in the installation and maintenance of solar panels. *2017 IEEE IAS Electrical Safety Workshop (ESW)*, 1–5. https://doi.org/10.1109/ESW.2017.7914834

Xu, R., Yu, P., Abramson, M. J., Johnston, F. H., Samet, J. M., Bell, M. L., Haines, A., Ebi, K. L., Li, S., & Guo, Y. (2020). Wildfires, global climate change, and human health. *New England Journal of Medicine, 383*(22), 2173–2181. https://doi.org/10.1056/NEJMsr2028985

CLIMATE CHANGE IMPACT ON MENTAL HEALTH
Adrienne Wald EdD, MBA, RN, CNE, MCHES
Associate Professor
School of Health and Natural Sciences
Mercy College

INTRODUCTION

Climate change is widely recognized as a leading threat to global health with outcomes mental health professionals confront (Borque & Cunsolo, 2014; Crimmins, Balbus, Gamble, Beard, Bell, & Dodgen, 2016). According to the American Psychiatric Association, climate change poses a threat to public health, including mental health, and is widely recognized as a current and accelerating threat to psychological or mental health worldwide (APA, 2017; Clayton, Manning & Hodge, 2014; Clayton, Manning, Krysgman, & Speiser, 2017; Trombley, Chalpuka, & Anderko, 2017; Hayes, Blashki, Wiseman, Burke, & Reifels, 2018). Mental health includes emotional, psychological, behavioral, and social well-being and extends beyond addressing mental illness, mental problems, and mental health disorders to include states of mental wellness, emotional resilience, and psychosocial wellbeing (Butler et al., 2014; Hayes et al, 2018; WHO, 2017). The American Academy of Nursing identifies mental health as an urgent public health issue and recognizes the significant global impact of climate change on the mental health and well-being of individuals (Liu et al., 2020).

GENERAL TOLL OF CLIMATE CHANGE ON MENTAL HEALTH

The impacts of climate change on mental health can be direct or indirect. Direct impacts include acute effects of exposure to extreme weather disaster events such as floods, extreme heat, tornadoes, hurricanes, and wildfires. Indirect effects are due to more gradual, longer chronic exposures to climate– or weather–related disaster events such as droughts or rising sea levels, increasing average air temperature, vector-borne diseases, poor or unsafe air or water quality, deforestations, economic or food insecurity, and unsafe food (Cianconi et al., 2020; Clayton et al., 2014; Dodgen et al., 2016; Hayes et. al, 2018).

Additionally, the threat of climate change, or secondary exposure, is recognized as a "stressor" and leads to adverse impacts on individuals and populations threatening connections to place and identity (Dodgen et al, 2016). Figure I illustrates how climate change impacts health in the U.S. including mental health.

ACUTE MENTAL HEALTH TOLL OF EXPOSURE TO CLIMATE CHANGE-RELATED DISASTERS

The acute mental health impacts of climate change can be psychological trauma from the immediate exposure to climate change-related disasters, including exposure to flooding, wildfires, hurricanes, tornadoes, and extreme heat events (Berry et al., 2010; Cianconi et al., 2020). All of these climate change-related events are now occurring with greater frequency, severity, and intensity (APA, 2017; IPCC, 2018). Before, during, and after these disaster events potential mental health effects ranging from symptoms of mild anxiety or distress to extreme post-traumatic stress or severe psychological trauma, or exacerbation of underlying mental health conditions may occur (APA, 2017; Cianconi et al., 2020; Dodgen et al, 2016; Clayton et al., 2017).

An Illustration on How Climate Change Impacts Physical, Mental, and Community Health

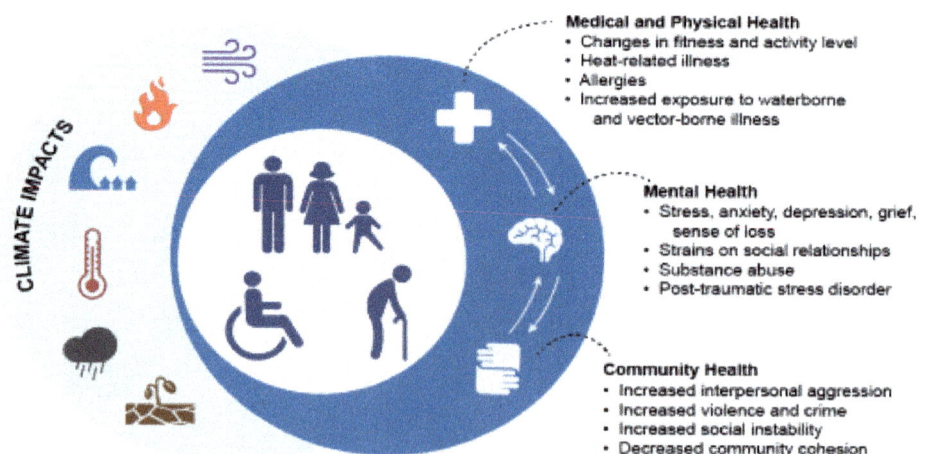

At the center of the diagram are human figures representing adults, children, older adults, and people with disabilities. The left circle depicts climate impacts including air quality, wildfire, sea level rise and storm surge, heat storms, and drought. The right circle shows the three interconnected health domains that will be affected by climate impacts--Medical and Physical Health, Mental Health, and Community Health.

Image source: U.S. Global Change Research Program. 2016. The impacts of Climate Change on Human Health in the United States: A Scientific Assessment.

Figure I: U.S. Global Change Research Program, 2016. The Impacts of Climate Change on Human Health in the United States: A Scientific Assessment. Reproduced as part of the public domain.

Those exposed to life-threatening extreme weather events are more likely to experience acute- and post-traumatic stress disorder (PTSD), depression, and anxiety (Dodgen et al., 2016; Galea, Nandi, & Vlahov, 2005). Impacts may also include somatic disorders, drug and alcohol abuse, higher rates of suicide, complicated grief, and elevated risk of child abuse (Cianconi, et al., 2020; Kessler, et al., 2008; Burke et al., 2018).

Climate disasters may impact individual and population mental health and psychological functioning, and may include strains on social relationships, domestic abuse, mental health emergencies, or may include a sense of loss, hopelessness, fatalism, and resignation, as well as a loss of autonomy and sense of control, and a loss of personal and occupational identity (APA, 2017; Cianconi et al., 2020; Clayton et al., 2014).

Data indicate that 25-50% of people exposed to an extreme weather disaster are at risk of adverse mental health effects. Up to 54% of adults and 45% of children suffer depression after a natural disaster (APA, 2017). There has been high rates of common mental health disorders and increased cases of new-onset mental health conditions among previously healthy individuals and those with pre-existing mental illness following hurricanes (Espinel, Kossin, Galea, Richardson & Schultz, 2019). Almost half (49%) of the survivors of Hurricane Katrina developed an anxiety or mood disorder, 1 in 6 (16.7%) developed PTSD, and suicide and suicidal ideation more than doubled (APHA, nd; Kessler et al., 2008; Lowe et al., 2013). Table 1 identifies those at high risk for adverse mental health outcomes.

Along with exposure to any of these events, several other risk factors for PTSD have been identified and are shown to be important across multiple studies (Galea et al., 2005). Those at risk of PTSD include:

- Women (shown to have a higher prevalence of PTSD after disasters than men)

- Those with preexisting or concurrent psychiatric comorbidity

- Those who have previously experienced traumatic events or substantial stressors

- Low social support has been shown to be a risk factor for PTSD

- Poor coping is a psychological characteristic that emerges as particularly predisposing to post-disaster PTSD (after psychiatric comorbidity has been accounted for)

- The potential role of television viewing as a correlate of post-disaster PTSD (Galea et al. 2005).

Those especially vulnerable to significant mental health impacts following a disaster may need urgent care and can present a significant challenge in an emergency context where pre-existing mental health services may have been destroyed or severely disrupted by the disaster (Fritze, Grant, Blashki, Burke & Wiseman, 2008).

Most individuals who suffer disaster-related psychological impacts from a traumatic event will recover over time (Bonanno, 2004). However, as many as 20% of individuals directly exposed experience chronic dysfunction which may not improve (Dodgen et. al., 2016). Recovery time varies for individuals after direct exposure. A 30% to 60% PTSD prevalence for victims of disasters, 5% to 40% for rescue workers, and 1% to 11% for the general population has been reported (Galea et al., 2005). Women are at greater risk for PTSD, as are individuals who have extreme guilt, anger, external locus of control, impaired coping ability, or a history of trauma. The severity of exposure to a disaster often predicts post-disaster symptoms; young and middle-aged adults are at greater risk for symptoms (Norris, 2002). For example, after Hurricane Andrew in Florida, 38% of children affected likely experienced PTSD at 3 months, with a decline to 18% at 10 months (USGCRP Global Change Research Program, 2016). Multiple risk factors contribute to poor psychological effects including physical injury, death of loved ones, property loss and displacement, among others (USGCRP, 2016). However, in some, positive psychological changes, or post-traumatic growth (PTG), is experienced as the result of successful coping with a traumatic event (USGCRP, 2016).

Consequences for mental health vary by type of extreme event, with unique impacts of specific disaster type and mental health consequences covering a wide range of disorders (Cianconi et.al., 2020). After extreme weather or other natural disaster events, there may be factors that constrain the ability to care for the mental health needs of affected people (Fritze, Blashki, Burke et al., 2008). Constraints may include:

- limitations in service capacity (resources and skills)

- high levels of immediate chaos

- widespread distress,

- and delays before essential services are reestablished (Silove & Steel, 2006).

In the aftermath of a climate change-related disaster the need for mental health services increases, while at the same time disruption in services or a reduced availability and accessibility of health services often occurs. Mental health nurses along with other health professionals are needed to provide evidence-based, trauma-informed, culturally competent care for those suffering from PTSD and other mental health conditions resulting from climate change-related events and exposures (Kameg, 2020; Nichols et al., 2020). Nurses and emergency mental health service professionals need a combination of interventions to meet the mental health needs of a distressed community, as well as the needs of those individuals who are traumatized, and those with severe mental illness (Rao, 2006).

Nurses in the emergency department (ED) should be prepared to address acute mental health trauma and to play a key role in assessment and screening of depression, suicide risk, anxiety, and substance abuse. The use of validated screening tools is important to identify acute mental health impacts from climate change-related events (Nichols et al., 2020). Documented surges in emergency department (ED) visits following climate change-related events require clinician attention to physical trauma as well as to mental health impacts (Sheikhbardisi, 2017; Wald, 2019). Evaluation and assessment, especially of those at increased risk of mental health impacts with careful attention to risk factors associated with specific climate change-related events (i.e.: those on psychiatric medications or those who are unhoused are at high risk during heat waves) are important. Additional education for clinicians may be necessary to ensure disaster planning and mental health care are addressed (Nichols et al., 2020; Veneema et al., 2017).

Surges in mental health-related visits to the ED following various types of climate change-related disasters are documented in both the acute and longer-term phases of these events (Nichols et al., 2020). Nurses in the ED should also be prepared to offer referrals for patients to appropriate community resources and mental health professionals (Nichols et al., 2020). In the public health arena, nurses can assist individuals and the community with disaster planning and preparedness and help them prepare for mental health treatment beyond the disaster area should it be necessary (Veneema et al., 2017).

GRADUAL, LONGER-TERM CLIMATE CHANGE EFFECTS IMPACT ON MENTAL HEALTH

More gradual, chronic, and long-term mental climate change-related exposures of excessive heat or air temperatures due to rising environmental deforestation, droughts, or rising sea levels may be similar or may differ from consequences related to acute, direct exposures (Cianconi et al., 2020; Clayton, et. al., 2014; Clayton, et. al,

2017). Wildfires may cause polluted air or contaminated water from erosion (Dodgen, et. al., 2016). Flooding from sea level rise due to melting glaciers can cause adverse environmental conditions impacting mental and physical health. Coastal erosion due to increasing floods may cause fears of relocation or forced migration (Cianconi, 2020). Long droughts have been associated with elevated levels of anxiety, depression and suicide, and post-traumatic stress disorders (Dodgen, et. al., 2016). After a record drought in the 1980s, the suicide rate doubled, including more than 900 farmers in the Upper Midwest (APHA, nd).

Effects on physical health may occur and indirectly impact mental health: increased heat stress, physical injury, or disease may impact mental wellbeing. Food supply disruptions, food insecurity or water insecurity, or unsafe food or water supply affect individual and community wellbeing with economic damage that can affect the social fabric of communities (Berry et al., 2010). Major upheaval may disrupt social, economic, and environmental factors that promote mental health at the community level (Fritze, 2008). Also, economic insecurity and economic crisis may lead to an increase in suicide rates and other mental health disorders especially among working men. Strong correlations of economic and climatic variables with suicide were found in Europe with higher male (62.4%) vs. female (41.7%) suicide variability among men (Fountoulakis et al., 2016).

Recovery and the severity and distribution of mental health problems may be influenced by aspects of community—resources, cohesion, resilience, and external supports. The term resilience is frequently used in climate change response and can be defined as the ability of a person (or a community) to cope with, grow through, and transcend adversity (Hobfoll et al., 2015). With strong community support, communities appear to fare better than where less support is available. This suggests the importance of investing in community social ties to enhance resilience and improve mental health outcomes for communities affected by climate change (Berry, 2018; Cloverdale et al., 2018). Planned relocation, risk communication, violence prevention, public health education, individual and collective participation in environmental activism, advocacy, and conservation are some of the approaches associated with positive psychological outcomes. Also, some anxiety, worry, or concern about climate change can be adaptive. Taking pro-environmental actions and engaging in activism and advocacy may support mental health and serve as effective mental health interventions (Verplanken & Roy, 2013).

Impact of Higher Average Air Temperatures and Prolonged Extreme Heat

There is evidence regarding the impact of rising temperature on suicidality. Suicide rates increase during extreme heat. In Finland, suicide rates were found to be positively correlated with temperatures (based on historical records from 1751 to 1990), when a national suicide prevention program was put into place (Helama et al., 2013). Suicide rates were found to increase by 0.7%, and by 2.1% in Mexico, for every 1°C increase in average monthly temperature over a period of decades (Espinal et al., 2019). If there is no reduction in greenhouse gas emissions and temperatures continue to increase, climate change may cause between 9,000 and 40,000 additional suicides by 2050 in the US and Mexico (Espinal et al., 2019). Analysis of social media communications also indicates that depressive language and suicidal thought was correlated with increased temperatures suggesting a decline in mental well-being. Evidence also links extreme heat to aggressive behavior or violence, including homicides. Hsiang and colleagues found an increase in the likelihood of interpersonal violence of 4%, and of 14% in group violence, occurs with a temperature increase of one standard deviation (Hsiang et al., 2013). By 2050, projections of 2°C to 4°C of warming in locations worldwide may impact these behaviors, with higher rates of human conflict possible. Even higher possible temperatures, of up to 10°C increases in urban areas due the urban heat island effect, may contribute to a rise of summer violence in urban communities (Hsiang et al., 2013; Burke et. al., 2018).

Normal sleep onset and maintenance are triggered by a drop in core body temperature. Sleep is an essential function for overall well-being and for mental health with negative impacts of poor sleep on mood, depression, and cognition. Increased heat contributes to insomnia and sleep disturbances potentially aggravating many psychiatric problems and reducing coping abilities (Obradovich et al., 2017). Those in urban areas without access to air-conditioning or cool places when heat is trapped by high night-time temperatures, sleep disturbances may occur (Obradovich et al., 2017).

Table 1: Vulnerable Populations at Higher Risk or Adverse Mental Health Outcomes Due to Exposure to Climate- or Weather-Related Disasters*

Vulnerable Population*	General Risk	Specific Mental Health Risk(s)
Children	At particular risk for distress, anxiety, and other adverse mental health effects in the aftermath of an extreme event	Significantly more children than adults have shown continued PTSD symptoms more than two years post-disaster, and, in general, children are more likely to be impaired by a disaster with possible adverse childhood experiences (ACEs)
Emergency Workers & First-Responders	Increased risk for mental health consequences including substance abuse	PTSD rates have ranged from 13% to 18% up to 4 years after large scale response events; impact of more frequent and intense events increase stress and vulnerability
Women, Pregnant Women & Post-partum Mothers	Women have higher PTSD rates and other mental health conditions after disasters than men	Higher rates of domestic abuse after a disaster Access to clean air and water threaten health and nutrition may affect coping ability and health of pregnancy
Economically Disadvantaged	Disproportionately experience the most negative impacts	More fragmented overall health, lower mobility, reduced health care access, economic limitations for recovery
People Who Are Homeless	High rates of mental illness	Increased risk for PTSD Vulnerable to vector-borne illness Increased vulnerability to extreme heat due to isolation and care deficits
Older Adults	Increased risk due to physical and cognitive vulnerability and depression	Greater challenges facing trauma
Individuals with Pre-existing or Prior Mental Illness	Disruption of behavioral health services Threats of psychological trauma	Those on psychiatric medications that interfere with temperature regulation are particularly vulnerable to extreme heat
Other at-risk groups: Farmers, immigrants, indigenous people, & veterans	Lack of access to care and social connections, language and cultural barriers	Difficulty identifying mental health problems and limited access to care.

* Based on data from Dodgen, Donato, Kelly, La Greca, Morganstein, Reser & Ruzek, et. al (2016) Ch. 8: Mental health and well-being. The impacts of climate change on human health in the United States: A scientific assessment., U.S. Global Change Research Program, Washington, DC, 217–246. doi:10.7930/J0TX3C9H.
**Also, farmers, those with limited mobility, immigrants, those living in coastal areas, those from Indigenous communities or tribes and veterans are also expected to experience higher risk of poor mental health outcomes

Those with severe psychotic disorders or mental illnesses, substance abuse disorders, or cognitive impairments including dementias, may be challenged during extreme heat. Psychiatric patients and the unhoused are particularly vulnerable to the physical effects of heat events. Preexisting mental illness alone raises the risk of mortality during extreme heat events between two- and three- fold (Cooper, 2000). Those with mental illness may have diminished judgment or have less ability to care for themselves and are therefore more likely to experience heat stroke and other heat-related morbidity or mortality. Extreme heat can affect behavior and psychiatric conditions leading to feelings of agitation or listlessness. People with schizophrenia may have underlying impairments in thermoregulation, intrinsic to the disease, as indicated by many psychotic patients who wear multiple clothing layers on hot days. Also, some psychiatric medications including antipsychotics, anticholinergic antidepressants have the potential to impair the body's heat regulatory functioning; sweating and dehydration can increase lithium levels, putting patients at greater risk for dangerous toxicity during heat waves (Martin-Latry et al., 2007). Longer and more severe heat waves associated with climate change are likely to be associated with increasing mortality, homicide, suicide, physical assault, and spousal abuse (Anderson, 2001; Basu & Samet, 2002; Qi et al., 2009).

Public health nurses should plan preventive measures for the protection of vulnerable populations prior to, during, and immediately after extreme heat events including availability of cooling centers and warning systems (Ciancino, 2020; Wald, 2019). Emergency departments should prepare for surge in visit volume (Wald, 2019) and increased inpatient mental health service use, self-injurious behavior, and suicidality (Kameg, 2020).

At-Risk Individuals, Vulnerable Populations, and Climate Change Inequity

Mental illness and substance abuse disorders are high among those who are most vulnerable to the effects of extreme heat and other climate change-related events. Poverty, substandard housing, and lack of access to cool environments all contribute to increased vulnerability. Unhoused mentally ill people have little control over their environments, limited ability to protect themselves from heat exposures, and therefore they are at among the most vulnerable to mental health problems.

The burden of climate change is also expected to fall disproportionately on the poor, children, the older adults, women (especially pregnant people), and first responders. Thus, climate change is likely to widen health disparities of people already suffering from inequities such as poor health, poverty, lack of housing, mental illness, and food insecurity. The disproportionate effects on those of less economic privilege or lower social status therefore have social justice implications (Dodgen et. al, 2016; Doherty & Clayton, 2011).

Climate Displacement and Migration

According to the United Nations High Commissioner for Refugees (UNHCR) population migration linked to climate change is already happening. They report that each year since 2008, an average of over 20 million people have been forced to move because of weather-related events, such as floods, storms, wildfires or extreme temperatures (UNHCR, https://www.unhcr.org/en-us/climate-change-and-disasters.html). Many others leave their homes because of slower or more gradual events, such as droughts, rising sea level, or coastal erosion. In areas ravaged by heat waves, long-term drought, rising sea levels, eroding coastlines, with food insecurity due to insufficient agricultural production or loss of other food sources, or increased levels of poverty and interpersonal conflict and violence is leading to a humanitarian crisis. The only option may be to flee. People exposed to these various types of climate change-related problems are forced to adapt their homes or communities to make them habitable or to leave their homes or communities, forcing them to migrate (UNHCR). The terms climigration and climigrant were coined by Bronen (http://www.climigration.org/) to refer specifically to this type of migration to replace misuse of the term "refugee." According to the UNHCR (https://www.unhcr.org/en-us/climate-change-and-disasters.html) while "climate refugee" is often used in the media and by others, this phrase does not exist in international law. Per the UNHCR, a "refugee" is defined as a person who has crossed an international border "owing to well-founded fear of being persecuted for reasons of race, religion, nationality, membership of a particular social group or political opinion." Climate change affects people inside their own countries, and typically creates internal displacement before it reaches a level where it displaces people across borders. The term "climate refugee" is not endorsed by UNHCR, making it more accurate to refer to "persons displaced in the context of disasters and climate change" (UNHCR).

Displacement or migration as a response to climate change adaptation poses considerable mental health threats. Leaving home and often all belongings as a "climigrant" may lead to a range of mental health problems: depression, anxiety, PTSD, substance abuse, and interpersonal violence. Most vulnerable are the poor, the old, the young, women, those with pre-existing mental health conditions, and those with less education. Negative mental health effects are linked with this climate change-related migration due to disrupted community ties, potential exacerbation of conflict and political instability (Torres & Casey, 2017). For example, those exposed to sea level rise and coastal erosion are more likely to experience anxiety and interpersonal conflict with others in their community (Torres & Casey, 2017).

Nurses must become part of the voice at national and international levels to address the needs of people who are forced to migrate due to climate change. Nurses must advocate urgently for their immediate safety and health needs and for the resources to be available to support communities following migration. Availability of support and economic opportunities in receiving countries are linked to better mental health outcomes for newly arrived communities (Porter & Haslam, 2005).

THREAT OF CLIMATE CHANGE: AWARENESS OF CLIMATE CHANGE IMPACTS MENTAL WELLBEING

There may be subtle, indirect effects of climate change that may influence mental health in varying degrees. For some people, the accumulated effects of multiple stressors may mean the difference between a person being mentally healthy or becoming mentally ill (USGCRP, 2016). Of late, terminology has emerged to describe specific mental health effects of climate change threats as relates to mental health (Cianconi et al., 2020).

Eco-Anxiety

In 2017, the American Psychological Association (APA) urged recognition of the term "eco-anxiety" as a genuine source of mental distress; it is considered an existential anxiety related to concerns about the enormous impacts of climate change or "a chronic fear of environmental doom" (APA, 2017). There is now recognition that climate change awareness and media coverage of climate change impacts can cause and intensify stress and anxiety, adversely affecting mental health (APA, 2017). Descriptions of climate change events in the news and other media can influence a person's stress response and mental well-being (Hayes, et al., 2018). Even without any direct exposure to the effects of climate change there is a growing number of people of all ages and across many geographic areas of the world who are suffering negative mental health effects from the threat posed by climate change. According to a national survey conducted in 2018, almost 70% of people in the United States are worried about climate change, with 51% reporting they feel "helpless" (Leiserowitz et al., 2018). As awareness of the impact and potential harm and future risk from climate change has increased, there is growing anxiety and fear related to the uncertainty it creates. Young people are

especially vulnerable. A survey of Australian children reported that 25% feared that the world would end before they got older (Tucci et al., 2007). A recent survey of youth living in the United States found that over 70% believe climate change will be harmful to people in their generation. About 57% of those interviewed reported that climate change makes them feel afraid (Palinkas, 2019). As a result of eco-anxiety, people are becoming anxious about their future and the future of the planet as we currently know it.

Climate or eco-anxiety is not considered pathologic or a clinical anxiety disorder, rather it is viewed as a reasonable and healthy response to an existential threat (Cunsolo & Ellis, 2018) or "a constructive and adaptive response to a serious problem" (Verplanken & Roy, 2013, p. 4). However, while many may continue to function normally despite fear or anxiety about climate change, this anxiety is associated with reduced or threatened mental health (Castelloe, 2018; Pihkala, 2018). Panic attacks, insomnia, obsessive thinking, and/or appetite changes caused by environmental concerns have been self-reported (Castelloe, 2018). While some people are driven to act others may become overwhelmed and anxious and for some individuals, intense anxiety or panic render them unable to act (Usher et al., 2019). This "eco-paralysis" or becoming so distressed they are unable to act, can be misinterpreted as apathy or lack of concern (Albrecht, 2011). Significant psychiatric morbidity may be produced by climate change in the form of eco-anxieties. Ecopsychology has emerged as a field focused on treatment of eco-anxieties (Cianconi et al., 2020).

To manage eco-anxieties, the American Psychiatric Association offers recommendations for building individual self-resiliency:

- Fostering caring, trusting relationships that provide support and encouragement

- Not viewing problems as unsolvable

- Making achievable goals and moving steadily toward them

- Looking at problems in a wider context

- Practicing good self-care and focusing on a positive self-image

- Keeping personal connections with places and cultural ties when possible

- Avoiding isolation and trying to connect with like-minded people (APA, 2017).

Solastalgia or Eco-Angst: Sense of Loss of Place

Some people experience a sense of loss or distress as climate change permanently effects the landscapes where they live, imposing a mental health burden. Land destruction may weaken or eliminate the feeling of belonging and comfort gained from a sense of connectedness. Solastalgia is the distressing feeling of losing a valued natural place or environment that is important (Albrecht, 2005). The phenomenon of solastalgia may be experienced or characterized by a sense of desolation and loss experienced by people suddenly forced to migrate from their home environment or may be more gradual when it is due to slower onset of changes in the local environment. Eco-angst refers to the sense of distress people experience when valued natural environments are negatively transformed (Goleman, 2009; Albrecht, Sartore, Connor, Higginbotham, Freeman, et al., 2007).

Eco-grief: Loss of Connection to Nature and to Nature's Mental Health Benefits

There is evidence that contact with natural environments can improve mental health, function, and offer rehabilitative benefits (Bowler et al., 2010; Seymour, 2016) and further research is exploring these connections (Frumkin, 2017). The biophilia hypothesis suggests that humans have an innate desire for connection with the natural world and derive important psychological and well-being benefits from this connection (Wilson, 1984). However, climate change-related adverse environmental impacts are disrupting this connection. As a result, there are growing feelings of loss from changes to personally significant places including one's home, community, natural habitats, and precious ecosystems. This phenomenon is known as "ecological grief" (Cunsolo & Ellis, 2018). Witnessing degradation of the natural environment may lead to strong grief responses (Gordon, Radford, & Simpson, 2019). "Nature deficit disorder" a term credited to Louv (2005) similarly refers to the lack of connection with the natural world in an increasingly technologic and indoor word, particularly in children. Although it is not an official "diagnosis" it is a label used to convey the impact on children as they are increasingly deprived direct contact with nature during outdoor play (Driessnack, 2009). Nature deficit disorder is related to rates of youth obesity rates, attention-deficit disorder, as well as impaired social skills including increased violence. As well as alterations in mental health such as depression (Driessnack, 2009). Mental health nurses have a key role to play in reducing and responding to the distress related to climate change as they counsel and serve as role models for their patients and colleagues (Usher, Durkin, & Bhullar, (2019).

ADDRESSING MENTAL HEALTH IMPACTS IN NURSING PRACTICE, EDUCATION AND POLICY

Nursing leadership across the care spectrum is an important part of the emergency and ongoing response to climate change impacts (Espinel, 2019). Nurses, along with psychiatric nurse practitioners, working with other mental health and health professionals are needed to address the growing threat of climate change to mental health and wellbeing. It is anticipated that many individuals and communities will need help to build resilience, foster optimism, cultivate active coping, increase preparedness, and support social connections. Disaster events increase the need for a range of mental health services especially among vulnerable populations. There is a critical role for nurses to take preventive action and collaborate with public health, community, and emergency-preparedness partners to reduce population vulnerability, and to support people whose mental health has been affected by climate change impacts. There are crucial roles in education for preparedness and planning for possible disaster impacts as well as for prevention and interventions for those who develop or exacerbate mental health disorders (Veneema et al., 2019). Nurses can help individuals and communities build resilience for optimal recovery.

Nurse educators must incorporate mental health impacts of climate change into the curriculum to ensure future nurses are equipped to care for and advocate for patients and are trained to counsel them to further the response to climate change for individual and collective mental health (McDermott-Levy et al., 2018). Faculty in colleges of nursing and other nursing programs can participate in the Nurses Climate Challenge (https://nursesclimatechallenge.org/) and commit to leadership in integrating climate change content into the nursing curriculum.

In addition, an expert panel of national nursing education experts have developed consensus recommendations for the advancement of disaster nursing education in the United States. National nurse readiness for disasters related to climate change, human conflict, and emerging infectious diseases triggering an ever-increasing number of disaster events is envisioned. Thus, a global nursing workforce prepared with the knowledge, skills, and abilities to respond to any disaster or large-scale public health emergency in a timely and appropriate manner is needed. The panel offers a strong mandate and specific action steps for the advancement of disaster nursing education in the nation (Veneema et al., 2017).

Similarly, a policy brief by the Environmental and Public Health Expert Panel of the American Academy of Nursing addresses the importance of the essential role of nurses in reducing health impacts due to climate change and outlines dual policy recommendations for nurses (Leffers & Butterfield, 2018). Upstream policy recommendations include reducing pollution, building resilient communities, and increasing the public's understanding of the connection between health and climate health. Downstream policies focus on climate adaptation, disaster response, and the importance of preparing the nursing workforce to address the health consequences of climate change (Leffers & Butterfield, 2018). An emphasis on both adaptation and prevention with urgency in advancing mental health awareness in the context of climate change are the stated position of the American Academy of Nursing (Liu, et al., 2020).

Nurses have a professional and moral obligation to educate patients and populations to support individual action and policies to address climate change. Efforts to reduce greenhouse gas emissions, to advocate for efforts and policies to limit pollution and protect the environment, and taking personal action are important actions. Participation by nurses in the Nurses Drawdown (https://www.nursesdrawdown.org/) is an option for obtaining expertise, resources, and tools to empower nurses, patients, and communities. This initiative aims to support nurses to lead and engage in policy change and civil action to tackle negative climate change impacts on overall health, mental health, and wellbeing.

MENTAL HEALTH RESOURCES ON CLIMATE CHANGE IMPACTS

Videos

- Climate Change and Mental Health, Harvard T.H. Chan School of Public Health (2017) (9:56) https://www.youtube.com/watch?v=eUl2YkBTPnY

- Eco-Anxiety in Kids: Expert Weighs in (6:10) https://www.youtube.com/watch?v=GXtBaDDbm4E

- How Climate Impacts Mental Health (Solastgia explained) (3:12 minutes) https://www.youtube.com/watch?v=tXsrla5UnHo

- How Your Mental Health is Impacted by Climate Change (9:25 minutes) https://www.youtube.com/watch?v=CK_GUFr8r6M

- Sundarbans: The Next Climate Refugees, The Atlantic (9:44) https://www.youtube.com/watch?v=m0xD4lg2Vmg

Webinars

- Mental Health and Our Changing Climate: Impacts, Implications, and Guidance (March 29, 2017) (1:00.29) https://ecoamerica.org/research/#mentalhealth

PDFs/Links

- 101 Things You Can Do to Help Address Climate Change https://www.psychology.org.au/getmedia/2a2156ab-559c-4316-888a-a8cd82fcb780/101-things-you-can-do-climate-change_1.pdf

- Climate Psychology Alliance https://www.climatepsychologyalliance.org/

- Ecoanxious Stories https://www.ecoanxious.ca/

- Disaster Preparedness, Response, and Recovery https://www.samhsa.gov/disaster-preparedness

- Good Grief Network https://www.goodgriefnetwork.org/

- Making the Connection: Climate Changes Mental Health https://www.apha.org/~/media/files/pdf/topics/climate/climate_changes_mental_health.ashx

- Mental Health and Our Changing Climate: Impacts, Implications, and Guidance March 2017 https://www.apa.org/news/press/releases/2017/03/mental-health-climate.pdf

- Nurses Drawdown https://www.nursesdrawdown.org/

- Nurses Climate Challenge https://nursesclimatechallenge.org/

- U.S. Climate Resilience Toolkit

  - Steps to Resilience https://toolkit.climate.gov/#steps

  - Climigration toolkit.climate.gov/tool/climigration

Climate Change and Mental Health Position Statements

- American Psychiatric Association: Position statement on the impact of climate change on mental health and psychological well-being www.psychiatry.org

- American Psychological Association. Resolution on affirming psychologists' role in addressing global climate change www.apa.org

REFERENCES

American Psychiatric Association (2017). *Position statement.* https://www.psychiatry.org/patientsfamilies/climate-change-and-mental-health-connections/affects-on-mental-health

Albrecht, G., Sartore, G. M., Connor, L., Higginbotham, N., Freeman, S., Kelly, B., Tonna, H. S., & Pollard, G. (2007). Solastalgia: The distress caused by environmental change. *Australasian Psychiatry, 15*(S1), 95–98

Albrecht, G. (2011). Chronic environmental change and mental health. In *Climate Change and Human Well-Being: Global Challenges and Opportunities*, Weissbecker, I. (ed). Berlin: Springer SBM, 43–56.

Anderson, C. A. (2001). Heat and violence. *Current Directions in Psychological Science, 10*(1), 33-38.

American Public Health Association (APHA). (n.d.) *Making the connection: Climate changes mental health.* https://www.apha.org/~/media/files/pdf/topics/climate/climate_changes_mental_health.ashx

Basu, R., & Samet, J. M. (2002). Relation between elevated ambient temperature and mortality: A review of the epidemiologic evidence. *Epidemiologic Reviews, 24*(2), 90–202, https://doi.org/10.1093/epirev/mxf007

Berry, H .L., Bowen, K. & Kjellstrom, T. (2010). Climate change and mental health: A causal pathways framework. *International Journal of Public Health, 55*(2), 23–132. doi: 10.1007/s00038-009-0112-0.

Berry, H. L., Waite, T. D., Dear, K. B., Capon, A. G., & Murray, V. (2018) The case for systems thinking about climate change and mental health. *Nature Climate Change.* doi:10.1038/s41558-018-0102-4

Bonanno, G. A. (2004). Loss, trauma, and human resilience: Have we underestimated the human capacity to thrive after extremely aversive events? *American Psychologist, 59,* 20-28. http://dx.doi.org/10.1037/0003-066x.59.1.20

Bourque, F., & Cunsolo, W. A. (2014) Climate change: The next challenge for public mental health? International *Reviews in Psychiatry, 26,*415–422

Bowler, D. E., Buyung-Ali, L. M., Knight, T. M. & Pullin, A. B. (2010). A systematic review of evidence for the added benefits to health of exposure to natural environments. *BMC Public Health, 10,* 456.

Butler, C. D., Bowles D. C., McIver L, & Page L. (2014). Mental health, cognition and the challenge of climate change. *Climate Change Global Health, 26,* 251.

Burke, M., González, F., Baylis, P., Heft-Neal, S., Baysan, C., Basu, S., & Hsiang, S. (2018). Higher temperatures increase suicide rates in the United States and Mexico. *Nature Climate Change, 8*(8), 723-729. doi:10.1038/s41558-018-0222-x

Castelloe, M. (2018). *Coming to terms with ecoanxiety; Growing awareness of climate change.* Psychology Today. https://www.psychologytoday.com/au/blog/the-me-in-we/201801/coming-terms-ecoanxiety

Cianconi, P., Betrò, S., & Janiri, L. (2020). The impact of climate change on mental health: A systematic descriptive review. *Frontiers in Psychiatry, 11,* 74. https://doi.org/10.3389/fpsyt.2020.00074

Clayton, S., Manning, C. M., & Hodge C. (2014). *Beyond storms & droughts: The psychological impacts of climate change.* American Psychological Association & ecoAmerica.

Clayton, S., Manning, C. M., Krygsman, K., & Speiser, M. (2017). *Mental health and our changing climate: Impacts, implications, and guidance.* American Psychological Association & ecoAmerica.

Coverdale, J., Balon, R., Beresin, E. V., Brenner, A. M., Guerrero, A. P., Louie, A. K., & Roberts, L. W. (2018). Climate change: a call to action for the psychiatric profession. *Academic Psychiatry, 42,* 317-323. https://doi.org/10.1007/s40596-018-0885-7

Cook, C., Demorest, S. L., Schenk, E. Nurses and climate action. (2019). *AJN The American Journal of Nursing, 119*(4), 54-60.

Cooper, R. (2000). *Impacts of extreme heat on mental health.* Psychiatric Times.https://www.psychiatrictimes.com/climate-change/impacts-extreme-heat-mental-health

Crimmins, A., Balbus, J.L., Gamble, C.B., Beard, J.E., Bell, D., & Dodgen, R.J., et. al. (2016). *The impacts of climate change on human health in the United States: A scientific assessment.* Eds. U.S. Global Change Research Program. http://dx.doi.org/10.7930/J0R49NQX

Cunsolo A. & Ellis, N. (2018). Ecological grief as a mental health response to climate change-related loss. *Nature and Climate Change, 8,* pp. 275-281.

Dougherty, T. J. & Clayton, S. (2011). The psychological impacts of global climate change. *American Psychologist, 66*(4), 265–276.

Dodgen, D., D. Donato, N. Kelly, A., La Greca, J. Morganstein, J., & Reser, J., et. al (2016). Ch. 8: Mental health and well-being. In *The impacts of climate change on human health in the United States: A scientific assessment.* U.S. Global Change Research Program, pp. 217–246. doi:10.7930/J0TX3C9H.

Driessnack, M. (2009). Children and nature-deficit disorder. *Journal for Specialists in Pediatric Nursing, 14*(1), 73-5.

Espinel, Z., Kossin, J. P., Galea, S. Richardson, A. S., & Schultz, J.M. (2019). Forecast: Increasing mental health consequences from Atlantic hurricanes throughout the 21st century. *Psychiatric Services, 70*(12), 1165-67. Doi 10.1176/appi.ps.201900273

Fountoulakis, K.N., Chatzikosta, I., Pastiadis, K. et al. (2016). Relationship of suicide rates with climate and economic variables in Europe during 2000–2012. *Annals of General Psychiatry, 15*, 19.

Friedli, L. (2009). *Mental health, resilience and inequalities.* World Health Organization. http://www.euro.int/_data/assets/pdf_file/0012/100821/E92227.pdf

Fritze, J. G., Blashki, G. A., Burke, S., & Wiseman, J. (2008). Hope, despair and transformation: Climate change and the promotion of mental health and wellbeing. *International Journal of Mental Health Systems 2*, 13 https://doi.org/10.1186/1752-4458-2-13

Frumkin, H., Bratman, G. N., Breslow, S. J., Cochran, B., Kahn Jr, P. H., Lawler, J. J., ... & Wood, S. A. (2017). Nature contact and human health: A research agenda. *Environmental Health Perspectives, 125*(7), 075001. https://doi.org/10.1289/EHP1663

Galea, S., Nandi, A., & Vlahov, D. (2005). The epidemiology of post-traumatic stress disorder after disasters. *Epidemiologic Reviews, 27,* (1), 78–91, https://doi.org/10.1093/epirev/mxi003

Gordon, T. A. C. Radford, A. N., & Simpson, S. D. (2019). Grieving environmental scientists need support. *Science. 366*, 6462. 193. doi: 10.1126/science.aaz2422

Goleman, D. (2009, September 27). *The age of eco-angst.* New York Times. https://opinionator.blogs.nytimes.com/2009/09/27/the-age-of-eco-angst/?mcubz=1.

Gordon, T. A., Radford, A. N., & Simpson, S. D. (2019). Grieving scientists need support. *Science, 366*, 193.

Hayes, K., Blashki, G., Wiseman, J., Burke, S., & Reifels, L. (2018). Climate change and mental health: risks, impacts and priority actions. *International Journal of Mental Health Systems, 12*(28). doi:10.1186/s13033-018-0210-6

Helama, S., Holopainen, J., Partonen, T. (2013). Temperature-associated suicide mortality: Contrasting roles of climatic warming and the suicide prevention program in Finland. *Environmental Health Preventive Medicine, 18*, 349-355.

Hobfoll, S. E., Stevens, N. R., & Zalta, A. K. (2015). Expanding the science of resilience: Conserving resources in the aid of adaptation. *Psychological inquiry, 26*(2), 174–180. https://doi.org/10.1080/1047840X.2015.1002377

Hsiang, S., Burke, M., & Miguel, E. (2013). Quantifying the influence of climate on human conflict. *Science, 13*, 341:1235367.

Intergovernmental Panel on Climate Change. (2018). *Summary for policymakers of IPCC Special Report on Global Warming of 1.5°C approved by governments.* https://www.ipcc.ch/2018/10/08/summary-for-policymakers-of-ipcc-special-report-on-global-warming-of-1-5c-approved-by-governments/https://www.ipcc.ch/2018/10/08/summary-for-policymakers-of-ipcc-special-report-on-global-warming-of-1-5c-approved-by-governments/

Intergovernmental Panel on Climate Change. (2014). *Climate Change 2014: Synthesis Report, Summary for Policymakers. Contribution of Working Groups I, II and III to the Fifth Assessment Report of the Intergovernmental panel on Climate Change.* Core Working Team. Pachauri, R. K. & Meyer, L. A. (Eds). IPCC.

Kameg, B.N. (2020). Climate change and mental health: Implications for nurses. *Journal of Psychosocial Nursing, 58*(9), 25-30.

Kessler, R. C., Galea, S., Gruber, M. J., Sampson, N. A., Ursano, R. J., & Wessely, S. (2008). Trends in mental illness and suicidality after Hurricane Katrina. *Molecular Psychiatry, 13*(4), 374–384. https://doi.org/10.1038/sj.mp.4002119

Leffers, J. & Butterfield, P. (2018). Nurses play essential roles in reducing health problems due to climate change. *Nursing Outlook, 66*(2), 210-213.

Leiserowitz, A., Maibach, E., Rosenthal, S., Kotcher, J., Ballew, M., Goldberg, M., & Gustafson, A. (2018). *Climate change in the American mind: December 2018. Yale University and George Mason University.* Yale Program on Climate Change Communication.

Liu, J., Potter, T., & Zahner, S. (2020). Policy brief on climate change and mental health/well-being. *Nursing Outlook, 68*, 517-522.

Louv, R. (2005). *Last child in the woods: Saving our children from nature-deficit disorder.* Algonquin Books.

Lowe, S. R., Manove, E. E., & Rhodes, J. E. (2013). Posttraumatic stress and posttraumatic growth among low-income mothers who survived Hurricane Katrina. *Journal of Consulting and Clinical Psychology, 81*(5), 877–889. https://doi.org/10.1037/a0033252

Martin-Latry, K., Goumy, M. P., Latry, P., Gabinski, C., Bégaud, B., Faure, I., & Verdoux, H. (2007). Psychotropic drugs use and risk of heat-related hospitalisation. *European Psychiatry, 22*(6), 335-338.

McDermott-Levy R., Jackman-Murphy K. P., Leffers J. M., & Jordan, L. (2018). Integrating climate change into nursing curricula. *Nurse Educator, 44,* 43–47. doi: 10.1097/NNE.0000000000000525

Nichols, P., Breakey, S., White, B. P., Brown, M. J., Fanuele, J., Starodub, R., & Ros, A. V. (2020). Mental health impacts of climate change: Perspectives of the ED Clinician. *Journal of Emergency Nursing, 46*(5), 590-599.

Nurse, J. Basher, D., & Bone, A. (2010). An ecological approach to promoting population mental health and well-being—A response to the challenge of climate change. *Perspectives in Health, 130*(1), 27-33.

Nurses Climate Challenge. https://nursesclimatechallenge.org/

Nurses Drawdown. https://www.nursesdrawdown.org/

Nobel, J. (2007, April 9). *Eco-anxiety: Something else to worry about* [Electronic version]. The Inquirer. http://www.philly.com.

Norris, F. H. (2002). Psychosocial consequences of disasters. *PTSD Research Quarterly, 3*(2), 1-8.

Obradovich, N., Migliorini, R., Mednick, S., & Fowler, J. H. (2017). Nighttime temperature and human sleep loss in a changing climate. *Science Advances.* https://advances.sciencemag.org/content/3/5/e1601555.

Palinkas, L.A. (2019, December 2). *One of the most overlooked consequences of climate change? Our mental health.* Environmental Health News. https://www.ehn.org/how-climate-change-affects-mental-health-2641458829.html.

Pihkala, P. (2018). Eco-anxiety, tragedy, and hope: Psychological and spiritual dimensions of climate change. *Zygon, 53*(2), 545–569.

Porter, M., & Haslam, N. (2005). Predisplacement and postdisplacement factors associated with mental health of refugees and internally displaced persons: A meta-analysis. *JAMA, 294*(5), 602–612. doi:10.1001/jama.294.5.602

Qi, X., Tong, S., & Hu, W. (2009). Preliminary spatiotemporal analysis of the association between socio-environmental factors and suicide. *Environmental Health, 8,* 46. doi:10.1186/1476-069X-8-46

Rao, K. (2006). Psychosocial support in disaster-affected communities. *International Review of Psychiatry, 18*(6):501-505.

Seymour, V. (2016). The human–nature relationship and its impact on health: A critical review. *Frontiers in Public Health.,4,* 260. doi:10.3389/fpubh.2016.00260

Sheikhbardsiri, H., Raeisi, A., Nekoei-Moghadam, M., & Razaei, F. (2017). Surge capacity of hospitals in emergencies and disasters with a preparedness approach: A systematic review. *Disaster Medicine and Public Health Preparedness, 11*(5), 612-620. doi: 10.1017/dmp,2016.178

Silove D., & Steel Z. (2006). Understanding community psychosocial needs after disasters: Implications for mental health services. *Journal of Postgraduate Medicine, 52,*121-125.

Torres, J. M., & Casey, J. A. (2017). The centrality of social ties to climate migration and mental health. *BMC Public Health, 17,* 600. https://doi.org/10.1186/s12889-017-4508-0

Trombley, J., Chalupka, S. & Anderko, L. (2017). Climate change and mental health. AJN *The American Journal of Nursing, 117*(4), 44-52. doi: 10.1097/01.NAJ.0000515232.51795.fa

UNHCR (n.d.). *Climate change and disaster displacement.* https://www.unhcr.org/en-us/climate-change-and-disasters.html.

Tucci, J., Mitchell, J., and Goddard, C. (2007). *Children's fears, hopes and heroes: Modern childhood in Australia.* Australian Childhood Foundation.

USGCRP (2016). *The impacts of climate change on human health in the United States: A scientific assessment.* Crimmins, A.J., Balbus, J.L., Gamble, C. B., Beard, J.E., Bell, D., Dodgen, R.J., Eisen, N., Fann, M.D., Hawkins, M, S.C., Herring, L., Jantarasami, D.M., Mills, S., Saha, M.C., Sarofim,J. & Ziska, Eds. U.S. Global Change Research Program, Washington, DC, 312 http://dx.doi.org/10.7930/J0R49NQX

USGS.(2006, February). *Fact Sheet 2006-3015. USGS Science Helps Build Safer Communities Wildfire Hazards—A National Threat.* https://pubs.usgs.gov/fs/2006/3015/2006-3015.pdf

Usher, K., Durkin, J. & Bhullar, N. (2019). Eco-Anxiety: How thinking about climate-related environmental decline is affecting our mental health. *International Journal of Mental Health Nursing, 28,* 1233–1234. doi:10.1111/inm.12673

Veenema, T. G., Lavin, R. P., Griffin, A., Gable, A. R., Couig, M. P. & Dobalian, A. (2017). Call to action: The case for advancing disaster nursing education in the United States.

Journal of Nursing Scholarship, 49, 688-696. doi:10.1111/jnu.12338

Verplanken B., & Roy, D. (2013). "My worries are rational, climate change is not": Habitual ecological worrying is an adaptive response. *PLoS ONE, 8*(9), e74708. https://doi.org/10.1371/journal.pone.0074708

Wald, A. (2019). Emergency department visits and costs for heat-related illness due to extreme heat or heat waves in the United States: An integrated review. *Nursing Economic$, 37*(1). 35-48.

Watts, N., Amann, M., Ayeb-Karlsson, S., Belesova, K., Bouley, T., Boykoff, M., ... & Costello, A. (2018). The Lancet Countdown on health and climate change: from 25 years of inaction to a global transformation for public health. *The Lancet, 391*(10120), 581-630.

Watts, N., Amann, M., Arnell, N., Ayeb-Karlsson, S., Belesova, K., Boykoff, M., ... & Montgomery, H. (2019). The 2019 report of The Lancet Countdown on health and climate change: ensuring that the health of a child born today is not defined by a changing climate. *The Lancet, 394*(10211), 1836-1878.

Weir, K. 2016. Climate change is threatening mental health. *Monitor on Psychiatry, 47*(7), 28. https://www.apa.org/monitor/2016/07-08/climate-change

Wilson, E.O. (1984). *Biophilia.* Harvard University Press.

World Health Organization. (1948). *Preamble to the Constitution of the World Health Organization as adopted by the International Health Conference.* New York, pp. 19–22.

World Health Organization. (2017). *Mental health.* http://www.who.int/mental_health/en/

A SYSTEM RESPONSE TO OUR CLIMATE EMERGENCY: INTERPROFESSIONAL EDUCATION

Teddie Potter PhD, RN, FAAN, FNAP
Clinical Professor
Director of Planetary Health
School of Nursing
University of Minnesota

INTRODUCTION

Any nurse who has cared for a patient in multi-system failure knows that the patient's survival depends on the full participation and collaboration of an interprofessional team. The pulmonologist, cardiologist, nephrologist, and skilled intensive care nurse cannot turn the situation around on their own. They must work together, each bringing their own unique knowledge and a commitment to collaborate on behalf of the patient. Complex systems like the human body require systems solutions; likewise, the climate emergency is a system crisis and therefore requires highly effective interprofessional and interdisciplinary collaboration. We cannot restore the health of the planet on our own.

BACKGROUND

If we think of planet Earth as a patient, there is evidence that this "patient" is in multi-system failure. From pollinator collapse, massive biodiversity loss, and ocean acidification, to the growth in population that outpaces our available resources, we are seeing the impact that humans have on the health of the planet. In fact, our impact is so great that this epoch is now known as the Anthropocene (Whitmee, et al., 2015).

One of the most immediate, and serious, "symptoms" of this planetary multi-system failure is climate change or more appropriately, the climate emergency (American Public Health Association, 2019). In fact, the World Health Organization (WHO) recognizes that, "Climate change is the greatest threat to global health in the 21st century" (WHO, n.d.). This climate emergency is a symptom of systemic failure; siloed disciplinary thinking has prevented us from seeing the intricacies of the connected ecosystem that our lives depend on. Our policies have failed to protect population health and our health profession curriculum has failed to prepare professionals for the health impacts of a collapsing planetary ecosystem.

Both the Intergovernmental Panel on Climate and Climate Change (IPCC) report, Global Warming of 1.50 C (2018), and the 4th National Climate Assessment (U.S. Global Change Research Program, 2018) indicate the window to prevent the most catastrophic impacts of climate change is rapidly closing. The enormity and severity of the climate crisis and the direct experience of climate related disasters is leading to increased mental health and wellbeing challenges including post-traumatic stress disorder (Boscarino, Hoffman, Adams, Figley, & Solhkhah, 2014) and eco-anxiety (Albrecht, 2011). These symptoms can be seen in patients, families, and communities and also in the health professionals and first responders who care for people in the midst of a climate related disaster.

One of the antidotes to despair is working on a solution in collaboration with others. In the words of the Planetary Health Alliance (n.d.)

Everything is connected — what we do to the world comes back to affect us, and not always in ways that we would expect. Understanding and acting upon these challenges call for massive collaboration across disciplinary and national boundaries to safeguard our health.

We are connected and our greatest hope for a solution to the climate emergency is interdisciplinary collaboration and partnership-based interprofessional practice.

AN INTERPROFESSIONAL APPROACH TO THE CLIMATE EMERGENCY

In the report, Crossing the Quality Chasm: A New Health System for the 21st Century, the Institute of Medicine (2001) recognized the growing complexity of health challenges and the care system. The report acknowledges, "Cooperation among clinicians is a priority. Clinicians and institutions should actively collaborate and communicate to ensure an appropriate exchange of information and coordination of care" (p. 4). Similarly, interprofessional education and collaborative practice (IPECP) offer the best chance of effectively addressing the complexities of the climate emergency.

The World Health Organization (WHO, 2010) further defines the unique nature of interprofessional collaboration:

Many health workers believe themselves to be practicing collaboratively, simply because they work together with other health workers. In reality, they may simply be working within a group where each individual has agreed to use their own skills to achieve a common goal. Collaboration, however, is not only about agreement and communication, but about creation and synergy. Collaboration occurs when two or more individuals from different backgrounds with complementary skills interact to create a shared understanding that none had previously possessed or could have come to on their own (p. 36).

Solving the climate emergency will require the "shared understanding" that collaboration affords.

But even collaboration needs further refinement. Eisler and Potter (2014), warn that collaboration can exist even in societies and organizations that orient toward hierarchies of domination. What we really want to work toward is networks that orient toward partnership. Key elements of hierarchies of domination include rigid ranking, scarcity thinking, and a high degree of shame, blame, and fear. Whereas, relationships that orient toward partnership are recognizable by members feeling valued and respected; communication flows both ways, instead of only top down; there is a sense of abundance; and leaders employ a "power with" rather than "power over" approach (Eisler & Potter, 2014). Partnership-based interprofessional collaborative practice offers the best model to disrupt some of the old patterns that have created the climate emergency in the first place.

Partnership practice acknowledges that one profession or discipline does not hold all the knowledge that is required to address systemic challenges such as the climate emergency. Partnership practice involves open communication across disciplinary boundaries with particular emphasis on inclusion of groups traditionally ignored or marginalized. In partnership-based networks, members respectfully dialog about possible solutions and do not rank one aspect of the system as being more important than other aspects of the system; i.e. the health of the planet is not superseded by the needs and wants of humans. In a partnership approach fear, shame, and blame are minimized, and in their place, we see hope and possibility. In that possibility is the possibility of a healthy planet and a healthy future for us all.

REFERENCES

Albrecht, G. (2011). Chronic environmental change: Emerging "psychoterratic" syndromes. In I. Weissbecker (Ed.), *Climate change and human well-being: Global challenges and opportunities* (pp. 43–56). Springer.

American Public Health Association. (2019). *Climate change.* https://www.apha.org/topics-and-issues/climate-change

Boscarino, J., Hoffman, S., Adams, R., Figley, C., & Solhkhah, R. (2014). Mental health outcomes among vulnerable residents after Hurricane Sandy. *American Journal of Disaster Medicine, 9,* 107–120.

Eisler, R., & Potter, T. (2014). *Transforming interprofessional partnerships: A new framework for nursing and partnership-based health care.* Sigma Theta Tau International.

Institute of Medicine. (2001). *Crossing the quality chasm: A new health system for the 21st century.* (Report brief). National Academies Press.

Intergovernmental Panel on Climate Change [IPCC]. (2018). *Global warming of 1.50 C.* https://report.ipcc.ch/sr15/pdf/sr15_spm_final.pdf

Planetary Health Alliance. (n.d.). *Our health depends on our environment.* https://planetaryhealthalliance.org/

U.S. Global Change Research Program. (2018). *4th national climate assessment: Volume II- impacts, risks, and adaptation in the United States.* https://nca2018.globalchange.gov/

Whitmee, s., Haines, A., Beyrer, C., Boltz, F., Capon, A., Ferreira de Souza Dias, B. Ezeh, A., Frumkin, H., …Yach, D. (2015). Safeguarding human health in the Anthropocene epoch: Report of the Rockefeller Foundation—Lancet Commission on planetary health. *The Lancet, 386,* 1973-2028.

World Health Organization [WHO]. (n.d.). *WHO calls for urgent action to protect health from climate change.* https://www.who.int/globalchange/global-campaign/cop21/en/

World Health Organization [WHO]. (2010). *Framework for action on interprofessional education and collaborative practice.* Geneva, Switzerland: WHO Press.

EXTREME WEATHER: HEAT STROKE SIMULATION
Kathryn P. Jackman-Murphy, Ed.D, MSN, RN, CHSE
Director, RN/BSN Program
Charter Oak State College

INTRODUCTION

Climate Change and extreme weather events are incidents that nurses need to integrate into their assessment and plan of care for all patients. The use of simulation in nursing education is now common in the preparation for practice and provides opportunities for nursing students and nurses alike to practice providing care for populations and illnesses they may not come in contact on a daily basis. Participants are able to perform skills and actively learn in a standardized manner without risk of harming actual patients. Simulation also provides opportunities for "do overs," where the learner is able to participate in another scenario after debriefing and apply the knowledge learned from the previous experience. Debriefing is an important component to the learning of simulation (Lavoie &. Clarke, 2017). Debriefing questions are provided with simulation scenarios.

The following simulations are for older adult, pregnant, pediatric, and young adult (occupational risk) patients. There are details for the older adult scenario that could be adapted for the other patient populations. The ANHE Education Workgroup would be very interested in sharing any adaptations you have developed.

PATIENT OVERVIEW

Geriatric Patient

Henry Murphy is a 72-year-old African American male with a past medical history which includes COPD, hypertension, and high cholesterol. He is a retired toolmaker who lives in an urban area in a small 3rd floor apartment with his wife Jean.

It has been quite warm over the past few days, with temperatures over 90 degrees with high humidity. The Murphys have limited funds and worry about the cost of running fans and air conditioning throughout the day to cool their apartment. In addition, there have been episodes of "brown-outs" in the Murphy's community. This has limited electricity to their home and the air conditioner does not run during these periods.

Social: Henry and Jean had one son who was killed in an automobile accident 10 years ago. They have a daughter-in-law Sandra, who is a nurse and one grandson, Sam who lives a few hours away. They try to be as involved and supportive to Henry and Jean Murphy as they can.

Henry is concerned about Jean because she is experiencing frequent memory lapses. He has assumed much of the household duties from his wife, such as cooking and cleaning. Henry's strength and endurance is limited due to his COPD. He has had several admissions for COPD exacerbations, and he spends much of his limited energy caring for and watching over his wife.

Henry Murphy Home Medications			
Advair diskus	250mcg/ 50mcg	inh	Q am/pm
Lisinopril	12.5 mg	po	Daily
Lopressor	50 mg	po	Daily
ASA	81 mg	po	Daily
Crestor	20 mg	po	Every evening
Singular	10 mg	po	Every evening

Pregnant patient

Patrice is a 28 year old female (G1-T0-P1-A1-L1) who is in her 8th month of an uncomplicated pregnancy. She began prenatal care as soon as she realized she was pregnant (8 weeks) and has maintained her appointments and medical recommendations (i.e. medications), only missing one appointment in her 5th month.

It has been quite warm over the past few days, with temperatures over 90 degrees with high humidity. Patrice and her husband have a limited income and they worry about the cost of running fans and air conditioning throughout the day as they have so many expenses to prepare for the new baby (i.e. crib, diapers, etc.). Additionally, to conserve energy, the town has had "brown-outs," where electricity has been limited to their home at times.

Patrice has come for a scheduled clinic visit. She walked to the appointment. Patrice tells the nurse that she has been feeling tired and dizzy and has leg cramps. Patrice stated that she must be "getting out of shape, I'm so big."

Social: Patrice lives with her husband in a three-family house, on the second floor, near her health provider's office. Her mother and father live on the first floor, and the 3rd floor is rented to a long-term tenant. She is able to walk to appointments instead of obtaining a ride or paying for a taxi/Uber. She works as an office assistant in a large company in the area and has health insurance coverage for prenatal visits and the delivery of the baby. She lives with her husband, Mark, who is supportive and both are looking forward to meeting their new baby.

Patrice Home Medications			
Prenatal Vitamin	I tablet	po	Q am
Ferrous Sulfate	235 mg	po	Q am

Pediatric Patient

Ryan is a 4-year-old who lives with her parents, Patrice and Mark, in an urban area near the health care provider's office. Their residence is a three-family house. Ryan's family live on the second floor of the house and his grandparents live on the first floor. The third floor is rented to a long-term tenant.

Ryan has not been feeling well over the past few days, complaining of nausea and leg cramps and her parent(s) are concerned about her complaints and take her to be evaluated by the health care provider. Ryan has a history of mild asthma, no hospitalizations, but has occasional wheezing that is treated with a rescue inhaler (Albuterol) as needed. Patrice, Ryan's mother, reports that dust and mold trigger Ryan's asthma.

It has been quite warm over the past few days, with temperatures over 90 degrees with high humidity. The family has limited income and worry about the cost of running fans and air conditioning throughout the day. The city has had periodic "brown-outs," where electricity has been limited to their home at times. During the brown-outs, Ryan's family is unable to use their air conditioner and fans.

Social: Ryan likes to play outside with her friends in the neighborhood. She also goes to the summer program in the neighborhood park. She lives with her parents in an urban area, and her mom is pregnant with her second child. Ryan is looking forward to meeting her new baby brother or sister and starting kindergarten in the next school year.

Ryan Home Medications			
Albuterol 90 mcg	2 puffs with spacer	inhalation	Every 4 hours as needed for wheezing

Young adult (outdoor worker)

Alex is a 19-year-old, working over the summer as a camp counselor at a local park for children in the neighborhood. He presents to the camp's first aid office after complaining of being very dizzy after a spirited softball game — counselors vs. campers. He also is complaining of a headache, abdominal discomfort-some "cramping" and nausea. He denies any medical issues/history and had a physical for college in which no issues were noted. He is accompanied by Pat, another camp counselor, who is concerned about Alex and related that she thinks Alex may have "passed out for a few seconds" and not just dizzy as Alex stated.

Social: Alex is home for the summer from college where he is majoring in theater. He is living on the camp property while camp is in session. His parents live one hour away and are expected shortly.

Alex Home Medications			
None			

SUPPLIES LIST

- Hi Fidelity Simulation with the following parameters
- Vital signs Temp 100.5
- Pulse 102 slightly thready
- RR 24-breath sounds with diffuse mild inspiratory and expiratory wheezing thru-out
- BP 102/50
- O2 Sat 91% R/A
- Spray bottle with water to simulate sweating
- Urinal with 100 mL dark urine

ROLES

- Nurse
- Observer (see checklist)
- Daughter-in-law or grandson
  - You live about 45 minutes away and cannot physically check on them every day, but stay in contact via phone and visit as much as possible.
  - You are very concerned about Henry and his condition. Henry has been tired lately and having difficulty caring for himself and his wife. He's been having difficulty for several weeks and you know he avoided getting care as he is more concerned for his wife, Jean. She is with your family while Henry is in the hospital. Jean seems to be more confused since she has been away from Henry and her home.
  - You are visiting hoping to reassure Henry and be supportive.

	Scenario Progression Outline Henry Murphy			
Time	**Monitor Settings**	**Pt./Manikin (Actions)**	**Student Nurse Interventions (Events)**	**Cue/Prompt**
Begin	Initial State: Patient in the Emergency Room/ Clinic with HOB elevated approx. 45 degrees. VS 100.5-102-24-102/50, O2 91% R/A, sweaty	Use only for Henry "I knew I was in trouble when I was at home, I couldn't breathe…but I didn't want to leave Jean" Henry relates his usual BP is much higher- about 140/80	Nurse(s) enter room, wash hands, introduces self to patient and family member/support person if present, and identifies patient. Obtains vital signs T-100.5-102-24-102/50, O2 91% R/A	Role member providing cue: Family member/support person chats with patient. Discussing how Jean, Henry's wife is doing. Be reassuring that she is doing fine, but anxious to see Henry and doesn't understand why she can't be home.
00:10	100 mL of dark urine at bedside	States he doesn't have pain, but has had leg cramps and a bit of a headache over the past few days, as well as some abdominal discomfort and nausea-so it has been a challenge to eat/ drink	Nurse(s) ask if Henry has any pain Nurses begin assessment Noting poor skin turgor, dry mucous membranes, small amount of dark colored urine Nurses review I and O over past day or so **Nurse assesses for signs of heat-related illness**	
00:15		Patient is a bit irritable, impatient with assessment Discusses that it is hard to drink "enough", he's watching over Jean- making sure she is okay and reminding her to eat and drink	Identifies symptoms of heat-related illness Heat cramps • Heavy sweating • Painful muscle cramps or spasms Heat exhaustion • Heavy sweating • Weakness • Fatigue • Headache • Dizziness • Nausea or vomiting • Fainting • Irritability • Thirst • Decreased urine output Heat stroke • Very high body temperature • Altered mental state • Throbbing headache • Confusion • Nausea • Dizziness • Hot, dry skin or profuse sweating • Unconsciousness	

			Scenario Progression Outline	
			Henry Murphy (Continued)	
Time	**Monitor Settings**	**Pt./Manikin (Actions)**	**Student Nurse Interventions (Events)**	**Cue/Prompt**
		Henry asks what he can do to feel better and not get sick again	**Nurse assesses for risk factors for heat-related illness** • Vulnerable population (elderly) • Urban environment • Physical activity (caring for self and wife) • Limited social network • Age • Historically underrepresented/person of color • No central AC cooler • Living alone • Co-morbidities (HTN, COPD) • Fixed income • Direct exposure to sun **Nurse provides education** • Maintain indoor temperature not higher than 82 degrees • Eating fresh fruits/vegetables (light, easy to digest foods) • Stay hydrated - drinking water or beverages without caffeine, sugar, or alcohol throughout the day • Avoid fats in high humidity • Air conditioning/community centers • Taking cold showers, bath or body wash • Contact with families/others • Rest breaks • Wear protective clothing • Wear loose, light colored clothing • Supply of power • Water/cooling area • Know signs and symptoms of heat stress • Stay out of the sun • Minimize physical activity • Use fans/air conditioners or cooling centers **Nurse collaborates with other health care professionals** • Social Service consult • VNA • Location of calling centers • Possible free transportation to cooling centers	Role member providing cue: Family member/support person chats with patient. Discussing how Jean, Henry's wife is doing. Be reassuring that she is doing fine, but anxious to see Henry and doesn't understand why she can't be home.

OBSERVER CHECKLIST
To be completed by observers and discussed in debriefing

Proposed correct treatment	Performed	Notes/Comments- Be sure to note specifics
Performs hand hygiene		
Introduces self to patient		
Identifies patients with 2 identifiers		
Utilizes therapeutic communication techniques		
Identify non-therapeutic communication techniques		
Completes Vital Signs		
Initiates head to toe assessment		
Performs head to toe assessment		
Modifies plan of care based on interaction sight client i.e. performs focused assessment		
Identifies symptoms of heat-related illness Heat cramps • Heavy sweating • Painful muscle cramps or spasms Heat exhaustion • Heavy sweating • Weakness • Fatigue • Dizziness • Nausea or vomiting • Fainting • Irritability • Thirst • Decreased urine output Heat stroke • Very high body temperature • Altered mental state • Throbbing headache • Confusion • Nausea • Dizziness • Hot, dry skin or profuse sweating • Unconsciousness		

Proposed correct treatment	Performed	Notes/Comments- Be sure to note specifics
Identifies contributing factors to heat stress • Vulnerable population (elderly) • Urban environment • Physical activity (caring for self and wife) • Limited social network age • Historically underrepresented/person of color • No central AC cooler • Living alone • Comorbidities (Htn, COPD) • Fixed income • Direct exposure to sun		
Instructs patient on methods for heat stress prevention • Maintain indoor temperature not higher than 82 degrees • Eating fresh fruits/vegetables (light, easy to digest foods) • Stay hydrated-drinking water or beverages without caffeine, sugar or alcohol throughout the day • Avoid fans in high humidity • Air conditioning/community centers • Taking cold showers, bath or body wash • Contact with families/others • Rest breaks • Wear protective clothing • Wear loose, light-colored clothing • Supply of power • water/cooling area • Knows signs and symptoms of heat stress • Stay out of the sun • Minimize physical activity • Use fans/air conditioners or cooling centers		
Interdisciplinary collaboration • Social Service consult • VNA • Location of cooling centers • Possible free transportation to cooling centers		

DEBRIEFING QUESTIONS
Outcomes:
1. Student(s) will recognize symptoms of heat-related illness and employ proper treatment
2. Student(s) will instruct patient/family regarding strategies to avoid future issues with heat related illness (heat cramps, heat exhaustion, and heat stroke, and death)
3. Student(s) will effectively communicate with patient, their support person, and other team members

POSSIBLE QUESTIONS TO GUIDE DEBRIEFING:
1. What were the priority problem(s) for this patient?

2. What were your goals for this patient?
3. What intervention(s) did you plan for these problems?
4. Were the intervention(s) effective?
5. How did you use effective communication with this patient?
   A. With their family member?
   B. With other members of the team?
6. How did you modify your plan of care based on the interactions and assessments with this patient?
7. What is your evaluation towards the goals you developed for this patient?

8. What would you do differently next time to meet these goals?

REFERENCES

Centers for Disease Control (CDC). (2016) *Climate change and extreme heat: What you can do to prepare.* www.cdc.gov/climateandhealth/pubs/extreme-heat-guidebook.pdf

Gamble, J. L., Hurley, B. J., Schultz, P. A., Jaglom, W. S., Krishnan, N., & Harris, M. (2013). Climate change and older Americans: State of the science. *Environmental Health Perspectives, 121*(1), 15–22. http://doi.org/10.1289/ehp.1205223

Harlan, S. L., Declet-Barreto, J. H., Stefanov, W. L., & Petitti, D. B. (2013). Neighborhood effects on heat deaths: social and environmental predictors of vulnerability in Maricopa County, Arizona. *Environmental Health Perspectives, 121*(2), 197–204. http://doi.org/10.1289/ehp.1104625

Hess, J., Saha, S. & Luber, G. (2014). Summertime acute heat illness in U.S. emergency departments from 2006 through 2010: Analysis of a nationally representative sample. *Environmental Health Perspectives, 122*(11), 1209-1215.

Lavoie, P., & Clark, S. (2017). Simulation in nursing education. *Nursing, 47(7),* 19-20.

Okwuofu-Thomas, B., Beggs, P. J., & MacKenzie, R. J. (2017). INTERNATIONAL PERSPECTIVES: A comparison of heat wave response plans from an aged care facility perspective. *Journal of Environmental Health, 79*(8), 28-37.

Perera, F. (2017). Multiple threats to child health from fossil fuel combustion: Impacts of air pollution and climate change. *Environmental Health Perspectives; 125*(2), 141-148.

CLIMATE CHANGE AND HUMAN MIGRATION
Sheila Stone, MSN, RN, CNE
ANHE Fellow 2019–2020

Nurses address complex, nonstable, and interacting stressors to human systems every day in extremely varied practice settings. Nurses deeply understand that health breakdowns result from interaction of multiple forces that overwhelm system adaptation and resilience. Nurses also know that addressing health crises in isolation, without addressing the interactions of causes and conditions, can result in solutions that are ineffective or even harmful (Neuman & Fawcett, 2002). The intersection of climate change, human migration, and human health is one such complex issue. It is increasing in importance, and aspects of it will become part of every nurse's practice. This section is intended to provide context, background, and resources for nurses to understand and apply nursing knowledge and skills for the benefit of our patients on multiple levels.

Climate-related migration has been part of the human story since the beginning of the species, and this is reflected in religious, mythological, and archaeological records (DeMenocal & Stringer, 2016). In modern times, climate change has become a leading cause of human migration (Benko, 2017, Burkett, 2009; Climate and Migration Coalition 2018 a, Groundswell, 2019; Institute for the Study of Diplomacy, 2017). In the first half of 2020, weather-related disasters displaced 9.8 million people and are the leading cause of new internal migrations worldwide. (IDMC, 2020, cited in Migration Data Portal, 2020). Although the developed world is currently a receiving location for international climate migrants, that is forecasted to change in the next few decades as the effects of global warming expand in severity and geographic range. Meanwhile, climate change and accompanying internal migration is already occurring in even the most stable economies.

Climate change complicates everything about human migration. Climate change differs from previous contexts in its geographic scope; the complex network of institutions in global society that is threatened; and the irreversible and urgent nature of the crisis. Some related issues with clear health implications include food and housing, social stability and social safety nets, violent conflict over natural resources, and health-related human rights (McLeman, 2020; McMichael, 2020; Smith-Cannoy, 2019). **Food security is compromised by short- and long-term climate effects**. Many Central American migrants claim food insecurity. Throughout the world, local agriculture is the direct source of food survival for at least 80% of rural residents, who lack access to global food markets (Campbell et. al., 2016) and are thus experiencing increased hunger. Climate-related crop yields, and therefore, human health, are directly affected by wildfire, drought, floods, and changing seasonal rainfall patterns. Cash and commodity crops are also affected, which lowers income and employment. These effects are already being felt worldwide (Baez et al., 2017; Climate Impact Map, 2021; Shaw, 2020; World Bank, 2018). Large monoculture crops are failing (NBC, 2019), and pivoting to other agricultural programs is difficult and expensive for several reasons: the need for large infrastructure investments, historical colonial land patterns, and the international scale of supply chains and marketing.

The availability of clean, suitable water for agriculture is decreasing due to weather changes and sea level rise. Water pollution is increasing, due to floods; typhoons; increased pests and, therefore, pesticides; and groundwater salinization related to coastal erosion and sea-level rise, which causes upstream river, irrigation canal, and wastewater treatment facility flooding. Feed and forage for livestock have become scarce and more expensive in parts of the world, including the United States. Fisheries and indigenous local cultural foodways, and large and small economies dependent on them, are also challenged by these forces.

Sea level rise is affecting habitability and, therefore, migration patterns. One third of the global population lives near a coast (Miller, 2017). Sudden extreme weather, such as typhoons, tornadoes, and hurricanes, has increased in geographic spread and severity. Changing weather patterns mean new locations are vulnerable. Storms stay in one place longer, increasing local wind and precipitation damage in some areas, and drought in others. Storms cause direct health effects via trauma, drowning, electrocution, and hypothermia, and indirect health effects via their impact on housing, healthcare facilities, energy, transportation, and workforce availability. Agricultural land is also submerged by river basins backing up and by coastal erosion. Up to one third of Bangladesh, for example, is at risk (Naser et al., 2019; Vidal, 2018). Small island nations and far northern indigenous lands are shrinking and even disappearing under rising sea levels caused by polar ice melt, raising international questions of nationhood, culture, and legal and financial responsibility (Noy, 2017).

Climate-related flooding also affects low-income coastal and river-adjacent housing in the United States (Flavelle, 2020; Herrmann, 2017; Holtz, 2019; Milman, 2020). This can be rapid-onset, as in sudden floods and hurricanes, or slower; for example, the increased frequency of basements flooding in the Gulf Coast and coastal Northeast. Residential water intrusion impacts electrical access and safety, property value, and health, for example increased mold, allergens, and unsafe food, medication, and property storage. Recovery from floods is influenced by economic disparities in terms of both initial and ongoing ability to invest in infrastructure and housing stock, as well as loss of labor due to trauma and temporary or permanent relocation. Also, seawalls and similar investments by high-resource communities may inadvertently direct water flow toward adjacent communities (Flavelle, 2020).

Climate change has well-established effects on human health. These areas are discussed in detail in the chapter by Anderko and Chalupka in the Climate and Health section in this text. These effects include heat-related morbidity and mortality, water- and vector-borne disease spread, decreased energy supplies and raw materials for individuals and health systems, wildfire and impaired air quality, cardiovascular and lung disease, cancer, occupational exposure to heat and to chemicals that combine differently at higher temperatures, and inability to meet healthcare infrastructure and emergency preparedness needs, as well as hunger, drowning, crowding, and mental health impacts related to environmental change (United States Centers for Disease Control, 2020).

Climate-related costs for health care will rise. Causes include increased need for outpatient care, decreasing availability of raw materials for devices and medications, and lost wages from increased illness (Limaye, V., 2019; Limaye et al., 2019)). Increased health care costs stress local and national budgets and create social instability (Limaye, Max, Constible, & Knowlton, 2019; Smith-Cannoy, 2019). These costs contribute to people's sudden or longer term needs and plans to migrate to more life-sustaining locations; they also impact health outcomes for individuals and societies (McMichael, 2020; Schwerdtle, Bowen, & McMichael, 2018; Shultz et al., 2019).

Climate change affects the availability of natural resources, and thereby affects and is affected by resource-related violence (Burrows & Kinney, 2016; Brzoska, 2019; Climate and Migration Coalition, 2018b; Hsiang, Burke, & Miguel, 2013; Thompson, 2019; Reuveny, 2008). Even functional governments can fail to address this issue in the face of immense needs caused by climate change. Food insecurity destabilizes societies (Smith-Cannoy, 2019). Areas of increasing violent conflict include urban systems,

transportation, health care, indigenous rights, international commerce, marine resources, and land ownership and use (IRC, 2019; Nicholas & Breakey, 2019). Internal migration to urban areas due to agriculture failure often precedes civilian violence in the receiving areas, and migrants without land and community are vulnerable, leading to cross-border migration (Abel et al., 2019; Sheller, 2018; Smith-Cannoy, 2019). Migrants are vulnerable to both state and nonstate violence (Bower & Olson, 2018;). Also, the conversion of forest to agricultural land affects and is affected by ecosystem health (Carr, 2009).

Climate migration is often conceptualized, in the United States and other countries, as a national and societal security risk. (Climate and Migration Coalition, 2019; Miller, 2017; Miller, 2019; Randall, 2018). This has led to specific priorities in funding for climate change adaptation. The individuals and nations most affected by climate change are not generally the entities most responsible for emitting greenhouse gases (Burkett, 2009). Divisions between environmentally secure and environmentally exposed individuals, communities, and nations are increasing (Sheller, 2018). To manage this conceptualization, governments have instituted policies, processes, and agreements. A brief overview of these follows.

GOVERNMENTAL RESPONSES

It is important to understand some of the legal and political background against which our patients' lives play out.

The terms "climate migrant" and "climate refugee" have no legal definitions, so they offer no legal status or protection. This lack of definition impairs accurate data collection, impeding planning and international cooperative agreements (Randall, n.d.[a]; Randall, n.d. [b]). The terms "climate-related displacement" and "environmental migrant" likewise lack universal definition. In the current global political climate, there is widespread resistance to adding any more legal reasons for cross-border migration (Keyes, 2019; Keyserlingk, 2018; McAdam, 2017; Randall, n.d. [c]). To assist in progressing on these issues, a number of useful frameworks have been developed, including those related to human migration, climate drivers of migration, and climate response. Here are a few of them.

Human migration varies along several spectra. These include voluntary/forced, planned/urgent, fast/slow, temporary/permanent, high/low agency, high/low resource, and internal/cross-border (international) (Climate and Migration Coalition, 2018 a). Proposed **categories of climate-linked human migration** include all of the above, plus driver-related factors such as habitability, resource conflict, and food and water scarcity. Additional categories include "trapped," those who want to leave but cannot, and "planned relocation of whole communities" (Ferris & Weerasinghe, 2020; Warner et al., 2013), including in the United States (Lewis, 2019).

The UN climate talks and the Paris Agreement of 2015 mentioned climate migration, but are not binding and neither addresses internal migration. The talks in 2018 built on that framework and made more concrete, but still nonbinding, recommendations for global cooperation in several areas, including data collection (Climate and Migration Coalition, 2018d; Climate Outreach, 2016). The 2019 UN climate talks in Madrid were notable for the failure to progress on a proposal for a global "climate damage fund" (United Nations OHCHCR; Rowling, 2019). One hopeful note is that the United States has now rejoined the Paris climate agreement and there is a mention of climate migration in this statement of intent from U.S. President Joseph Biden, so there will be a U.S. task force (Aton, 2021).

TERMINOLOGY AND DEFINITIONS

It is important to understand the meanings of specific terms to understand the challenges that climate migrants face.

A "refugee" meets the conditions of the 1951 Convention Relating to the Status of Refugees (Geneva convention). These conditions include "real" risk of harm to an individual, by the government, based on belonging to a "protected class" of individuals. A "refugee" is outside of their destination country when they apply' an "asylum seeker" applies for humanitarian resettlement under the refugee convention but is inside the destination country when they apply. Both these categories are making legal claims for humanitarian protection.

There have been various unsuccessful attempts to update the definition of "climate refugee." One stumbling block has been the difficulty of proving specific governmental causes in the case of climate-displaced people (Huggel et al., 2015; Keyserlingk, 2018), although that is being addressed in political, legal, and scientific research (e.g. Aton, 2021; Burkett 2009; Huggel et al., 2015).

A "migrant" is anyone who is moving to a new residence and represents a spectrum of situations. "Internally displaced persons" are migrants moving involuntarily within their own national borders. A "stateless" person is not considered a national by any nation; examples might be born during migration, or failed refugee or asylum case with no permission to reenter the country of origin. "Circular migration" refers to people who have two or more homes; it can be occupational or economic. Circular migration has long been used by agricultural workers and is ever more common in the context of climate related agricultural failure. The principle of "non-refoulement" states that "a person should not be returned to a country where they face serious threats to life and freedom" (IOM, 2019b; UNHCR, 2017; 2021). An "economic migrant" leaves their home solely for financial reasons. Again, the distinction between "climate-caused" or "climate-related" and "economic" migration is not universally defined—how far, or how frequently, does the water need into the house to come before it is a reason to move?"

The current scope of climate migration: It is hard to gather accurate data regarding climate displacement, since we lack definitions, tools, and surveys and since climate displacement is often only part of a complex, interacting process, which may lack a legally precipitating cause (Randall, n.d. a; Randall, n.d. b). Projections of numbers of climate migrants range from 150–300 million by 2050: a number of people equal to the fifth (or possibly fourth) largest country in the world. (Keyserlingk, 2018). People who live in the 48 least developed countries in the world are five times more likely to die in a climate-related disaster than those living in the rest of the world (Ciplett, Roberts, & Cahn, 2015; Miller, 2017). According to one estimate, in 2016 anthropogenic climate change displaced 10–26 million people globally, disproportionately from the global south and low-emitting countries. In 2019, the total number of international migrants was at least 272 million (United Nations Department of Economic and Social Affairs, 2019).

This is not just an international issue that will affect migration TO the United States; these effects will also be felt within the United States (Climate Impact Lab, 2021; U.S. Global Change Research Program, 2014). Internal migration will occur, and in some projected scenarios, people will be trying to migrate north from the United States to Canada (Shaw et al., 2020).

Human rights violations are both drivers and results of displacement. Climate change–related human rights violations are novel in scale and scope and are tightly interwoven with international development, aid, and commerce. There are many areas of overlap, including displacement of former refugees by current refugees, temporary flight in cases where the refugee's home is not rebuildable, repeated loss displacement, and vulnerability during travel (IRC, 2019; Sheller, 2018; Smith-Cannoy, 2019). For example, national greenhouse gas reduction strategies may conflict with land rights (McLeman, 2020; Smith-Cannoy, 2019). Fatal Journeys reports that at least 16,000 people died crossing international borders between 2014 and 2019 (IOM, 2019a; 2020). The industries that extract fossil fuels to run our cities have negative consequences on places that we think of as distant (Sheller, 2018).

The U.S. response to climate change has been characterized as an "armed lifeboat" (Ross-Brown, 2013). Most research and resources addressing climate change in the United States have gone to the military sector. Energy resources are a major component in geopolitics. The Department of Defense was planning for climate change as early as 1993 (DOD, 1994) and funds and resources have been allocated to a military response to climate migration since the United States government began addressing this issue (Miller, 2017; National Intelligence Council, 2006; Ross-Brown, 2013; Schwartz & Randall, 2003; US GAO, 2019). This includes equipment, training, research and development, and personnel and personnel maintenance (Miller, 2017; 2019).

The U.S. immigration system has become ever more militarized and restrictive (American Immigration Lawyers Association, 2021; Davis & Shear, 2019). U.S. immigration laws have been heavily politicized since their beginning in the late 1800s (Kerwin, 2018; McNeill, 2020). The immigration system includes the State Department, which issues visas (permission to cross borders), the Department of Justice, the Immigration and Nationality Act, residence and citizenship permissions, the Department of Homeland Security, Customs and Border Patrol, and Immigration and Customs (ICE). Categories of the United States immigration system affected by changes accelerated in the last four years include work- and family-based permissions, per-country ceilings, refugees, asylees, and deferred deportation programs such as Temporary Protected Status (TPS) and Deferred Action for Childhood Arrivals (DACA).

All of these interlocking systems are complex and expensive and have been further expanded in the last four years (American Immigration Council, 2019; American Immigration Legal Council, 2020). This has prevented resources from flowing toward climate mitigation, adaptation, or resilience, both in the United States and abroad (Gustin & Henninger, 2019). Instead, resources have been focused on military defense against immigrants and immigration (Miller, 2017; Miller, 2019; Whitehead, 2014). The U.S. budget for immigration is 27 times higher than it was 30 years ago (American Immigration Council, 2020) and has increased by 133,567% since 1980 (Miller, 2019). Although the United States spends millions of dollars on foreign aid, most of that money is spent on border security and policing (Miller, 2017; Miller, 2019).

The border itself poses human rights concerns, as normal laws don't apply in border zones (Kawakubo, 2020; Walia, 2013). In the last few years, the U.S. border zone has expanded to 100 miles from the border, including 65% of the U.S. population (Miller, 2019; Misra, 2018). "Interior enforcement" has provided new powers, including targeted surveillance and warrantless searches, to border patrol agents far away from the border. This expansion of power has been justified through appeals to common beliefs about the migrant population. Common narratives about migrants include that they are opportunists, security threats, victims, political pawns, economic drains, criminals, and unassimilable aliens.

NURSING IMPLICATIONS

Nurses can take action on multiple levels: as individuals, as nursing professionals, and as American citizens. In choosing and engaging in action, various facets of this human rights crisis should be considered. These include the challenge/opportunity spectrum; the complex, historical, intersectional, global, and urgent nature of this crisis; the scope of influence; various frameworks, such as economic, political, health, humanitarian, justice, and security perspectives; and considerations for nursing practice.

Some international legal organizations have released overarching **conceptual frameworks for environmental migration**, including the concept of the uncompensated wrong (Burkett, 2009) and a proposed humanitarian framework for environmental migrants (Kalin & Weerasinghe, 2017), partially operationalized for further work in the IOM and United Nations initiatives discussed in the previous section. Solutions ranging from local to global will be needed. It is essential to realistically assess the climate adaptive capacity of "remain in place" solutions and to objectively consider both collective and individual safety and survival. Global disparities in the interdependent rights "to a home" (Manuel, 2018) and "freedom of movement" (Sheller, 2018) are among human rights that influence conflicting political approaches to global climate change.

As Zenju Earthlyn Manuel (2018, p. 8) writes, "It looks like homelessness is happening to particular groups, but it is happening to all. We are in a free fall toward the unknown. Our whole species is faced with homelessness."

Nurses can serve as informed political advocates. Advocacy includes promoting policies that facilitate a decrease in individual and collective contributions to climate change. This includes recognizing the disproportionate impact of the United States and the healthcare sector's significant production of greenhouse gases. The healthcare sector has a unique responsibility and opportunity to act. The healthcare field has a healing mission and has committed to "do no harm," yet its operations contribute significantly to climate change and, as a result, to the very diseases it is trying to treat. The healthcare sector's greenhouse gas emissions make up 9.8% of the U.S. total; if it were its own country, healthcare would rank 13th in the world for greenhouse gas emissions, more than the United Kingdom (Eckelman et al., 2020; Eckelman & Sherman, 2016). Specific healthcare efforts to ameliorate this impact include Healthcare Without Harm (2021), Nurses Climate Challenge (2021), Nurses Drawdown (Project Drawdown, 2021), Planetary Health (Planetary Health Alliance, 2021), Practice Greenhealth (2021) and local interventions that make global warming reduction behaviors accessible and feasible.

While mitigating climate change in the ways above is important, nurses also can be involved in climate adaptation and resilience efforts. This is where there is the greatest need for nurses to understand climate migration.

Nurses can advocate for migrants' human and health rights, including recognition of the impact of climate change on human migration. For example, migrants are heavily represented in healthcare settings, and many have a wealth of knowledge and experience that is either untapped or is tapped without recognition or reimbursement (American Immigration Council, 2018; 2020). Healthcare professionals can actively support their migrant coworkers and patients and intervene if they witness individual and systemic discrimination in the workplace or community (McNeill, 2020).

Nurses can also become more aware and share their knowledge about migrant health risks and the link between climate change and migration in local communities. In migrant-heavy workplaces, such as those in the food service, cleaning, agricultural, and manufacturing industries, health risks may include mandatory overtime; unsafe or broken equipment; heat, chemical, and infectious disease exposure; sexual harassment; and inadequate protective supplies. In some workplaces there are separate healthcare facilities for migrants, which potentially increases their risk of abuse and inferior health care. In some of these situations, migrants and healthcare workers alike are afraid to speak up about health risks, knowing that retaliation has occurred in the form of physical and legal threats. Nurses working in these settings, and in detention facilities, need and deserve professional support to uphold professional standards by substantively addressing these issues, either within the systems or, in some cases, by "whistle-blowing."

Nurses can be aware of basic best practices for caring for migrant patients, and advocate in their spheres for their implementation. Specific best practices for migrant health care for nonspecialist providers in the United State include prioritizing screening, accommodation, and knowledge of local resources, and implementing measures to ensure that health information is not misunderstood. Climate migrants are dealing with losses, not only of previous roles and resources, but of the very landscape of "home". It is important to recognize and respond to grieving, and work with and support the strengths that have made it possible for them to arrive to our care settings. Nurses are positioned by education and work roles to effectively both assess and respond with to these strengths and challenges. For more information about environmental risks for migrating people, please see the Immigrants and Refugees section in the Vulnerable Population unit.

CONCLUSION

Climate change, human migration, and human health crises intersect in ways that can be overwhelming. However, the intersectionality of this situation means that many opportunities exist for nurses to apply our compassion, knowledge, and determination toward effective action. We know that moving forward one step at a time can lead to transformation. The very foundations of our profession rest on caring combined with knowledge, hard work, and moral courage. Nurses can care effectively for the health of climate migrants and communities by understanding more about the causes and conditions that have led to their suffering. As practice Greenhealth (2021) states, "Efforts aimed at protecting and improving our health will not succeed without addressing the social, economic, and ecological catastrophes that largely underpin the health, safety, and happiness of individuals and communities worldwide."

The knowledge and resources presented in this article and bibliography is intended to provide context for understanding and thus working with the climate migration related health issues that are certain to arise in each nurse's practice.

The author of this section would like to acknowledge to following people for their comments and support in this work: Nancy Chaney, Chris Fasching Maphis, Barbara Gottlieb, David Holland, Katie Huffling, Kaira Jewel Lingo, Gene Locke, Ruth McDermott-Levy, Matthew Paterson, Nancy Rudner, Barbara Sattler, Marcy Schneck, Eva Stitt, Jennifer Jacoby Anne Trippeer, Erica Uhlman, and Stephanie Marshall Ward.

REFERENCES

Abel, G. J., Brottrager, M., Cuaresma, J. C., & Muttarak, R. (2019). Climate, conflict, and forced migration. *Global Environmental Change, 54*, 239–249. https://doi.org/10.1016/j.gloenvcha.2018.12.003

American Immigration Council (2018, January 17). *Special report: Foreign-trained doctors are critical to serving many US communities.* https://rb.gy/ei1yuo

American Immigration Council (2019, October 10). *How the United States immigration system works [Fact Sheet].* https://www.americanimmigrationcouncil.org/research/how-united-states-immigration-system-works

American Immigration Council (2020, August 6). *Immigrants in the United States [Fact Sheet].* https://www.americanimmigrationcouncil.org/research/immigrants-in-the-united-states

American Immigration Lawyers Association (2021, February 17). *Tracking notable executive branch action.* https://www.aila.org/advo-media/agency-liaison/tracking-notable-executive-branch-action

Aton, A. (2021, February 8). *Biden pushes U.S.—and the world—to help climate migrants.* Scientific American. https://www.scientificamerican.com/article/biden-pushes-u-s-and-the-world-to-help-climate-migrants/

Baez, J., Caruso, G., Mueller, V., & Niu, C. (2017). Droughts augment youth migration in northern Latin America and the Caribbean. *Climatic Change, 140*, 423–435. https://doi.org/10.1007/s10584-016-1863-2

Benko, J. (2017, April 19). *How a warming planet drives human migration.* The New York Times. https://www.nytimes.com/2017/04/19/magazine/how-a-warming-planet-drives-human-migration.html

Bower, E., & Olson, J. (2018, December). *Women on the move in a changing climate: A discussion paper on gender, climate, and mobility.* Sierra Club & UN Women. https://contentdev.sierraclub.org/sites/www.sierraclub.org/files/program/documents/Women-Climate-Report.pdf

Brzoska, M. (2019). Understanding the disaster-migration-violent conflict nexus in a warming world: The importance of international policy interventions. *Social Sciences, 8*(6), 167. doi:10.3390/socsci8060167

Burkett, M. (2009). Climate reparations. *Melbourne Journal of International Law, 10*(2).

Burrows, K., & Kinney, P. (2016). Exploring the climate change, migration and conflict nexus. *International Journal of Environmental Research and Public Health, 13*(4), 443. doi:10.3390/ijerph13040443

Campbell, B. M., Aggarwal, P. K., Corner-Dolloff, C. A., Girvetz, E. H., Loboguerrero, A. M., Ramirez-Villegas, J., Rosenstock, T., Sebastian, L. S., Thornton, P. K., Wollenberg, E., & Vermeulen, S. (2016). Reducing risks to food security from climate change. *Global Food Security, 11*, 34–43. doi.10/1016/j.gfs.2016.06.002

Carr, D. (2009). Population and deforestation: Why rural migration matters. *Progress in Human Geography, 33*(3), 355–378.

Ciplet, D., Roberts, J. T., & Cahn, R. (2015). *Power in a warming world: The new global politics of climate change and the remaking of environmental inequality.* MIT Press.

Climate Impact Lab. (2021). *Climate Impact Map.* http://www.impactlab.org/map/#usmeas=absolute&usyear=1981-2010&gmeas=absolute&gyear=1986-2005

Climate and Migration Coalition. (2018 a). December 4, 2018. *Climate change and migration 101.* https://www.youtube.com/watch?v=-Xq7QEdV1B0&t=5s

Climate & Migration Coalition (2018b). December 10, 2018. *Hot wars: climate change and conflict.* https://www.youtube.com/watch?v=PiMCxTaxZ8I&t=1843s

Climate and Migration Coalition. (2018c). December 16, 2018. *Migration and displacement at the climate talks.* https://www.youtube.com/watch?v=3XOTcY6weYU

Climate and Migration Coalition. (2019). July 25, 2019. *Security, for who?* https://www.youtube.com/watch?v=i5LNiESyD1I

Climate Outreach. (2016, December 14). *Fixing climate-linked displacement: are the climate talks enough?* https://www.youtube.com/watch?v=m4L-hzBeBlg&feature=emb_imp_woyt

Davis, J. H. & Shear, M. D. (2019). *Border wars: Inside Trump's assault on immigration.* Simon & Schuster.

deMenocal, P., & Stringer, C. (2016). Climate and the peopling of the world. *Nature, 538,* 49–50. https://doi.org/10.1038/nature19471

Department of Defense, United States. (2015, July 23). *Congressional report: National implications of climate change.* https://archive.defense.gov/pubs/150724-congressional-report-on-national-implications-of-climate-change.pdf

Department of Homeland Security, United States. (2012). *Climate change adaptation roadmap.* https://rb.gy/fxxjzz

Eckelman, M. J. & Sherman, J. (2016, June 9). Environmental impacts of the U.S. health care system and effects on public health. *PLoS ONE, 11*(6), e0157014. https://doi.org/10.1371/journal.pone.0157014

Eckelman, M. J., Huang, K., Lagasse, R., Senay, E., Dubrow, R., & Sherman, J. D. (2020, December). Health care pollution and public health damage in the United States: An update. *Health Affairs, 39*(12). https://www.healthaffairs.org/doi/10.1377/hlthaff.2020.01247

Ferris, E. & Weerasinghe, S. (2020). Planned relocation as a protection tool in a time of climate change. *Journal on Migration and Human Security, 8*(2), 134–149. doi: 10.1177/2331502420909305

Flavelle, C. (2020, August 26, 2020). *U.S. flood strategy shifts to 'unavoidable' relocation of entire neighborhoods.* The New York Times. https://www.nytimes.com/2020/08/26/climate/flooding-relocation-managed-retreat.html

Gardiner, S. M. (2011). *A perfect moral storm: The ethical tragedy of climate change.* Oxford University Press.

Groundswell. (2019, March 19). *New report says climate change could force millions to move within their countries* [YouTube video]. https://m.youtube.comwatch?feature=emb_logo&v=d6ijhQn_ww4&time_continue=11

Gustin, G. & Henniger, M. (2019, July 9). *Central America's choice: Pray for rain or migrate.* NBC News. https://www.nbcnews.com/news/latino/central-america-drying-farmers-face-choice-pray-rain-or-leave-n1027346

Healthcare Without Harm. (2021). https://noharm-uscanada.org/HealthyClimate

Herrmann, V. (2017, August). *The United States climate change relocation plan: What needs to happen now.* The Arctic Institute. https://www.thearcticinstitute.org/wp-content/uploads/2017/09/The-United-States-Climate-Change-Relocation-Plan_2017.pdf

Holtz, J. (2019, March 19). *Managed retreat due to rising seas is a public health issue.* UW News. https://www.washington.edu/news/2019/03/19/managed-retreat-due-to-rising-seas-is-a-public-health-issue/

Hsiang, S.M., Burke, M., & Miguel, E.. (2013). Quantifying the influence of climate on human conflict. *Science, 341*(6151), 1235367. doi: 10.1126/science.1235367

Huggel, C., Stone, D., Eicken, H, & Hansen, G. (2015). Potentials and limitations of the attribution of climate change impacts for informing loss and damage discussions and policies. *Climatic Change, 133*(3): 453–467. DOI:10.1007/s10584-015-1441-z

IDMC. (2020). *Migration Data Portal.* Institute of Migration.

Institute for the Study of Diplomacy, Edmund A. Walsh School of Foreign Service, George Mason University. (2017, April). *New challenges to human security: Environmental change and human mobility.* Georgetown University.

International Organization for Migration (IOM). (2019a). *Fatal journeys: Missing migrant children.* https://publications.iom.int/system/files/pdf/fatal_journeys_4.pdf

International Organization for Migration (IOM). (2019b). *Glossary on Migration.* Rhttps://publications.iom.int/system/files/pdf/iml_34_glossary.pdf

International Organization for Migration (IOM). (2020). *World migration report 2020.* https://www.iom.int/wmr/

International Rescue Committee (IRC). (2019, September 27). *Rescue facts: How climate change affects refugees.* https://m.youtube.com/watch?time_continue=4&feature=emb_logo&v=VcmVSfHvlTk

Kalin, W. & Weerasinghe, S. (2017). *Environmental migrants and global governance: Facts, policies, and practices.* International Organization on Migration.

Kawakubo, F. (2020). Privatizing border security: Emergence of the border-industrial complex and its implications. *Public Voices, 17*(1), 32-38.

Kerwin, D. (2018). From IIRIRA to Trump: Connecting the dots on the current US immigration policy crisis. *Journal on Migration and Human Security, 6*(3), 192–204. doi:10.1177/2331502418786718

Keyes, E. (2019). Environmental refugees? Rethinking what's in a name. *North Carolina Journal of International Law & Commercial Regulation,* 462–486.

Keyserlingk, J. G. (2018) *Immigration control in a warming world*. Imprint Academic.

Lewis, A. S. (2019). *The Drowning of Money Island: A forgotten community's fight against the rising seas threatening coastal America*. Beacon Press.

Limaye, V. (2019, September). *Bitter pill: The high health costs of climate change [Fact Sheet]*. National Resources Defense Council (NRDC). https://www.nrdc.org/resources/bitter-pill-high-health-costs-climate-change

Limaye, V. S., Max, W., Constible, J., & Knowlton, K. (2019). Estimating the health-related costs of 10 climate-sensitive U.S. events during 2012. *GeoHealth, 3*, 245– 265. https://doi.org/10.1029/2019GH000202

López-Carr, D. & Marter-Kenyon, J. (2015). Human adaptation: Manage climate-induced resettlement. *Nature, 517* (7534), pp. 265-7.

Manuel, Z. E. (2018). *Sanctuary: A meditation on home, homelessness, and belonging*. Wisdom Publications.

McAdam, J. (2017, June 6). *Seven reasons the United Nations Refugee Convention should not include "climate refugees."* The Sidney Morning Herald. https://www.smh.com.au/opinion/seven-reasons-the-un-refugee-convention-should-not-include-climate-refugees-20170606-gwl8b4.html

McLeman, R. (2020, December) *How will international migration policy and sustainable development affect future climate-related migration?* Transatlantic Council on Migration, Migration Policy Institute. https://www.migrationpolicy.org/research/international-migration-policy-development-climate

McMichael, C. (2020, June). Human mobility, climate change, and health: Unpacking the connections. *The Lancet: Planetary Health, 4*(6), e217–e218. https://doi.org/10.1016/S2542-5196(20)30125-X

McNeill, T. (2020, September 2020). *The long history of xenophobia in America*. TuftsNow. https://now.tufts.edu/articles/long-history-xenophobia-america

Miller, T. (2017). *Storming the wall: Climate change, migration, and homeland security*. City Lights Books.

Miller, T. (2019). *Empire of borders: The expansion of the US border around the world*. Verso.

Milman, O. (2020, December 1). *Climate crisis to triple flooding threat for low-income US homes by 2050*. The Guardian. https://www.theguardian.com/environment/2020/dec/01/climate-crisis-triple-flooding-threat-low-income-us-homes-by-2050

Misra, T. (2018, May 14). *Inside the massive U.S. 'border zone'.* Bloomberg CityLab. https://www.bloomberg.com/news/articles/2018-05-14/mapping-who-lives-in-border-patrol-s-100-mile-zone

Naser, M. M., Swapan, M. S. H., Ahsan, R., Afroz, T., & Ahmed S. (2019). Climate change, migration and human rights in Bangladesh: Perspectives on governance. *Asia Pacific Viewpoint, 60*(2), 175–190.

NBC News. (2019, July 8.) *How climate change drives migration*. YouTube.

Neuman, B. & Fawcett, J. (2002). *The Neuman Systems Model* (4th ed.). Prentice-Hall International.

Nicholas & Breakey (2019). The economics of climate change and the intersection with conflict, violence, and migration: Implications for the nursing profession. *Nursing Economics, 37*(1) 23 – 34.

Noy, I. (2017). To leave or not to leave? Climate change, exit, and voice on a Pacific island. *CESifo Economic Studies, 63*(4), 403–420. doi: 10.1093/cesifo/ifx004

Nurses Climate Challenge. (2021). https://nursesclimatechallenge.org/

Planetary Health Alliance (2021). *Planetary health*. https://www.planetaryhealthalliance.org/planetary-health

Practice Greenhealth. (2021). *Sustainability solutions for healthcare*. https://practicegreenhealth.org/

Project Drawdown (2021) *Nurses Drawdown*. https://www.nursesdrawdown.org

Randall, A. (n.d.[a]) *Climate refugee statistics: how many, where, and when?* https://climatemigration.org.uk/climate-refugee-statistics/

Randall, A. (n.d.[b]) *Environmental refugees: who are they, definition, and numbers*. https://climatemigration.org.uk/environmental-refugees-definition-numbers/

Randall, A. (n.d.[c]). *Why governments will eventually, reluctantly, back migration as climate adaptation*. https://climatemigration.org.uk/governments-back-climate-migration-adaptation/

Randall, A. (2018). *Migration is a successful climate adaptation strategy: opinion*. Al-Jazeera. https://www.aljazeera.com/opinions/2018/3/11/migration-is-a-successful-climate-adaptation-strategy

Reuveny, R. (2008). Ecomigration and violent conflict: case studies and policy implications. *Human Ecology, 36*, 1–13 DOI 10.1007/s10745-007-9142-5

Ross-Brown, S. (2013, September/October). *Armed lifeboat: Government's response to natural disaster.* Utne Reader. https://www.utne.com/politics/natural-disaster-zm0z13sozros

Schwartz, P. ,& Randall, D. (2003), *An abrupt climate change scenario and its implications for United States national security.* Homeland Security Digital Library. https://www.hsdl.org/?abstract&did=444312

Schwerdtle, P., Bowen, K., & McMichael, C. (2018). The health impacts of climate-related migration. *BMC Medicine, 16*(1). doi: 10.1186/s12916-017-0981-7.

Shaw, A., Lustgarten, A., & Goldsmith, J. W. (2020, September 15). *New climate maps show a transformed United States.* ProPublica. https://projects.propublica.org/climate-migration/

Sheller, M. (2018). *Mobility justice: The politics of movement in an age of extremes.* Verso Press.

Shultz, J.M., Rechkemmer, A., Rai, A., & McManus, K.T. (2019). Public health and mental health implications of environmentally induced forced Migration. Disaster Medicine and Public health Preparedness 13 (2). 116-122. doi: 10.1017/dmp.2018.27 Smith-Cannoy, H. (Ed.) (2019). *Emerging threats to human rights: Resources, violence, and deprivation of citizenship.* Temple University Press.

Thompson, B. (2019, October 15). *Climate change and displacement: How conflict and climate change form a toxic combination that drives people from their homes.* The UN Refugee Agency USA. https://www.unhcr.org/en-us/news/stories/2019/10/5da5e18c4/climate-change-and-displacement.html

UNHCR. (2017, June). *Key concepts on climate change and disaster displacement.* https://www.refworld.org/docid/594399824.html.

UNHCR. (2021). *The 1951 Refugee convention.* https://www.unhcr.org/en-us/1951-refugee-convention.html.

United Nations Department of Economic and Social Affairs (2019, December 17). *The number of international migrants reaches 272 million, continuing an upward trend in all world regions, says UN.* UN DESA News. https://www.un.org/development/desa/en/news/population/international-migrant-stock-2019.html

United Nations OHCHCR. (2015) Understanding human rights and climate change. Submission of the Office of the High Commissioner for Human Rights to the 21st Conference of the Parties to the United Nations Framework Convention on Climate Change. https://www.ohchr.org/Documents/Issues/ClimateChange/COP21.pdf

United States Centers for Disease Control. (2020). *Climate and health: Climate effects on health.* https://www.cdc.gov/climateandhealth/effects/default.htm

U.S. Global Change Research Program. (2014). *Future climate.* https://nca2014.globalchange.gov/highlights/report-findings/future-climate

U.S. Government Accounting Office (US GAO) (2019, January). *Climate change activities of selected agencies to address potential impact on global migration.* https://www.gao.gov/assets/700/696460.pdf

Vidal, J. (2018, January 4). *Boats pass over where our land was: Bangladesh's climate refugees.* The Guardian.

Walia, H. (2013). *Undoing border imperialism.* AK Press.

Warner, K., Afifi, T., Kälin, W., Leckie, S., Ferris, B., Martin, S. F., & Wrathall, D. (2013, June). *Policy brief: Changing climate, moving people: Framing migration, displacement, and planned relocation.* UN University: Institute for Environment and Human Security (UNU-EHS).

Whitehead, J. (2014, June 17). *Has the department of homeland security become America's standing army?* River Cities' Reader. https://www.rcreader.com/commentary/has-department-homeland-security-become-americas-standing-army

World Bank. (2018, March). *Groundswell: Preparing for internal climate migration.* https://www.worldbank.org/en/news/infographic/2018/03/19/groundswell---preparing-for-internal-climate-migration/

ADVANCING THE CLIMATE CHANGE AGENDA FOR NURSING IN FINLAND

Iira Titta, MSN, RN
Doctoral Candidate, Department of Nursing Sciences
University of Eastern Finland

INTRODUCTION:

Like every country, Finland and its population are experiencing the health impacts of climate change. Nurses can take a leading role in addressing climate change in the Finnish health sector. This includes the impact on the healthcare system, addressing gaps in nursing education, generating the evidence to influence health outcomes, and advocacy and collaboration to advance a climate change agenda that addresses health.

THE HEALTHCARE SYSTEM

Like all healthcare systems, the Finnish healthcare system will face challenges as a result of climate change. To effectively address and prevent these risks, social and healthcare services must take proactive measures to adapt to the changing climate (Meriläinen et al., 2021). The potential to advance healthcare adaptation to climate change's health effects is growing in Finland. This includes developing health and social care units to prepare for disruptions caused by extreme weather events, improving citizens' awareness of the health risks of climate change and their readiness to respond to them, and tracking the effects of weather and climate using data collection systems in the environment and health sectors (Mäkinen et al., 2019).

EDUCATION AND AWARENESS

To foster sustainable healthcare practices, nursing education programs in Finland must incorporate climate change and environmental sustainability into their curricula. By integrating climate change-related topics, such as the health impacts of climate change, sustainable healthcare practices, and climate change resilience, nursing students will be equipped with the necessary knowledge and skills to address climate change-related challenges in their future practice. Additionally, continuous professional development programs and workshops on climate change and sustainability should be provided to practicing nurses, empowering them to become champions of climate action within their healthcare settings (Goodman, 2011; Savell & Sattler, 2012; Lilienfeld et al., 2018; Tiitta et al., 2020).

RESEARCH AND EVIDENCE

Robust research is vital to inform evidence-based policies and interventions to address climate change and its impact on health. Nursing researchers in Finland should prioritize conducting studies that explore the links between climate change and health outcomes, develop innovative strategies to mitigate climate-related health risks, and evaluate the effectiveness of interventions aimed at promoting climate resilience in healthcare settings. The findings from such research can be used to advocate for policy changes and guide the development of sustainable healthcare practices that minimize the carbon footprint of healthcare delivery systems (Polivka & Chaudry, 2018; Tiitta et al., 2020).

ADVOCACY AND COLLABORATION

Nursing organizations and professional associations in Finland should actively advocate for climate action and collaborate with other stakeholders to influence policy development. By engaging in public campaigns, lobbying for sustainable healthcare policies, and participating in interdisciplinary collaborations, nurses can amplify their voices and contribute to the development of climate change-friendly healthcare systems as well as addressing the health impacts of climate change upon the population. Collaboration with policymakers, environmental organizations, and other healthcare professionals can facilitate the integration of climate considerations into healthcare policies, practice guidelines, and quality improvement initiatives (Kurt, 2017; ICN, 2018; Lilienfeld et al., 2018; Butterfield et al., 2021).

CONCLUSION

Moving the climate agenda forward for nursing in Finland requires a multifaceted approach encompassing education, research, advocacy, and collaboration. By integrating climate change and sustainability into nursing education, conducting relevant research, advocating for policy changes, and collaborating with diverse stakeholders, nursing professionals can drive positive change in healthcare systems, promote climate change resilience, and mitigate the health risks associated with climate change.

REFERENCES

Butterfield, P., Leffers, J., & Díaz Vásquez, M. (2021). Nursing's pivotal role in global climate action. BMJ : British Medical Journal (Online), 373. https://doi.org/10.1136/bmj.n1049

Goodman, B. (2011). The need for a 'sustainability curriculum' in nurse education. *Nurse Education Today*, 31(8), 733-737.

International Council of Nurses (ICN). 2018. *Nurses, climate change and health.* https://www.icn.ch/sites/default/files/inlinefiles/PS_E_Nurses_climate%20change_health.pdf

Kurth, A. E. (2017). Planetary health and the role of nursing: A call to action. *Journal of Nursing Scholarship*, 49(6), 598–605. https://doi.org/10.1111/jnu.12343

Lilienfeld, E., Nicholas, P. K., Breakey, S., & Corless, I. B. (2018). Addressing climate change through a nursing lens within the framework of the United Nations Sustainable Development Goals. *Nursing Outlook*, 66(5), 482–494. https://doi.org/10.1016/j.outlook.2018.06.010

Meriläinen, P.; Paunio, M.; Kollanus, V.; Halonen, J.; Tuomisto, J.; Virtanen, S.; Karvonen, S.; Hemminki, E.; Kuusipalo, H.; Koivula, R.; Mäkelä, H.; Huusko, S.; Voutilainen, L.; Huldén, L.; Raulio, S.; Keskimäki, I.; Partonen, T.; Mänttäri, S.; Viitanen, A-K.; Kangas, P.; Sarlio, S.; Lyyra, K.; Viljamaa, S.; Mukala, K. (2021). Climate change in the healthcare and social welfare sector: Climate change adaptation plan of Ministry of Social Affairs and Health (2021–2031). *Publications of the Ministry of Social Affairs and Health*, 2021, 36. https://julkaisut.valtioneuvosto.fi/bitstream/handle/10024/163643/STM_2021_36.pdf?sequence=1&isAllowed=y

Polivka, B.J., Chaudry, R.V. (2018). A scoping review of environmental health nursing research. *Public Health Nursing*, 35, 10–17. https://doi.org/10.1111/phn.12373

Savell, A. D., & Sattler, B. (2012). Infusing environmental health concepts into an existing nursing course. *Nurse Educator*, 37(6), 268–272

Tiitta, I., McDermott-Levy, R., Turunen, H., Jaakkola, J.,& Kuosmanen, L. (2020). Finnish nurses' perceptions of the health impacts of climate change and their preparation to address those impacts. *Nursing Forum.* https://doi.org/10.1111/nuf.12540

CLIMATE CHANGE, HEALTH, AND EQUITY
Adelita G. Cantu, PhD, RN
Associate Professor
University of Texas Health San Antonio
School of Nursing

It has been reported that climate change is one of the greatest public health threats that we face today. The consequences of climate change have been well documented. These include morbidity and mortality from intense heat, asthma exacerbation, and mental health issues related to displacement due to severe weather events.

However, we know that these health issues do not affect every community equally. For instance, African Americans have a 36% higher rate of asthma incidents and are 3 times more likely to die or visit the emergency room from asthma-related complication than non-Hispanic Whites (Hoerner & and Robinson, 2008). Native American and Alaskan Native communities lack access to clean, potable drinking water at higher rates than others. Warmer water temperatures may exacerbate already-high rates of diarrhea-associated hospitalizations for Native American and Alaskan Native children (Singleton, et al., 2007). Nearly 1 in 2 Latinos live in counties with poor air quality. Latino children are twice as likely to die from asthma as non-Latino Whites, and Latino children living in areas with high levels of air pollution have a heightened risk of developing Type 2 diabetes (Morello-Frosch, et al, 2009).

Equity refers to the act of being fair and impartial. Health equity means that everyone has a fair and just opportunity to be as healthy as possible. However, due to systemic barriers, many marginalized communities are more susceptible to the health effects of climate change, despite their having contributed less to the mechanisms responsible for climate change. Many of these systemic issues are historic, such as the past racist redlining practices, which was the mid-20th-century practice by banks and insurers to concentrate African Americans and other underrepresented homeowners within certain neighborhoods. Many of the nation's historically redlined districts "now contain the hottest areas" in the United States, according to data collected from 108 cities across the country (Hoffman, Shandas, & Pendleton, 2020). As a result, residents of those areas face a disproportionate risk of heat-related mortality and health impacts associated with heat and carbon pollution.

Another example of this inequity is tree canopies. The benefits of trees are well known, not only for the shade that is provided but trees are vital as a force against climate change as they remove carbon dioxide, a greenhouse gas, from the atmosphere. However, a map of tree cover among major cities is also a map of historically underrepresented, low-income neighborhoods as they usually do not have trees due to lack of investment in historically underrepresented, urban neighborhoods. African Americans are more likely to live in neighborhoods with few trees and more heat-trapping pavement (Morello-Frosch, et al, 2009). The rate of heat-related deaths in African Americans is 150–200% greater than that for non-Hispanic Whites (Morello-Frosch, et al, 2009).

Many cities across the nation are now developing climate adaptation and mitigation plans. These plans must acknowledge that, due to historic racist policies, not all community members contribute equally to climate change, nor have the same resources or capabilities to protect themselves from its negative effects. Currently, San Antonio, TX, the SA Climate Ready Plan is using a climate equity framework that will prioritize communities burdened the most by climate change and those most vulnerable to it. Climate equity will ensure that these communities will play a central role in the just transformation of the institutional systems that have created the unequal burden of climate impacts. This will be operationalized by a screening tool that will be used to measure the equitable nature of all adaptation and mitigation strategies going forward. The themes include 1) access and accessibility; 2) affordability; 3) cultural preservation; 4) health, and 5) safety and security (SA Climate Ready, 2019, pg 58).

Nurses play an important role in advocating for and with historically underrepresented communities that are experiencing the inequitable impacts of climate change. Nurses must also educate policymakers about the health impacts of climate change, the greater risk for low-income communities of color, and assure that this is addressed in climate change adaptation plans.

REFERENCES

Hoerner, J. A., & and Robinson, N. (2008). *A climate of change: African Americans, global warming, and a just climate policy for the U.S.* The Environmental Justice and Climate Change Initiative. http://urbanhabitat.org/files/climateofchange.pdf.

Singleton, R. J., Holman, R. C., Yorita, K. L., Holve, S., Paisano, E. L., Steiner, C. A., ... & Cheek, J. E. (2007). Diarrhea-associated hospitalizations and outpatient visits among American Indian and Alaska Native children younger than five years of age, 2000–2004. *The Pediatric*

Infectious Disease Journal, 26(11), 1006–13. https://doi.org/10.1097/INF.0b013e3181256595

Morello-Frosch, R., Pastor, M., Sadd, J., Shonkoff, S. (2009). *The climate gap: Inequalities in how climate change hurts Americans & how to close the gap.* http://dornsife.usc.edu/assets/sites/242/docs/ClimateGapReport_full_report_web.pdf.

Hoffman, J. S., Shandas, V., & Pendleton, N. (2020). The effects of historical policies on resident exposure to intra-urban health: A study of 108 US urban areas. *Climate, 8*(1), pp. 1-15. https://www.mdpi.com/2225-1154/8/1/12/htm

American Forests. 2021. *Tree equity in America's cities.* https://www.americanforests.org/our-work/urban-forestry/

City of San Antonio City Council. (2019). *SA climate ready: A pathway for climate action and adaptation.* https://www.sanantonio.gov/Portals/0/Files/Sustainability/SAClimateReady/SACRReportOctober2019.pdf

CLIMATE JUSTICE FOR ADVANCING JUST-RELATIONS AND RESPONSIBILITIES FOR PLANETARY HEALTH

De-Ann Sheppard PhD(c) MScHQ
Nurse Practitioner
Independent Indigenous Nurse Researcher
Mi'kma'ki

Jessica LeClair, PhD(c), MPH, RN
Clinical Instructor
University of Wisconsin - Madison
School of Nursing

Robin Evans-Agnew, PhD, RN,
Associate Professor, Nursing and Healthcare Leadership
University of Washington Tacoma

Climate change is already happening, and those who are least responsible for this human- caused catastrophe will be under the greatest threat. Nurses encounter individuals and populations impacted by climate injustice. In this section, we explain the importance of nursing action for advancing just Relations[1] and Responsibilities for Planetary Health. We follow the wisdom of Māori nursing theorist Irhapeti Ramsden in approaching this work through the lens of Cultural Safety. Dr. Ramsden Teaches us to capitalize Cultural Safety as a first way of being observant on how power operates to erase the ways of knowing of the Maori and other Indigenous peoples. In addition, we explain the Global Nurse Agenda for Climate Justice and provide short examples to stimulate discussion, debate, and love as action in this and future generations of nurses.

Let us begin with a story. Stories are vital to our response to climate injustice: they help us integrate multiple ways of knowing. They provide us an inclusive way to share our urgency with others. The tribes of the Pacific Northwest have great Respect for the Salmon. Roger ,Fernandes is a storyteller from the čʔéɬxʷaʔ nəxʷsʌ́áy̓əm Lower-Elwha S'Klallam Tribe who gave us permission to share his version of the story of the Salmon Boy (Sčánnəxʷ Swiʔqúʔiɬ) (Fernandes, Personal communication May 24, 2023). Roger teaches storytelling at universities and in local schools. Story-telling is an oral

tradition and pedagogy that allows the listener to hear what they hear and everyone leaves with their own experiences of meaning and interpretation. Demonstrating Respect and ethical practice, we acknowledge that this is how we heard the story from Roger. He tells us that to save the Salmon is to save ourselves. These stories are powerful teachers and every time we hear them we learn something new.

There was a boy who disobeyed his Elders. He had been taught that when he finished eating a salmon, he was to return the bones back to the water to show Respect to the Salmon People and to use those bones so they could come back. One time when he was following other children from the Longhouse back down to the water to return the bones he decided he was too tired to go, and he threw the bones into the bushes saying to himself, "no one will ever know". Later that day he was playing down by the water on a big rock, and he slipped and fell into deep water, and he would have drowned if someone had not saved him. The Salmon People saved him, and they took him down to their village under the ocean where they were kind to him, fed him, and gave him warm blankets. All he had to do everyday was to play with the Salmon children. The boy was so happy he said to himself "I want to stay here, live here, I will never go back to the land".

But one day something happened that changed everything. He was playing with the Salmon children when he noticed a little Salmon girl hiding in the rocks out of sight of the others, playing by herself. He wondered why she wasn't playing with the others, and then finally he saw her try to walk out, and she was wincing and dragging one leg, because it had no bones in it, she tried to raise an arm, but it flopped sideways because there were no bones in it. Right away that boy knew what had happened. The bones he had thrown away never made it back to the Salmon People so that little girl was in pain, that little girl could not play with the others because of him.

And right then he knew he had to do something, so he went back to the Salmon People and asked permission to return to the land to tell them what he had learned. The Salmon People agreed but warned him that he would never be able to return, never be able to play in their village again. He thought hard and decided he would still go, because it was very important. And they took him back and he walked out of the water into his village. The people saw him coming and they saw he was

---

[1] Note on Capitalization: Indigenous scholars resist colonial grammatical structures and recognize ancestral knowledge by capitalizing references to Indigenous Ways of Knowing (Younging, 2018). Respect, Relations and Responsibilities are capitalized to acknowledge Indigenous Mi'kmaw Teaching of our collective Responsibilities to m'sit no'ko'maq (All our Relations). Respect for Land, Knowledge Keepers, Elders and the names of Tribes, including the Salmon People, and Indigenous institutions such the Longhouse are also denoted with capitals. For more see Table 1, Evans-Agnew et al., 2023.

alive when they had believed him to be drowned and would never return home to them again. As they ran to greet and hug him, he put his arms up and said "stop!" He told them he was no longer the naughty little boy that he once was, he told them he had important things to tell them. "The things we do on the land", he told them, "affect the things that live in the water. We must Respect and protect the house of the Salmon People". And this is what that little boy told his people of the time he lived with the Salmon People in their villages under the ocean. And that is all of the story called Salmon Boy and there are many ways to tell this story from different tribes but it is always the same, a boy returns to teach his people something he learned from the Salmon People to tell them something he learned.

Nursing is more than caring for a body, it is about communicating our Respect for the person and their ways of Relating and healing with the Land. We capitalize Land as a way of showing Respect for "all aspects of the natural world: plants, animals, ancestors, spirits, natural features, and environment (air, water, earth, minerals)" (Redvers, 2020, p.90). Much of this ANHE textbook is instruction for a deeper Respect for the environment. For us, nursing is about having Respect for the Land and the Relations that people have with their family, their community, and the Land in which they live. For example, the Salmon Boy in the story realizes the importance of his interconnection with the Land after seeing the consequences of his dis-Respect to his people and to the Salmon People. Returning to his village he committed to sharing his story and model to others the importance of Respect.

Irhapeti Ramsden's Māori nursing theory of Cultural Safety is centered on the experiences of the Māori and the theft of their Land and livelihood by the colonizing and capitalist practices of the British Empire (Ramsden, 2002). The focus of Cultural Safety is on the nurse and their actions that perpetuate ideologies of oppression such as colonization and white supremacy. Beginning with self-reflection, Cultural Safety challenges the nurse to identify *and take action to change* not only ourselves, but those economic, ecological, political, and social structures that are causing the person, family, and community to not feel safe. An important theoretical distinction is that the power to decide if care is safe (or not) is held by the person, family and community. Simply put, the nurse must Respect the people, the Land, and the agreements made between them.

Climate change is one of multiple unjust threats to *Good*[2] Relations with the Land: caused by extractive and colonial ideologies of domination and corporate capitalism and maintained through various patterns of violence that threaten Planetary Health (Faerron Guzmán et al., 2021). The consequences of these ideologies are unjust because those corporations and nations who have contributed the most to pollution suffer less than those persons, communities, and nations who have contributed the least (Lilienfeld et al., 2018; Shue, 1992). Consider people already dispossessed of shelter and living on streets in our communities: not only do they already have first-hand knowledge of their insecure relations with the Land and from surviving environmental threats, but when a climate change event occurs, they will be the first to experience the impacts. All people who have been marginalized from participating fully in decisions regarding how we live on the Land are frontline communities first affected by changes in Planetary Health (International Climate Justice Network, 2002). Another group affected are those that live on the "fencelines" of polluting industries and toxic dumps. A climate event such as a storm or smoke from a forest fire will have a cumulative impact on the health of a fenceline community (Radavoi, 2015).

Frontline and fenceline communities have long understood these oppressions and have been leaders in resisting patterns of white supremacy, colonialism, human supremacy, patriarchy, and corporate capitalism through the struggle for environmental justice. In 1991 the First National People of Color Environmental Leadership Summit, attended by over 1,100 people from every state and Puerto Rico, identified racist land use policies and the right to live, work, go to school, play, and worship in a clean and healthy environment in 17 principles for environmental justice (First National People of Color Environmental Leadership Summit, 1991). While it is considered widely to be a founding document of the Environmental Justice Movement, it is also a founding document for Planetary Health and Climate Justice. The first of the 17 principles affirms "the sacredness of Mother Earth, ecological unity and the interdependence of all species, and the right to be free from ecological destruction" (Commission for Racial Justice, 1992). This is why the story of Salmon Boy is so appealing because it reminds us of the many interconnected pathways between people and the environment, the importance of listening to and centering the voices of frontline and fenceline communities, and for respecting the Land.

---

[2] 'Good' is a term, used in many Indigenous circles, to set an intention to conduct ourselves and our work harmoniously. In Nursing this would align with Cultural Safety.

In 2021 the Alliance of Nurses for Healthy Environments convened an international steering committee to define Climate Justice and describe a Global Nurse Agenda (CJ Agenda) for action. This committee had included six nursing organizations from Canada, the US, and Latin America and began with centering the voices of nurses around the world and listening to frontline and fenceline communities[3]. They developed and curated a Climate Justice Podcast series with nurses in Chile, Colombia, Canada, Finland, Kenya, Oman, Uganda, Tasmania, and the United States (US). Members appraised the findings from a large street survey of urban and rural residents living in marginalized communities on their coping with environmental threats, and included one committee member's (Evans-Agnew) youth-guided photovoice investigation on Nurse Actions for Climate Justice with frontline teens living in the Pacific Northwest.

Members of the Climate Justice in Nursing Steering Committee drafted and then published a definition of Climate Justice as the "social, racial, economic, environmental, and multi-species justice issues of the climate crisis through centering the experiences and ways of knowing in frontline and fenceline communities and safeguarding the rights of Nature to achieve Planetary Health" (LeClair et al., 2022, p.S257). They then developed the CJ Agenda modeling it after the classic Bali Principles for Climate Justice (International Climate Justice Network, 2002) with a preamble setting out factual claims as the basis for nursing action, followed by five domains (Economic, Ecological, Ideological, Political,

and Social) and 33 principles for action. Launching this CJ Agenda at the 26th meeting of the United Nations Congress of Parties on climate change (COP26), they solicited feedback from the ANHE nursing community, adjusted the text, and then published the CJ Agenda on their website in January 2022 (ANHE, 2022). Steering committee members helped with dissemination of the CJ Agenda at national and international nursing conferences.

A small group went on to publish these principles. They sought leadership from L'nu nursing scholar De-Ann Sheppard[4] (Mi'kmaw) who encouraged the group to speak with Elder Dr. Albert Marshall (Mi'kmaw) to deepen engagement and thinking on how nurses should apply the CJ Agenda. This work resulted in a publication (Evans-Agnew et al., 2023) and a refinement of the CJ Agenda into 36 principles (Table 1).

Our conversations with Elder Albert taught us about the importance of the relationship when integrating our ideas with Indigenous Ways of Knowing Planetary Health. This work coincided with the publication of "The Determinants of Planetary Health: An Indigenous Consensus Perspective" and a global group of Indigenous scholars, practitioners, land and water defenders, respected Elders, and Knowledge-Keepers (Redvers, et al, 2022). In this text, they emphasize how the integration of multiple Ways of Knowing counteracts colonial understandings of time and science (Redvers et al, 2022). Their framework identified Indigenous determinants for planetary health nested within three levels of relationships: Mother Earth (respect for feminine/ancestral knowledge),

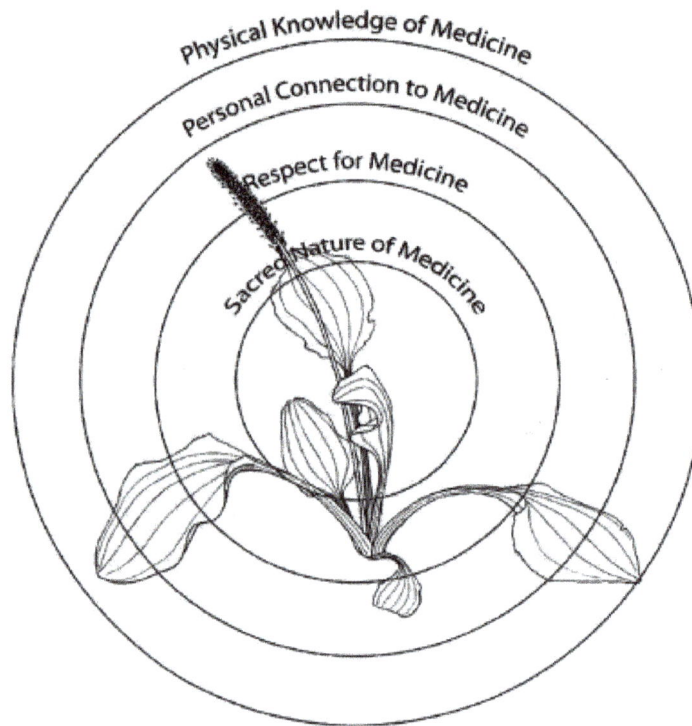

Figure 1 Elder Murdena's ways of knowing Mi'kmaw medicine

Image Acknowledgement: Elder Murdena Marshall
http://www.integrativescience.ca/Activities/

---

[3] Frontline communities are those that are often the first to experience the impacts of climate change and whose members have important insights and skills in coping and policy solutions (International Climate Justice Network, 2002. Fenceline communities are groups living close enough to an industrial or toxic environment to experience harm from the associated pollution and are at elevated risk for further harm from climate events (Radavoi, 2015).

[4] Atlantic Region Representative to the Canadian Association of Nurses for the Environment.

Table 1

Domain	Principles*
Economics and Health	1. Engage nurses across all sectors to lead climate change and environmental initiatives.
	2. Design and maintain circular economies in the greening of health systems and other systems for providing basic needs.
	3. Expose corporate actions that advance or maintain climate injustice and recognize the ecological debt multinational corporations owe the Planet.
	4. Hold institutions accountable for transfer of loss and damage resources for recovery.
	5. Direct the allocation of resources for climate resilience to frontline and fenceline communities.
	6. Establish partnerships with communities for adaptation in sustainable food, water, and agricultural practices.
	7. Demand safe working conditions for farmworkers, fisherfolk, and other frontline workers.
	8. Support a decarbonized, inclusive, equitable, and Just Transition for economies that encompasses a Planetary Health framework.
Ecology and Health	9. Develop deep practices in meaningfully engaging the self and others with the environment to advance ecological respect, healing, environmental and Planetary Health, environmental stewardship, and justice.
	10. Monitor and translate ecological assessment data on human-related risks and impacts to communities and systems.
	11. Adopt the conception of Indigenous communities for the rights of Nature to maintain its ability to recover and defend herself from the actions of human beings.
	12. Apply the precautionary principle in decision making related to introducing new technologies and employing old and untested technologies.
Ideologies and Health	13. Affirm the sacredness of Nature, ecological unity, and the interdependence of all species.
	14. Confront worldviews that center racism, classism, sexism, ageism, ethnocentrism, and anthropocentrism.
	15. Advance environmental health, Planetary Health, and human rights in nursing, public health, and healthcare education systems.
	16. Apply ways of knowing health beyond the boundaries of empirical knowledge to consider non-hierarchical and relational orientations towards understanding rupture and repair.
	17. Adopt (w)holistic orientations to the intertwining of health, environment, and humans toward Indigenous ways of knowing and care for life.
	18. Promote the transformation and updating of nursing ethics codes in every Nation within the frameworks of the Nursing Code of Ethics of the International Council of Nurses.

interconnecting determinants (humans, community relationships, science) and those determinants at the level of Indigenous Peoples (Land rights, language, health, Elders & children). There are important ways nurses should prepare themselves for action on Climate Justice and Planetary Health. Elder Albert and his (late) wife Elder Murdena have inspired the movement toward integrative medicine in Canada and in Planetary Health, bringing together both Indigenous and Western scientific ways of knowing (Integrative Science, nd). Integrative

science uses visuals to help explain concepts. Elder Murdena developed a drawing to explain ways of knowing Mi'kmaw Medicine (Figure 1) which helped us understand the ways of knowing Climate Justice.

The outer circle in the figure indicates our *Physical Knowledge of Medicine*. This is often the place where the power of western nursing science is at its greatest and where the science on climate change has had the most impact in changing minds and alerting the world to the

Table 1 (cont)

Domain	Principles*
Politics and Health	19. Adopt the 17 United Nations Sustainable Development Goals and the Decade of Action for achieving them at local, national and international levels.
	20. Lead adaptation and mitigation efforts in partnership with policymakers and communities on the frontlines of environmental degradation.
	21. Affirm democratically accountable government roles in the environment and support leadership of affected communities in the processes to address climate change.
	22. Support transparent and democratic practices for governmental decision making regarding climate justice including whistleblower actions against corruption.
	23. Organize for infrastructure system change (food, water, air, earth) through participatory action approaches.
	24. Transform international and national migration, immigration, asylum, and resettlement policies from concerns for border security to concerns for mitigating the human and ecological impacts of climate migration and advancing migrant health and adaptation in sending and receiving countries.
	25. Assure the interdependence of biodiversity and human health is represented in policies.
	26. Take collective action integrating western science with Indigenous knowledge holders to decolonize systems and address the effects of colonization.
	27. Lead social, economic, and environmental health for the well-being and sustainability of populations.
Social Systems and Health	28. Involve and participate with communities in climate justice actions through assessment, planning, activism, mitigation, adaption, & restoration.
	29. Design healthy social systems, such as through active transportation, green energy, and healthy and sustainable food ways.
	30. Improve responsiveness of healthcare and population health systems to climate events, including health system coding for climate-change.
	31. Develop and promote emancipatory social and relational systems and practices for intergenerational, intercultural, transdisciplinary, and international collaboration.
	32. Learn from Indigenous frames for social systems: living well together, being kind hearted and caring, and communicating honestly.
	33. Identify and mitigate the environmental, social, and mental health risk factors to which climate migrants are exposed as a result of their displacement and insertion in new contexts.
	34. Advocate for Universal Health Coverage and renew commitments to primary health care.
	35. Transform access to Nature for marginalized populations.
	36. Grow environmental consciousness through transformative experiences in embodied land-based, art-based, storytelling, drumming, and dancing.

*These principles were revised from the original by the Global Nurse Agenda for Climate Justice steering committee on 11-20-2022.

threat. Still at this level, we must also be observant of the other ways our patients and communities physically know Medicine. Working inward, the next circle of Knowing is Relational, our understanding of our *Personal*

Connection as nurses to *Medicine* and the ways in which we build Relations with others and the Land. This is a specialized area of nursing work, navigating social, emotional, mental, and environmental health in all our Relations. At the *Respect for Medicine* circle, we are challenged to consider justice in these Relations with the Land and consider actions that embody this Respect in the struggle for dignity, rights, and self-determination not just for humans, but also for Nature. The inner circle of Ways of Knowing medicine is the *Sacred Nature of Medicine*, those privately shared Relations with the Land and Medicine which bind groups of people together with the Land in ceremonial sharing for *Good*. The Sacred Nature of Medicine is the hardest for the nurse to connect with as an outsider, given that they are private, and require ancestral knowledge (Redvers et al. 2022).

To be able to comprehend the multiple levels in Elder Murdena's Ways for Knowing Mi'kmaw medicine, both individually, and [w]holistically, Elder Albert urged us to employ a Mi'kmaw concept known as *Etuaptmumk* or two-eyed seeing (Bartlett et al., 2012). *Etuaptmumk* values all perspectives and initially may seem simple, however, as you deepen your understanding and begin to see the nuances essential to Climate Justice nursing practice, you appreciate the gifts it brings. It helps us overcome our sense of powerlessness to act against the colonial matrix of domination, because when we witness a local injustice, we can - at the same time - comprehend how this event is interconnected with the whole, including ourselves. *Etuaptmumk* helps us Respect the plurality of ways of knowing in our patients and communities. *Etuaptmumk* helps us transcend western conceptions of time when we work across generations in building Relations and actions for justice. *Etuaptmumk* is a practice of Cultural Safety, where we recognize and act to address oppression, while simultaneously reflecting on our own biases and oppressions of others. *Etuaptmumk*, we feel, is the Knowledge that Salmon Boy brings back to his village.

Another Mi'kmaw verb, which we hope inspires nursing action to address Climate Justice and demonstrates the 'Why' for writing the CJ Agenda, is Ksaltultinej (love as action). Ksaltultinej is the only way to resist the internal and external forces of colonialism, supremacy and corporate capitalism: those oppressive structures in nursing that privilege Western Science and attempt to erase the importance of the Land. The "Mi'kmaw teachings of Etuaptmumk and Ksaltultinej call forth Responsibilities to act, and in doing so move us into a space of potential to resist [these] colonizing forces" (Sheppard, 2020, p.1).

Figure 2: "Hospital Design"

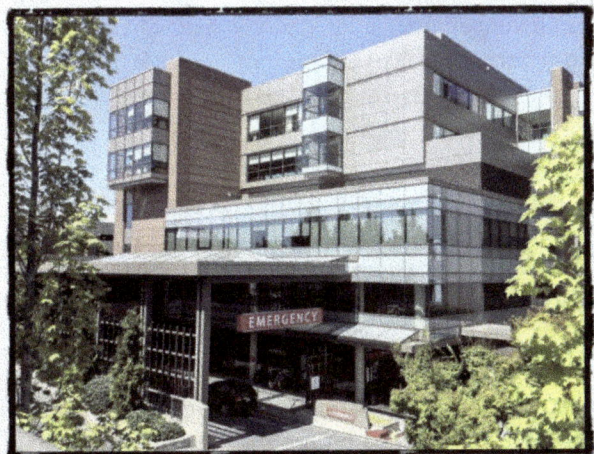

CHA: Hospital Design

You see a big building for emergencies and cars, it looks generally big and all that but in reality, once you enter it's like more cramped it's more like it's more small space it's not as like as big and spacious as shown in the outside. I think this can harm us because it is just a one location, that like many people would have to like try to get here, or need to drive here, which would harm the environment as well. I think there would be another alternative possibility that if hospitals were more spread apart to help everyone in the neighborhood all around the community: so that they wouldn't have to go too far and that they could just take bus, walk, or ride a bike to get to the clinic. So that it's closer and safer for them so that they wouldn't have to drive all the way over here which led to more problems to their environment and led to more problems.

Figure 3: "Sewer"

AD: Sewer

This is a sewer, which is next to a salmon stream. It's very disgusting it probably hasn't been cleaned in a long time. A lot of people don't pay attention to the sewers, and it smells really bad. And this is affecting the river. And it is letting harmful chemicals into the water, where salmon are swimming, and we eat those fish, and that's really bad for us and them. And also, it kills them. And we won't have fish like salmon anymore. it goes into the ocean and the harms fish, and it travels around the world It's not only affecting us, it affects everyone. People have a lot of waste and we just like to throw away stuff. And to things we love: like fishes and deer and other wildlife. We have this problem, because we have a lot of things that we don't need. And so what ends up happening is, it gets wasted and all this waste goes into these rivers. We have to stop buying unnecessary things. I think that one way we could maintain this sewer is maybe we could have people come in and clean and make sure it doesn't go into the ocean.

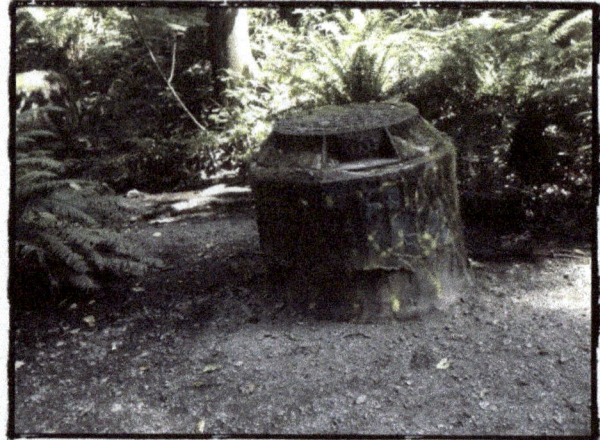

The obvious conflict for nurses as they confront the ravages of climate change and a Planet under multiple human-caused threats is the challenge of protecting frontline and fenceline communities from being further harmed in the choices we make to improve Planetary Health. Simply put, how will the working families who depend on the corporate industries of extraction (oil, plastics, chemical, precious metals, construction) be supported in the transition away from these industries? For example, in this era of climate change, the cycle of colonialism is driving more precious metal extraction for batteries in our electric cars. No amount of new technology invented to address climate change will mitigate the structures that inflict oppression and suffering. The Climate Justice in Nursing Steering Committee elected to embrace the concept of a Just Transition. A Just Transition calls for moving from an extractive mindset (dig, burn, dump) to a regenerative mindset (care, cultivate, cooperate) across local, national, and international systems (Evans-Agnew & Aguilera, 2022; Just Transition Alliance, nd). The values filter for the Just Transition (Just Transition Alliance, nd) inspired the five domains for nursing action in the CJ Agenda: shift economic control to community; advance ecological restoration; lift ideologies of racial justice and social equity; democratize wealth and workplace through political action, relocating production and consumption;

and retain and restore cultures and traditions for social health.

The CJ Agenda is an entry point for nurses to consider and imagine ways to advance Planetary Health in their locations, on their Land. The 36 principles provide suggestions for a variety of actions including research, education, advocacy, policy, and practice (ANHE, 2022; Evans-Agnew et al., 2023). They help us think of the multiple perspectives and settings for action through the application Etuaptmumk and Ksaltultinej. We provide brief examples aligned to the five domains of the CJ Agenda below in order to stimulate dialogue and generate Ksaltultinej. We illustrate each one with a photo and phototext provided by the Climate Justice in Nursing Steering Committee and the "Lakewood Teens for Climate justice" photovoice project (ANHE, 2022).

Economics: Principle #2, Design and maintain circular economies in the greening of health systems and other systems for providing basic needs (Figure 2).

Health care system facilities are significant climate polluting industries. Nurses witness first-hand the burden that plastic waste places on fenceline communities through incineration or dumping. There are several efforts that nurses can get involved in at hospitals and other facilities (Healthcare without Harm) and at their nursing training programs (Nurses Climate Challenge School of Nursing Commitment) that provide tools and resources for moving to circular economies in these systems: employing strategies to refuse, reduce, reuse, repair, and recycle resources, as well as climate mitigation and adaptation strategies.

Ecology: Principle #10, Monitor and translate ecological assessment data on human-related risks and impacts to communities and systems (Figure 3).

As this ANHE textbook indicates, nurses are increasingly being called on to appraise ecological assessment data from the testing and monitoring of water, soil, air quality, and climate predictions. Just like communicating complicated health protocols to patients and public health issues communities, nurses will need to be able to translate indicators of Planetary Health for the people and communities they provide care. Nurse educators on our Climate Justice in Nursing Steering Committee, especially those in Latin America, are calling for more integration between nursing education programs and the environmental sciences (Orostegui Santander, 2020; Palmeiro-Silva, et al., 2021).

Ideology: Principle #17, Adopt (w)holistic orientations to the intertwining of health, environment, and humans toward Indigenous Ways of Knowing and care for life (figure 4).

This textbook entry is concerned with listening to the wisdom of Mi'kmaw Elders and nurses. In the figure, the teen who took the photo of Yakama, Umatilla, and Nez Perce tribes on horseback has connected us to a fundamental (and Indigenous) ideology of reciprocity "they used, and they also gave". Integrative science is intended to offer a safe place for nurses with western viewpoints to begin to unpack their ideological constraints and to enter Relationships with Indigenous ways of knowing and Respect for Planetary Health. The most important way of knowing for the outsider here is Respect (see figure 1), and as such the nurse, when considering how to weave their understanding within another Indigenous conception must pay Respect to the original keepers of this Knowledge and not to pan-Indigenize. Name the Tribe, the Elder, the People who are teaching you this; pay them the Respect of naming them.

Politics: #19. Adopt the 17 United Nations Sustainable Development Goals and the Decade of Action for achieving them at local, national and international levels (Figure 5).

Competition between hospitals and healthcare systems may not make our cities more sustainable in the face of climate change, as competition can encourage hospitals to expend resources and energy to build identical and therefore redundant facilities (e.g. building fountains or

Figure 4: "Horses"

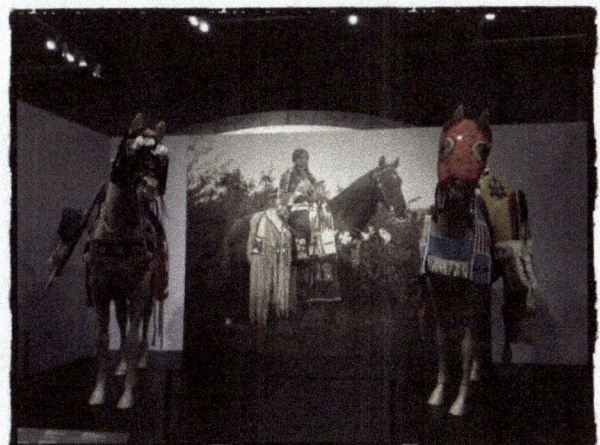

CHA: Horses

These are horses and clothing from the Yakama, Umatilla, and Nez Perce Native American tribes and Nations who live in our state. I think, as you can tell here like you can see bags and clothing. You can tell they used horses back then to travel to wherever they needed to go or whatever they needed to get, and also hunting as well. This was another use of transportation without using, as we know, cars and airplanes. Probably the best thing was that Native Americans used without hurting the environment, because they used and they also gave because since they were more into nature than other people were. This was a big benefit for a long time: they helped, took care of, and treated the earth as though it was its own thing. Maybe we can use different types of transportation. Not saying that we should stop using like cars and all that, but maybe we can use alternatives like buses or walking or bikes and skateboards as well to reduce the chemicals and harmful things. If we didn't use cars as transportation as much and used other means of transportation, we could be in a more sustainable environment. We can teach others and do change ourselves.

Figure 5: "Fountain"

TH: Fountain

This water fountain is outside of a hospital. This water fountain can be harmful for us. Because if we have an emergency, we have to go around the fountain. And I also think they put the fountain in there because they're trying to make the hospital look nice, putting a bunch of flowers around the hospital and having a fountain in front of it. So, I think they're trying to make the hospital look better and try to compete with other hospitals, so more people can go to their hospital and not other hospitals. What we should do, I think, is not care what our hospital looks like on the outside. Just because one hospital has a bunch of flowers and a fountain outside of it and the other one doesn't, it doesn't matter how it looks like on the outside because either way you're going to be treated the same way at either Hospital.

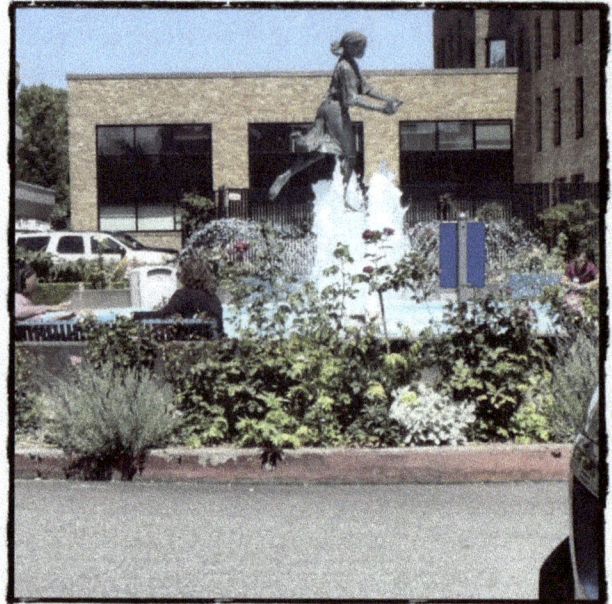

Figure 6: "Litter"

TJ: Litter

This is by a salmon stream. I was walking, taking pictures and I realized that there was a lot of litter and trash around the trails. I was trying to look around to see if there were any trash cans or signs, but there wasn't any trash cans on the trail. People get encouraged to throw their trash anywhere. And I think a lot of people that go there and they see that there's already trash there that kind of gives them like the green light to just leave their trash there because they're like, "Oh well no one else is doing it, no one comes and picks it up, we should just leave our trash here". So I think it's important if the park managers, the people that run the place or own that property to invest in putting trash cans and putting signs to encourage people to take care of the planet, and take care of the trails in the parks. Not just remodel but replace stuff and make it more eco friendly for the people that go there so its clean for all the people that are going to go there to hike.

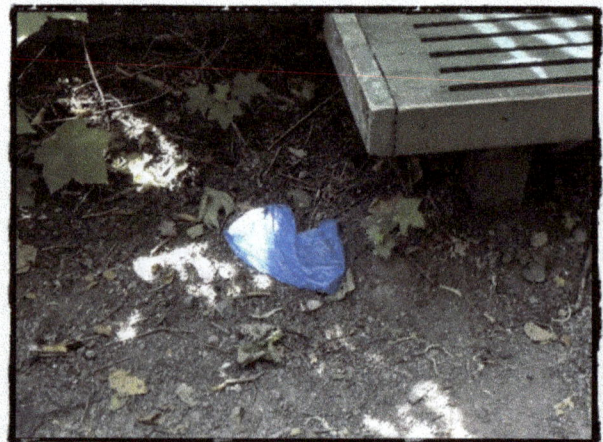

cancer "centers"). Nurses looking to frame their Climate Justice work in political action would do well to begin within the framework of the United Nations (UN) Sustainable Development Goals (SDGs). The SDGs provide 17 arenas for action (including climate) on a political stage and assume the interrelationship of the social determinants of health and our environment (Lilienfeld et al., 2018, United Nations, 2015). The origins of the UN climate change work is in the global movement for sustainability (Agyeman et al., 2002, Evans-Agnew et al., 2023). By investigating one or two of these actions, nurses can have something important to say in local and regional political movements concerning planning and development.

Social: #32. Learn from Indigenous frames for social systems: living well together, being kindhearted and caring, and communicating honestly (Figure 6).

We need to transform the way we work together as nurses. In the US we benefit from a broad range of opportunities for nurses, and yet we eat our young, we apply an artificial hierarchy to the health professions, and we experience burnout working in oppressive systems because we are using extractive mindsets in our social systems (Pagano, 2021). Just like the teen who took this photo observed, "no-one else is doing it [picking up our trash].. So we should just leave our trash here", social systems break down if we do not apply a value frame as a basis for beginning our work together. The struggle for Planetary Health and Climate Justice will be dangerous and taxing, nurses will need to work with humans and with Nature - Msit No'ko'maq (Mi'kmaw - All my Relations). Our strength will come from the ways we team up with others, across professions, disciplines, and ecosystems to sustain our efforts and practice Cultural Safety.

CONCLUSION

In this chapter we began with our interpretation of the story of Salmon Boy (Sčánnəxʷ Swiʔqúʔiɫ) to better understand what we now must do in the name of Climate Justice and Planetary Health. We have outlined a background and communicated the urgency of the need for advancing Climate Justice and Planetary Health in our work as nurses. We listened to Elder Albert Marshall and the wisdom of Mi'kmaw Ways of Knowing medicine through Etuaptmumk and Ksaltultinej. We listened to the voices of frontline youth who were asked what nurses should do for Climate Justice. We explored some of the history of how an international group of nurses, convened by the Alliance of Nurses for Healthy Environments, considered first the voices of frontline and fenceline nurses and communities from around the world, and then applied Ksaltultinej to suggest 36 actions for Climate Justice. We explained the ways nurses can make change today, just like Salmon Boy, to return to our villages, committed to sharing our stories and inspiring action in ourselves and others.

REFERENCES

Agyeman, J., Bullard, R. D., & Evans, B. (2002). Exploring the nexus: Bringing together sustainability, environmental Justice and Equity. *Space & Polity*, 6(1), 77–90. https://doi.org/10.1080/13562570220137907

Alliance of Nurses for Healthy Environments. (2022). *Climate justice agenda for nursing.* https://envirn.org/climate-justice-agenda-for-nursing/

Bartlett, C., Marshall, M., & Marshall, A. (2012). Two-Eyed Seeing and other lessons learned within a co-learning journey of bringing together indigenous and mainstream knowledges and ways of knowing. *Journal of Environmental Studies Science*, 2, 331-340. Doi: 1007/s13412-0120

Evans-Agnew, R. A. & Aguilera, J. (Accepted). Climate justice is environmental justice: System change for promoting planetary health and a just transition from extractive to regenerative action. *Health Promotion Practice.*

Evans-Agnew, R. A., LeClair J., & Sheppard D.M. (2023). Just-Relations and Responsibility for Planetary Health: the global nurse agenda for climate justice. *Nursing Inquiry*, (Online ahead of print), 1-16. DOI:10.1111/nin.12563

Faerron Guzmán, C. A., Aguirre, A. A., Astle, B., Barros, E., Bayles, B., Chimbari, M., El-Abbadi, N., Evert, J., Hackett, F., Howard, C., Jennings, J., Krzyzek, A., LeClair, J., Maric, F., Martin, O., Osano, O., Patz, J., Potter, T., Redvers, N., … Zylstra, M. (2021). A framework to guide planetary health education. *The Lancet - Planetary Health*, 5(5), e253–e255. https://doi.org/10.1016/S2542-5196(21)00110-8

First National People of Color Environmental Leadership Summit, (1991). *17 principles of Environmental Justice. First National People of Color Environmental Leadership Summit Washington, DC.* https://www.ejnet.org/ej/principles.pdf.

International Climate Justice Network (2002). *The Bali Principles of Climate Justice.* Corpwatch. https://www.corpwatch.org/article/bali-principles-climate-justice.

Just Transition Alliance (n.d.). *Just Transition Framework.* https://jtalliance.org/

Health Care Without Harm, (nd). *Healthcare Without Harm: Leading the global movement for environmentally responsible healthcare.* https://noharm.org/

LeClair, J., Evans-Agnew, R.A., & Cook, C. (2022). Defining climate justice in nursing for public and planetary health. *American Journal of Public Health*, 112(S3): S256–S258. https://doi.org/10.2105/AJPH.2022.306867

Lilienfeld, E., Nicholas, P. K., Breakey, S., & Corless, I. B. (2018). Addressing climate change through a nursing lens within the framework of the United Nations Sustainable

Development Goals. *Nursing Outlook*, 66(5), 482–494. https://doi.org/10.1016/j.outlook.2018.06.010

Nurses Climate Challenge (nd). Nurses Climate Challenge: US, Canada, & Europe. https://nursesclimatechallenge.org/

Orostegui Santander, M. A. (2020). *Elemento teórico del cuidado ecosistémico en el campo de la enfermería desde un enfóque curricular ecoformador.* Doctoral Dissertation, Simón Bolívar University, Barranquilla, Colombia. https://hdl.handle.net/20.500.12442/6899

Pagano, M. P. (2021). *Understanding health care in America: culture, capitalism and communication.* Routledge.

Palmeiro-Silva, Y. K., Ferrada, M. T., Ramírez Flores, J., & Santa Cruz, I. S. (2021). Cambio climático y salud ambiental en carreras de salud de grado en Latinoamérica. *Revista de Saúde Pública*, 55(17), 1-8. https://doi.org/10.11606/s1518-8787.2021055002891

Radavoi, C. N. (2015). Fenceline communities and environmentally damaging projects: An asymptotically evolving right to veto. *Tulane Environmental Law Journal*, 29(1), 1–29.

Ramsden I. M., (2002). *Cultural safety and nursing education in Aotearoa and Te Waipounamu.* Doctoral Dissertation, Victoria University, Wellington, NZ.

Sheppard, D. (2020). Getting to the heart of cultural safety in Unama'ki: Considering Ksaltultinej (love). *Witness*, 2(1), 51–65. https://doi.org/10.25071/2291-5796.57

Shue, H. (1992) 'The unavoidability of justice', in A. Hurrel and B. Kingsbury (Eds). *The international politics of the environment: Actors, interests and institutions*, pp. 373–97. Clarendon Press.

United Nations, (2015). *A/RES/70/1 - Transforming our world: the 2030 Agenda for Sustainable Development.* http://www.un.org/ga/search/view_doc.asp?symbol=A/RES/70/1&Lang=E

Younging, G. (2018). *Elements of Indigenous style: A guide for writing by and about Indigenous peoples.* Brush Education. https://www.brusheducation.ca/books/elements-of-indigenous-style

INTRODUCTION

The well-placed recent focus on structural issues that have contributed to racial and ethnic inequities, particularly in health and healthcare, have strengthened the importance of nurses intervening on the social determinants of health. Many of those structural issues are policies that in many ways contribute to factors that lead to health disparities. Nurses are uniquely educated and positioned to advocate for policies that improve the health of populations and communities through the creation of policies that place health in the forefront. The nursing process, though commonly applied in the clinical practice setting, provides the foundation for advocacy and policy in a broader setting. According to Gallup polls, nurses are the most trusted professionals and therefore play a critical role in shaping policies aimed at protecting the public. This section contains chapters that will demonstrate how the steps in the nursing process, assessment, diagnosis, implementation and evaluation, are readily transferable to the policy arena. In addition this section will also provide guidance, through stories, on how nurses can, and should, engage in advocacy initiatives to shape broader public health policy at the organizational, local, state and federal levels. Strategies for advocacy are discussed; these include building coalitions and influencing policy through legislative lobbying for environmental health policies.

USING NURSING PROCESS TO GUIDE ADVOCACY FOR ENVIRONMENTAL HEALTH

Aislynn Moyer, DNP, RN
Director of Nursing
Penn State Milton S. Hershey Medical Center
Hershey, PA

The nursing process is one of the first, and arguably most important, frameworks a nurse will ever learn. The key elements of assessment, diagnosis, planning, implementation, and evaluation guide everything that nurses do regardless of the area in which they practice. It is the very act of assessing and diagnosing patients with nursing problems that allows a nurse to best advocate for the patients he or she cares for. It only makes sense then that the same process would guide the way in which nurses advocate for themselves, and the larger nursing profession. Additionally, nurses can advocate for individuals and families, populations, policies, legislation, and environmental justice.

Advocacy can be defined as the act of supporting a cause (Merriam-Webster, 2014). The important piece of the definition is the act of supporting the cause. It is one thing to agree with a cause or a process, but to support it through an act is where advocacy is born. Many nurses have particular passions within the profession but are unsure of how to advocate for them. The nursing process is the natural guide to successful advocacy.

ASSESSMENT

The first step in the nursing process is assessment. A thorough assessment takes into account both objective and subjective data that then helps the nurse better understand the problem. It is important to gather as much data on a specific topic so that advocacy can be successful. Not understanding every side of an issue can be a big mistake. When an opponent of the issue raises a concern or a neutral party asks a question, the nurse advocate must be prepared to address the concern. This is not to say that the nurse advocate must know everything, but he or she should have a baseline comprehensive understanding of all sides of the issue. What is most important is that the nurse advocate understands how the issue impacts the profession of nursing.

DIAGNOSIS

Assessment leads naturally to the second step in the advocacy process: diagnosis. Diagnosing the problem requires the nurse advocate to step away from the collected data, form themes, and determine the root problem. It is important during this step to remember that the data collected is evidence of a problem. It is the problem that must be identified to successfully advocate for a solution. For example, if one were to advocate for all residents in a particular area to recycle but no recycling programs were easily accessible (pick up, drop off centers, etc.) the true problem would not be addressed. The advocacy would need to focus on recycling programs first.

PLANNING

The planning phase of advocacy comes naturally to most nurses in clinical practice. Once the problems are identified, there are usually specific actions that need to take place. This is not the case with advocacy, as many nurses are not sure how to take action for advocacy. As the old saying goes, knowledge is power. Education is always a good starting point. Think about who needs to understand the problem. Once education starts, others will begin to ask questions and challenge ideas. The nurse advocate must be able to discuss the given issue from all sides. In planning for advocacy there may not always be a clear direction to take. This is why it is important to stay open minded and be ready for opportunities. Always be willing to talk to those around you about your concerns; you never know who you may be talking to or what connections that person may have.

IMPLEMENTATION

The implementation phase of advocacy is continuously evolving and requires multiple skills.

Be ready. As mentioned in the planning phase, there may be new opportunities that present themselves so the nurse advocate should always be ready. It is important to get the information out to the public and key people who need to know about it such as legislators, agency leaders, and other nurses.

Do not be shy; be assertive. Using the knowledge the advocate has gained, it is important to not be shy. Write letters to newspapers, government officials, large organizations, and nursing journals. Post information to blogs and other social media outlets. Call in to radio or television shows that are discussing related topics. Offer to speak on the topic at local schools, conventions, or town hall meetings. Remember that how the advocate presents themselves verbally and in writing, will determine how much weight others put on the information being shared.

Be professional. Be sure to always be professional and objective. Do not get into arguments but rather state facts and allow others to share their opinions. If the advocate knows the problem well, they will already be expecting what those on the other side of the issue may say.

Be persistent. If important people with action power only hear about the issue once in a while, they tend to not put much weight to it.

Collaborate with others. The more decision-makers hear a message, the more they will be aware of the issue and possible solutions. Nurse advocates display their leadership by partnering with existing groups and requesting others' support for nurses engaged in advocacy. The foremost nursing organization that advocates for environmental health is the Alliance of Nurses for Healthy Environments (ANHE). The Policy/Advocacy Forum of ANHE can be found at https://envirn.org/policy-advocacy/

The following Table lists examples of environmental organizations that nurse advocates can partner with to reduce environmental health risks and promote healthy communities.

Organization name	Website	Organizational purpose
Safer Chemicals, Healthy Families	http://saferchemicals.org/	A national effort to protect families from toxic chemicals
Environmental Working Group (EWG)	http://ewg.org/	Empowers people to live healthier lives in a healthier environment. EWG drives consumer choice and civic action with breakthrough research and an informed public
Environmental Defense Fund (EDF)	http://edf.org/	We think differently about how to solve environmental problems, working across disciplines and with diverse groups of people
Health Care without Harm (HCWC)	https://noharm.org/	An international coalition of hospitals and health care systems, medical professionals, community groups, health-affected constituencies, labor unions, environmental health organizations and religious groups leading the global movement for environmentally responsible heath care
Center for Health, Environment, and Justice	http://chej.org/	Mentors a movement, empowering people to build healthy communities, and preventing harm to human health caused by exposure to environmental threats
Physicians for Social Responsibility (PSR)	http://www.psr.org/environment-and-health/	PSR's Environment and Health Program addresses toxics and global warming — challenges to life and well-being that pervade the entire planet

EVALUATION

Contrary to how it may seem, evaluation is not the end of the nursing process, but rather a checkpoint along the way. It is also a necessary step in the advocacy process. It is important that the nurse advocate take time to reflect on the advocacy that has been done and determine how to move forward. The nurse advocate should ask themselves questions: Is there more information that needs to be collected? Are there people or groups that I have not yet reached out to? What change has taken place in regards to this issue? What change is left? What other initiatives exist that support this cause? Can we partner together? Always go back and relook at assessment, diagnosis, planning, and implementation to see if anything needs to be updated or changed. This step is crucial in keeping your advocacy relevant.

Part of evaluation is also celebrating where you have come. Even if big change has not occurred, celebrate the fact that people were educated who previously did not fully understand the issue. Each small win contributes to bigger change. Do not be discouraged but rather be encouraged to keep pressing forward.

CONCLUSION

The nursing process becomes the subconscious guiding force behind all that nurses do. The same can be said for advocacy. By taking one's time to thoughtfully move through each phase, the nurse advocate can develop a successful plan of advocacy. Remember advocacy is a form of action. Find others who are passionate about the same topics and join together to take action. Advocacy is a powerful tool that can be used to transform people and guide change. Why wait? Get started today!

REFERENCE

Merriam-Webster. (2014). *Advocacy.* http://www.merriam-webster.com/dictionary/advocacy

COALITION BUILDING: A POWERFUL POLITICAL STRATEGY

Anne Hulick, JD, MS, RN
Director
Connecticut Clean Water Action
Coordinator
Coalition for a Safe and Healthy Connecticut

Hacah Boros, MSN, RN
Coordinator of Environmental Health
Connecticut Nurses' Association

Mary Jane Williams, PhD, RN
Professor Emeritus
Central Connecticut State University

Nurses are the most trusted professionals according to Gallup polls year after year (Gallup Poll, 2016). We hear this a lot. So what does it mean and how do we utilize the public's trust to advocate for policies that improve health for all citizens? The fact is that nurses are viewed by the public as highly educated healthcare practitioners that truly have their clients' best interest at heart. Patients trust us to advocate for them at the bedside, in the clinical setting and broadly, in the public arena. Unfortunately, nursing education does not often include courses or practicums on how nurses can advocate for more health protective policies. As a result, we don't view ourselves as the powerful leaders that we really are. We advocate daily with physicians and other members of the health care team but somehow don't think we are qualified to talk to lawmakers—who usually know far less than you do about nursing and healthcare. So can nurses play a role in shaping policy? It seems like a daunting task and one that most nurses are not comfortable with. And yet, we are from the very beginning, educated to advocate for patients. The irony is that while we may not think of ourselves as proficient at advocating with policy makers for laws that protect the health of citizens, nurses are uniquely positioned—and educated—to do just that!

So, how do we transfer the skills that we've learned and applied at the bedside to our state houses to be effective advocates for improving health? How do we acknowledge the trust placed in us by the public to make a difference on a broader scale? In this chapter, the reader will

- review the theoretical underpinnings and skills gained in our nursing education that are readily transferable to advocating for public policies to improve health for all citizens,

- learn how to apply those skills outside of the traditional healthcare setting, and

- learn to incorporate the leadership skills of team or coalition building to enhance the nurses' capacity to effect change on a broader scale.

Our professional role as advocates started with Florence Nightingale. Florence Nightingale was a strong nurse advocate who shaped the delivery of healthcare and health policy. She recognized the value of collecting and analyzing data to improve outcomes and to effectively communicate with leaders to help implement changes that improved health outcomes. She worked with supporters, colleagues and policymakers to enact broad social change (Mason et al., 2007, p. 14).

Since this time, the professional role of nurses includes competence in advocacy. The ANA Revised Code of Ethics for Nurses with Interpretive Statements states the nurse is expected to collaborate with "other health professionals and the public in promoting community, national, and international efforts to meeting health needs" and to shape social policy (Mason et al., 2007, p.36).

The International Council of Nurses (2008) states "nurses have an important contribution to make in health services planning and decision-making, and in development of appropriate and effective health policy. They can and should contribute to public policy related to preparation of health workers, care delivery systems, health care refinancing, ethics in healthcare and determinants of health." It is essential that the nurse recognize the concept of "upstream thinking" of primary prevention that addresses the notion that to protect the health of an individual, it is imperative to see the person holistically (Butterfield, 2002).

Despite this, nurses often don't recognize the skills and preparation gained through their nursing curriculum that enables them to serve as professional, credible advocates outside of the traditional clinical setting. Our educational preparation usually does not include practicum opportunities that allow us to apply the very same skills used in a hospital or clinical setting advocating for what is best for our patient to the statehouse or the board room where we advocate for public policies to improve health care systems. This is unfortunate as nurses often don't recognize that they are highly skilled advocates in these settings. Nurses often shy away from taking advantage of these opportunities and lose out on utilizing our collective power for transformative change (Patton, 2015).

NURSING PROCESS

How do we become more comfortable transferring the skills and expertise we gain from our practice to non-traditional settings where we can influence policy? It might not seem readily apparent but the nursing process that we use every day provides a strong framework for advocating for policy at the state house or other non-traditional setting. Without even thinking about it, nurses are adept at assessing the situation, developing a plan, implementing and evaluating that plan to achieve desired outcomes.

Lesson Applied

As a critical care nurse and nursing director, the nursing process was something that became second nature in my daily practice. Without thinking, I would assess my patients, develop and implement plans and evaluate outcomes. As a director, I would do the same—assess the situation, develop a plan to implement a new program on the units, implement the plan in collaboration with other members of the health care team and evaluate how it all went. This all changed when I had the opportunity to go to meetings at our state house to discuss concerns about the health impacts of exposure to chemicals. I found that I was nervous and unsure of how or what to say and lacked confidence in my ability to talk to legislators despite being knowledgeable on the subject. What I found, after reflecting on the meeting, was the nursing process applied here as well. I realized that during the meeting, I assessed the legislators' knowledge base and level of support and this guided how we proceeded during the meeting. Intuitively, we were able to gauge our discussion and develop a plan for next steps. This awareness helped to build confidence for future meetings, our advocacy work and our evaluation of next steps.

COMMUNICATION

From the start, nurses are taught effective communication skills in order to interact with patients, family members, and other members of the health care team. We are used to speaking with physicians to advocate for what we think is best for our patients—even when the physician or other member of the health care team may not agree. We are educated to take complex issues and explain them to different audiences and we are good listeners. Nurses are also used to giving organized reports to on-coming shift personnel which turns out to be a very effective template for advocating for policy changes with legislators.

Talking to policy makers or legislators is no different. Generally, nurses are much more educated on patient care, health issues, the health care system and relevant policies than most lawmakers. As we do in the clinical setting, nurses should incorporate peer-reviewed research and evidence-based practice when advocating for policy changes. Nurses' credibility as informed health professionals goes a long way in influencing policymakers that often have little experience with the health care issues you are working to address. Policy makers are often very busy with multiple issues from multiple constituents. Here again, nurses are highly skilled to communicate effectively in these types of situations. The practice of giving a report to another healthcare practitioner in advocating for a patient readily transfers to communicating with legislators. Nurses often use a consistent format to present the situation, background, assessment and resolution needed for a patient. Advocating for a change in policy fits this format nicely.

Lesson Applied

When I first started working as a nurse lobbying for more health protective chemical policies—like banning bisphenol-A from recyclable containers including baby bottles and infant formula containers, I was unsure what to say to legislators that I would see at the state house. I found they would often not have much time and somehow, I assumed that they knew more than I—after all, they were legislators. However, I always introduced myself, stated I was a nurse and explained that BPA is a synthetic chemical that disrupts hormones and is particularly harmful to infants and young children. Depending on the legislator's questions and time, I'd provide some background and hand them a research fact sheet that explains the problem and I'd end by asking for their support of the bill to ban BPA in these products. I realized that this method of communicating was no different than speaking with a physician or health care practitioner when I felt a patient needed an order for pain medication.

WORKING IN TEAMS

Nurses are critical members of the health care team, working with both licensed and unlicensed personnel to achieve the patient's goals. By virtue of our academic preparation, we learn to work collaboratively, to delegate, to supervise and to build effective working relationships with co-workers. Working with other team members, we identify patients' needs and work to achieve patient care goals. Nurses utilize leadership skills to coordinate patient care and advocate on behalf of the patients and families that they serve. These skills are vital to the work of advocacy and crucial to building coalitions—an important vehicle for advancing policy and one that will be discussed in more detail.

Nurses, often without recognizing it, are uniquely qualified and have critically important roles as advocates outside of their traditional work setting. Our knowledge and expertise, use of the nursing process, communication and leadership skills and our ability to work effectively in teams are the foundations for being effective leaders in health policy and advocating for changes that broadly impact public health. Providing mentoring and academic opportunities to practice these skills in non-traditional settings are needed to expand nurses' involvement in shaping policy at the local, state and federal levels.

COALITIONS - POWERFUL VEHICLES FOR CHANGE

Coalitions are groups of individuals and groups that come together around a common interest and agree to work together to achieve agreed upon goals (Berkowitz, 2007). Coalitions are actually a lot like health care teams —individuals with different backgrounds working to achieve patient care goals. These teams can be extremely effective or sources of frustration if the dynamics of the group are not managed well or mutual respect and a sense of team is lacking. In this section, we'll discuss what makes a coalition successful and share a case study in which nurses have led a successful coalition working to advocate for more health protective chemical policies.

COMPONENTS OF A COALITION

Mason, Leavitt and Chaffee suggest that successful coalitions have four common ingredients—leadership, membership, resources and serendipity or opportunity (2007, p.137). Leaders who can facilitate open dialogue; work with coalition members to tap into individual skills, comfort levels and expertise; and foster camaraderie and a sense of team are critical to a successful coalition. A leader who inspires others, creates a vision and organizing plan for the work, and facilitates sharing of the workload helps to build and sustain a passion for keeping coalition members engaged. The work of the coalition often arises from a problem or issue that is not easily solved within routine structures or methods. It is incumbent upon the leader to be able to help shape and articulate a winning strategy, build consensus, and communicate often so that all members feel included and empowered.

While the leader has an important role, successful coalitions utilize a shared governance framework and structure rather than the typical organizational structure that most are used to working in. While shared governance models have been typically implemented in

health care and academic settings, this framework is well suited for coalitions. While there are numerous definitions of shared governance, the concepts of partnership, accountability, equity and ownership are fundamental (Anthony, 2004). A shared governance structure means that accountability for outcomes is shared, that all members are on equal footing and decisions are made by consensus rather than a majority vote. This structure may be viewed as inefficient and cumbersome by some at first. However, proper facilitation and supporting individual members as they learn and grow in this work environment yields a strong commitment to the team, a sense of empowerment, and pride in the accomplishments of individual members and the group as a whole. Coalition partners that collaborate in this manner "demonstrate their willingness to enhance each other's capacity for mutual benefit and a common purpose by sharing risks, responsibilities, resources and rewards" (Himmelman, 2001).

Membership

When people come together to discuss collaborating on an issue, community problem or the need for policy change, the first step is to identify who else should be involved. Building diverse groups of individuals helps strengthen a coalition, build the base and power of the group, and promote a cohesive and unified vision. Reaching out to all stakeholders in the process is an important first step. Members of the coalition often represent various groups that lend strength and capacity to the overall mission. Again, similar to working in health care teams, nurses are used to working with members from different academic disciplines and yet are competent to coordinate the care plan for their patients. Similar skills apply when working with diverse coalition members. Here again, it is important to recognize and solicit the input of all coalition members, evaluate their skills and contributions to the work and achieving the goal, utilize this information to collectively develop a plan for achieving the goal and, together, implement the plan. Coalition membership may change for a variety of reasons including shifting priorities for coalition group members and individuals, funding, capacity to continue to support the coalition, and individual life choices. It is important to acknowledge this as a normal part of a Coalition's life cycle and to work to continue to build and strengthen relationships with new stakeholders, continue to develop coalition leaders, empowering them to their full capacity, and to stay focused on the overall goal.

STRUCTURE

The structure of the coalition may vary depending on the work, the membership, and the resources. Some coalitions may have a formal steering committee that almost serves as a board or advisory group along with other committees to achieve certain aspects of the work such as marketing and social media and advocacy. Other coalition structures may not be as formalized, with members assisting with all aspects of the work. No matter the structure, it is important for the leader and the members to assure that the principles of shared governance and the overall campaign are moving forward. While these structures are often not as formalized as those in a typical health care setting, the inherent nature of nurses' ability to apply the nursing process provides a valuable framework for routinely assessing and revising the plan. Nurses work collaboratively with other members of the team to gain consensus on adapting to changes, while still working towards the overall strategic goal.

COALITION MEETINGS

Nurses frequently interact with other members of the health care team as they are planning for and taking care of patients. These interactions help to build trust, promote collegiality and a sense of common purpose, and serve as the mechanism to achieve the goal—what is best for the patient. The same principles apply in coalitions though there are struggles. Regular meetings and communications are critically important for coalitions yet often challenging as members have regular jobs and other priorities. Face to face meetings allow coalition members to further develop personal relationships, a sense of belonging, and ownership for achieving the goal of the coalition. Using on-line meeting scheduling technologies help to schedule meetings at times that are best for all coalition members. See http://doodle.com/. In addition to in-person meetings, regular conference calls enable members to stay connected and develop short-term goals and activities that build the coalition's momentum. A combination of these formats is vital to establishing an overall identity and sense of purpose and structure for coalition members. Also these meetings help provide a framework for getting work done by busy coalition members. Coalition leaders must work hard to develop and strengthen relationships and a sense of "esprit de corps" outside of the traditional workplace setting.

RESOURCES

Coalitions may not have a lot of resources like funding or marketing or communications departments; so the membership of the coalition is often the most valuable resource. Members are involved for a reason—a common passion or vision. There is nothing more powerful and it is critical that this energy is tapped into and utilized to its fullest capacity. Each member brings unique skills and abilities to the team, which the leader must tap into, develop and rely on. Empowering members of the coalition so that they are contributing and growing in their roles helps to achieve and sustain momentum and builds the power of the coalition far beyond what a marketing or communications department might be able to do.

Members of the coalition also serve as the best marketers of the coalition and the goal that the group is working on. Using social media, setting up on-line invitations to events, sharing the day to day work on websites, Facebook and other sites, helps to build the campaign, expand name recognition and engage others in the coalition's work.

NEXT STEPS

Now that you have the coalition's goal in mind, the key stakeholders involved and a structure and processes for getting the work done, what are next steps? Again, our basic nursing preparation serves us well. Developing a campaign plan with a coalition is not all that different from developing a plan of care for a patient with other members of the health care team—and nurses do this with great skill.

The coalition plan or campaign plan is really no different in that it includes the team's assessment of problems and barriers, identifying stakeholders and developing a plan that lays out the key steps and accountabilities that ultimately lead to achieving the goal. The plan is often laid out so that it provides a long-term view of all the steps and processes needed to achieve the goal and is intended to be a working document that is revised, updated and modified along the way. More on campaign planning can be found here: http://knowhownonprofit.org/campaigns/campaigning/planning-and-carrying-out-campaigns/planning.

PROMOTING THE COALITION

The importance of building name recognition and promoting the work of the coalition cannot be underestimated. Doing this well assures that current members will stay engaged and energized, new members will be attracted, decision-makers will be aware of the objectives and goals of the coalition, and a momentum for success will be developed and shored up for the long haul—even when the going gets tough. Everyone wants to be on a winning team so it is important to convey the message that you are winning or at least, achieving concrete positive steps towards a win even if you are not winning right now. It is critical that you keep the coalition in the news and in the forefront of people's minds.

How do you promote the Coalition with limited resources and capacity? Fortunately, using social media is a great first step. Setting up a campaign website and Facebook page can make a huge difference in sharing the coalition's name and goal as well as serve as a vehicle for 'action-alerts' and mobilizing people to events. Encouraging coalition members to write letters to the editor and opinion editorials are also great ways to share the coalition's priorities develop coalition leaders and show a diversity of members that support the cause. Also, it is helpful to identify contact members of key media outlets who will receive press advisories and releases from the coalition. Reaching out to members of the media to build relationships and educate them on the issues that the coalition is working on also goes a long way to building momentum for your campaign. Here again, nurses are well suited to promote communications and marketing of the coalition's work. Typically, printed letters and opinion pieces need to be short, concise and compelling, much like the routine communication skills that nurses use to advocate for patients' needs. Similarly, when talking with reporters and other members of the media, nurses are highly credible and adept at framing the issue and the means to resolve the problem. Gaining comfort talking with members of the media is really no different than talking with other members of the health care team and is a valuable skill for nurses to utilize when working with coalition partners on policy initiatives.

While social media is a great tool, there is nothing more important in building and sustaining a coalition than building true relationships. Coalition leaders should invest time in personal connections, reaching out to new members and groups and understanding the value of supporting mutually beneficial work. A new group that may be interested in the Coalition's mission will likely appreciate and remember an offer to attend the group's meeting or event. Helping new members or groups with things that they need builds a symbiotic relationship that strengthens a coalition. Staying connected with personal phone calls, thank you notes or meeting for coffee go a long way to help new members and groups feel engaged in the coalition and build a sense of team, even when members are not physically working together on a daily basis

RESOURCES FOR COALITION BUILDING
- Beyond Intractability: Coalition Building
- Developing Effective Coalitions: An Eight Step Guide

- Community Tool Box: Starting a Coalition

CASE STUDY: The Coalition for a Safe and Healthy CT

In 2007, members of the Connecticut (CT) Nurses' Association, CT Nurses Foundation, the CT Public Health Association, the CT Coalition for Environmental Justice, Connecticut, CT Citizens Action Group, CT Clean Water Action and ConnPIRG, came together to discuss the growing body of evidence linking exposure to toxic chemicals in consumer products with the rise in many diseases. None of these organizations were working on this issue at the time yet, key leaders of these groups recognized a need to collaborate to raise awareness and to develop campaign strategies to press for more health protective policies at the state and federal level. During the initial meetings, a decision was made to form a coalition of like-minded organizations and member groups and to map out a plan to educate policymakers and citizens across Connecticut. It also provided an opportunity for the organizing groups to share resources, garner expertise, and set short term and long term goals to address environmental issues in a coordinated proactive manner. It provided an opportunity to bring a more powerful voice to the legislative process. The Coalition provided a more organized effort as we approached issues considered relevant to changing policy at the state level.

Coalition leaders identified that focusing on the presence of toxic chemicals such as lead and phthalates in toys would serve as a great way to elevate the profile of the issue, garner media attention and generate public support. Giving presentations at events, schools, and meetings all over the state helped to get the word out and to establish the Coalition's identity. These forums were also effective at engaging new members and building momentum for a winning campaign to pass a law in Connecticut restricting lead and phthalates in toys!

The Coalition continued to build on this success by working with national experts and partners to identify other chemicals like bisphenol-A (BPA), a commonly used chemical found in polycarbonate plastic (like baby bottles), thermal receipt paper and the lining of aluminum cans. BPA is also a hormone disruptor and strongly linked to breast cancer, reproductive disorders, insulin resistance and diabetes. In 2009, the Coalition expanded its grassroots campaign, added new members, organized several high profile events to garner media attention and successfully passed a landmark bill banning BPA from recyclable containers and infant formula containers! This was a huge win against extraordinary odds and tremendous opposition from the industry lobbyists. No other state had successfully banned BPA this broadly and Connecticut was now leading the way!

The Coalition has stayed together and grown stronger through in-person meetings, weekly conference calls, and using consensus-based decision making in all of its work. A strong focus on developing individual members' interests and leadership skills helps to keep people feeling good about their contributions even as they fluctuate over time and as other commitments come up. Coalition partners continue to work hard on outreach, engaging new members, providing education, and engaging with media outlets and policy makers to press for on-going reform. Frequent updates to the website and social media help to keep citizens engaged and active in Coalition activities.

REFERENCES

Anthony, M., (January 31, 2004). Shared governance models: The theory, practice, and evidence. *Online Journal of Issues in Nursing, 9*(I). www.nursingworld.org/MainMenuCategories/ANAMarketplace/ANAPeriodicals/OJIN/TableofContents/Volume92004/No1Jan04/SharedGovernanceModels.aspx.

Berkowitz, B., & Wolf, T. (2000). *The Spirit of the Coalition.* American Public Health Association. Cited from Mason, D; Leavitt, J and Chaffee M; (2007) *Policy and Politics in Nursing and Health Care,* 5th edition p. 135.

Butterfield, P. G. (2002). Upstream Reflections on Environmental Health: An Abbreviated History and Framework for Action. *Advances in Nursing Science,* 25(I), 32–49. http://nursing.wsu.edu/Research/PDFs/Upstream_Reflections_on_Environmental_Health__An.6%20(1).pdf.

Gallup. (2016). *Honesty/Ethics in Professions.* http://www.gallup.com/poll/1654/honesty-ethics-professions.aspx.

Himmelman, A.T. (2001). On coalitions and the transformation of power relations: Collaborative betterment and collaborative empowerment. *American Journal of Community Psychology,* (29)2:278.

International Council of Nurses. (2008). *Participation of nurses in health services decision making and policy development.* http://www.icn.ch/images/stories/documents/publications/position_statements/D04_Participation_Decision_Making_Policy_Development.pdf.

Mason, D., Leavitt, J., & Chaffee, M. (2007). *Policy and politics in nursing and health care* (5th ed.). W. B. Saunders Company.

Patton, R.M., Zalon, M. L., & Ludwick, R. (Eds.). (2015). *Nurses making policy: From bedside to boardroom.* Springer Publishing Company.

CASE STUDY IN ENVIRONMENTAL HEALTH ADVOCACY
Sarah B. Bucic, MSN, APRN-BC Member, Nurses Healing Our Planet (NHOP)
Delaware Nurses' Association

It started with Styrofoam. The hospital cafeteria was under renovation and suddenly all plates and trays went from paper to Styrofoam. As a staff nurse and founder of Nurses Healing Our Planet (NHOP), Michelle Lauer took notice of the change and was concerned by the seemingly endless heaps of non-recyclable garbage being generated. Spurred by participation in the hospital's shared governance council as well as returning to school for her Master's in Nursing Science degree, Michelle felt empowered and compelled to get involved in changing hospital policy on recycling. She joined the 'green team' that was forming in the hospital and started learning about environmental nursing.

After a positive discussion with the Director of Nursing Education, Michelle was encouraged to reach out to the nursing staff for help in hospital waste reduction. Several volunteers, with a similar vision, agreed to participate in her efforts. To better understand the scope of the problem, the group followed the hospital trash trucks to the landfill. It was an eye opening experience as they noticed the landfill was filled to capacity. Turns out, hospitals in the United States produce more than 5.9 million tons of waste annually and often have not developed recycling strategies or green teams. This spurred the nurses to develop and implement a hospital-wide recycling program that started with placing recycling receptacles at the hospital. Eventually five baby units began to recycle baby bottles and, in the emergency room, one-time use items such as urinals, bedpans and emesis basins were changed from plastic to a durable cardboard.

The group agreed that environmental health issues should not be limited only to the waste the hospital generated but should be a state-wide effort. This led to the formation of Nurses Healing Our Planet (NHOP), an ad-hoc committee of the Delaware Nurses Association in 2007. "We were really on a roll," said Michelle.

Flushing or pouring down the drain was the standard practice for medication disposal which resulted in contaminated drinking water. One of the first projects for NHOP was to provide another means for the public to dispose of unused/unwanted medications. NHOP members worked with the Drug Enforcement Agency (DEA) to hold the first pharmaceutical drug take back events in the state of Delaware. These events became successful due to the support and effort of State and Federal agencies, pharmacists and many volunteers. The take back events created public awareness of contamination of the drinking water caused by pharmaceuticals, how best to dispose of medications, and discussions about management of controlled substances. Many other states were moving in the direction of safe drug disposal at the time of these events. This led to national drug take back events coordinated by the Drug Enforcement Agency. Each year, spring and fall, drug take back events across the country eliminate thousands of pounds of drug waste from entering the nation's water supply and reduce risk of drug abuse.

NHOP received grant funding from the Campaign for Safer Cosmetics to increase awareness of toxics in personal care products among nurses and the public. The Campaign for Safer Cosmetics is a broad based coalition whose mission is, through public advocacy, to eliminate drugs known to cause cancer, reproductive harm and other adverse health impacts in cosmetics and personal care products. Through public education, NHOP crisscrossed the state advocating for safer products and elimination of cancer-causing chemicals. Nurses Healing Our Planet was very busy in 2009. The group developed a partnership with the University of Maryland Nursing Environmental Health Education Center. Through this relationship, NHOP members learned about an array of other environmental health issues that required attention at the State and National levels. NHOP nurses attended the Clean Med conference that year and collaborated with other nurses at the conference to send postcards requesting that cows, providing milk for a common brand of yogurt, not to be treated with growth hormone. One year later, the yogurt maker announced it would no longer make yogurt with milk from cows treated with recombinant bovine growth hormone (RBGH).

Concurrently, in Delaware, a coal burning power plant was being proposed for development. NHOP nurses testified against the power plant and in favor of a wind farm as an alternative energy source. Citizens for Clean Power and NHOP partnered for a grassroots campaign against the coal plant proposal, citing health effects of the coal and gas power plants. The efforts included letters to the newspaper and testifying before the regulatory body. Fortunately the outcome was the proposal did not move forward and Delmarva Power, the local utility, now factors in the health effects on how they generate electricity.

At this time, NHOP learned about babies being born "pre-polluted." A study showed an average of 200 industrial compounds, pollutants and other chemicals in umbilical cord blood of 10 newborn babies, with a total of 287 chemicals found in a study group. Of the 287 chemicals found in umbilical cord blood, 180 cause cancer in humans or animals, 217 are toxic to the brain and nervous system, and 208 cause developmental problems. The dangers of exposure to these chemicals in combination have never been studied (EWG, 2005). An NHOP nurse worked at changing hospital policy by replacing plastic products with phthalates-free products in the NICU. At this time, nationally these products were being removed from IV bags and tubing in the hospital setting.

NHOP also met with Delaware congressional legislators regarding the Safer Chemicals Act of 2011. NHOP recognized that Federal law does not adequately protect Americans from toxic chemicals. These chemicals are being found in makeup, personal care products and items used everyday. The primary law responsible for ensuring the safety of chemicals, called the Toxic Substance Control Act (TSCA), was passed in 1976 and has not been updated since. The law is so weak that the U.S. Environmental Protection Agency (EPA) has only been able to require testing on less than 2% of the more than 80,000 chemicals that have been on the market since TSCA was adopted (Denison, 2009). NHOP continues to meet with our U.S. Senators regarding the Chemical Safety Improvement Act (CSIA) S.1009. As drafted, the CSIA would not deliver the critical elements of meaningful public health and environmental protection. NHOP believes the bill should not move forward unless fundamental issues are fully addressed as outlined by Safer Chemicals Healthy Families.

In 2010, NHOP became aware of Bisphenol-A (BPA), which is a hormone-disrupting chemical. BPA can mimic or block hormones and disrupt the body's normal functions and is found in baby bottles, sippy cups, the linings of food cans, and in paper register receipts. BPA is also found in medical devices and equipment such as plastic flasks, beakers and containers. BPA can leach, especially when heated, from products into food and drinks (Calafat, 2009). Monitoring studies find the chemical in more than 90% of the adult population (Calafat, 2008). With this information, members of NHOP worked with local legislators, some who were Registered Nurses, to pass a Resolution, which enumerated and recognized the health concerns related to BPA.

One year later, members of NHOP worked on helping Delaware become the 10th state to implement a ban on BPA in children's products by getting support letters,

going to meetings and educating legislators about the harms of BPA. Working with State Senators and Representatives who were Registered Nurses greatly accelerated the bill's movement and NHOP learned a lot about the legislative process in the interim.

The BPA ban passed unanimously in both House and Senate but members of NHOP had to prepare testimony about BPA and its effects should the legislature ask for more information. The bill's sponsors requested NHOP members to be present each time the bill was presented in a committee meeting or voting sessions should testimony be required or questions asked. This required a number of NHOP trips to Legislative Hall. NHOP quickly formed collaborations with Natural Resource Defense Council, the Mid-Atlantic Center for Children's Health and the Environment, Delaware Chapter of the American Academy of Pediatrics, Physicians for Social Responsibility, the Breast Cancer Fund, and the Consumers Union. Many provided support letters and some came in person from Washington D.C. in case testimony was necessary. In June 2011, the Governor of Delaware signed into law a ban on BPA in children's products. The ban prohibits manufacturers from selling or offering to sell any children's product containing BPA. Knowingly selling products with BPA intended for children under age 4 designed to be filled with food or liquid, is now a Class A Misdemeanor in Delaware. It was especially exciting to see that in 2012, when the FDA banned BPA from baby bottles and sippy cups nationally due to a request from the American Chemistry Council, the American Chemistry Council directly cited the number of state bans that had passed as a reason for requesting the FDA ruling (FDA Regulations, 2013; Safer States, 2013).

There are limited ways for the general public to safely dispose of mercury thermometers and thermostats. In 2011, NHOP organized a dual county mercury return in collaboration with the Delaware Division of Public Health and two local hospitals where mercury thermometers were collected, in exchange for a digital thermometer, and safely disposed of by the Division of Public Health. Overall, 10 pounds of liquid mercury was collected. Delaware Division of Public Health provided the electronic thermometers and disposed of the mercury waste free of charge. Collaborations are key in environmental health!

NHOP hosted an environmental health nursing conference in 2011 featuring our Secretary of Natural Resources in Delaware. NHOP invited nursing students, as we know that the next generation of nurses will need to understand the context in which they and their patients will be living and working.

In 2011, along with other environmental groups, NHOP requested the Governor of Delaware to create a Comprehensive Energy and Climate Change Plan.

NHOP members have testified in Washington D.C. for the American Nurses Association on the Clean Air Act to keep it strong for the health of their patients and the public. NHOP has participated in stroller brigades in Delaware and Washington D.C. and two nurses have been Delaware Clean Air Ambassadors on behalf of the American Nurses Association. There are also a number of nurse luminaries in the NHOP group.

NHOP continues to follow and support progress being made on uncovering the health effects of hydraulic fracturing (fracking) and flame-retardants. Flame retardants, used for over 30 years, can be found in consumer electronics, furniture, and mattresses and find their way into blood, breast milk, and umbilical cord blood impairing memory, learning, and behavior in laboratory animals at very low levels. They may also affect thyroid hormones and reproduction. Most at risk are developing fetuses, infants, and young children (Washington Toxics Coalition, 2005).

Through 2014 and beyond, NHOP will continue to participate in work groups, such as the Delaware plastic bag workgroup, which discussed options of plastic bags, educates nurses and the public on environmental concerns that affect health, partners with environmental groups such as the Delaware Sierra Club and give talks on energy, air quality and their health effects.

NHOP writes an environmental article for each publication of the Delaware Nurses Association quarterly newspaper, The Reporter. Our group continues to write op eds and letters to the editor and most importantly be the voice for the health of our patients when environmental issues arise.

REFERENCES

American Nurses Association (ANA). (2007). *ANA's principles of environmental health for nursing practice with implementation strategies.* http://www.nursingworld.org/mainmenucategories/workplacesafety/healthy-nurse/anasprinciplesofenvironmentalhealthfornursingpractice.pdf.

Calafat, A. M., Weuve, J., Ye, X., Jia, L.T., Hu, H. Ringer, S., Huttner, K. & Hauser, R. (2009). Exposure to bisphenol A and other phenols in neonatal intensive care unit premature infants. *Environmental Health Perspectives, 117*(4), 639–644. http://www.ncbi.nlm.nih.gov/pmc/articles/PMC2679610/.

Calafat, A. M., Ye, X., Wong, L.Y., Reidy, J.A., Needham, L. L. (2008). Exposure of the U.S. population to bisphenol A and 4-tertiary-octylphenol: 2003-2004. *Environmental Health Perspectives, 116*(1), 39–44. http://www.ncbi.nlm.nih.gov/pmc/articles/PMC2199288/.

Denison, R. (2009). Ten essential elements in TSCA reform. *Environmental Law Review, 39,* 10020-10028. http://www.edf.org/sites/default/files/9279_Denison_10_Elements_TSCA_Reform_0.pdf.

Environmental Working Group (2005, July 15). *Body burden: The pollution in newborns: A benchmark investigation of industrial chemicals, pollutants and pesticides in umbilical cord blood.* http://www.ewg.org/research/body-burden-pollution-newborns.

FDA. (2013). *FDA Regulations No Longer Authorize the Use of BPA in Infant Formula Packaging Based on Abandonment; Decision Not Based on Safety.* http://www.fda.gov/Food/NewsEvents/ConstituentUpdates/ucm360147.htm.

Practice Greenhealth. (2014). *Waste: Background.* https://practicegreenhealth.org/topics/waste.

Safer Chemicals Healthy Families. *The Toxic Substances Control Act.* http://saferchemicals.org/legislative-update/.

Safer States. (2013, January 17). *Updates on the fight against BPA.* http://www.saferstates.com/assets/BPA-policy-history.pdf.

Washington Toxics Coalition. (2005) *Toxic flame retardants (PBDEs): A priority for a healthy Washington, A toxic free legacy coalition fact sheet.* http://watoxics.org/files/pbde-factsheet/at_download/file.

CHEMICAL POLICY REFORM
TOXIC CHEMICALS IN THE ENVIRONMENT:
EFFORTS TO CONTROL AND REGULATE

Jeanne Leffers, PhD, RN, FAAN
Professor Emeritus
University of Massachusetts Dartmouth

Katie Huffling, DNP, RN, CNM, FAAN
Executive Director
Alliance of Nurses for Healthy Environments

The issue of hazardous chemical exposure is a serious concern for nursing practice, education, research and advocacy. In the United States, efforts to regulate chemical safety have not been effective. The vast majority of the more than 80,000 chemicals developed during the past sixty years have not been evaluated for safety to humans. However, during that time, a large number of chemicals have been implicated as possible causes of a variety of health conditions such as cancer, reproductive health issues including birth defects, neurological conditions such as autism, and learning disabilities, and chronic diseases such as cardiovascular disease, pulmonary diseases and diabetes.

The first legislation to control chemicals was the Toxic Substances Control Act of 1976 (TSCA). TSCA was enacted with the purpose of controlling harmful chemicals but has not been an effective law to protect humans. Further, it was the only major piece of environmental legislation never updated.

During the past few years, US legislators have proposed changes to the law. The late Senator Frank Lautenberg first introduced a bill in 2005 to improve the federal government's surveillance, testing and control of chemicals for safety. In April 2011 Senators Senator Frank Lautenberg (D-NJ) Senator Inouye (D-HI) and Senator Kirsten Gillibrand (D-NY) introduced the Safe Chemicals Act but this bill died in Congress and was not enacted. Later efforts such as the Chemical Safety Improvement Act were not enacted. This bill would have limited individual state's power to enact stronger laws, creating weaker chemical standards and putting human health at greater risk.

On March 10, 2015, Senators Udall (D-NM) and Vittner (R-LA) introduced S.697. The Senate passed this on December 17, 2015. Congressman John Shimkus (R-IL) introduced the TSCA Modernization Act in the House and it passed 398 to 1 on June 22, 2015. As these bills were different approaches to the same issue, the bills were sent into Conference Committee where members of the Senate and House negotiated a final bill that would be voted on in both Houses. On May 24, 2016, the House of Representatives voted to pass a bipartisan House-Senate agreement of the Frank R. Lautenberg Chemical Safety for the 21st Century Act, HR 2576 by a margin of 403-12. The US Senate then passed this on June 7, 2016 and the act was signed into law by President Barack Obama on June 22, 2016.

According to Safer Chemicals Healthy Families, the new Lautenberg Act gives the EPA new authority to strengthen chemical safety and protection of the health of the people living in the United States. However, as EPA is only mandated to address 30 chemicals within the first 3.5 years after enactment, the pace with which unsafe chemicals will be addressed will be very slow. The law:

- Requires EPA to regulate a chemical based solely on its health and environmental impacts. This replaces TSCA's burdensome cost-benefit safety standard—which prevented EPA from banning asbestos.

- Establishes a minimum enforceable schedule and requires EPA to "begin safety reviews on 10 chemicals within 180 days of enactment and then another 20 chemicals from the high priority list within 3.5 years."

- Expedites action on persistent, bioaccumulative, and toxic (PBT) chemicals;

- Explicitly requires protection of vulnerable populations like children and pregnant people.

- Gives EPA enhanced authority to require testing of both new and existing chemicals.

- Sets judicially enforceable deadlines for EPA decisions.

- "[R]equires that manufacturers substantiate the basis for claiming chemical identity as confidential and creates a deadline for EPA review of confidential business information (CBI) claims." Under the new law, EPA can now share information with states and health and environmental professionals as long as confidentiality is maintained.

- Still has no minimum health and safety data requirements for new chemicals; however EPA must make an affirmative finding that the chemical is not likely "to present an unreasonable risk before a company can begin to manufacture."

- States can regulate a chemical until the EPA designates it a "High-Priority" chemical. The state's regulation will then be pre-empted until EPA decides on its restrictions (a process that can take 2-3 years). (Safer Chemicals, Healthy Families, 2016)

While the health and advocacy community did not achieve many of the health protective policies that they had worked to include in TSCA reform, this bill is an improvement over TSCA and the June 22, 2016 signing was an historic event.

Concern for issues such as chemical policy reform does not end with the passage of this Act into law. Nurses, citizens and advocacy groups continue to advocate for better policies to protect human health. For example, the advocacy group Safer Chemicals, Safer Families is a coalition that represents millions of individuals from citizens to health care professionals. More than 450 organizations are represented in the coalition. Of these 16 are nursing organizations including the Alliance of Nurses for Healthy Environments (ANHE), the American Nurses Association, the National Association of Hispanic Nurses, the American College of Nurse Midwives, and state nurses associations from Connecticut, Delaware, Idaho, Maryland, Massachusetts, Ohio and Washington state.

The coalition seeks to achieve:

5. A well-educated public that can use its power as both citizens and consumers effectively. (Strong federal and state policies to protect the public from toxic chemicals.)

6. Strong corporate policies to substitute safer chemicals for those that are already known to be toxic.

7. A well-educated public that can use its power as both citizens and consumers effectively (http://saferchemicals.org/what-we-want/)

The Safer Chemicals, Safer Families coalition offers information for the public such as their section on chemicals and health as well as action plans such as the Stroller Brigade and the Mind the Store campaign.

Many nurses have been active in chemical policy reform for a number of reasons: to protect themselves, their patients and their families from chemicals that cause adverse health effects personally and for their offspring. Physicians for Social Responsibility (PSR) conducted a biomonitoring study of 12 doctors and 8 nurses to determine their exposures to hazardous chemicals. The report, Hazardous Chemicals in Health Care: A Snapshot of chemicals in Doctors and Nurses notes an average of 24 chemicals in their bodies, including those known or suspected to be carcinogens, endocrine disruptors, or neurotoxicants.

The nurses of the Alliance of Nurses for Healthy Environments (ANHE) have been working to support safer chemical policies with their advocacy efforts to protect vulnerable populations, preserve state's rights, establish deadlines and timetables, ensure adequate data, act on the worst chemicals and support the right to know. In addition to chemical policy reform, ANHE nurses work across all areas of environmental health as advocates for safer energy sources, climate action, healthier communities, and use of safer products among others.

Resources:

1. Nurses Chemical Policy Toolkit

2. Safer Chemicals, Healthy Families

REFERENCES

Safer Chemicals, Healthy Families. (2016). *An Abbreviated Guide to the Frank R. Lautenberg Chemical Safety for the 21st Century Act.* http://saferchemicals.org/get-the-facts/an-abbreviated-guide-to-the-frank-r-lautenberg-act-chemical-safety-in-the-21st-century-act/

ANATOMY OF A LEGISLATIVE MEETING

Aislynn Moyer, DNP, RN
Director of Nursing
Penn State Milton S. Hershey Medical Center

Legislative meetings are a great opportunity to talk directly with decision makers of local, regional, and national governments. These meetings help educate and guide government leaders on important topics. Legislative leaders base their decisions on what they currently know and understand. This makes it important that nurses, and others, educate leaders on specific topics so that they can make truly informed decisions. Knowing the importance of meeting with legislative leaders is only the beginning. Before one can ever attend a meeting, it is imperative to understand the anatomy of such a meeting.

BEFORE THE MEETING

First and foremost before a legislative meeting, you must schedule the meeting. It is next to impossible to show up unnoticed and spend time with a legislative leader. Take time to schedule the meeting. Secondly, be sure to do all necessary homework. If the topic of the meeting is something that has already been discussed in legislative circles, be sure to understand all sides of the issue. It is also important to fully understand the message that you want to bring. Having evidence and personal stories to back your message is also helpful. Thirdly, the message should be condensed. Legislative meetings tend to be brief and you must be prepared to make all your important points in a timely fashion. This takes preparation ahead of time to be sure you do not miss anything. Although you can never guarantee that the legislative leader will read it, you can send information ahead of time or bring written materials with you. The fourth step to prepare for the meeting is to be on time. With such brief meeting times schedule, being even a few minutes late can result in not meeting with the leader at all.

DURING THE MEETING

Once inside a legislative meeting, begin to develop a relationship. Introduce yourself, what you do, and what brings you to the meeting. Be sure to stick to the message you want to send. Do not start talking on a tangent or switching issues. Take notes! If important information related to another issue is mentioned, write that down to follow up on later. Stay objective and truthful. If you are asked a question you do not know, say you do not know, but you will find out! Word your message in a way that is not threatening or critical of specific people or government parties. Allow time for questions so you can be sure the legislative leader understands your message. Before leaving the meeting, be gracious for the time and thank the leader for meeting with you. This helps build the relationship.

AFTER THE MEETING

Legislative relationships should never end with the meeting. Always follow-up. If there was information you did not know during the meeting, research it and follow up with the leader. Send a letter or email or make a phone call thanking the leader for their time and reinforcing the key point of the message. Offer yourself for questions if the leader has any. Make sure to keep in contact with the leader. Legislative leaders keep track of how many points of contact people make with them. Having just one or two is not enough to make a strong statement. This is why developing a relationship is so important.

CONCLUSION

Legislative meetings are an effective way to advocate and educate legislative leaders on important issues. In order to ensure successful meetings, care must be taken to prepare for the meeting. With specific action before, during, and after the meeting, a relationship can be built that will be key in having your voice heard.

ACTS OF NURSING ADVOCACY
Kathryn P. Jackman-Murphy Ed.D., MSN, RN, CHSE
Director, RN/BSN Program
Charter Oak State College

Nurses have been ranked as the most trusted profession for the past 18 years according to Gallup polls. In the most recent poll, 85% of Americans rate nurses as having high levels in honesty and ethics (Reinhart, 2020). Nurses are the most trusted profession and we must use our collective voice to advocate for those we serve. Our voices as health professionals carry more weight now than ever before. Our patients and communities trust that we advocate for their health.

The Alliance of Nurses for Healthy Environments (ANHE) Policy and Advocacy Workgroup has monthly calls to discuss current policy issues and the critical role that nurses can play in advocating to protect public health and the environment. These discussions lead to actions that elevate the voice of nursing on some of the most pressing issues of our time including climate change, access to health care, environmental impacts and toxic chemical pollution. Please see the ANHE website (www.envirn.org) for the date and times for these calls-all are welcome to join!

Opportunities for Acts of Advocacy can happen in our everyday lives. These opportunities can be large or small, but each one can have a positive impact towards a healthier environment. We have highlighted a few stories of nurses in action towards advocating for their families, community, patients, and themselves.

Adelita Cantu PhD, RN
Associate Professor
University of Texas Health San Antonio
School of Nursing

Childhood asthma is the most common chronic disease in children. Although childhood asthma is the same asthma that adults get; children often have different and more intense symptoms due to their particular sensitivity when exposed to allergens such as pollen and chemicals. Childhood asthma disproportionally affects children that live in low income communities and children of color. Current data reports that 16% of African American children have asthma compared to 6% of Whites. Also Hispanic children with asthma are twice as likely to visit the Emergency Room as Whites. https://minorityhealth.hhs.gov/omh/browse.aspx?lvl=4&lvlid=60 and https://www.cdc.gov/vitalsigns/childhood-asthma/index.html.

Often asthma attacks mean missed school days which can translate to poor academic progress further widening the disparities in academic achievement between communities of color and White non Hispanic communities.

As a public health nurse and an Associate Professor at the University of Texas Health Science Center in San Antonio School of Nursing, I have been aware for many years that pediatric asthma cases in the city have been alarmingly high, especially among low income, historically underrepresented children. In 2017, the childhood asthma hospitalization rate for Bexar County was 14.8 per 10,000 population. In our city, non-Hispanic African Americans experience high hospitalization rates than non-Hispanic whites and Hispanics. The rates of asthma hospitalizations are almost five times higher in children than adults. In 2018, I began to work with a group of health professionals, hospital administrators, school districts, health insurance companies and community stakeholders to form the South Texas Asthma Coalition with the goal of reducing asthma hospitalizations through better management.

The Coalition implemented a program called SA Kids B.R.E.A.T.H.E. (Building Relationships, Effective Asthma Teaching in Home Environments). https://www.sanantonio.gov/Health/HealthServices/Asthma

The Coalition advocated to our city council to fund this program which used the community health worker model to go to the homes and work with families of children with asthma to assist in asthma management. This approach allows the community health worker, using a perspective of social determinants of health, to address all the barriers to asthma management. These include health literacy, medication management, developing an asthma care plan in collaboration with the schools and assisting the parents or caregivers in reducing exposure to asthma triggers. Referrals are made to SA Kids B.R.E.A.T.H.E. by health care providers, local schools and hospitals and the community health workers conduct home visits where screening of the home environment and social determinants of health are conducted. The community health worker continues to meet with the family for 6 months to guide them through an asthma management plan.

Using community health workers is an evidence-based method of health promotion and health education that is widely used throughout the globe. Advocating to use this approach to tackle some of the most challenging health issues is an important role that nurses can play.

Jeanne Leffers, PhD, RN, FAAN
Professor Emeritus
University of Massachusetts Dartmouth
College of Nursing and Health Sciences

Nurses can develop advocacy skills in a variety of ways. As a long-time nursing educator, I recognized that advocacy was essential to student competencies and integrated into many nursing courses I taught including public health, policy, environmental health and nursing leadership. Beginning students learned to advocate for patients and for safe practice settings. More advanced students recognized that their professional role must include advocacy in practice. So, many years ago when I completed my own baccalaureate education I began the journey to build advocacy skills. A common statement we hear as nurses is that a nurse must be "at the table" or in places where decisions are made. It is a learning process to develop skills to do so.

Early in my career I learned first-hand that policies can be changed with effort and advocacy when with a few other nurses and new mothers, advocated for family centered care for women who delivered their babies by cesarean section. At the time I was a certified childbirth educator and witnessed the difference in the experience that we prepared expectant mothers to anticipate and the reality for those who delivered their child with cesarean section birth. In 1975, all of the hospitals in the Washington, D.C. area had more restrictive birth policies for those having cesarean births regarding holding the baby at birth, having a support person including their significant other in the delivery room and the option of having the newborn stay in their hospital room. A group of childbirth educators representing the four childbirth education organizations in the Washington, D.C. area came together to advocate for change. Through our advocacy efforts and visiting the appropriate administrator at each local area hospital with a maternity unit, we were successful in cesarean delivery policy changes at 7 hospitals within a six-month time period. That confirmed to me the power of nurses to make a difference through advocacy.

My efforts through the ensuing years to make change in many areas of nursing education or practice included both direct efforts through letter writing; contact with elected officials; serving on the board of directors of a health center, family service center and visiting nurse agency; and joining with other nurses to write policy papers and position statements. However, I as a nursing educator also strongly believed that the classroom was a significant way to build advocacy. If students left their nursing programs with the firm belief in their ability to make a difference to not only the patients in their care, but also to population health, the practice setting, patient outcomes, and nursing interventions through their advocacy, my efforts would be broader and more significant.

As my public health nursing focus broadened to include global health and environmental health I found that I needed more knowledge and skills to advance my advocacy work. This included participation in many programs, workshops and conferences on these topics as well as completing a global health course and environmental health course in an MPH program. I joined with other nurses as we met and developed the Alliance of Nurses for Healthy Environments (ANHE) and with a group of nurses in my own state of Rhode Island to build our Environmental Health Task Force, which was formally the Rhode Island State Nurses Association (RISNA) becoming the ANA-RI. We collaborated with other RI organizations, schools and elected officials to advance environmental health in nursing.

My most significant role as an advocate was as a member of the Environmental Protection Agency's (EPA) Children's Health Protection Advisory Committee (CHPAC) where my background as a nurse, public health nurse, and leader who had experience in pediatrics, public health, national nursing organizations, and environmental health education, research and advocacy led to my selection. During my five years as a member of CHPAC, we wrote letters with our professional advisement to the EPA Administrator on such children's health topics as the social determinants of health, prenatal exposures to hazardous substances, farmworker protection, lead poisoning, national ambient air quality, chemical toxicants in water, pesticides, food, toys and other chemical exposures. We were also asked to review the United States Global Change Research Program draft report, The Impacts of Climate Change on Human Health in the United States: A Scientific Assessment where we made our recommendations in a letter to the Administrator. This role reinforced to me that as nurses our voices are significant and necessary to advance health for all. No other professional group brings the same unique skills and experience as nurses do.

My advice to all nurses and nursing students to advance their skills and experience in advocacy whether in policy development or change, services on advisory committees of boards can be summed up in the following:

3. Recognize your responsibility and power as a nurse to make a difference.

4. Begin where you have both passion for and knowledge of the issue.

5. Learn as much as possible about both the pros and cons of the issue.

6. Select a place to begin your efforts be it a letter to the editor, to an elected official, to the administrator of your workplace or an organization of which you are a member.

7. Seek out other nurses who can help you by working together or building a coalition.

8. Act. Take the first step and keep going to make the difference!

Each step becomes easier as you gain the skills and success to move forward. Remember you can serve in an advocacy role in nursing practice, research, education as well as the policy arena. The ultimate role of research is to improve practice while education is essential to becoming a strong advocate.

Mary Jane Mongillo Williams, PhD, RN
Professor Emeritus
Central Connecticut State University

Over the last five decades nursing evolved from a subservient, nearly all female profession to an autonomous, diverse profession. My education as a nurse began in the early sixties, our class of 31 was all female and was taught to respect the authority of the administration and the physicians who provided medical care for our patients.

During my first summer as a nursing student, I worked charge on nights on a thirty-four-bed surgical unit. It became immediately evident that I needed to advocate for my patients if I expected them to have the best care possible. I also realized that I had to be assertive and persistent in my communication with physicians and hospital administration – there were concepts not fostered in nursing diploma programs in the 1960's.

Over the next two years I devoted my time to being the best nurse possible. I studied and prepared for the practice setting. Nursing became my life.

Upon graduation, I went to work on a Medical Surgical floor, progressed to practice in the first Intensive Care Unit and decided it was time to go back to school. I completed a Bachelor's degree in Psychology and took a Head Nurse position in a local hospital on a General Medical Unit. During my time on this unit I developed my advocacy skills, along with a strong voice for my most vulnerable patients. I was often challenged by the nursing

leadership and physicians regarding my requests, but in the end my requests were honored and my patients received the care and treatment appropriate for their diagnosis.

It was during this clinical experience I learned to use available science and current research to ensure my arguments for change were as strong as possible. Over the following twenty plus years, I studied, I practiced and I moved from clinical practice into nursing education. My practice was always guided by the current theory and current research.

I have participated in my professional organization since becoming an RN and during my tenure as President of the Connecticut Nurses Association, I attended a meeting at American Nurses Association in Washington, D.C. The Executive Director and I met with the leadership of multiple national environmental groups. It was an exciting conference and I went back to Connecticut energized about the importance of the natural environment on public health. I was especially interested because the town I grew up in was a super fund site – meaning it received money from the Federal Government to clean up industrial pollution. Our water had been contaminated by solvents recovery and we had to borrow water from a nearby city.

In collaboration with the Executive Director of CT Nurses Association we bought together all of the environmental groups in CT. We developed a coalition to advocate for environmental health, which evolved into the "Coalition for a Safe and Healthy Connecticut", currently under the excellent leadership of Anne Hulick. JD, MSN, RN. This experience and the advocacy related to the environment was my first concrete experience advocating at the state level.

However, over the past 25 years I have been the spokesperson for nursing policy at the state level. I was drafted in 1997 when the Chair of Government Relations became ill. I felt totally unprepared. I was so nervous during the first few times I testified that I thought I would be physically ill. However, I managed to control my anxiety and I soon realized that as a nurse with a strong educational background in nursing theory, science and practice, I was more knowledgeable about the issues we were discussing then the individuals listening to my testimony.

My advice to all nurses interested in the advocacy role - we are all extremely well prepared by our education and practice to be strong policy advocates at the state and national level. What I found most useful was the knowledge I gained by virtue of education and practice. As an advocate, we all need to:

- Establish a sound base of knowledge related to the issue.

- Utilize current research and science to support your issue.

- Draw on your nursing education to support your issue, such as:

  - Theoretical Knowledge

  - Research Skills

  - Knowledge of Science

  - Assessment Skills

  - Communication Skills

  - Presentation Skills

  - Group Skills

These are just a few of the many concepts and skills that your nursing education affords you and help in a policy environment. Nurses bring to the policy table the most unique set of skills as a health care provider profession. We are exposed to life and death situations daily. We deal with all levels of administration and a variety of physiological and psychological challenges as part of our daily routine. We are taught to be proactive and we are the backbone of the profession.

The knowledge and skills we have make us the best overall advocates in multiple settings, the most important as I see it is in the policy arena. You must develop a "THICK SKIN", politicians are not always gracious, nor are they always open to our suggestions and the expertise we bring to the table. But they often quickly learn to respect the research applicable to the legislation they are attempting to craft.

I have enjoyed every moment of my policy work at the state level. It has been one of the most satisfying experiences in my career and it resulted in the development of great respect for the profession and what we bring to the table as advocates for relevant issues.

Kathryn P. Jackman-Murphy Ed.D., MSN, RN, CHSE
Director, RN/BSN Program
Charter Oak State College

I was completing my master's degree at the University of Hartford when I was introduced to environmental health (EH). One of our projects was to present information on EH on several topics including personal care products, water and pesticides to several nursing groups. During this time I learned the use of pesticides had some serious concerns, including neurodevelopmental disorders such as attention-deficit hyperactive disorder, autism spectrum disorder (Saffron, 2020), cancer, asthma, diabetes (Kim, 2017) and childhood poisoning (EPA, 2017).

I was working as a public health nurse and was aware of pending state legislation regarding regulating the regular, scheduled application of pesticides in kindergarten-12 grade schools. I knew children are more susceptible to the effects of chemicals as pound for pound, they breath more air, drink more fluids, eat more food than adults (Pesticide Action Network, n.d.), their bodies were still growing and developing, as well as their hand-to-mouth behaviors to explore their world (American Academy of Pediatrics, 2020). I was very concerned about this possible legislation allowing the regular application of these chemicals of concern, regardless if they were needed and expose not only children but also the faculty, staff, visitors and community members to these potentially harmful products. But what actions could one person take that would make an impact?

I was asked to present nursing at Career Day at a local middle school and I was thrilled to be able to share information about the career that I love with the students. When I arrived, I found that one of the other presenters was a state legislator who would be considering the pesticide bill! Like most academics, I traveled with my flash drive and all of my academic information. One file was a collection of drawings by Yaqui Indian children, an indigenous group from Mexico. This seminal study demonstrated the effects of pesticides by comparing the drawings of 4-5-year-old children (Guillette, 1998). The two groups were similar genetic backgrounds, diets, water mineral contents, cultural patterns, and social behaviors, with the only difference being exposure to agricultural pesticides. The study found the children who had been exposed to pesticides had decreased stamina, gross and fine eye-hand coordination difficulties, memory deficits, and a decreased ability to draw a person as compared to a peer of similar age from the group that had not been exposed to pesticides. The children who had not had pesticide exposure had far more detail in their drawings, while the children that had been exposed to pesticides pictures were at times quite difficult to decipher they were of a person.

I had these pictures on my flash drive! I was able to quickly go to the library before meeting the children and print several of these pictures. Now, to approach my representative! We both were waiting in the queue to speak about our careers-I had my chance! I introduced myself as a pediatric nurse and was interested in environmental health. I told him about the dangers of pesticides and that I did not want the legislation to pass. I showed him the children's drawings. while I explained the study and pointed out the differences in the different sets of figures. I offered to be available for other questions and as I finished, I reinforced my ask: Not to vote for this legislation. He seemed very interested and took the drawings with him at the closure of the event. I found out later that he voted against the regular schedule application of pesticides in K-8 schools!

I remembered the important points that had been taught to me from the very beginning by Dr. Barbara Sattler and Brenda Afzal RN: Say you are a nurse, tell them what you want and why it is important. Success!

My take-aways from my first act of advocacy were: it was easier than I thought, it was powerful to be able to talk with my legislator-the person who represents me in government and to tell them what I wanted them to do for myself, my family and my community. I would do it again-and I have!

REFERENCES

Guillette, E. M. (1998, June). An anthropological approach to the evaluation of preschool children. *Environmental Health Perspectives, 106*(6), 347-353. https://ehp.niehs.nih.gov/doi/pdf/10.1289/ehp.98106347

Kim, K. H. (2017). Exposure to pesticides and the associated human health effects. *The Science of the Total Environment,* 525–535.

Pediatrics, A. A. (2020). *Protecting children from pesticides: information for parents.* Healthychildren.org: https://healthychildren.org/English/safety-prevention/all-around/Pages/Protecting-Children-from-Pesticides-Information-for-Parents.aspx

Pesticide Action Network. (n.d.). *Children.* http://www.panna.org/human-health-harms/children

Reinhart, R. J. (2020, January 6). *Nurses continue to rate highest in honesty, ethics.* Gallup. https://news.gallup.com/poll/274673/nurses-continue-rate-highest-honesty-ethics.aspx

Saffron, J. (2020, March). *Environmental factor.* National Institute of Environmental Health Sciences. https://factor.niehs.nih.gov/2020/3/science-highlights/brain-development/index.htm

US Environmental Protection Agency. (2017, October 27). *Reduce your child's chances of pesticide poisoning.* https://www.epa.gov/safepestcontrol/reduce-your-childs-chances-pesticide-poisoning

NURSES AND HEALTH POLICY: INTERVENING MACROSCOPICALLY AS ENVIRONMENTAL HEALTH ADVOCATES

Joanne F. Costello, MPH, PhD, CNSPH-BC
Professor
Rhode Island College School of Nursing

Nurses advocate in significant ways to protect individuals and families from environmental hazards. For example, nurses have worked in community settings with individual families of lead poisoned children in health clinics, screening for lead levels over 5 micrograms per deciliter and providing health education to assist parents to secure an environment free of paint dust and chips. Other nurses in acute care settings provide lifesaving respiratory treatments and pharmaceuticals to adults who suffer from severe environmentally triggered asthma. These nurses work directly with patients to provide education and intervention that prevents illness and injury and restores health. The following case illustrates how nurses and nursing students can have a strong impact on health policy to improve health outcomes.

The role of educating and intervening to restore health when environmental agents threaten harm is, of course, essential to nursing practice and facilitates positive health status in people across the lifespan (ANA, 2015). It is important nursing work that prevents illness and injury and restores physical, social, and psychological wellness in individuals and families. Clinical intervention and counseling and education, common nursing roles, are frequent in our healthcare system, but are not the most efficient use of resources and do not provide the greatest potential impact at a population level. Interventions impacting families and individuals for whom services are provided are called microscopic interventions.

Frieden's Health Impact Pyramid (2010), seen in Figure 1, illustrates the amount of resources required relative to the impact on health outcomes. According to this model, the two categories which have the least amount of impact on outcomes and yet require the greatest amount of resources for the intervention are clinical interventions and education and counseling, seen at the top of the pyramid. These are considered to be tertiary prevention interventions, with a focus upon minimizing complications and harm after the illness or injury has already occurred. The greatest impact with the least amount of resources required to promote health is upstream prevention at the base of the pyramid in the socioeconomic factors category. Lack of sanitation and

Figure 1. Health Impact Pyramid (Frieden, 2010)

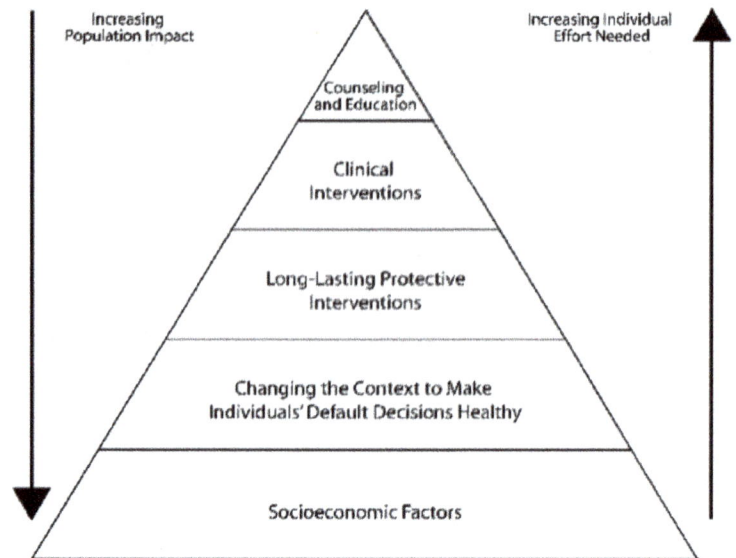

increased exposure to environmental hazards are examples of risk factors that may be mitigated with interventions that change socioeconomic status such as improving access to education, both of which affect critical social determinants of health such as housing and nutrition. These are considered to be health promotion and primary prevention interventions, occurring prior to any health issues already being present, and are the most efficient use of resources.

Advocacy through health policy interventions impacting on the lower categories of the pyramid are the most effective and efficient actions that will have the greatest impact on the greatest number of the population. An example of the most impactful intervention at base of the pyramid would involve promoting changes in socioeconomic factors such as advocating for legislation raising the minimum wage which would allow families to live in healthier housing. The intervention at the second level of the pyramid that would have strong impact with a small amount of resources is making default decisions healthy. Assuring through regulation that lead is not in paint products as was done in 1978 in the United States is an example of this level of intervention. The unhealthy choice is eliminated by the health policy in this case. The third level of the pyramid, providing long lasting protective interventions, are interventions such as standardizing lead screenings for children at 1 and 5 years old or mandating lead screening routinely for children living in high risk zip codes.

Interventions that demonstrate a large impact to a significant segment of the population such are those that are achieved using health policy initiatives are called macroscopic interventions. Martins (2015) provides a clear illustration of the difference between microscopic and macroscopic approaches. She notes that macroscopic nursing approaches examine interfamily and intercommunity themes of health and illness in contrast to microscopic interventions which examine individual response to health and illness. The focus of the macroscopic approach is on modifying social, economic, and environmental factors impacting health and illness, often through social and political action. In contrast, the focus of the microscopic approach is on modifying individual behavior to promote health (Martins, 2015).

Policy actions that impact on the base of the pyramid of social factors such as investments of a large amount of resources in housing, nutrition, and human services are more common in Europe. The United States, in contrast, invests a disproportionate amount of funds in the upper part of the pyramid on costly complex health care interventions that impact once disease has already occurred (Butler, Matthew, & Cabello, 2017).

C. E. Winslow, founder of Yale School of Public Health, created a definition of public health in 1920 that still is the gold standard today. His emphasis upon health policy as a tool to promote the public's health is demonstrated in the definition which includes the need for the "development of the social machinery which will ensure to every individual in the community a standard of living adequate for the maintenance of health; organizing these benefits in such fashion as to enable every citizen to realize his birthright of health and longevity" (Kemper, 2015). This definition reflects the awareness that the barriers to individuals alone without societal infrastructure to improve their own health can often be insurmountable and that public policies can offer opportunities for significant population health changes that have far reaching and sustainable impact.

ADVOCATING FOR HEALTH POLICY: LEAD POISONING IN RHODE ISLAND

Rhode Island has some of the oldest housing stock in the country. It the smallest state in the United States with a history of industrial labor, a high rate of immigration, and a high population density. These factors contribute to the reason that lead paint in older homes is the primary source of childhood lead poisoning (Rhode Island Department of Health, 2020). The Geographic Information Systems (GIS) map to the right demonstrates variation in the age of properties in the state, illustrating areas where children are at highest risk for lead poisoning which is linked to high levels of poverty (Holler, 2016).

Figure 2 Percentage of Housing Built Prior to 1980 (Holler, 2016)

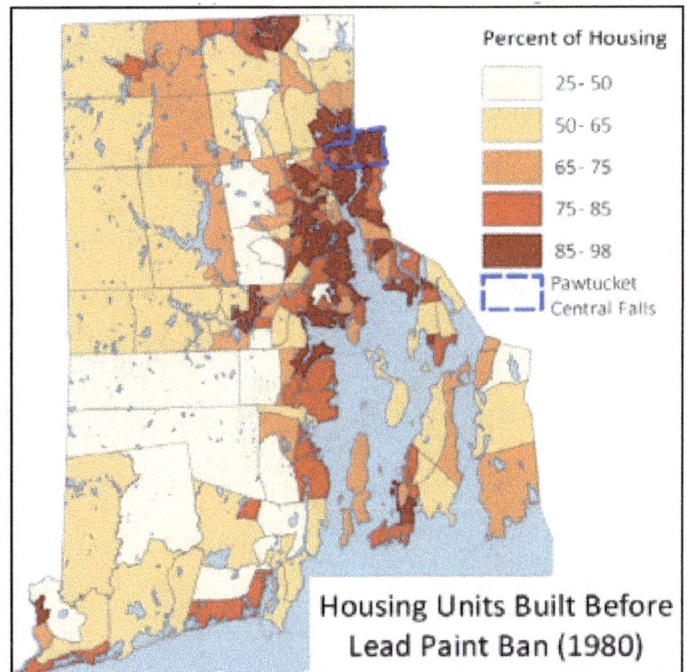

Housing built before the 1978 regulation of lead paint poses serious risks to human health, especially to pregnant people and children. Hauptman, Bruccoleri, and Woolf (2017) report that exposure of children to environmental lead in dust, paint, water, and other sources continue to pose serious health risks for children. Prevention of exposure is the optimal strategy requiring healthcare providers and advocacy groups to join in efforts to protect children from this serious threat.

Lead poisoning is a serious preventable childhood health issue causing irreversible brain damage leading to "an increased risk for behavioral problems, decreased cognitive abilities, and lower academic performance" (RI KIDSCOUNT, 2020). It also causes a variety of other serious health issues including decreased hearing, delayed puberty, and kidney damage. Significant negative academic impact has been demonstrated by even low levels of lead poisoning, with greater negative impact correlating to higher lead levels. RI KIDSCOUNT (2020) reports:

"The most significant declines in academic performance occurred among children with the highest blood lead levels and those living in the four core cities. Children with lead exposure are also at increased risked for absenteeism, grade repetition, and special education services."

The GIS map of Rhode Island below shows geographically the average percent of children who were lead poisoned in the state from 2002-2015 (Holler, 2016).

Figure 3 Average Percentage of Lead Poisoned Children by RI Location 2012-2015

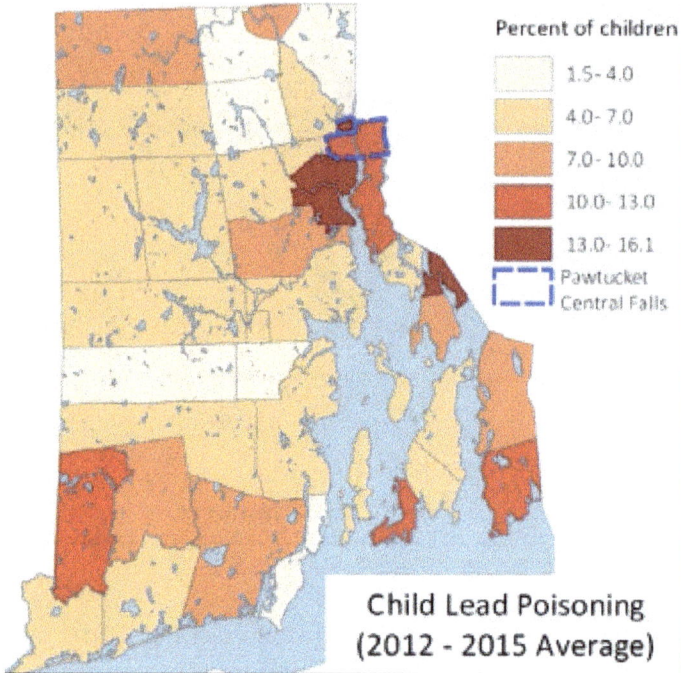

Child Lead Poisoning (2012 - 2015 Average)

(Holler, 2016)

The highest levels of lead poisoning in the state are seen in Rhode Island's core cities of Central Falls, Pawtucket, Providence, and Woonsocket, areas where more than 25% of children in Rhode Island live in poverty and where high numbers of children are from historically underrepresented backgrounds. The high numbers of children affected and dramatic disparities in who was impacted was a catalyst to state activists including nurses. Health professionals, advocates for children's health, congregations predominantly comprised of members from historically underrepresented groups, environmental justice groups, anti-poverty groups, and grass roots groups of families who were affected partnered with the Department of Health to form a strong coalition to combat this serious health issue affecting mainly children living in poverty from brown and black families.

A group of undergraduate nursing students in a community health nursing clinical practicum and I enthusiastically joined this coalition and were committed to engaging in an intervention that would shift the tide in favor of the affected kids. I had served on the Board of Directors of the Childhood Lead Action Project for

several years, acting as Vice President and then President of the Board. The Board was diverse and composed of key members of the community including affected parents, attorneys, nurses and physicians, realtors, clergy, politicians, and bankers. I was able to introduce my students to these members and others in the community who were committed to the goal of reducing childhood lead exposure. My work on the Board of Directors provided an important perspective and allowed me to connect the students and network with other health activists who had similar goals in our community.

I engaged my students in the process through their public policy assignment, which gave them the opportunity to learn about the epidemiology of the issue, consequences to society, and to obtain real life experience in the legislative process. This assignment is a well-developed learning activity in the students' undergraduate community/public health nursing course. Public policy activity has been part of the curriculum at our program for over twenty-five years and has significantly increased the political astuteness of students (Byrd et al., 2012) and inspired many graduates to continue to be health activists throughout their careers.

State legislation was sponsored in both the RI House and Senate to influence health policy on a macroscopic level by requiring lead safe certificates for rental housing where most cases of lead poisoning were found to occur. This proposed legislation faced significant opposition from landlords and realtor groups. During the time the law was being considered by the legislature, the undergraduate nursing students and I appeared on a local radio program to educate the audience on the risks of lead poisoning and the benefit of laws that would require

Figure 4 Percentage of Children Entering Kindergarten with Elevated Lead Levels 2003-2020

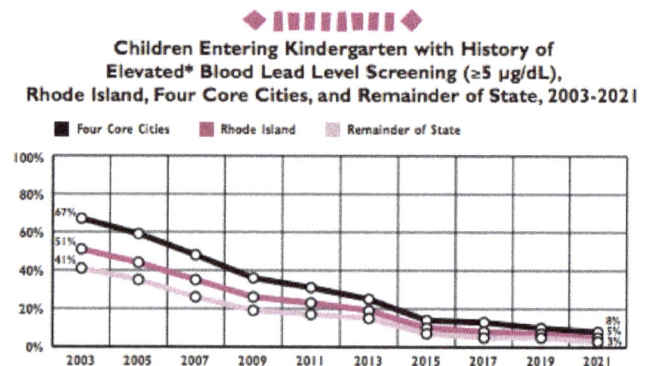

(RI KIDSCOUNT, 2020)

Table 23. **Lead Poisoning in Children Entering Kindergarten in the Fall of 2021, Rhode Island**

CITY/TOWN	NUMBER TESTED FOR LEAD POISONING	CONFIRMED WITH BLOOD LEAD LEVEL ≥5 µg/dL	
		NUMBER	PERCENT
Barrington	184	3	*
Bristol	151	5	*
Burrillville	129	3	*
Central Falls	300	26	8.7%
Charlestown	51	0	*
Coventry	289	7	*
Cranston	772	26	3.4%
Cumberland	352	6	*
East Greenwich	148	2	*
East Providence	491	16	3.3%^
Exeter	47	0	*
Foster	29	0	*
Glocester	63	1	*
Hopkinton	67	4	*
Jamestown	24	1	*
Johnston	241	4	*
Lincoln	213	7	*
Little Compton	15	1	*
Middletown	213	4	*
Narragansett	50	3	*
New Shoreham	16	2	*
Newport	265	20	7.5%^
North Kingstown	254	3	*
North Providence	331	3	*
North Smithfield	100	3	*
Pawtucket	833	46	5.5%
Portsmouth	146	4	*
Providence	2,636	226	8.6%
Richmond	39	2	*
Scituate	91	2	*
Smithfield	141	3	*
South Kingstown	200	8	*
Tiverton	132	3	*
Warren	83	2	*
Warwick	751	15	2.0%^
West Greenwich	30	0	*
West Warwick	325	7	*
Westerly	164	4	*
Woonsocket	539	23	4.3%^
Unknown Residence	*1*	*NA*	*NA*
Four Core Cities	*4,308*	*321*	*7.5%*
Remainder of State	*6,597*	*174*	*2.6%*
Rhode Island	*10,906*	*495*	*4.5%*

(RI KIDSCOUNT, 2020)

The Childhood Lead Project was founded by a strong, and committed social worker who valued interdisciplinary collaboration and the nursing discipline's contribution to this important work. This group along with other policy activists were responsible for passage of the Lead Hazard Mitigation Law (Lead Hazard Mitigation Law, 2012) which requires landlords to disclose lead hazards, maintain properties to keep them safe, and obtain a certificate of conformance to demonstrate lead safe status. This macroscopic intervention in which nurses and nursing students played a crucial role and has had a tremendous impact on reducing the number of children who have suffered from childhood lead poisoning. The graph below in Figure 4 demonstrates the dramatic reduction in cases of childhood lead poisoning from 2003-2020 from 67% to 8% of children living in the 4 core cities.

Clearly, many years of costly efforts at tertiary microscopic care did not come close to making the impact that this macroscopic intervention made. I have been involved with the Childhood Lead Action Project for the past thirteen years and have engaged large numbers of undergraduate and later graduate students in advocacy related to this issue. As new issues arise, such as COVID-19 which has caused more children to be in their unhealthy home environments for longer exposure and has decreased the number of children who are regularly screened, my students and I adapt to barriers and change our focus. The work is still not complete with disparities continuing to exist in the core cities. In 2020, 226 (8.6%) of children -226 too many-entering kindergarten in Providence had levels of lead greater than 5 micrograms/deciliter. The figure to the right shows the disparate variance in burden in Rhode Island's 39 cities and towns.

lead safe housing. We attended coalition meetings and educated legislators and the public about the data. We provided testimony for the RI state legislature at hearings as professionals who had directly seen the impact of lead poisoning. We participated in a press conference in support of the legislation which illustrated the number of kids affected by lead poisoning with children's handprints on a long banner.

Since the legislative intervention which significantly improved, but did not eliminate, childhood lead poisoning in the state, nurses and nursing students have continued to advocate and intervene on the macroscopic level, testifying before the legislature to maintain enforcement funding for certificates of conformance, lobbying a refugee resettlement organization to require lead safe certificates for housing for new refugees settling in the state, advocating for water line replacements to be equitably distributed, and broadening the fight to affordable safe housing. The current president of the Board of Directors of Childhood Lead Action Project is a nurse with an MSN in Population/Public Health Nursing who continues to collaborate with diverse grassroots groups to advocate for healthy housing for the state's most vulnerable families. Nurses from all specialties and at all levels should supplement their microscopic practice and use their status as a member of the United States' most trusted profession to advocate for legislation, initiatives, and programs that have large and sustainable impact on populations, especially the policy that benefits those who may not be able advocate for themselves.

REFERENCES

American Nurses Association (ANA). (2015). *Nursing: Scope and standards of practice* (3rd ed.). American Nurses Association.

Butler, S.M., Matthew, D.B., & Cabello, M. (2017, February 15). *Re-balancing medical and social spending to promote health: Increasing state flexibility to improve health through housing.* Brookings Institute. https://www.brookings.edu/blog/usc-brookings-schaeffer-on-health-policy/2017/02/15/re-balancing-medical-and-social-spending-to-promote-health-increasing-state-flexibility-to-improve-health-through-housing/

Byrd, M., Costello, J., Gremel, K., Schwager, J., Blanchette, L., & Molloy, T. (2012). Political astuteness of baccalaureate nursing students following an active learning experience in public policy. *Journal of Public Health Nursing,* 1-11.

Freiden, T. R., (2010). A framework for public health action: The health impact pyramid. *American Journal of Public Health, 100*(4), 590-595.

Hauptman,M., Bruccoleri, R., and Woolf, A. D. (2017). An update on childhood lead poisoning. *Clinical Pediatric Emergency Medicine, 18*(3), 181-192.

Holler, J. (2016, July 26). *Health geography primer for Rhode Island Family Medicine.* https://www.josephholler.com/files/HealthGeogRI.pdf

Kemper, S. (2015, June 2). *C-E.A. Winslow, who launched public health at Yale a century ago, still influential today.* Yale News. https://news.yale.edu/2015/06/02/public-health-giant-c-ea-winslow-who-launched-public-health-yale-century-ago-still-influe#:~:text=%E2%80%9CPublic%20Health%20is%20the%20science,principles%20of%20personal%20hygiene%2C%20the

Lead Hazard Mitigation, Title 42 § 128-1 (2012). https://law.justia.com/codes/rhode-island/2012/title-42/chapter-42-128.1/

Martins, D. Thinking upstream: Nursing theories and population-focused nursing practice. In Nies, M.A. & McEwen, M., (Eds). *Community/Public Health Nursing.* Elsevier.

Rhode Island Department of Health. (2020). *Childhood Lead Poisoning.* https://health.ri.gov/data/childhoodleadpoisoning/

Rhode Island KIDSCOUNT Factbook (2020). *Children with lead poisoning.* http://www.rikidscount.org/Portals/0/Uploads/Documents/Factbook%202020/Individual%20Indicators/lead-poisoning-2020fb.pdf?ver=2020-04-03-103700-983

ENGAGING IN CIVIL DISOBEDIENCE: A PUBLIC STATEMENT TO INFLUENCE CLIMATE CHANGE POLICY

Ruth McDermott-Levy, PhD, MPH, FAAN
Professor
Co-Director, Mid-Atlantic Center for Children's Health and the Environment
Villanova University
M. Louise Fitzpatrick College of Nursing

The Superior Court of the District of Columbia, Criminal Division was the heading of the paper I was handed after paying a $50.00 fine. About two inches lower on the paper was the statement, "You have been arrested for the following offence: 22-1307 Crowding, Obstructing or Incommoding." I grabbed the paper and with a friend we got a ride back to our D.C. hotel where we were to attend that evening's social activities of the American Academy of Nurses Transforming Health Driving Policy 2019 Conference appropriately titled: "Our Social Responsibility to Health: Impact and Influence."

In 2019, actress and climate change activist, Jane Fonda was motivated to bring attention to the existential risk of climate change by hosting Fire Drill Fridays at the Nation's capital in Washington, D.C (Fonda, 2019). After many years of educating nurses; advocating for effective climate change policy with state and national lawmakers; writing op-eds about the health impacts of climate change and the related air pollution; and speaking at the Global Climate & Health Summit held in conjunction with COP24 in Katowice, Poland, I took a step I never imagined I would do as a nurse. I put on my lab coat and wrapped my stethoscope around my neck and joined four other nurses, clergy, climate activists, and celebrities, Jane Fonda and Ted Danson to make a public statement. It is important that nurses make a public stand because climate change is real and if left unchecked it will have detrimental effects on the health of all of us with the greatest impact on society's most vulnerable: the poor, older adults, children, pregnant people, outdoor workers, people of color, immigrants, refugees, and indigenous people (Huffling, 2020).

As a public health nurse, educator, and researcher it is critical that I communicate the risks of climate change to protect and preserve the health of those at risk: all of us. The science is there. In 2016, the U.S. Global Change Research Program, made of 13 federal agencies issued their federally mandated quadrennial report that detailed the human health impacts across the United States: very few paid attention, and very little changed. In 2018 the world's leading scientist of the UN Intergovernmental Panel on Climate Change (IPCC) issued the sobering report that we cannot rise above a global average temperature increase of 1.5° C. I thought that would capture the world's attention. Nothing changed.

The Scope and Standard of Nursing Practice (American Journal of Nursing, 2015) and our nursing license require that we advocate for the health of our patients. As a public health nurse that addresses environmental health risks, my patients are in communities, states, and regions. But with climate change, my patient seems to be the planet that sustains us. So, after doing everything I could to call attention to the climate crisis and influence U.S. climate change policy, I took a more public approach and joined others for Fire Drill Friday to engage in civil disobedience, also known as: 22-1307 Crowding, Obstructing, or Incommoding.

I did not do this lightly, as I mentioned I have been trying to "sound the alarm" with others for several years. So, before actually going to Washington I:

- Reflected on why I felt the need to participate in Fire Drill Friday.

- Spoke with an attorney who addresses occupational law.

- Reviewed the requirements of my home state board on nursing related to my nursing license and arrest.

- Learned about the procedures and what to expect related to the civil disobedience event.

- Discussed with my family and let them know my plans.

The event itself was well planned. We received detailed information in advance about what to expect, how to physically prepare (including being well hydrated and nourished the day before), what to bring and not to bring with us, and where to meet the day of the event. The early part felt like any environmental or climate rally I

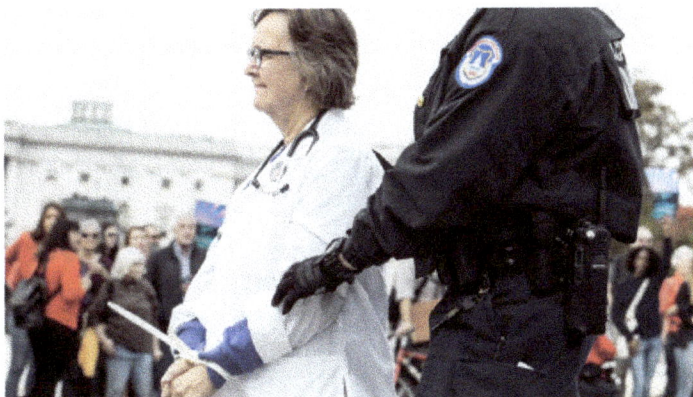

had attended in the past. At the end of the "rally portion", those of us who were willing to risk arrest moved into the street and did not move. The Capital police were very respectful and asked us to move. After three warnings, when we did not move, we were handcuffed and taken to be processed. For our group, processing took about 5 hours. We sat in a police warehouse and we were able to talk with the others sitting near us. Overall, it was a humbling experience of climate change solidarity.

After we were released, we quickly headed back to the hotel to get something to eat and get cleaned up for an evening of celebration at the conference. I quietly returned to my normal professional life. A few people heard about what had happened and were commenting. I was surprised and a bit panicked, that it would get out that I had been arrested. After all, I had never been arrested before. I quickly learned, that is the whole point of civil disobedience. It is a public display to make a political statement. Civil disobedience is used to peacefully highlight an injustice, to undo a wrong. If nurses, the most trusted profession by the public, are willing to take the time to call public attention to a matter that affects our health, maybe others will pay attention. So, now I share my arrest, including a letter to my state board of nursing explaining why I did what I did and why more nurses must make a stand for our health. Our arrest was shared on social media and a quick photo of the nurses getting arrested made the national news. I have found that I get different responses. Some people congratulate me. Others ask why I got arrested. When asked I respond, "It is an opportunity to educate more people and help them make a link between air pollution, energy choices, and climate change policies and their health."

Civil disobedience is one of the last ways to influence policy, it is used when other more traditional methods have failed. However, nothing could be more important than addressing climate change and the associated health risks. Nurses do have a social responsibility to impact and influence health.

REFERENCES

American Nurses Association (ANA) (2015). *Nursing: Scope and standards of practice (3rd ed.).* American Nurses Association.

Fonda, J. (2019, December 5). *We have to live like we're in a climate emergency. Because we are.* The New York Times. https://www.nytimes.com/2019/12/05/opinion/jane-fonda-climate-change.html

Huffling, K. (2020). Our house is on fire. Join us in the streets. *Public Health Nurse, 37*(1) 1-2. https://doi-org.ezp1.villanova.edu/10.1111/phn.12704

Intergovernmental Panel on Climate Change (n.d.). *Special Report: Global Warming of 1.5°C.* https://www.ipcc.ch/sr15/

U.S. Global Climate Research Program (2016). *The Impacts of Climate Change on Human Health in the United States: A Scientific Assessment.* Crimmins, A., J. Balbus, J.L. Gamble, C. B. Beard, J. E. Bell, D. Dodgen, R. J. Eisen, N. Fann, M.D. Hawkins, S. C. Herring, L. Jantarasami, D. M. Mills, S. Saha, M. C. Sarofim, J. Trtanj, and L. Ziska, (Eds.). U.S. Global Change Research Program. 312 pp. http://dx.doi.org/10.7930/J0R49NQX

Unit VIII:
Theory and Research

INTRODUCTION

Since the early days of professional nursing practice, nurses have been observing and analyzing environmental data. Nurses have used their findings to influence the care they provide. In the 1850's Florence Nightingale subscribed to the health theory of the time, miasma. Miasmatic theory held that "bad air" was responsible for diseases such as cholera and chlamydia. Of course, now we know that is incorrect. But, it took people willing to look at the problem differently, ask questions of those exposed, and conduct further research to advance our understanding of the impact of the environment on our health. Technological advances, such as the microscope, helped as well.

The scientific community, including nurses, has made observations and analyzed data to accurately identify what is happening related to human health and the environment. Over time the theories that frame our understanding of a problem have changed. Advancing our knowledge of how our environment influences our health does not occur unless we formally examine a problem through research methods. Nurses at all levels of practice are positioned to make observations, collect data, and analyze data regarding the environmental impact on the health of individuals, families, communities, and nations.

This unit describes the work of nurses who are engaged in environmental health research and environmental health theories and models to frame nursing research.

APPLICATION OF THE ECOJUSTICE EDUCATION THEORETICAL FRAMEWORK TO NURSING PRACTICE

Kristi Jo Wilson PhD, RN, FNP-BC, CAFCI
Assistant Professor of Nursing
University of Michigan-Flint
School of Nursing

While promoting and maintaining health, nursing care also creates pollution (about 5,500 tons daily or 2 million tons a year) and 20% of that pollution (400,000 tons) is hazardous (Anthony, 2015). Ironically, this is in contrast to the major concepts held within the foundational documents of nursing. For instance, Standard 7 and Standard 17 in The American Nurses Association Scope and Standards of Practice (ANA, 2015) contains language that supports ethical practice and the support of environmentally sound practices.

Although nursing education constructs sound values and attitudes in future nurses, like caring that is free of bias and strong patient advocacy, educators do not connect the dots when it comes to nursing and environmentally sound practices. For instance, outcomes in nursing education are successful completion of the NCLEX-RN passage rates and behaviors that contribute to sound patient care; however, consideration of the environment is not a strong priority of measurement. In addition, the American Association of Colleges of Nursing's (AACN) Baccalaureate Essentials (2008) that informs nursing curricula, does not include specific measures of environmental health. Although the Essentials are under revision, there are no specific indicators that environment and nursing will be strongly interrelated as the environment is described within the context of nurse and patient (AACN, 2019).

As a holistic profession, nurses must consider the connection of human beings and environment and bring about change in behaviors that contribute to waste and environmental concerns. The American Holistic Nurses Association (AHNA) describes holistic nursing as "all nursing practice that has healing the whole person as its goal" (AHNA, 2019, para 1) and the person as whole includes the consideration of human beings as embedded within the environment (AHNA, 2019). Author Wendell Berry (1995) reminded us of this notion when writing about health as embedded within a larger system: "To be healthy is literally to be whole; to heal is to make whole" (p. 87).

The Flint Michigan Water Crisis highlights the interdependence that is required among human beings and the environment. One cannot have true health if we are mired in toxic relationships and a polluted environment. In other words, human beings and environment have to be in an interdependent relationship in order to recognize wellness. I have always counted the area of Flint, Michigan as my environmental commons. An environmental commons is filled with relationships with the environment that includes air, animals, rocks, soil and water (Bowers, 2006; Martusewicz, Edmundson & Lupinacci, 2015). For as long as I can remember, I have enjoyed activities within the commons that include walking by the Flint River and taking in the smells and sounds of the local fresh fruits and vegetables at the Flint Farmers Market. The importance of this relationship became real to me during the Flint Water Crisis. The poisoned river exposed the interdependence between human beings and the natural world. Not only do human beings rely on this body of water, but so do animals and wildlife like trees, soil, and plants. The consideration for the natural world is one of the tenets of an environmental commons, where all life can be affected as a result of a disregard of the social and ecological systems that we depend upon.

Theoretical frameworks such as The Ecojustice Education (EJE) theoretical framework help to deepen the awareness of connection to the environment and therefore the idea of what is health. The EJE framework reminds us that human beings cannot be separated from a larger entity, as we are fully dependent on a complex, interdependent system (Wilson, 2017). Unlike many approaches in nursing education that combine social and environmental issues into separate and distinct spheres, this framework operates from the position that social problems and environmental degradation emerge from the same foundational causes. A cultural ecological analysis (part of the EJE theoretical framework) helps to expose those causes because it examines the intersection between social and ecological problems and traces a deep history so that nurses can understand why things are the way they are today. Although there is no formal diagram to represent the framework, a tree with roots creates a strong metaphor or symbol for the EJE framework.

By looking at the diagram of a tree and applying the EJE theoretical framework, nurses can unpack the concept of health by becoming aware that health is constructed within socioeconomic, political, cultural, and ecological contexts that affect how personnel in the medical and nursing fields practice (see picture below). The deep history represents the roots of nursing and the branches represent the way things are today as situated in socioeconomic, political, cultural, and ecological contexts.

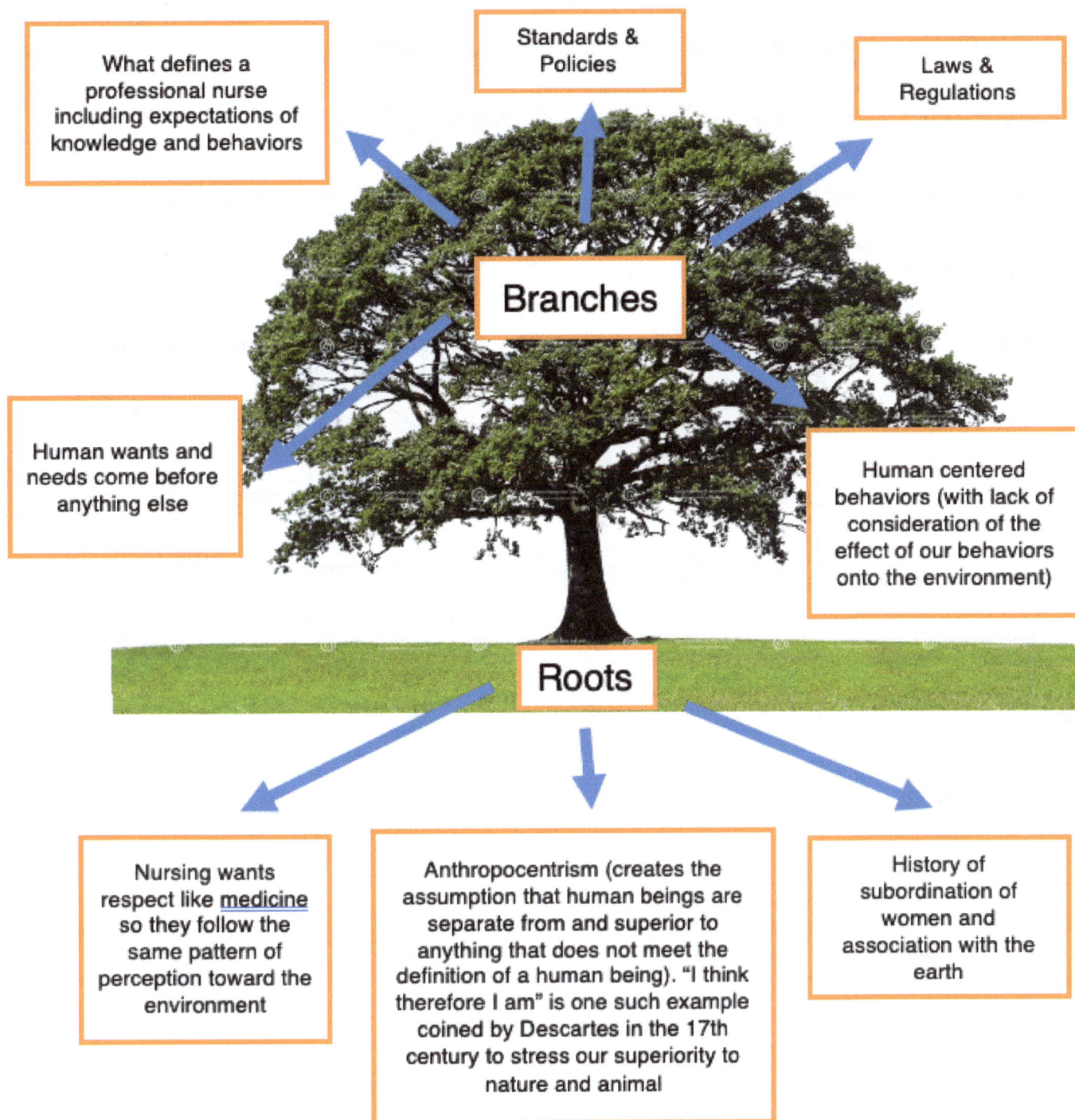

Branches

What defines a professional nurse including expectations of knowledge and behaviors

Standards & Policies

Laws & Regulations

Human wants and needs come before anything else

Human centered behaviors (with lack of consideration of the effect of our behaviors onto the environment)

Roots

Nursing wants respect like medicine so they follow the same pattern of perception toward the environment

Anthropocentrism (creates the assumption that human beings are separate from and superior to anything that does not meet the definition of a human being). "I think therefore I am" is one such example coined by Descartes in the 17th century to stress our superiority to nature and animal

History of subordination of women and association with the earth

For example, the hospital culture is concerned with infection prevention and the use of gloves is recommended. However, as nurse researchers have noted, the use of gloves is not necessary in all cases and contributes to the toxicity in the environment due to its petroleum-based origins of the gloves that are intended to support patient care (Grose & Richardson, 2015; Wilson, Prieto, Snigleton, O'Connor, Lynham & Loveday, 2015).

When the nurse is functioning from an Ecojustice Educational (EJE) Framework there can be a holistic perspective that addresses socioeconomic, political, cultural, and ecological contexts in which the nurse practices. For example, there are specific actions that nurses can take to improve the environment and thus promote the health of those in the nurse's care. Consider the following questions to ask yourself during patient care and the resources that are available:

1. Consider using gloves for patients only when necessary. Ask yourself, "Do I have to wear gloves if I'm taking vitals and the patient is clean and dry?" Know the facts about what diseases are transmissible through bodily fluids and which fluids are vectors for the disease.

2. Become aware of the disposal practices of plastic or toxic items in your workplace. Are they recycled or thrown in the general waste? What is the problem with disposing them into the general waste?

3. Review the guidelines for the disposal of pharmaceutical items in your workplace. How certain are you that they won't end up in the water supply?

4. Educate yourself, your coworkers and patients on the need to be aware of environmental concerns that cause illness in humans or develop a "local eco-medical literacy" (Adlong & Dietsch, 2015, p. 20). One example is knowing that climate change and temperature increases can lead to food borne illnesses such as salmonellosis (Adlong & Dietsch, 2015). Another example is understanding that climate change is correlated with increasing incidents of allergies and asthma (D'Amato et al., 2015) and tend to affect human beings who live in economically depressed areas (McDermott-Levy, Jackman-Murphy, Leffers & Jordan, 2019; MacMunn, 2018).

5. Think of ideas to make products reusable. A reusable product cuts down on the energy needed to create a new product. For example, one nurse advocated for new patient slippers made of cotton scraps instead of cotton that is processed (Sattler & Choiniere, 2011). Another nurse suggested isolation gowns that are washable and items that were once assumed as single use can be reused safely such as oximeter probes, compression sleeves, and blood pressure cuffs (Schenk, 2017).

6. Become aware of food waste in your organization. Americans on average throw away 161 billion pounds of food each year (Aubrey, 2019). This statistic includes places where nurses work like hospitals and extended care facilities. Wasted food leads to an increased emission of methane, a gas that contributes to climate change. In addition, growing food requires land that is made available from deforestation in order to create space to grow food.

7. Inquire about the type of energy used at your workplace. The more fossil fuels used, the more dangerous gases are emitted to the environment that erode the ozone layer and lead to climate change. For example, the Alliance of Nurses for Healthy Environments (ANHE) in partnership with the Climate for Health, created a fact sheet that helps signify the specific actions nurses can take to support the environment (Cook, 2018).

8. Seek to understand that values within our culture that create hierarchization and exclusivity and lead to ecological crises. With this awareness, relationships that were once normalized or seen as that's just the way it is, will be questioned, seen as unethical and challenged by nurses. For instance, when nurses assume that a person who is admitted with a history of drug abuse is "faking it," "manipulative," or "drug seeking", it makes it easier for nurses to define them as someone who does not deserve their full attention or care. These assumptions feed into our actions of not fully advocating for the patient through rationalization that the patient is less than and not worthy of empathy and care. This separation of "us" and "them" feeds into other relationships and events such as the lack of consideration of something non-human and therefore perceived as less than (e.g., water) in comparison to human beings. The loss of connection embedded in these values and behaviors lead to the degradation of ecosystems that we depend upon and this is what happened in the Flint Water Crisis.

9. If you are a nurse educator, think about the overall purpose of nursing education. David Orr (2004) stressed that all education is environmental because the effects of our actions are not separate from the environment. Nurse educators are called to create a platform of learning that includes the ideas as described in the suggestions above in order to transform thinking and open students' minds up to the inter-relationality of environment and nursing.

A grounding in EcoJustice education can support nurses' understanding that becoming aware of the inner workings and values of their healthcare organization and getting involved in changes that support the environment will help reduce waste and affect change. After all, individual changes are powerful but changes at the institutional level affect change at a greater expanse. In order to accomplish the suggested tasks, nurses must reflect on their idea of what nursing is including the responsibilities that go along with the profession.

Given their scientific acumen and priority of caring and connecting with patients, nurses are in a prime position to be seen as experts on what attitudes and behaviors among human beings can create health in all members, including the more-than-human-world that includes the water, animals, soil, air, and plants (Abrams, 1997). The EcoJustice Education theoretical framework is one way to challenge the assumptions in nursing and open nurses up to the risk of learning and embracing this broader perspective on health and thus be catalysts for change in nursing and nursing education. The immediate and long-range impact of that change bodes well for the health of the Earth as well as ALL of its inhabitants (Wilson, 2017).

REFERENCES

Abrams, D. (1997). *The spell of the sensuous: Perception and language in a more-than-human-world.* Vintage Books.

Adlong, W., & Dietsch, E. (2015). Nursing and climate change: an emerging connection. *Collegian, 22*(1), 19-24.

American Association of Colleges of Nursing (2008). *The Essentials of Baccalaureate Education for Professional Nursing Practice.* American Association of Colleges of Nursing.

American Association of Colleges of Nursing (2019). *Healthy work environments.* https://www.aacn.org/nursing-excellence/healthy-work-environments?tab=Patient%20Care.

American Holistic Nurses Association (2019). *What is holistic nursing?* https://www.ahna.org/About-Us/What-is-Holistic-Nursing.

American Nurses Association (ANA) (2015). *Scope and standards of practice* (3rd ed.). American Nurses Association.

Anthony, S. (2015). *How much waste do hospitals generate?* https://www.medassureservices.com/blog/hospitals-medical-waste/.

Aubrey, A. (May 23, 2019). *To reduce food waste, FDA urges best if used by date labels.* The Salt, NPR. : https://www.npr.org/sections/thesalt/2019/05/23/726079350/to-reduce-food-waste-fda-urges-best-if-used-by-date-labels.

Berry, W. (1995). *Health is membership in. Another turn of the crank.* (pp. 86–109). Counterpoint.

Bowers, C. A. (2006). *Revitalizing the commons: Cultural and educational sites of resistance and affirmation.* Rowman & Littlefield.

Cook, C. (July 24, 2018). *Nursing advocacy for clean energy and climate solutions.* https://www.envirn.org/nursing-advocacy-for-clean-energy-and-climate-solutions/.

D'Amato, G., Holgate, S.T., Pawankar, R., Ledford, D. K., Cecchi, L., Al-Ahmad, M., …Annesi-Maesano, I. (2015). Meteorological conditions, climate change, new emerging factors, and asthma and related allergic disorders. A statement of the World Allergy Organization. *World Allergy Organization Journal, 8*(25). doi: 10.1186/240413-015-0073-0.

Grose, J. & Richardson, J. (2015). Can a sustainability and health scenario provide a realistic challenge to student nurses and provoke changes in practice? An evaluation of a training intervention. *Nursing & Health Sciences, 18*(8), 256–261 doi: 10.1111/nhs.12241

McDermott-Levy, R., Jackman-Murphy, K. P., Leffers, J. M. & Jordan, L. (2019). Integrating climate change into nursing curricula. *Nurse Educator, 44*(1), 43-47.

MacMunn, A. (December 6, 2018). *15 health and medical groups strongly oppose EPA's proposal to weaken carbon pollution limits on new power plants.* https://www.lung.org/about-us/media/press-releases/15-health-and-medical-groups.html.

Martusewicz, R. A., Edmundson, J., & Lupinacci, J. (2015). *EcoJustice education: Toward diverse, democratic, and sustainable communities* (2nd ed.) New York, NY: Routledge.

Martusewicz, R.A. & Wilson, K. (2017). Health as holism. In Martusewicz, R.A. (Ed.), *A pedagogy of responsibility: Wendell Berry for EcoJustice Education.* Pp. 136 – 153. New York, NY: Routledge.

Orr, D.W. (2004). *Earth in mind: On education, environment and the human prospect.* Island Press.

Sattler, B., & Choiniere, D. (2011). Environments & health: The greening of a major medical center. *The American Journal of Nursing ,111*(4), 60-62.

Schenk, B. (2017). *Reducing the environmental effects of healthcare and nursing practice.* https://envirn.org/reducing-the-environmental-impacts-of-healthcare-and-nursing-practice/.

Wilson, K. (2017). *An EcoJustice Analysis of Nursing Education* (Doctoral dissertation). ProQuest Dissertations and These Global (10618978).

Wilson, J., Prieto, J., Singleton, J., O'Connor, V., Lynham, S. & Loveday, H. (2015) The misuse and overuse of non-sterile gloves: Application of an audit tool to define the problem *Journal of Infection Prevention, 161,* 24-31.

THE INTEGRATIVE MODEL FOR ENVIRONMENTAL HEALTH AND THE MODIFIED INTEGRATIVE MODEL FOR ENVIRONMENTAL HEALTH

Ruth McDermott-Levy, PhD, MPH, RN, FAAN
Professor
Co-Director, Mid-Atlantic Center for Children's Health and the Environment
Villanova University
M. Louise Fitzpatrick College of Nursing

The Integrative Model for Environmental Health (IMEH), developed by Dixon and Dixon (2002), provides a useful framework for environmental health programs and research. The model has four environmental exposure domains: 1) Physiological, 2) Vulnerability, 3) Epistemological, and 4) Health Protection. These four environmental domains are linked by diffuse boundaries within each domain; thus, the domains are not discrete, and phases of a research project may address more than one domain. The domains are iterative and rely on one another to identify, understand, and address an environmental health risk or exposure. This also speaks to the complexity and the necessity of an interdisciplinary approach to environmental health problems (Dixon & Dixon, 2002).

The *physiological domain* addresses the physiological processes and impact that environmental exposures. It addresses the question, "What is the problem?" (Dixon & Dixon, 2002, p. 45). There are four elements within the physiological domain: agents, exposure, incorporation, and health effects. The agent is the environmental toxin or toxicant that can cause a health risk. Examples of an agent are particulate matter air pollution, pesticides, PFAS, a virus, or radiation. The *exposure* is the contact the agent has with the human being. The exposure can be dermal, ingestion, or respiratory routes. *Incorporation* is the accumulation of the agent in the body, the physiological response, and monitoring the agent. Finally, the *health effects* refer to the outcome of the agent, exposure, and incorporation leading to acute or chronic illness, a latency period, or death. Areas such as the toxicology of the environmental exposure, the epigenetic impact, biomonitoring, and physiological symptoms from the exposure would be considered in the physiological domain.

The *vulnerability domain* is concerned with the multiple factors and characteristics that influence the environmental health risks of individuals, families, communities, and populations. This domain would include the confluence of environmental justice, health disparities, and the social determinants of health. Examples that would be included in the vulnerability domain would be a child who lives with parents who smoke in the home; an incineration plant within a low-income community; or an island nation that is experiencing sea-level rise with climate change. The vulnerabilities of environmental justice communities would also be highlighted within the vulnerability domain of the IMEHR framework.

The *epistemological domain* addresses what individuals, families, communities, or populations know and what they need to know related to environmental health risks. This domain examines people's awareness and how people learn about and understand environmental risks and the impacts on their health. This is an area that nursing has played an important role in communicating the evidence regarding an environmental agent and its risk upon human health.

The *health protective* domain includes the actions that people take to respond to an environmental health risk or exposure. Within this domain there are three elements: 1) people's *concerns about the health risk*; 2) their *sense of efficacy* or their confidence in their ability to address the health risk; and 3) the *actions* that they will take in response to an environmental health risk. This domain is closely associated with the way that nurses deliver educational interventions to individuals, families, and communities. Nurses assess learners' existing knowledge or understanding of the health problem; nurses determine the learners' ability to take action; and nurses provide evidence-based actions to make changes to improve environmental health.

The IMEH has been used in a variety of research and environmental health educational programming. Macdonald (2004) used the IMEH to analyze the SARS outbreak in Toronto, Canada. Larsson et al. (2006) used the framework to understand the perceptions of environmental health concerns of rural community leaders. Harnish et al. (2006) used the IMEH to guide research related to rural parents' understanding of environmental health risks for their children. Perron and O'Grady (2010) used the model to organize an integrative literature review of lead poisoning in children and McDermott-Levy (2016) relied on the IMEH to structure a community based participatory research project for environmental health education in a fracking community.

Polivka and colleagues (2013) used the model for a community based participatory research project with urban neighborhoods. Following focus groups to understand the needs of the community, the investigators determined that the IMEH should be modified to demonstrate the community's vulnerabilities and there should be a greater link to demonstrate that the physiological domain informs the epistemological domain, thus making the model much more iterative. Additionally, the investigators changed an epistemological domain element from social knowledge to social understanding and added societal characteristics to the vulnerability domain to reflect the influence of public policy upon communities addressing environmental health risks. These changes yielded the Modified IMEH which has utility for community based environmental health research.

The Integrative Model for Environmental Health and the Modified Integrative Model for Environmental Health have utility for environmental health programs and research. This model and its modified version highlight the ways in which nurse address health risk by understanding the vulnerabilities of the population, examining the physiological impacts, including the existing evidence, and developing a plan to address the environmental health risks.

REFERENCES

Dixon, J. K., & Dixon, J. P. (2002). An integrative model for environmental health research. *Advances in Nursing Science, 24*(3), 43–57.

Harnish, K. E., Butterfield, P., & Hill, W. G. (2006). Does Dixon's integrative environmental health model inform an understanding of rural parents' perceptions of local environmental health risks? *Public Health Nursing, 23*(5), 465–471.

Larsson, L. S., Butterfield, P., Christopher, S. & Hill, W. (2006). Rural community leaders' perceptions of environmental health risks: Improving community health. *AAOHN Journal, 54*(3), 105–112.

Macdonald, M.T. (2004). From SARS to strategic actions reframing systems. *Journal of Advanced Nursing, 47*(5), 544–550.

McDermott-Levy, R. (2016). *Evaluation of Environmental Health Education Resources for Residents of Unconventional Oil and Gas Development Communities in Pennsylvania.* Conference proceedings, American Public Health Association Meeting, Denver, CO. https://apha.confex.com/apha/144am/meetingapi.cgi/Session/49253?filename=144am_Session49253.html&template=Word

Perron, A., & O'Grady, K. (2010). Applying Dixon and Dixon's integrative model for environmental health research toward a critical analysis of childhood lead poisoning in Canada. *Advances in Nursing Science, 33*(1), E1–16

Polivka, B. J., Chaudry, R., Crawford, J. M., Wilson, R. & Galos, D. (2013). Application and modification of the integrative model for environmental health. *Public Health Nursing, 30*(2), 167-76. doi: 10.1111/j.1525-1446.2012.01050.x.

NURSES DRAWDOWN: EVIDENCE-BASED STRATEGIES FOR NURSING
Sara Kramer, BSN, MS, RN
Worcester State University

Nurses Drawdown is a project in collaboration with the Alliance of Nurses for Healthy Environments (ANHE) and Project Drawdown. Project Drawdown is an initiative that began in 2014 to identify scientifically based solutions to reduce, or drawdown, greenhouse gas emissions. As stated by the Project Drawdown project, "drawdown is the future point in time when levels of greenhouse gases in the atmosphere stop climbing and start to steadily decline. This is the point when we begin the process of stopping further climate change and averting potentially catastrophic warming. It is a critical turning point for life on Earth" (drawdown.org/drawdown-framework, 2021).

Nurses Drawdown moves the concept of Project Drawdown forward to include nursing and collaborative interdisciplinary interventions. The Nurses Drawdown carries on the mission of ANHE in promoting healthy people and healthy environments by educating and leading the nursing profession, advancing research, incorporating evidence-based practice, and influencing policy. It is important to develop Nurses Drawdown as nursing is the largest group of health professionals, with nurses and midwives accounting for nearly 50% of the global health workforce (World Health Organization (WHO), 2020). Therefore, nurses are in positions to significantly impact climate change (who.int, 2020). Nurses Drawdown is positioned to engage nurses from all regions of the world to work toward evidenced-based climate change actions (Nursesdrawdown.org, 2021).

The Nurses Drawdown website is a source for nurses to begin addressing climate change and to access evidence-based information, but Nurses Drawdown also offers inspiration from exemplars of the work that other nurses and midwives have done. The website provides videos and nurses testimonials. Actions described on the website at nursesdrawdown.org include five key areas that the organization has identified for drawdown: Food, Mobility, Gender Equity, Energy, and Nature-Based solutions. These five key areas were selected because they are pertinent to the work of nurses and exhibit the importance of human health and the health of the planet.

- Food: Committing to eating a more plant-based diet, use clean-burning cookstoves, and reduce food waste.

- Mobility: Promoting walkable cities, including improving bike infrastructure and mass transit.

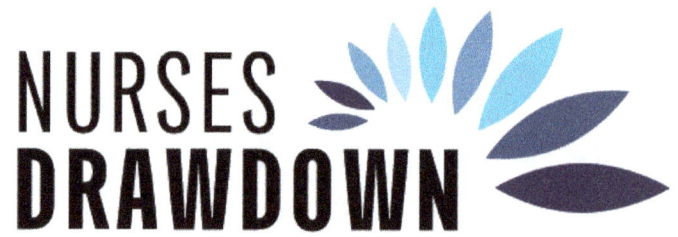

- Gender Equity: Supporting education for girls and access to family planning.

- Energy: Supporting a clean energy future by promoting energy efficiency and advocating for a transition to renewable energy.

- Nature-Based Solutions: Planting trees and protecting forests (nursesdrawdown.org, 2021).

These five focus areas are a way for nurses to get started in taking personal and professional action. Interested participants can learn more by clicking the "take action" tab and learn strategies to move their engagement in climate solutions forward.

Involving nurses in climate change action and enlisting their help in communicating messages is an important step toward mitigating the effects of climate change. Information and education are needed to help form a cohesive message that nurses can communicate to patients and other healthcare providers. Nurses are placed in positions where they work with people from all different backgrounds across the lifespan. This means that nurses can communicate messages to many different people of various backgrounds in communities (Leffers et al., 2016).

Preparing a nursing workforce to address climate change is important. In fact, public health nurses acknowledged that climate change threatened human health, with 65% of public health nurses noting that within twenty years health-related impacts of climate change would be considered serious (Polivka, Chaudry, and MacCrawford, 2012). However, the public health nurses also noted that they did not feel they had the tools or resources needed to address the issues related to climate change (Polivka et al, 2012).

Anaker et al. (2015) also described that nurses were not prepared to address environmental health issues, stating "daily work requires substantial effort, leaving neither time nor energy to consider environmental health" with patients' needs as the priority. Nurses' and other health professionals felt that they were unable to address climate change even if they viewed issues of sustainability important. The requirements of their work limited their

Permission for image use from Nurses Drawdown

REFERENCES

Anåker, A., Nilsson, M., Holmner, Å., & Elf, M. (2015). Nurses' perceptions of climate and environmental issues: a qualitative study. *Journal of Advanced Nursing, 71*(8), 1883–1891. https://doi.org/10.1111/jan.12655.

Cooper, J., & Goren, A. (2007). Cognitive dissonance theory. In R. F. Baumeister, & K. D. Vohs, *Encyclopedia of social psychology*. Sage Publications. https://gold.worcester.edu/login?url=https://search.credoreference.com/content/topic/cog.

DiNapoli, L., Gomez, J., Chi, K., Hanoch, N., Li, J., Goresko, J., Kim, J., & Yung, T. (2019). *Integrating Climate Change into the Nursing Curriculum.* https://www.sustainability.upenn.edu/sites/default/files/pdf/Final%20Report-Nursing%20Curriculum.pdf.

El Ghaziri, M., & Morse, B. (2020). Climate change in nursing curriculum: The time is now. *Journal of Nursing Education, 59*(11), 660. doi: 10.3928/01484834-20201020-14.

Leffers, J., McDermott-Levy, R., Nicholas, P. K., & Sweeney, C. F. (2017). Mandate for the nursing profession to address climate change through nursing education. *Journal of Nursing Scholarship, 49*(6), 679-687. https://doi.org/10.1111/jnu.12331.

Nurses Drawdown. (2021). *A project of the Alliance of Nurses for Healthy Environments and Project Drawdown.* https://www.nursesdrawdown.org/.

Polivka, B. J., Chaudry, R. V., & Mac Crawford, J. (2012). Public health nurses' knowledge and attitudes regarding climate change. *Environmental Health Perspectives, 120*(3), 321-5.

Project Drawdown. (2020, August 19). *Drawdown framework.* http://drawdown.org/drawdown-framework.

World Health Organization (2020). *Nursing and midwifery.* https://www.who.int/news-room/fact-sheets/detail/nursing-and-midwifery.

ability to address climate change. An increase in nurses' awareness of their role in climate change and health can help to build foundations for a more sustainable healthcare sector (Anaker et al., 2015).

Nurses Drawdown can be a valuable resource for nursing students, practicing nurses, nurse educators, and nurse scientists to learn, contribute to, and develop research questions to address climate change action. With more than twenty collaborating organizations from around the globe, Nurses Drawdown has global influence and brings about a platform for the organizations to engage together. Nurse Drawdown is an accessible tool to influence climate change education, climate action, and promote a healthier future for our planet and our patients.

BRIEF INTRODUCTION TO ONE HEALTH
David R. Wolfgang, VMD, MPH, DABVP Dairy,
Retired
Pennsylvania State Veterinarian

One Health is a collaborative effort of multiple disciplines — working locally, nationally, and globally — to attain optimal health for people, animals and the environment. "The One Health Initiative is a movement to forge co-equal, all-inclusive collaborations between physicians, osteopathic physicians, veterinarians, dentists, nurses and other scientific-health and environmentally related disciplines, including the American Medical Association, American Veterinary Medical Association, American Academy of Pediatrics, American Nurses Association, American Association of Public Health Physicians, the American Society of Tropical Medicine and Hygiene, the Centers for Disease Control and Prevention (CDC), the United States Department of Agriculture (USDA), and the U.S. National Environmental Health Association (NEHA). Additionally, more than 950 prominent scientists, physicians and veterinarians worldwide have endorsed the initiative" (One Health Initiative, 2019). One Health (formerly called One Medicine) is dedicated to improving the lives of all species—human and animal—through the integration of human medicine, veterinary medicine and environmental science.

One Medicine was a movement begun in the late 1990's into the early 2000's which focused on health issues that humans and domestic animals shared. Initially this concentrated on similar clinical diseases in humans and animals by examination of models, causality, zoonotic and emerging infectious diseases. This concept gained much exposure and popularity with the best-selling book Zoobiquity (Natterson-Horowitz, B. & Bowers, K., 2012).

It is increasingly recognized that for One Health to be effective, it must confront not only shared human and animal infectious diseases, but also the effects of toxic chemicals, malnutrition, trauma, climate change, declines and extinctions of species, and underlying societal drivers of these problems. The One Health approach promotes collaborations between clinicians, biomedical research scientists, public health laboratories, and environmentally related disciplines, who will work with others in agriculture, business, government and the broader society to address a broad array of emerging disease issues and thereby protect human, animal, and ecosystem health.

To better understand One Health it is important to be able to describe relationships between determinants of health and health outcomes in a very broad sense. It is

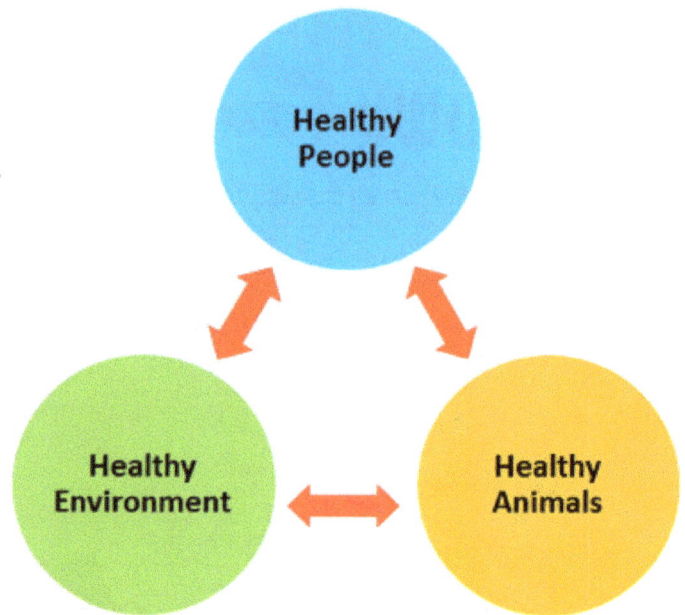

appreciated that the health of human populations is critical. Elements of public health and epidemiology are essential to achieve this goal. It is impossible to truly understand One Health without a grasp of epidemiology, epidemiological studies, and how health of individuals and populations can be affected by changes in society, domestic and wild animals, as well as the built and natural environments. In a majority of One Health epidemiology studies many more environmental components are included than have been traditional in earlier public health research.

Singular focus on people and their health can miss important clues and early indicators of environmental hazards and injuries that can foreshadow impending health challenges for society. A classic example is the documented effects endocrine (hormone) disruptors in the environment have had on amphibians. Amphibians have had the most precipitous decline of all vertebrate species since the last global survey in 2004 (Orton, F. & Tyler, C.R. 2015). The potential extent and deleterious effects these ubiquitous chemicals might have in people are just now beginning to be recognized (National Institute of Environmental Sciences, 2019).

Infectious diseases are probably the area in One Health that has received the most study and interest. It is nearly impossible to listen to the news each day and not hear of health cases involving communicable disease of some nature. These cases frequently have zoonotic, food safety, antibiotic resistant or emerging disease components (CDC, 2017). In these more complex cases, practitioners need to understand infection patterns in terms of risk factors, transmission dynamics, and evolution of the causative agent. A One Health prospective can help provide a more comprehensive understanding of the principles of infectious disease epidemiology and strategies for disease control and prevention.

The health of current and future generations depends on wise decisions today. A growing population needs potable water, a nutritious diet, and a sustainable environment. Chemicals, natural and man-made, add impacts both intended and unintended on the food system as well as ecosystem (CDC, 2018). Creation of man-made structures and intrusions for agriculture and commerce fragment feral environments and wild populations making wild populations more vulnerable. Speed and distance by which people, animals, and products are moved globally make it easy to transport novel infectious disease agents and invasive species (CDC, n.d.). As human numbers grow and more resources are drawn from the Earth, it is imperative that systems be in place to ensure the vibrancy and resilience of our home. One Health is an initiative which can promote collaboration between health practitioners and scientists to more efficiently solve current health problems. One Health is also a preventative strategy which can help ensure the future health of people, animals and the environment is enhanced and sustainable.

SUGGESTED BOOKS

Atlas, R. M. and Maloy, S. (2014). *One health — People, animals and the environment.* American Society of Microbiology Press.

Nadakavukaren, A. (2011). *Our global environment: A health perspective (7th ed.)* Waveland Press Inc.

Rabinowitz, P. M. & Conti, L. A. (2009). *Human-animal medicine. Clinical approaches to zoonoses, toxicants and other shared health risks.* Saunders.

Sala, O.E., Meyerson, L. A., & Parmesan, C. (2009). B*iodiversity Change and Human Health.* Island Press.

REFERENCES

Centers for Disease Control (CDC). (n.d.) *Zoonotic Diseases: How do germs spread between animals and people?* https://www.cdc.gov/onehealth/basics/zoonotic-diseases.htm

Centers for Disease Control (CDC). (2017). *Consumption of raw milk.* www.cdc.gov/foodsafety/rawmilk/raw-milk-index.html

Centers for Disease Control (CDC). (2018). *Harmful Algal Bloom (HAB)-associated illness.* https://www.cdc.gov/habs/illness-symptoms-freshwater.html

National Institute of Environmental Health Sciences. (2019). *Endocrine disruptors.* https://www.niehs.nih.gov/health/topics/agents/endocrine/index.cfm

Natterson-Horowitz, B., & Bowers, K. (2012). *Zoobiquity.* Knopf Doubleday.

One World-One Medicine-One Health. (2019). *One health initiative.* http://onehealthinitiative.com/

Orton, F., & Tyler, C. R. (2015). Do hormone-modulating chemicals impact on reproduction and development of wild amphibians? *Biology Review, 90,*1100 – 117. https://doi.org/10.1111/brv.12147

NURSE RESEARCHERS
Kathryn P. Jackman-Murphy Ed.D., MSN, RN, CHSE
Director, RN/BSN Program
Charter Oak State College

The Alliance of Nurses for Healthy Environments (ANHE) has several workgroups that nurses can join to become actively involved in the work of improving the health of the environment. This diverse group of nurses not only has a variety of nursing experience-both in tenure and areas of practice, but also in their focus areas of environmental health they champion.

The focus of ANHE's Research Workgroup is to frame and support an agenda for enabling nurses to solve environmental challenges to health through the creation of new knowledge. The Research Work Group provides excellent resources, support, and mentorship for all researcher experience levels – from novice to expert. The ANHE Research Work Group benefits from close partners working in advocacy, practice, and education. Critical research questions arise from these relationships and the resulting research agenda reflects the most current and pressing challenges of our profession. The workgroup meets monthly and all interested are encouraged to attend.

The members of the Research Committee demonstrate their commitment to environmental health in their research and the publication of their findings. Below are some examples of the wonderful nurse researchers involved in this workgroup, their areas of research and some of their publications. Come join us!

NURSE RESEARCHER: JESSICA CASTNER, PHD, RN-BC, FAEN, FAAN

Dr. Castner is the Editor-in-Chief of the Journal of Emergency Nursing and founding owner and principal of Castner Incorporated, a woman-owned small business research institute. Dr. Castner obtained her PhD from the University of Wisconsin-Milwaukee, MSN with a public health nursing focus from University of Missouri-Columbia, and her BSN from Marquette University. Dr. Castner has also completed advanced research training through NIH/NINR's intramural Summer Genetics Institute and Big Data Bootcamp. As a nurse scientist, Dr. Castner has been recognized as a Fellow in the Academy of Emergency Nursing and American Academy of Nursing for a unique and enduring contribution to the specialty by pioneering the integration of environmental health research, emergency nursing, and data science expertise.

Clinically, Dr. Castner is a board certified Asthma Educator (AE-C) and emergency nurse (CEN).

Describe how you discovered ANHE and your interest in the organization:

I learned about ANHE from Dr. Barbara Sattler's keynote presentation at the Midwest Nursing Research Society's annual conference, and personal recommendations to engage from Drs. Laura Anderko and Barbara Polivka.

What is your research interest area?

My research program centers on multi-level environmental determinants of health and health emergency outcomes including inhaled toxicants, telehealth, disaster preparedness, healthy occupational environments.

With over 50 manuscripts in peer-reviewed journals, Dr. Castner's research can be found at the following link: https://bit.ly/2JWnnf7.

NURSE RESEARCHER: DORIAM ESPERANZA CAMACHO RODRÍGUEZ

Brief bio-please include where you went to nursing school, and schools for advanced degrees.

• Nurse, Cooperative University of Colombia Campus Santa Marta

• Specialist in quality management and health auditing, Cooperative University of Colombia Campus Santa Marta

• Master's in quality, Safety and Environment Management, Viña del Mar University

• Doctorate in Nursing, University of Carabobo

Describe how you discovered ANHE and your interest in the organization

I discovered ANHE through an internet search six years ago. This network inspired me to work in research in the area of environmental health and invite colleagues from my country (Columbia) to become interested in the subject.

What is your research interest area?

My area of interest in research is children's environmental health and right now I am in the process of publishing the products of my doctoral thesis entitled "Theoretical Model of Integral Care for the Promotion of Child Environmental Health: A Vision from the Nursing Professional."

Some examples of Doriam's work:

- Systematic review of the promotion of children's environmental health: its objective was to identify the relationship between environmental attitudes and behaviors in nursing students of a Colombian University.

- Application of environmental bioethics in the professional practice of nursing: To identify how environmental bioethics is applied in the professional practice of nursing: http://www.revenfermeria.sld.cu/index.php/enf/article/view/1644/428

- Systematic review of children's environmental health promotion: The purpose of this study was to identify the interventions aimed at the promotion of children's environmental health available in the literature and their relationship with the conditions and requirements to achieve health according to the Ottawa Charter: https://revistas.unimagdalena.edu.co/index.php/duazary/article/view/2500/1943

NURSE RESEARCHER: LISA M. THOMPSON, RN, FNP, PHD, FAAN

Lisa is an Associate Professor in the School of Nursing, with a secondary appointment in the Department of Environmental Health at Rollins School of Public Health. Before arriving at Emory in 2017, I was a faculty member in the School of Nursing at UC San Francisco from 2008-2017. I received my RN, MSN degrees and my FNP post-master's certification at San Francisco State University in 1996. I received my MS and PhD at University of California, Berkeley in 2008.

How did you discover ANHE and what is your area of interest in the organization?

I discovered AHNE in 2017 after moving to Emory. I attended a nursing conference and met nursing faculty who work in Environmental Health. We began to collaborate together, and published a paper (Castner, J., Amiri, A., Rodriguez, J., Huntington-Moskos, L., Thompson, L. M., Zhao, S., & Polivka, B. (2019). Advancing the symptom science model with environmental health. Public Health Nursing, 36(5), 716-725). I am currently co-chair of AHNE's research working group with Luz Huntington-Moskos. I attend the climate change working group meetings too.

What is your research interest area?

I spent the past 16 years working on research projects related to household air pollution in rural Guatemala, starting as a graduate student at UC Berkeley on an NIH-funded randomized stove intervention study on infant pneumonia (RESPIRE trial). RESPIRE was the first-ever randomized intervention trial to measure reductions in childhood pneumonia from an introduced chimney stove intervention. The RESPIRE study provided a wood-burning chimney-stove to over 500 randomized households. We measured personal exposures among women and children and found that while we were able to reduce kitchen levels by 90%, personal exposures were only reduced by 50-60%. My analysis of birth weight among infants enrolled in the RESPIRE study was the first publication at that time that measured air pollution levels among pregnant people instead of relying on self-reported exposure.

In 2017, I completed a study where I developed a theory-driven behavioral intervention strategy that allowed women to adopt and sustain the use of liquid petroleum gas stoves during pregnancy and infancy (NACER study) in rural Guatemala. Currently I am co-investigator on the HAPIN trial, an NIH and Gates-funded randomized controlled trial of a liquid petroleum gas stove, 18-month free fuel distribution and behavior change communication to promote adoption of clean cookstoves in half of 3,200 households in four countries (India, Guatemala, Peru, and Rwanda). This study aims to deliver rigorous evidence regarding potential health benefits in children during the first year of life, including low birth weight, preterm birth, stunting, severe pneumonia and early childhood development.

Some examples of Lisa's work:

- Thompson, L. M., Bruce, N., Eskenazi, B., Diaz, A., Pope, D., & Smith, K. R. (2011). Impact of reduced maternal exposures to wood smoke from an introduced chimney stove on newborn birth weight in rural Guatemala. *Environmental Health Perspectives, 119*(10), 1489-1494.

Article synopsis: Major constituents of solid fuel smoke, specifically carbon monoxide (CO), particulate matter (PM) and Polycyclic Aromatic Hydrocarbons ($PAHs$), are the same air pollutants found to contribute to adverse perinatal outcomes in ambient air pollution studies and tobacco studies. We have successfully conducted studies to measure urinary biomarkers of exposure to by-products of solid fuel combustion in rural Guatemala in the NACER study.

- Weinstein, J. R., Diaz-Artiga, A., Benowitz, N., & Thompson, L. M. (2019). Reductions in urinary metabolites of exposure to household air pollution in pregnant, rural Guatemalan women provided liquefied petroleum gas stoves. *Journal of Exposure Science and Environmental Epidemiology.* doi:10.1038/s41370-019-0163-0

Article synopsis: Understanding how to influence behavior change among new stove adopters is an important area of focus when introducing new clean stove technologies. Theory-driven interventions are the cornerstone to understanding adoption and sustained use of complex technologies.

- Thompson, L. M., Diaz-Artiga, A., Weinstein, J. R., & Handley, M. A. (2018). Designing a behavioral intervention using the COM-B model and the theoretical domains framework to promote gas stove use in rural Guatemala: a formative research study. *BMC Public Health, 18*, 1-17.

- Thompson, L. M., Hengstermann, M., Weinstein, J. R., & Diaz-Artiga, A. (2018). Adoption of liquefied petroleum gas stoves in Guatemala: a mixed-methods study. *EcoHealth, 15*, 745-756.

NURSE RESEARCHER: ADRIENNE WALD, EDD, MBA, RN, CNE, MCHES

Adrienne is an Associate Professor of Nursing at Mercy College in New York teaching undergraduate research and health promotion. She holds a doctorate degree (EdD) from Teachers College Columbia University focused on health behavior and nursing education; her MBA is in health care administration, and her BSN is from Boston University. Dr. Wald is a member of the American Public Health Association (APHA), active in the environmental and public health nursing sections, the American College of Sports Medicine (ACSM) as well as the Alliance of Nurses for Healthy Environments (ANHE), Sigma Theta Tau, and is a Fellow of the New York Academy of Medicine. Her expertise includes health education, health promotion, and primary prevention including obesity/weight management, tobacco control, physical activity, cancer prevention, and the impact of the environment on health behaviors. Her public health advocacy work has included serving as a state health promotion policy expert for the Society of Public Health Educators and as a member of the New York State and American Public Health Associations.

Describe how you discovered ANHE and your interest in the organization.

My introduction to ANHE was through a five-day writing retreat held on Martha's Vineyard held in 2017, organized by several AHNE members including Mary Jane Williams, Ruth McDermott-Levy, and Barbara Sattler. It was an inspiring few days brainstorming on environmental issues and areas of interest, and focusing on individual writing projects, sharing with and obtaining feedback from colleagues. It was also a fabulous opportunity to connect with true ANHE leaders doing important work on a variety of environmental advocacy, education, and research projects. In addition to the work done at the retreat, there was a fabulous spirit of collaboration, dedication, and lots of "good" fun! Upon my return from the retreat, I became much more involved in the work of AHNE and in bringing this work to my students and faculty colleagues, as well as engaging them in local and NYS advocacy for environmental policies.

What is your research interest area?

My research has focused on health-promoting behaviors, with a particular interest in mainly physical activity, as well as nutrition, and sleep behaviors in college students. More recently I am interested in extreme heat events due to climate change and their impact on public health and the health care system; now I am examining the intersection of extreme heat events and physical activity behaviors and sports events. I was pleased to present a webinar for the AHNE Research Group last year on my article published in Nursing Economics (see below).

Some examples of Adrienne's work:

- Wald, A. (2019). Emergency department visits and costs for heat-related illness due to extreme heat or heat waves in the United States: An integrative review. *Nursing Economic$, 37*(1), 35-48. http://www.nursingeconomics.net/necfiles/news/Climate_Change.pdf

- Wald, A. & Garber, C. E. (2017), A review of current literature on vital sign assessment of physical activity in primary care. *Journal of Nursing Scholarship*. doi:10.1111/jnu.12351. https://bit.ly/34cTkGy

- Wald, A., Muennig, P., O'Connell, K.O., & Garber, C.E. (2013). Associations between healthy lifestyle behaviors and academic performance in U.S. undergraduates: A secondary analysis of the American College Health Association's National College Health Assessment II. *American Journal of Health Promotion*, (May/June). DOI: 10.4278/ajhp.120518-QUAN-265. https://bit.ly/2WfuOQT

- Rooney, M., & Wald, A. (2007). Interventions for the management of weight and body composition changes in women with breast cancer. *Clinical Journal of Oncology Nursing, 11*(1): 41-52.

NURSE RESEARCHER: KRISTI JO WILSON

Kristi is a 1986 diploma graduate from Hurley School of Nursing in Flint, MI and completed her BSN in 1989. She obtained her family nurse practitioner/MSN degree from Michigan State University and became certified in 2001.

Kristi obtained her PhD in Educational Studies with a concentration in urban and nursing education from Eastern Michigan University in 2017. She is a full-time nurse educator at University of Michigan-Flint and also work in the acute care and the outpatient setting, consulting with endocrine patients and patients who need medical surgical management. Kristi is also a nurse practitioner who performs neuro-anatomical acupuncture after becoming certified in 1989.

Describe how you discovered ANHE and your interest in the organization

When I was directed toward ANHE due to my interests, I said "Where have you been all of these years? I thought I was alone as a nurse!" I am amazed at the courage and tenacity of these nurses who draw the connection between our bodies and the earth. They look beyond the way we were trained in nursing school (well at least I was) in that nursing school trained me to negate the environment and only focus on the environment of the nurse and the patient. I do not blame my teachers because they were so smart and dedicated. They taught me the way they were taught and were formed by the expectations of their profession. However, change is necessary and the risk of not changing is too great - for all of us.

What is your research interest area?

I am interested in EcoJustice Education (EJE). To further explain, the EJE framework reminds us that human beings cannot be separated from a larger entity, as we are fully dependent on a complex, interdependent system. Unlike many approaches in nursing education that combine social and environmental issues into separate and distinct spheres, this framework operates from the position that social problems and environmental degradation emerge from the same foundational causes and those causes are exposed through a cultural ecological analysis that examines the intersection between social and ecological problems.

Some examples of Kristi Jo's work:

- Wilson, K. (2022). Application of the EcoJustice Education theoretical framework in nursing practice. In McDermott-Levy, R., Murphy, K, Leffers, J, Cantu, A., Curtis, K, and Hulick, A. (Eds). *Environmental health in nursing*, (2nd ed.). Alliance of Nurses for Healthy Environments.

- Wilson, K. J. & Stanley, E. (2019). The crisis and the shutoffs: Reimagining water in Detroit and Flint, Michigan through an EcoJustice analysis. *Annual Review of Nursing Research, 38.*

- Linton, M. E., Wilson, K. J., Dabney, B. W., & Johns, E. F. (2020). Integrating environmental sustainability content into an RN-to-BSN program: a pilot study. *Journal of Nursing Education, 59*(11), 637-641.

THE NURSE'S ROLE IN ENVIRONMENTAL HEALTH THROUGH THE LENS OF THE THEORY OF HUMAN CARING WITH A HEALTHY DOSE OF FLORENCE NIGHTINGALE

Lisa Jordan PhD, RN, CNE

Kathryn P. Jackman Murphy Ed.D, MSN, RN, CHSE

There is a great deal of focus on the care of the client within the healthcare environment with the realization that it is vital that nurses consider the client's entire environment. The environment is defined by the American Nurses Association (ANA) as: the atmosphere, milieu, or conditions where one lives, works, or plays (2007). This broader definition helps set the foundation to protect the health of our clients, their families, ourselves, and the global community.

Nurses realize through the utilization of Jean Watson's Theory of Human Caring we can use the connections between human values of caring, social justice, and economics. This includes the spectrum of environments of caring and healing as our inner selves, schools, homes, businesses, communities, healthcare settings, institutions and governments. Nurses must be involved in each of these caring-healing environments and be committed to equity, inclusion, universal respect and environmental thriving (Rosa, Dossy, Koithan et. al., 2020). As nurses, we must manage each environment while uniting across our differences and similarities of our peers, clients and communities.

The Theory of Human Caring recognizes the connection between health, caring, poverty, justice, and peace (Watson, 2008). It is through this world view nurses establish the basis for caring not only for others, but also extending across our communities and the world. Caring is a central component of nursing (Turkel & Watson, 2004) and caring for each and every person, no matter the environment needs to be included in the practice of every nurse in order to create and maintain a healthy environment for all. A healthy environment, supports a healthy planet and essentially will help provide a caring and healing environment. An unhealthy environment and unhealthy planet is lacking in caring behaviors leading to the detriment of humanity.

Promoting the health of the environment is not a new concept in nursing, quite the opposite-it is embedded in the very foundation of nursing. Florence Nightingale, the founder of modern nursing started the path of protecting and improving the environment by calling on nurses to manage the environment by controlling light and noise, ensuring clean air and water, and maintaining the cleanliness of the patient's environment with the goal to promote health and healing (Nightingale, 1860). She believed a poor environment was detrimental to health and contributed to diseases and when the environment was improved, the patient would be in the best possible condition to improve and heal. Nightingale also addressed social injustices, advocated for policy for institutions, the public and communities to develop a moral, healthy and caring society for all citizens (Watson, 2008).

Nightingale demonstrated caring by altering the environment of the soldiers of the Crimean War to improve conditions and implementing seemingly simple changes such as adequate nutrition, preventing overcrowding of the wards, providing fresh air, clean bandages and hand washing to support the health and welfare of those in her care. She knew the importance of sharing the results of these changes by using statistics to communicate the effect of the changes and challenged stakeholders to support her institutions of care. For her work, Nightingale was ridiculed and not received positively by many involved in the care of the soldiers. For example, Dr. John Hall, head physician at the Scutari Hospital during the Crimean War called Nightingale a "petticoat imperieuse" (Florence the Woman, 2021) and reported her improvements to the care environment as harmful to the medical department (Hammer, 2020).

Nursing theorist Jean Watson (2012) calls on nurses to continue the work of human caring by advocating for improved global health and well-being and expanding the impact of human caring. Watson proposes that caring is the "highest form of ethical commitment to patients, families, communities, society, civilization, and planet Earth" (p. 58) noting the interconnection between human-to-human and human-to-environment relationships. The caring practices apply to all people, at all times, and transcend biological, physical, economic, geographic, religious, political, or social differences. Rosa, Dossey, Koitham et. al., (2020) notes Watson's theory demonstrates that the interconnectedness of humanity and human survival is linked to all aspects of the global environment including animal species and ecosystems.

Caring for all environments will help to create a healthy planet to ensure clean, pure air and water for each and every citizen. Nurses must work to protect vulnerable populations such as the very young, the very old, outdoor workers and those with comorbidities, such as mental illness and cardiac disease. These populations, along with the poor and underserved are more at risk of exposure and harm due to chemicals of concern, unclean water, and air. Children, whose organs are still developing and pound for pound eat more food, drink more fluids, breathe more air than adults, ingest more harmful substances. This result can lead to life-long effects of exposure such as asthma, diabetes or cancer. In fact in 1979 the Surgeon General Julius Richmond reported that environmental factors contributed directly or indirectly to nearly every major chronic disease and 20% of the deaths in the United States (U.S, Department of Health, Education and Welfare as cited in Gerber & McGuire, 2000). A healthy planet will support healthy people and populations, protected from harmful substances which create illness, disease and death. As nurses, we must acknowledge our vital role in caring for health and the health of the environment.

Human caring and environmental caring are in direct alignment with the American Nurses' Association's (2010) Scope and Standard of Practice that called for the inclusion of environmental health into nursing practice. The third edition published in 2017 further strengthened the nurse's role in environmental health and health of the environment in each practice setting. These documents provide a framework for environmentally healthy and safe nursing care, guided by the foundation of disease prevention and social justice, built on the foundational work of early nurse leaders including Florence Nightingale and Lillian Wald and continues to be applicable to our daily practice today.

It is the responsibility of every nurse to demonstrate care for the earth or earth caring in order to protect the fragile health of the environment to protect our health, the health of the planet and the health of future generations. Citing Watson in her article, Earth Caring, Eleanor Schuster echoed the importance of care and caring behaviors while highlighting the importance of interconnectedness across the Environment, Nursing, and Caring. Shuster challenged nurses to recognize how our earth can be damaged by the need for profit and to take personal responsibility to support our global home through advocacy for our patients and our world. Shuster further stressed that nurses could manage such care through an interprofessional approach and partner together to heal our environment and foster health (2013).

Nurses must demonstrate caring and support other nurses and healthcare professionals involved in the work of environmental health. All nurses must work together to improve the environment and continue the work of Florence Nightingale and Jean Watson to support the health and welfare of all citizens. Incorporating caring for the earth into our everyday practices will guide nurses to consider the impact of our decisions not only for the present but also the future of our world.

REFERENCES

Akerman, L. (2019). Caring science education: Measuring nurses' caring behaviors. *International Journal of Caring Sciences, 12*(1), 572-583.

American Nurses Association (Ed.). (2007). *Principles of environmental health for nursing practice with implementation strategies.* American Nurses Association

American Nurses Association. (2010). *Scope and Standards for Nursing Practice.* American Nurses Association

Florence the Woman. (2021). *Florence Nightingale 200 years.* https://www.florence-nightingale.co.uk/dr-john-hall-1795-1866/

Gerber, D. E., & McGuire, S. L. (2000). Teaching students about nursing and the environment: Part 2-Legislation and resources. *Journal of Community Health Nursing, 16*(2), 81-94

Hammer, J. (2020, March). *The defiance of Florence Nightingale.* Smithsonian Magazine: www.smithsonianmag.com/history/the-worlds-most-famous-nurse-florence-nightingale-180974155/

Nightingale, F. (1860). *Notes on nursing: What it is, and what it is not.* D. Appleton and Company.

Rosa, W. E., Dossey, B.M., Koithan, M., Kreitzer M. J., Manjrekar, P., Meleis, A. I., Makamana, D., Ray, F.A., Watson, J. (2020). Nursing Theory in the Quest for the Sustainable Development Goals. *Nursing Science Quarterly, 3*(2),178-182.

Schuster, E. A. (2012). Earth Caring. In Wolf, Z.R., *Caring in Nursing Classics: An Essential Resource* (pp. 445-449). Springer.

Turkel, M., Watson, J. (2014). Advancing Caring Science through International Collaboration and Partnerships. *International Journal of Human Caring, 18*(4), 65-65

Watson, J. (2012). Guest Editorial. *International Journal of Human Caring,16*(2), 5.

Watson, J. (2008). Social justice and human caring: A model of caring science as a hopeful paradigm for moral justice for humanity. *Creative Nursing,14*(2), 54-61.

www.ingramcontent.com/pod-product-compliance
Lightning Source LLC
Chambersburg PA
CBHW080354030426
42334CB00024B/2867